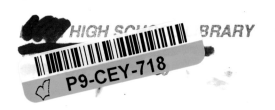

Encyclopedia of Plague and Pestilence

Copyright © 1995 by George C. Kohn

Facts On File, Inc.
460 Park Avenue South
New York NY 10016

Library of Congress Cataloging-in-Publication Data

Encyclopedia of plague and pestilence / editor, George C. Kohn.
    p. cm.
  Includes bibliographical references and index.
  ISBN 0-8160-2758-7 (acid-free paper) : $40.00
  1. Epidemics—History—Encyclopedias. I. Kohn, George C.
RA649.E53 1995
614.4'9'03—dc20   94-23135

Facts On File books are available at special discounts when purchased in bulk quantities for businesses, associations, institutions or sales promotions. Please call our Special Sales Department in New York at 212/683-2244 or 800/322-8755.

Printed in the United States of America

VB VC 10 9 8 7 6 5 4 3 2 1

This book is printed on acid-free paper.

ENCYCLOPEDIA OF PLAGUE AND PESTILENCE

Editor
GEORGE C. KOHN

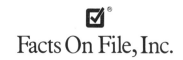

Facts On File, Inc.

AN INFOBASE HOLDINGS COMPANY

Editor
George C. Kohn

Contributors
Elizabeth Cluggish
Susan May Danseyar
Judith E. Estabrook
Michelle Foyt
Michelle H. Gosselin
Christina C. Kohn
George C. Kohn
Suzanne H. Nathanson
Rosalie C. Popick
Ashwinee Sadanand
Suzanne Solensky

CONTENTS

PREFACE

Humanity has always been vulnerable to and fearful of infectious disease, which has wrought misery, devastation, and havoc in lands throughout the world since ancient times. Bubonic plague, typhus, smallpox, cholera, yellow fever, influenza, scarlet fever, malaria, diphtheria, and poliomyelitis are some infectious diseases that have attacked whole communities or societies and caused dreadful epidemics—outbreaks of disease that have struck a large number of people in an area at the same time. An epidemic may also be called a pandemic when it spreads over a wide geographical area or through many countries of the world.

The scourge of epidemic disease retains an important place in the history of humanity. Times of pestilence have gravely interrupted human affairs and brought great suffering, which has often been described and reported in detail. Various peoples all over Europe were periodically decimated by visitations of bubonic plague between the fourteenth and seventeenth century. Smallpox and other diseases invaded and crippled the Aztec and Inca civilizations in Latin America in the sixteenth century, killing a high proportion of those who fell sick. Accounts of armies that were depleted or defeated by pestilential infection stretch back to the Middle Ages and the ancient world, and epidemics have frequently ruined the best-laid plans of military leaders, kings, and others.

And the danger posed by epidemic disease has not gone away; the ever-enlarging human population, rapid international transportation, disease resistance to medicines, insect resistance to insecticides, and medical complacency at times have all made new epidemics possible. New strains of old pestilences have also appeared.

The *Encyclopedia of Plague and Pestilence* is a compendium of geo-historical information about major, outstanding, and unusual epidemics in regions of the world from ancient times to the present. A comprehensive enumeration of all the epidemics known to have occurred could not possibly be accomplished in a single volume reference work like this; moreover, that was not my intention. I held the book to a limited number of noteworthy epidemics. Besides, there is attenuated historical (and epidemiological and pathological) interest in the constant repetition of facts of the same kind, namely the identification, cause, mode of transmission, and symptoms of various diseases (the index will direct readers to particular entries where these facts are presented). The book presents important facts about particular epidemics: when and where they started; how or why they occurred and spread; whom they affected; and what was the outcome or significance. The entries are concerned with cause and effect primarily, and only sequentially and minimally deal with epidemiology, pathology, and etiology. The active relationships between disease-causing parasitic organisms and human populations are left to explication in medical texts, journals, and other sources.

The encyclopedia's entries are listed alphabetically: **Afghan Influenza Epidemic of 1918,** . . . **Boston Smallpox Epidemic of 1666,** . . . **Canadian Typhus Epidemic of 1847,** . . . **Plague of Athens, Great,** . . . **Plague of Florence in 1630–33,** . . . **Rio de Janeiro Yellow Fever Epidemics of 1849–1902,** . . . **Shanghai Hepatitis Epidemic of 1988,** . . . **U.S. Poliomyelitis Epidemic of 1916,** . . . **Zanzibar Cholera Epidemic of 1869.** The book contains numerous "See," "q.v.," and "See also" cross-references, directing readers to related entries. Main entries having the same name but different dates are listed in chronological order, despite the fact that dates may not follow alphabetically (for example, **Asiatic Cholera Pandemic of 1846–63** precedes **Asiatic Cholera Pandemic of 1865–75,** which precedes **Asiatic Cholera Pandemic of 1881–96**); this imposes upon a mass of historical facts some kind of sequential order. The headings of entries that recount "plague epidemics" have been reduced to just "plague" (a term meaning both a specific epidemic disease and a calamitous disease epidemic); thus readers will find entry headings such as the **London Plague of 1563, Italian**

Plagues of 1477–79, Maltese Plague of 1675–76, and **Egyptian Plague of 1834–35.**

Included in each of the entries are some bibliographic sources in an abbreviated, "Further reading" reference at the end. These same sources and others are listed in a full, selected bibliography at the end of the book. Readers wishing to delve further into various epidemics will find these books and articles valuable. The encyclopedia also has a timetable of epidemics (those in the book) and the usual, general index as well as a geographical index, in which epidemics are arranged chronologically under a country (France, Russia, etc.), continent (Africa and Europe), or region (Caribbean and Scandinavia) connected with them. Also included are the broad, geographical terms Middle East, Oceania, and Latin America, as well as the historical term Ancient History.

Finally, I wish to thank the book's contributors, who helped me greatly with the work involved and who are listed separately on another page. An expression of thanks is also extended to Randy Ladenheim-Gil, Alexander Thorp, and Kathy Ishizuka and my publisher, Facts On File.

—George C. Kohn

A

Afghan Cholera Epidemics of the 1930s and 1940s
Cholera outbreaks of varying intensity that affected
Afghanistan in the 1930s and 1940s, originating almost always in India (the two countries shared a
common border until 1947). The first outbreak began
in July 1930 in the Kabul River valley. The towns of
Kabul, Jalalabad, and Charikar were soon infected.
The disease spread south to Ghazni, where 160 cases
were reported over two days. By August 1930 it had
arrived in Kandahar and Makur Kalat, where it was
particularly virulent; the epidemic subsided the following month.

During 1936–37 outbreaks of cholera occurred, but
details about them are scanty or not available. In
1938, however, Afghanistan reported a large epidemic. The infection was evidently introduced into
the country by nomadic tribes from the area of the
future Pakistan, and traveled rapidly from Afghanistan's southern province in June through the eastern
provinces to attack the capital, Kabul, in November.
Official Afghan reports listed 3,855 cholera cases
from June to December 1938. The fatality rate was 56
percent, with 2,141 persons dying from the disease
in 1938. The government launched a massive immunization program at the time, and almost 500,000
people were inoculated in the eastern region.

Nonetheless, epidemic cholera reappeared in Afghanistan in 1939. Officials, uncertain where it began, watched the disease move through the province
of Kandahar to Seistan in the southwest and then to
Herat in the north. Details of individual outbreaks
are not known; officially, 849 cholera deaths were
recorded in 1939. Two years later there were minor
outbreaks, mainly in southern Afghanistan; in 1946
officials recorded 35 cholera cases and 12 deaths
from this acute intestinal disease in the Gardez and
Orgun districts.

The government tried to establish and enforce
quarantine regulations along Afghanistan's eastern
border; it failed because of the difficulty in anticipat-
ing and controlling the movement of nomadic tribes,
whose members were often responsible for transmitting the infection from one place to another. Visitors
from a country where cholera was endemic were
required to produce proof of immunization, as were
Muslim pilgrims bound for the shrine of Mazar-i-
Sharif, in the north. Immunization was also enforced
in Afghanistan when an outbreak threatened.

Further reading: Pollitzer, *Cholera;* Simmons et al.,
Global Epidemiology.

Afghan Influenza Epidemic of 1918   Brief but severe visitation of the Spanish Influenza Epidemic of
1917–19 (q.v.) that struck Afghanistan in the fall of
1918. Little is known about how or where the outbreak first began, but it apparently peaked about the
same time as did the epidemic in northern India (see
INDIAN INFLUENZA EPIDEMIC OF 1918–19).

Influenza was first observed in Kabul (Afghanistan's capital) in early October 1918; over the next
fortnight, the disease spread quickly throughout the
city, affecting an estimated 80 percent of the people.
Initially, the case fatality rate was not noticeably
high, but in the third week of October it mounted
rapidly; some 60 to 80 persons reportedly perished
from influenza in and around Kabul every day, and
nearly 100 deaths occurred each day during the last
ten days of October.

The epidemic continued to spread throughout Afghanistan with shocking virulence until the end of
the first week of November 1918. Afterward, having
infected much of the population, influenza dissap-
peared as quickly as it had arrived. About 10,000
persons were reported to have died from the flu in
Kabul and the vicinity in the four weeks ending
November 8, 1918. See also PERSIAN INFLUENZA EPI-
DEMIC OF 1918.

Further reading: *Reports on Public Health and Medical Subjects, No. 4.*

Afghan Smallpox Epidemic of 1970–72   Series
of smallpox outbreaks over a three-year period in
Afghanistan, which led to increased government
support for the World Health Organization–spon-

sored smallpox surveillance and eradication program.

In 1970, 21 of Afghanistan's 28 provinces reported 1,044 cases of smallpox in 83 separate outbreaks. Of these, 156 cases (15 percent of the total) were reported from Kabul's (the capital city's) poorer areas, and the incidence of smallpox was rising. At least five of the outbreaks occurred within the confines of the Infectious Diseases Hospital in Kabul. Alarmed, the Afghan authorities swung into action and launched an intensive vaccination campaign in the city during the winter of 1970–71.

The number of outbreaks increased to 107 in 1971, but actual smallpox cases declined to 736. The following year, the number of outbreaks and cases fell sharply, with only 11 provinces reporting any incidence. In the first six months of the year, ten provinces reported 196 cases in 39 outbreaks. After June 1972, smallpox incidence was detected only in the southern provinces of Oruzgan, Kandahar, and Zabul. In September, the last indigenous cases were reported from Oruzgan. Later that year, Zabul reported one outbreak and Kandahar two outbreaks, but upon investigation these were found to have been imported from Pakistan. The surveillance and eradication strategy launched by the World Health Organization thus appeared to have achieved its objective within a span of 36 months.

Further reading: Fenner et al., *Smallpox and Its Eradication*.

African AIDS Epidemic Catastrophic epidemic of AIDS (acquired immunodeficiency syndrome) in parts of Africa since 1987; expected to kill an estimated 500,000 persons a year by the end of the twentieth century. The deadly disease, for which there is no vaccine, no cure, and no proven effective treatment at this time, has a crippling effect on the human immune defense system. The most dominant feature of AIDS is extreme wasting and weight loss, earning it the name "slim disease" in Uganda, the worst hit nation in Africa and the heart of the epidemic.

Epidemiologists and other researchers are still debating the origin of the human AIDS virus. One theory holds that the virus existed undetected in human beings for countless centuries, most likely in isolated African villages. Because a person can harbor the AIDS virus for years before dying from it and because rural Africans contract numerous diseases that frequently kill them at an early age, the virus could have been infecting people for a very long time without any notice until recently. Another theory states that the virus "jumped" into human beings from infected African monkeys relatively recently;

viruses in the monkeys are genetically similar to the human immunodeficiency virus (HIV), which is proclaimed to be the cause of AIDS. (However, scientists have reported cases of people who suffer from an AIDS-like condition and yet have no trace of HIV in their body.) Alleging that AIDS originated in Africa angers many blacks and whites, who feel that this essentially blames Africa for the AIDS problem.

Almost certainly the AIDS virus has been silently spreading in sub-Saharan Africa since the mid-1970s. In 1980 Kigali (Rwanda's capital) and Kinshasa (Zaire's capital) were the first African cities recognized to have epidemic problems, and by 1982 Uganda to the north and Zambia to the south reported AIDS epidemics. The deadly virus spread itself primarily by heterosexual intercourse among urban people having multiple partners. Infected female prostitutes were (and still are) the main factor in the transmission of the virus among most Africans. (In Europe and the United States, AIDS spreads primarily among homosexual and bisexual men and intravenous drug users; a key factor is the practice of anal intercourse, during which small fissures or tears may occur in the anal canal, which allow the virus, carried in semen, to enter the bloodstream of the receptive partner.)

By June 1988 a total of about 11,000 AIDS cases were reported in 43 African countries, and by July 1991 the cumulative number of cases from 52 African countries was almost 93,000. At the time the countries of North Africa reported few cases of AIDS, but places like Uganda, Rwanda, Zaire, Kenya, Malawi, Burundi, Ethiopia, and Tanzania in Central and East Africa were severely affected. The epidemic moved then into West Africa (notably the Ivory Coast, Ghana, and Cameroon), and reported cases began to escalate throughout the continent. Many of the patients began contracting a deadly form of tuberculosis (TB), a degenerative lung disease, causing more alarm (airborne TB bacteria threaten AIDS patients and healthy persons as well).

By 1993 the World Health Organization (WHO) reported an estimated 7.5 million persons infected with HIV in sub-Saharan Africa, who were expected to develop either AIDS or AIDS-related complex (ARC), a term used to describe a condition involving evidence of immunodeficiency, swollen glands, recurrent fever, weight loss, or a combination of these symptoms. In 1994 researchers reported as many as 30 different strains of HIV that often escape conventional tests used to detect their presence in blood (the new strains, first isolated in Cameroon, had not yet been detected in the United States). According to the WHO, AIDS cases had not yet reached a plateau in Africa, where an estimated ten million persons were expected to be infected by the mid-1990s. Researchers in other organizations had gloomier projections, envisioning an explosive spread of the disease, particularly in Asia, far surpassing sub-Saharan Africa in the number of AIDS cases.

Further reading: Koch-Weser and Vanderschmidt, *The Heterosexual Transmission of AIDS in Africa*; World Health Organization, *Weekly Epidemiological Records*; Joseph, *Dragon Within the Gates*.

African and Asian Conjunctivitis Pandemic of 1969–71

Extensive pandemic of acute hemorrhagic conjunctivitis (AHC) that began in Africa and spread throughout Asia and to parts of Europe between 1969 and 1971. Known by a variety of names, including Apollo 11 disease, Bangla Joy disease, Singapore epidemic conjunctivitis (see SINGAPORE CONJUNCTIVITIS EPIDEMICS OF 1970–80), picornavirus epidemic conjunctivitis, and epidemic hemorrhagic conjunctivitis, AHC affected millions of people during and after this pandemic. After a 24-hour incubation period, the virus causes congestion, swelling, watering, and pain in the eyes. Subconjunctival hemorrhage is the most distinctive symptom. The cornea can be affected, but rarely in a serious way. Recovery is rapid and usually begins by the third day in treated cases unless there are complications. During the pandemic, a new enterovirus—later designated as enterovirus type 70 (E70)—was isolated as the main causative agent.

The pandemic reportedly began in an eastern suburb of Accra, the capital of Ghana in West Africa, in June 1969. From September 1969 to February 1970, it spread like wildfire along the coast to Nigeria, Cameroon, and the Ivory Coast. Togo, Dahomey (Benin), Liberia, and Sierra Leone were infected between February and June 1970, Gambia in October, and Senegal between September and December 1970. The epidemic peaked in Morocco (137,991 cases were treated) during December 1970–January 1971 before spreading to Algeria, Tunisia (February), Kenya (the disease arrived by sea in April 1971 and infected a coastal city and then Nairobi in late 1971 and early 1972), and Libya (summer of 1971). There were unconfirmed reports of an AHC epidemic in the United Arab Republic (Egypt and Syria) during 1971–72, but the earliest recorded epidemics there occurred in 1972–73.

Some scholars believe that the pandemic had a second focus in Java, Indonesia, some 13,000 miles away. Muslim pilgrims returning from Mecca may have been the only link between Indonesia and Saudi Arabia. Indonesia's capital, Djakarta, suffered an epidemic of AHC during April–September 1970. Between July and December 1970, the virus attacked Bali and eastern and central Java. Over the next year, most of Indonesia was infected.

In the densely populated countries of Southeast Asia, the virus spread rapidly. Tiny Singapore suffered two epidemics of AHC—the first in September 1970 and the second in June 1971—during both of which AHC crossed over to infect Malaysia before the month was over. India was invaded by a large and widespread epidemic (see INDIAN CONJUNCTIVITIS EPIDEMIC OF 1971), affecting major cities like Bombay, Calcutta, Lucknow, Amritsar, Pune, Madras, and New Delhi between April and June 1971. Later in the same year, outbreaks of AHC were reported from Thailand (June), Cambodia, Hong Kong, Taiwan, Korea, and the Philippines.

Japan's first wave of AHC epidemics occurred in 1971; the island of Kyushu was struck in August, the city of Tokyo in October and the city of Sapporo in December and January 1972. In addition, in 1971, small outbreaks were reported from Moscow (summer) and Rotterdam and London (September 1971).

During the September 1970 epidemic in Singapore and in subsequent epidemics in Hong Kong and Malaysia, a new strain of the coxsackie virus A24 (CA24) was incriminated as the cause of the pandemic. From 1972 to 1979, AHC continued to erupt in epidemic form in many countries all over the world.

Further reading: Melnick, ed., *Progress in Medical Virology*; Evans, ed., *Viral Infections of Humans*.

African Cholera Pandemic of 1989–91

Serious outbreaks of cholera throughout the continent of Africa between 1989 and 1991, infecting about 210,000 persons and killing at least 25,000 of them. The *Vibrio el tor* bacterium was then cholera's main infectious agent in Africa, where it was spread by human carriers, by infected food, water, and feces, and by flies. Causing diarrhea, dehydration, colicky abdominal pain, nausea, vomiting, and sometimes coma, the acute intestinal disease quickly became epidemic in places where there was a breakdown in, or lack of, sanitation.

In 1989 nearly three quarters of the world's cholera cases were reported in 16 African countries—35,606 cases. Africa accounted for a large majority of all cholera cases reported to the World Health Organization from 1970 to late 1991, when the pandemic on the continent subsided but continued to rage in some areas.

Lusaka, the capital city of Zambia in south-central Africa, recorded scores of deaths from cholera in February–March 1989; physicians there, however, claimed that fatalities were considerably higher, that dead people were quickly buried without being reported. The disease spread north to Kitwe and other towns in Zambia's Copperbelt, where hundreds contracted it, and health officials provided instructions to the inhabitants for disposal of garbage, which was seldom picked up at regular intervals. Garbage was often thrown in an open pit close to doorways of houses in Kitwe, where each household also dug a pit for a latrine. People were further instructed to boil water, which came out of outdoor communal taps and was frequently polluted; cholera could also spread easily around open-air markets where the vendors lived closeby in mud brick houses.

Outbreaks also occurred in 1989 in Mozambique, Angola, Niger, Rwanda, Tanzania, and Malawi, where a catastrophic epidemic began in October. In addition, the island country of São Tomé and Príncipe, located in the Gulf of Guinea off West Africa, reported nearly 4,000 cases of cholera in 1989, the first time the disease was known to have broken out there. That year, increasing experience in treating cholera patients and the widespread use of oral rehydration significantly helped reduce the case-fatality rate, and yet prevention of cholera remained difficult because the modes and vehicles of transmission varied from country to country. Commonly transmitted by water, it also was carried by foods such as millet and rice sold by street vendors everywhere, as well as by raw and inadequately cooked seafood harvested from cholera-infested waters. Furthermore, traditional native funeral practices, such as cleaning cholera victims' colons before burial, helped contribute to the spread of the disease.

In 1990 there were 39,211 cholera cases reported in Africa, and in 1991 the total number of African cases soared to about 135,000, of which 16,700 were fatalities. (In comparison, the number of cholera cases in the Peruvian Cholera Epidemic of 1991–92 [q.v.] was more than 400,000 but the fatality rate was less than one percent.) Zambia, Nigeria, and Ghana (where the disease became very serious in 1991) reported increased outbreaks for a period; despite medical progress with rehydration therapies, Africa's death rate from cholera worsened due to the lack of access to life-saving oral rehydration salts (ORS). Also, armed conflicts in some countries during the epidemics contributed to delayed or incorrect management of cholera cases.

Further reading: "Cholera—Worldwide, 1989," *Journal of the American Medical Association;* "Cholera in Africa: Lessons on Transmission and Control for Latin America," *The Lancet.*

African Influenza Epidemic of 1890 See EUROPEAN INFLUENZA PANDEMIC OF 1889–90; ASIATIC INFLUENZA PANDEMIC OF 1889–90.

Albenga Meningitis Epidemic of 1815 Important, isolated Italian outbreak of cerebrospinal meningitis (CSM), occurring in the Ligurian seaport of Albenga on the Gulf of Genoa in 1815. CSM first appeared in Geneva, Switzerland, in 1805, and later erupted in the coastal cities of Nice, France, and Genoa, Italy, which lie to the west and east respectively of Albenga. Though remotely situated on the seaboard of the Ligurian Alps, Albenga had some trading ties by land and sea to Nice and Genoa, and apparently the acute bacterial disease was carried by infected traders and others from these places to Albenga. (The infectious bacterium *Neisseria meningitidis [Neisseria intracellularis]* is commonly spread by direct contact, through droplets or mucus, by sneezing or coughing.)

Morbidity of CSM in Albenga was high—about 70 percent—with hundreds of persons suddenly ill with fever, intense headaches, nausea, vomiting, and stiff necks; convulsions were common in children. About 80 percent of the stricken suffered from bleeding and pulmonary complications, which led to death. CSM remained confined to the valley region of Albenga and did not spread southward to the nearby ports of Imperia and San Remo. These valley regions bordering the Gulf of Genoa had little or no contact with each other, according to some sources; and it is well known for CSM to break out in small isolated epidemics. Later in 1815, the Albenga epidemic was reported by three Italian physicians in separate medical publications.

Further reading: Foster and Gaskell, *Cerebro-Spinal Fever;* MacNalty, *Epidemic Diseases of the Central Nervous System.*

Algerian Malaria Epidemic of 1941 See CONSTANTINE MALARIA EPIDEMIC OF 1941.

Algerian Relapsing Fever Epidemic of 1943–46 Acute epidemic of louse-borne relapsing fever in Algeria, North Africa, killing about 2,000 of the 31,847 persons reported infected.

Relapsing fever, caused by a spirochete (bacterium) called *Borrelia recurrentis,* entered Algeria from Libya, where it had affected the Jaba as-Sauda area of the Fezzan desert region since late 1942. Penetrating westward into northern Algeria in 1943, this spirochetal disease (spread by lice) struck the territory of Touggourt and the town of Biskra; about 2,700 people contracted the disease, characterized by high fever lasting two to nine days, and some 250 persons perished in these places. Many Algerian localities failed to report the sickness, which at first assumes symptoms common to other febrile diseases; thus, recorded cases in Touggourt and Biskra were believed to be a small part of the total incidences.

In November 1944 the disease moved into the northern Algerian department (district) of Constantine, evidently coming from neighboring Tunisia, where it had prevailed since late 1943. About three quarters of Algeria's population lived in the three northern departments of Constantine, Alger, and Oran (which were then overseas provinces of France), where the infection spread because of undernutrition, a high degree of lice infestation, and lack of soap. The epidemic reached its peak in Constantine in March–April 1945 and in Oran in July of that year.

From Oran, relapsing fever moved west into Morocco and, by the end of 1945, had claimed the lives of about 1,000 people in Algeria's northern regions. There were some reports that as many as 400,000 people were infected in 1944–45. Northern Algeria experienced sporadic outbreaks in 1946, when 3,156 persons were recorded as infected with the disease.

The southern territories of Algeria (comprising 85 percent of the country's land area but sparsely populated) recorded 9,991 cases of relapsing fever in 1946, when the epidemic struck and subsided. Overall mortality ranged from three to ten percent during the epidemic period in Algeria. To curb the disease's spread, systematic lice disinfestation of the populations in the diseased areas was employed; antibiotics also contributed to the reduction in fatalities. See also MOROCCAN RELAPSING FEVER EPIDEMIC OF 1945–46.

Further reading: Hartwig and Patterson, *Disease in African History*; Simmons et al., *Global Epidemiology*.

Algerian Typhus Epidemic of 1942–44   Epidemic louse-borne typhus fever that killed 12,840 out of approximately 52,000 infected people in Algeria, North Africa, during World War II. Some sources have said that actual infections from 1942 to 1944 may have been as high as 260,000 cases. Outbreaks of typhus in Algeria had occurred at irregular intervals since 1868 (when a serious epidemic struck), with the most recent (prior to 1942) in 1936–38. World War II caused much social upheaval, overcrowding, and unsanitary conditions in most of North Africa; these conditions were favorable for the spread of classic typhus fever, caused by the infectious organism *Rickettsia prowazeki* and transmitted by the body louse *Pediculus humanus humanus* (which is infected by feeding on a typhus patient's blood).

In February 1942, when cold weather required the wearing of garments easily infested with lice, discouraged washing, and prolonged the survival of rickettsiae in lice feces, the disease spread quickly through Algeria's three northern departments of Alger, Oran, and Constantine (areas where three quarters of all Algerians lived). Men and women of all ages were infected, and all races were affected, with morbidity proportionally greater among Arabs and Berbers (a Caucasoid people of North Africa, most of whom consider themselves Muslims). About 38,000 typhus infections were reported in 1942, with about 11,000 fatalities (almost 30 percent). The mortality rate was highest among white Europeans—30 to 50 percent—whereas among the Algerian native groups, who were continuously exposed to typhus, the mortality ranged from ten to 20 percent. The epidemic declined considerably with the beginning of warm weather in 1942, but it was on the rise again the following winter (clothing, bedding, and dust containing dry, infected lice feces may remain infectious for many months, passing into human wounds).

During the winter of 1943, relapsing fever (another louse-borne infection, distinct from typhus but also attributed to wartime) concurrently broke out in Algeria, causing more misery for the people in the following months. Typhus was again widespread in 1943, particularly in the towns of Télagh and Ammi Moussa and the valley of Cheliff in Oran. It also severely struck the inhabitants in the Aures Mountains in southern Constantine and those in the Laghouat, Ziban, and Chellala regions in the Territoires du Sud (Southern Territories). These areas reported a total of 11,362 typhus cases and about 1,600 human deaths within three months.

Morbidity declined significantly throughout Algeria in 1944, with a mortality rate of about ten percent (2,409 typhus cases with 240 deaths). Algerian civilians were the main victims of the three-year epidemic, which also affected the North African countries of Egypt, Morocco, and Tunisia. Thousands of U.S. and other foreign troops stationed in Algeria during the war were given inoculations with the highly effective Cox-Craigie typhus vaccine; very few cases and no deaths from typhus occurred among U.S. troops. Because of preventive measures taken by Algerian authorities, including the disinfestation of infected clothing with DDT powders and the mass immunization of people in infected areas, the incidence of typhus declined to only 99 cases in 1949.

Further reading: Ackerknecht, *History and Geography of the Most Important Diseases*; Spink, *Infectious Diseases*.

Angolan Smallpox Epidemic of 1864–65   Most serious smallpox outbreak to strike what is now Angola (then called Portuguese West Africa) in the nineteenth century. Confined mainly to Angola's northern region, the contagious viral disease affected about a third of the population and killed more than 25,000 people in one year.

In February 1864 smallpox-infected passengers aboard a ship apparently from Portugal carried the disease to the northern Angolan port of Ambriz (Ambrizete). Prior to 1864, smallpox had been endemic in parts of the country; for instance, in 1687 a severe outbreak of the disease had threatened the Portuguese slave trade there. In 1864 smallpox moved southward along the coast to Luanda, the capital of Angola, which became the focal point of the epidemic by mid-1864.

As thousands of persons contracted the deadly "pox," a disease that can blind and disfigure many, entire village populations fled from Luanda and the district. In their flight, sick Angolans carried the virus to other parts of the country, unwittingly infecting others. From Luanda, smallpox moved inland along the caravan route to the eastern cotton-growing area of Malange, an important trade station, where large quantities of wax, cotton, ivory, gum, and copper were abandoned because of native fears and deaths from the epidemic. Farther east, the town of Cassange, fearful of contagion, suspended trade with Malange during this period.

Smallpox also spread by seamen from Luanda to the island of São Tomé and the coastal town of Novo Redondo in Angola. It also reached central Angola's Bié plateau in 1865 and the Herero tribal people in South-West Africa (Namibia) that same year. Commerce in northern Angola declined further when another smallpox outbreak occurred in 1865 and copper mining activities were halted due to depopulation from the disease.

During the beginning of the epidemic, in April 1864, explorer Joaquim Rodríguez Graca, who had opened up Angola's eastern region, died from smallpox on his farm there in Golungo Alto. Another famous explorer in Central Africa, Lásió Magyar, also succumbed to smallpox in Angola's Bié region in 1864. North of Angola, the French colony of Gabon suffered a less serious smallpox outbreak during this time, but there is no evidence that it was related to Angola's. Smallpox's rampage in the northern section of Angola resulted in much of the population being shifted to the southern section.

Further reading: Hopkins, *Princes and Peasants: Smallpox in History;* Shurkin, *The Invisible Fire.*

Antonine Plague (Plague of Galen) Epidemic, perhaps of smallpox or measles, brought back to the Roman Empire by troops returning from campaigns in the Near East. Beginning in A.D. 165, it raged throughout Asia Minor and much of Europe for 15 years, claiming the lives of two Roman emperors—Lucius Verus, who died in 169, and his co-regent Marcus Aurelius Antoninus, who ruled alone until

his own death in 180. Nine years later the disease broke out again, noted the ancient Roman historian Dio Cassius, and caused up to 2,000 deaths a day at Rome.

Under Emperor Verus, the imperial troops had gone to the east when Parthian forces attacked Armenia. The Romans' defense of their eastern lands was hampered as the troops succumbed to the disease. Worse still were the epidemic's effects in the rest of the empire. Many towns and villages, both in Italy and the provinces, lost all their inhabitants, according to the ancient Spanish writer Paulus Orosius. Sweeping as far north as the Rhine, the disease even infected Germanic and Gallic peoples outside the empire's borders. For the past few years these northern groups had been pressing southward in search of more land to sustain their growing populations. With their own ranks thinned by the epidemic, the Romans found themselves unable to push the tribes back. An attack against one group, the Marcomanni, had to be postponed until 169 because the imperial troops were cut down by the disease.

During the epidemic, in 166, the great Greek physician and writer Galen left Rome to go home to Asia Minor. Some scholars have accused him of fleeing for fear of the disease, but others, noting that he returned to Rome in 168 when summoned by the emperors, have defended him against these charges of cowardice. As unclear as Galen's motives is his description of the epidemic, found in the treatise *Methodus Medendi.* Only fever, diarrhea, and inflammation of the pharynx are mentioned, as is a skin eruption, sometimes dry and sometimes pustular, appearing on the ninth day of the illness. The scanty information left by Galen prevents us from determining the exact nature of the disease, but many scholars have diagnosed it as smallpox. According to U.S. professor William McNeill, the Antonine Plague and the Plague of Cyprian (qq.v.) were outbreaks, one of smallpox and one of measles (not necessarily in that order), that devastated Mediterranean-area populations with no previous exposure—or immunity—to either disease.

Like Galen, Emperor Marcus Aurelius was away from Rome, though for a much longer time. From 167 on he commanded his legions near the Danube, trying with only partial success to stave off attacks by the Germanic peoples across the river. To console himself in the lonely hours at camp, Marcus wrote his *Meditations,* one passage of which (IX.2) claims that even the pestilence around him is less deadly than falsehood, evil behavior, and lack of true understanding. While dying from the disease, Marcus (whose family name, Antoninus, was given to the epidemic) is said to have uttered these last words:

"Weep not for me; think rather of the pestilence and the deaths of so many others."

Further reading: Marcus Aurelius, *Meditations;* McNeill, *Plagues and Peoples;* Zinsser, *Rats, Lice and History.*

Ashanti Influenza Epidemic of 1918 Offshoot of the worldwide Spanish Influenza Epidemic of 1917–19 (q.v.), killing about 9,000 native people in Ashanti (central Ghana), two percent of the total population. The reported fatalities listed only those who had received European medical care; in many cases, dead bodies removed for burial in native villages were never recorded.

Ashanti was a powerful, militaristic West African native kingdom prior to the British takeover of it in 1896. Little is known about diseases there before Anglo-colonization, but the kingdom seemed not to have suffered high death rates from disease in the previous two centuries. On September 8, 1918, influenza entered Kumasi, the Ashanti capital, when sick African soldiers from a British regiment returned home from World War I. That month the infection spread rapidly through Ashanti, forcing the government to close all schools and major roads, to confine soldiers to their barracks, and to discourage groups from congregating and citizens from traveling. But to the east of Kumasi, many contracted the flu in October and spread it northward. Ashanti's chief commissioner recorded that from six to 20 persons perished from it each day during the first six weeks of the epidemic.

Central Ashanti was hardest hit, having some 4,500 fatalities in this most populous region with good transportation facilities that allowed greater movement of people. In Kumasi alone, an estimated 800 Africans died—four percent of the capital's total population of some 20,000. Often the medical personnel became too ill with flu to help native patients. In the southern Ashanti region, about 2,500 lives were lost, mostly in Obuasi, where the gold fields were closed on October 11 when African workers refused to show up for mining after three European miners died from the flu. The mortality was less severe in other Ashanti regions, with about 1,500 deaths reported in the western part and some 500 in the northern part. The epidemic finally waned after mid-December 1918.

Further reading: Collier, *The Plague of the Spanish Lady;* Hartwig and Patterson, *Disease in African History.*

Ashanti Plague of 1924–25 Grave outbreak of plague that afflicted 166 persons, mainly in the Ashanti capital city of Kumasi, where 90 persons succumbed to bubonic plague, 29 to pneumonic plague, and 21 to septicemic plague from mid-June to mid-September 1924.

Most likely, plague was imported to the Ashanti people from the nearby Gold Coast (Ghana) colony of Sekondi, where plague was raging in March–April 1924. Infected train passengers and cargo carried the disease from Sekondi to Kumasi, an inland railroad terminus. The first bubonic case was a worker living near the railroad cargo shed who was bitten by a plague-carrying flea. Other men working in Kumasi fell victim, despite anti-plague vaccinations of some 2,000 people there. Seven men living in the same compound in the city's native Zongo extension died; several of them had engaged in trade in the railroad shed, where they either received an infective flea bite or associated with plague-infected persons. By mid-June 1924 Kumasi was placed in quarantine, and soon an additional 103,000 anti-plague vaccinations were administered. But 48 more plague cases occurred in the overcrowded Zongo extension, where sanitary facilities were extremely poor.

The epidemic raged in the rat-infested Zongo market but much less so in Fanti New Town, another part of Kumasi, which was relatively clean and modern. More than 80 percent of the plague cases occurred in the Zongo sections of the city.

When no new cases of plague were reported by mid-September 1924, the quarantine in Kumasi was lifted. However, there was a brief outburst of the disease there in mid-November, and the city was then placed under quarantine for 11 days. The following month the nearby town of Bekwai reported one plague case. The epidemic was thus confined mainly to Kumasi for an entire year and lasted officially until 1925. See also GHANIAN PLAGUE OF 1908.

Further reading: Gregg, *Plague: An Ancient Disease in the Twentieth Century;* Hartwig and Patterson, *Disease in African History.*

Asian Influenza Pandemic of 1957–58 Massive epidemic of influenza that quickly enveloped most areas of the world within six months of its first outbreak in Kweichow (southwest China) in early February 1957. Some scholars believe it originated in Vladivostok in 1956. Globally, the pandemic affected 10 percent to 35 percent of the population, but the overall mortality rate (about 0.25 percent) was considerably lower than in many epidemics. (See ASIATIC INFLUENZA PANDEMIC OF 1889–90; SPANISH INFLUENZA EPIDEMIC OF 1917–19; INDIAN INFLUENZA EPIDEMIC OF 1918–19; HONG KONG INFLUENZA PANDEMIC OF 1968.)

From southwest China, the virus spread to Hong Kong and Singapore in April, where it was identified as a major new subtype, H2N2, of the Asian A2 influenza virus, capable of wreaking havoc across the world. Japan was infected in early May. The Japanese epidemic occurred in two waves: the first, from May to July, and the second, from September to December. In quick succession, Indonesia, the Philippines, India, Australia, Pakistan, Iran, and Yemen were infected. In the Pacific region, children and young adults were severely afflicted.

Iraq, Egypt, Sudan, and other areas in Africa were invaded (through shipboard outbreaks) in July as was the west coast of South America and, subsequently, the rest of the continent. Much of Central Europe, Rumania, Greece and the British Isles came under attack in August and September. Scandinavia and North America were affected in October. The United States and the United Kingdom were the worst hit. By November 1957, almost every country in the world had been affected by the pandemic.

About two days after being infected, the patient complains of a headache, starts shivering and coughing. Abruptly, the fever increases, the headache intensifies and the patient develops a severe body ache. Except in the most severe cases, fever does not last beyond two to three days, but there is a heavy nasal discharge and the cough worsens. Even when the fever is gone, the cough and lassitude can persist. Some patients develop complications—respiratory, cardiovascular, or neurological. (Early research of this subtype had established that it could cause fatal pneumonia.) During this pandemic, neurological complications of various kinds were reported from many countries. The second wave produced greater mortality. The H2N2 virus strains continued to cause global outbreaks until early 1968. See also BRITISH INFLUENZA EPIDEMIC OF 1957–58; U.S. INFLUENZA EPIDEMIC OF 1957–58.

Further reading: Leslie, ed., *Asian Medical Systems;* Henschen, *The History of Diseases;* Stuart-Harris et al., *Influenza: The Viruses and the Disease;* Kilbourne, *Influenza.*

Asiatic Cholera Pandemic of 1817–23

First great cholera pandemic of the nineteenth century; unprecedented in its fury, it affected almost every country in Asia.

While early cases of cholera were reported from Purneah in Bihar (state in northeast India) in early 1816, the pandemic is believed to have originated in the town of Jessore (near Calcutta) in August 1817 (see INDIAN CHOLERA EPIDEMIC OF 1817–18). A civil surgeon, reporting on the high incidence of a severe gastrointestinal disease among his patients, drew attention to the source of contagion—contaminated rice. Amidst attacks of vomiting and diarrhea thousands of people collapsed and died, including hundreds of British soldiers transiting through Bengal. Cholera then spread rapidly across the country and, in December 1818, arrived in Sri Lanka (Ceylon).

Meanwhile, the infection was transmitted to the Afghan and Nepalese soldiers fighting against British troops along India's northern borders. Traversing the overland route, cholera arrived in Burma (Myanmar) and Thailand (see THAI CHOLERA EPIDEMIC OF 1820). Almost simultaneously, it was seaborne to Sumatra, Java (see INDONESIAN CHOLERA EPIDEMIC OF 1821), the Philippines, China (see CHINESE CHOLERA EPIDEMIC OF 1820–22), Japan (see JAPANESE CHOLERA EPIDEMIC OF 1822), and the southeast Asian mainland.

British troops, arriving in Muscat (in Oman) in 1821 to put an end to the slave trade, brought cholera with them. From Muscat, it was carried by the slave traders along the eastern coast of Africa to Zanzibar. Basra, at the head of the Persian Gulf, was invaded in 1821. Shortly thereafter, it traveled upstream to Baghdad and also infected an invading Persian army. Syria, Anatolia, and the port of Astrakhan in southern Russia were also infected (see ASTRAKHAN CHOLERA EPIDEMIC OF 1823). An exceptionally severe winter in 1823–24 ensured that cholera did not spread beyond the Caspian Sea into Europe.

The rapidity and virulence with which the disease struck entire populations took everyone by surprise. Subsequently, cholera became endemic in most of the Asian countries and continued to wreak havoc in many parts of Russia. This pandemic marked the first recorded spread of the disease outside India and affected hundreds of thousands of people. Those which followed were more widespread in their impact.

Further reading: Marks and Beatty, *Epidemics.*

Asiatic Cholera Pandemic of 1826–37

Second cholera pandemic, which, like the first (see ASIATIC CHOLERA PANDEMIC OF 1817–23), originated in the province of Bengal in northeast India. Unlike the first pandemic, this one also penetrated countries in Europe and on the North American continent and is considered by many to be the greatest cholera pandemic of the nineteenth century. It is important to note, however, that scholars have disagreed about when this pandemic ended and the next one began.

The pandemic began in 1826 with outbreaks in the Ganges River delta of Bengal (see INDIAN CHOLERA EPIDEMIC OF 1826–27). It then traveled up the Ganges River and entered Punjab province. Simultaneously, it spread along the regular routes to quickly extend over most of India. From Lahore in the northwest, cholera used the caravan routes to reach Kabul and Balkh in Afghanistan and crossed over into Russian territory at Bukhara in 1827. In 1828, cholera reached Chiva and was carried by the Kirghese hordes to Orenburg (Chkalov, Russia) at the southern tip of the Ural Mountains in August 1829.

In late 1829, Tehran in Persia (Iran) was infected, apparently via Afghanistan (see PERSIAN CHOLERA EPIDEMIC OF 1829–30). Moscow was invaded in August 1830 and, by 1831, the epidemic had infiltrated Russia's main cities and towns. Russian soldiers brought the disease to Poland in February 1831 and from there its transmission was very rapid. Hungary was struck in June 1831 (reportedly some 250,000 cases, about 100,000 deaths) and, in Germany, Berlin (August 1831) and Hamburg (October 1831) reported cholera outbreaks. By now all the Baltic ports were reeling under the impact of the disease. In the north, cholera spread into Finland and Sweden. Vienna was infected in the same year, but the Austrian authorities were better prepared to deal with the outbreak, having received advance warning of its arrival. Everywhere, panic-stricken governments introduced desperate measures to deal with the disaster.

In October 1831, cholera entered England and Wales (more than 21,500 persons died in both countries from the disease) and Scotland (9,500 deaths) despite the strict quarantining of ships and merchandise. The cities of London and Glasgow were particularly hard hit. By March 1832, Ireland was invaded (25,000 deaths). France was struck in 1832 as well. In the same year, Irish immigrants to Canada and the United States carried cholera with them. Cholera attacked Havana, Cuba, in February 1833, killing more than 8,000 inhabitants, and arrived in Mexico where, by August, it had claimed some 15,000 lives.

While the disease continued to ravage most of Europe, it was also spreading rapidly in another direction. In the spring of 1831, pilgrims from Mesopotamia (modern Iraq) and the Arabian Peninsula brought cholera to Mecca, site of Islam's holiest shrine, at the time of the annual *Hadj* (pilgrimage). Within three weeks, nearly 3,000 Muslim pilgrims returning home from Mecca died of the disease. Mecca was thereafter regularly invaded by cholera epidemics until about 1912. Another branch of the epidemic infected Syria and Palestine, while a third offshoot crossed into Cairo (July 1831) and quickly infected the Nile River delta. Thirty-thousand human deaths were reported from Cairo and Alexandria over a 24-hour period. Muslim pilgrims also brought cholera into Tunis in 1831. Over the next few years, Ethiopia, Somaliland, Zanzibar, and, subsequently, other countries in North Africa (Algeria and Sudan) were invaded.

An English ship transported cholera into Portugal early in 1833. Spain, even with its strict enforcement of quarantine measures, was infected in August 1833. In December 1834, the epidemic reached Marseilles, France. The rest of southern France and most of Italy were attacked over the following two years. In 1837, cholera reached Malta, killing about 3,000 people in a few months.

Little is known about the cholera pandemic's journey east of India. Apparently, traces of the first pandemic had lingered in Indonesia and the Philippines until 1830. Cholera was also reported from China in 1826 and 1835 (at Canton), from the Straits Settlements (Malaysia and Singapore) in 1826, and from Japan in 1831. Cholera continued to erupt in various parts of India throughout the 1830s.

In England, the pandemic prompted the passage of the landmark Public Health Act and the Nuisances Removal Act in 1848. See also BRITISH CHOLERA EPIDEMIC OF 1832, U.S. CHOLERA EPIDEMIC OF 1832.

Further reading: Marks and Beatty, *Epidemics;* Longmate, *King Cholera.*

Asiatic Cholera Pandemic of 1846–63

Third in a series of cholera pandemics (see ASIATIC CHOLERA PANDEMIC OF 1817–23, ASIATIC CHOLERA PANDEMIC OF 1826–37) that began in India and spread over many countries.

The outbreaks that led to this pandemic actually began much earlier—in fact, just as the second pandemic was subsiding over Europe. In 1837, there was a resurgence of cholera in the Lower Bengal region. It gradually spread west, reaching Kabul in Afghanistan in 1839. Early in 1840, cholera once again erupted in Lower Bengal. Troops assembled here en route to military duty in China transported the disease to Britain's Straits Settlements and, in July 1840, to China, where cholera raged for two years. It then spread east to the Philippines and west along the trade routes from Canton to Burma and across Central Asia to Bukhara (see RUSSIAN CHOLERA EPIDEMIC OF 1829–31) in 1844. One arm spread into Iran in 1845 and then as far north as Derbent on the Caspian Sea. Another arm penetrated Afghanistan, then east into the Punjab before branching out southwest to Karachi and southeast to Delhi.

Meanwhile, in 1845, cholera reappeared in Lower Bengal and spread rapidly south to Madras and Sri Lanka and west to Bombay. In May 1846, it was carried across shipping routes to Aden, Jedda, and much of the Arabian coast. It then entered Iraq and reinvaded Iran (see PERSIAN CHOLERA EPIDEMICS OF 1846–63) in the summer and Baghdad in September 1846, before progressing north along the Tigris and Euphrates rivers. In November 1846, cholera struck Mecca (see MECCA CHOLERA EPIDEMIC OF 1831), killing over 15,000 people in and around the city.

After a brief lull during the winter of 1846–47, cholera erupted again in April 1847 in Derbent, spread along the Caspian coast to Astrakhan (see ASTRAKHAN CHOLERA EPIDEMIC OF 1823) and north along the Volga River. It also broke out in Tbilisi in July, and continued west to the Black Sea and beyond (Constantinople was infected late in 1847) and northwest past the Caucasus range into the heart of Russia. The Orenburg (Chkalov) region was also breached (perhaps via the Ural River) as, apparently, was Tobolsk in Siberia. It reached Moscow in September 1847 and, when winter arrived, was nearing Olgopol and Riga in Latvia.

Early in 1848, cholera exploded all over Europe, extending from Norway in the north to England, Scotland, and Ireland in the northwest, to Spain in the southwest, and to the Balkan countries in the east. Muslim pilgrims returning to Egypt from Mecca in 1848 brought cholera with them. Its reappearance in Constantinople caused outbreaks in Syria, Palestine, and, possibly, Iran.

Cholera entered the United States through Staten Island (New York) and New Orleans. From New Orleans, it spread north along the Mississippi River and west into Texas.

The spring of 1849 began with another round of cholera explosions. France and Italy were infected, as were Algeria and Tunisia in North Africa. England suffered a virulent onslaught; at its height, the epidemic claimed some 1,000 lives a day. In May 1849, cholera began spreading rapidly from foci in New York City and New Orleans until most of the United States east of the Rockies was affected. Canada, already struck by sea from Europe, was also attacked by cholera overland from the United States. Mexico was similarly attacked, and a ship carried the disease from New Orleans to Panama late in 1849.

In 1850, there was a severe cholera attack in Egypt and along coastal North Africa. Most of Europe, including areas affected in 1849, was once again infected. For the first time, Sweden and Denmark and the Maltese and Ionian islands were affected. Mainland Greece remained untouched, as in 1837.

Also in 1850, cholera reached California overland and by sea (from Panama). In South America, Colombia and parts of Ecuador were infected. Cuba and Jamaica suffered severely in 1850 and 1851. From Cuba, cholera was transported to Grand Canary Island in May 1851, where it caused 9,000 human deaths in a very short period. Morocco was also plagued in 1851, but cholera was relatively quiescent in Europe except for outbreaks in Poland, Silesia, and Pomerania (German-Polish region on the Baltic). Cholera reemerged in Poland in 1852 and spread into the adjoining Russian provinces and Prussia.

Meanwhile, in 1848–49 cholera had renewed its onslaught in India and, after an outbreak in 1852, embarked on its traditional voyage to the west via Iran and Iraq. In 1853, northern Europe, the United States, Mexico, and the West Indies suffered outbreaks.

This phase of the pandemic represents a complicated mixture of local eruptions and fresh importations of the disease, and its course is not easily traceable. Cholera was fairly widespread in northern Europe in 1854; England, in particular, suffered acutely, but southern Europe was more severely affected. Troop movements from southern France (during the Crimean War) carried cholera to Greece and Turkey. Farther west, it raged through much of the United States, Canada, Mexico, Colombia, and many islands in the West Indies. Though a bad year for cholera, 1854 was also crucial; English physician John Snow's experiments in London showed that contaminated water was an important factor in the spread of cholera.

In 1855, the onslaught continued with some new areas added to the list. Cholera spread from the Arabian Peninsula into Syria and Asia Minor (Turkey). Among the other countries affected were Egypt, Sudan, Morocco, the Cape Verde Islands, Italy, and the adjoining areas of Austria and Switzerland, as well as Venezuela and Brazil.

Between 1856 and 1858, Spain and Portugal were the only European countries to be seriously affected; Central America and Guiana in northern South America were also hit.

In 1852, cholera spread east to Indonesia and later invaded China and Japan (see JAPANESE CHOLERA EPIDEMICS OF 1858–59 AND 1862) in 1854; it became a serious concern in the East in 1857–59. The Philippines were infected in 1858 and Korea a year later.

During this pandemic, the tiny island of Mauritius in the Indian Ocean suffered four outbreaks; neighboring Réunion suffered one. In East Africa, the island of Zanzibar became an important focus of the disease. From here, cholera spread to Mozambique, Madagascar, the Comoro Islands, and Uganda. Ethiopia, first invaded by the disease in 1853, suffered serious outbreaks in 1855 and 1858.

Throughout the 1850s, cholera repeatedly flared up in India. In 1859, an outbreak in Bengal once again led to the transmission of the disease along the usual routes to Iran, Iraq, Arabia, and northwest into Russian territory. Outbreaks were simultaneously reported from Sweden, Denmark, western Prussia, the Netherlands, and Spain. Some ports in Morocco and Algeria were also infected via Spain in 1859. In the early 1860s, cholera was also reported from India, Japan, and Iran.

Further reading: Pollitzer, *Cholera;* Marks and Beatty, *Epidemics.*

Asiatic Cholera Pandemic of 1865–75   Fourth cholera pandemic of the nineteenth century (see ASIATIC CHOLERA PANDEMIC OF 1846–63) and perhaps the most widespread of them all.

In 1863, cholera once again broke out in the Lower Bengal region and spread throughout India. Unlike the previous pandemics, it did not follow the traditional routes across Afghanistan and Persia (Iran) and the Caspian Sea ports into Europe. Rather, Indian Muslim pilgrims visiting Mecca (see MECCA CHOLERA EPIDEMIC OF 1831) reportedly introduced it directly into the Middle East. It is not clear when this introduction occurred, but it caused a massive outbreak in May 1865. Of the 90,000 pilgrims gathered in Mecca, at least 30,000 were struck by cholera either there or in nearby Jedda (Jidda) in western Arabia. Returning home, the Muslim pilgrims spread the disease throughout the Arabian Peninsula, to Iraq (Mesopotamia), Syria, Palestine, and across the Red Sea to Suez and Alexandria in Egypt.

From Alexandria, cholera was transported by refugees all over Egypt, and much Mediterranean traffic and trade ensured its entry into the seaports of Istanbul (July 1865), Smyrna (Izmir), Ancona, and Marseilles. From Istanbul (Constantinople), cholera was distributed all over Turkey, south to Cyprus, Rhodes, and a few Ionian islands, and northwest into Bulgaria, Rumania, and the former Austrian province of Bucovina (Bukovina). Russia was also breached in several provinces, but the infection did not spread much farther until 1866.

Sicily and southern Italy became infected via Ancona, and Paris and much of France were attacked in September 1865. In 1866, cholera resurfaced in parts of France, but in 1867, there were only minor incursions in French territory. Spain suffered an invasion in July 1865 that subsequently led to outbreaks in Portugal. Cholera's invasion of England and Luxembourg in 1865 was not severe. However, the situation in Luxembourg turned virulent in 1866, spreading cholera to Germany's Rhineland-Palatinate and Westphalia in 1866–67.

After a brief lull during the winter of 1865–66, cholera erupted once again in Europe early in 1866 and coursed rapidly through the continent, aided by military movements. It spread extensively in Russia, claiming 90,000 human lives in 1866. Russia was again struck in 1867 but not as severely. The Scandinavian region (except Sweden, which had 4,503 deaths) escaped serious infection in 1866. Germany endured terrible losses (about 115,000 deaths in Prussia alone) as did Austria (80,000 deaths), Hungary (30,000 deaths), the Netherlands (20,000 deaths), and Belgium (30,000 deaths). Cholera also broke out in Italy in 1866 and the next year was devastating; a series of epidemics, including one in Sardinia, brought the Italian death toll for 1867 to 130,000. In Great Britain, about 15,000 died from cholera. Introductions from Italy caused small outbreaks in Switzerland and some other European localities.

Cholera spread extensively from various points in Africa. From Jedda it crossed the Red Sea to the ports of Suakin and Massawa and moved into Ethiopia. Somaliland reported a severe epidemic in 1865 caused by a direct importation from Bombay (via Aden). Traveling south from Ethiopia, the disease reached Zanzibar in 1869 (70,000 deaths) and Mozambique in May 1870; from here it moved to Madagascar, the Seychelles, and the Comoro Islands. Tunisia was apparently infected through Sicilian smugglers and Algeria (via France) in 1865. The Algerian outbreak of 1867 claimed some 80,000 lives. Morocco was infected by pilgrims in 1865 and had an epidemic in 1868. The disease spread from here to countries in French West Africa, Gambia, and Portuguese Guinea (Guinea-Bissau).

Many West Indian islands suffered epidemics during 1865–70: Hispaniola (1866), St. Thomas (1868), and Cuba (1867–70). Guadeloupe, invaded via Marseilles, lost 12,000 of its 150,000 residents in 1865–66.

The United States was attacked either in 1865 or 1866 (see U.S. CHOLERA EPIDEMIC OF 1866). R. Pollitzer (see below) believed that the infection arrived in New York from Le Havre, France, in autumn 1865 but did not become epidemic until spring 1866. Newly extended railway lines and troop movements caused the rapid spread of cholera to parts of Louisiana (about 12,000 lives were lost in New Orleans), Texas, and other southern states, and as far west as Albuquerque, New Mexico. National cholera mortality for that year was estimated at 50,000 deaths, far lower than during previous epidemics. In 1867, other U.S. cities suffered minor outbreaks. New Orleans and vicinity were struck severely again in 1873.

Between 1866 and 1868, the disease traveled from New Orleans into Nicaragua and Honduras. Paraguayan troops who were battling both the disease and joint Argentinian-Brazilian forces in April 1866 transported it to Corrientes, Argentina. From there it spread (1867) along the Parana River into Buenos Aires (December) and Uruguay (1868). It also spread overland from Argentina into Bolivia and Peru (considered cholera's first invasion of South America's west coast). Cholera was rampant in southern Brazil (via Paraguay) in 1867 and 1868.

Russia continued to suffer the ravages of cholera in 1868–69; an epidemic of moderate intensity rocked the city of Kiev in August 1869. Thirty-seven Russian provinces were attacked by cholera in 1870; it was particularly intense in 1871 in European Russia and in the southern Siberian cities of Tobolsk and Tomsk, where about 130,000 lives were lost. The disease was also virulent in southern and western Russia in 1872, and the death toll was just as high as in 1871.

The Black Sea ports of Rumania, Bulgaria, and Turkey (notably Istanbul and Trabzon) were invaded via Russia in 1871, as were Finland, Sweden, Prussia, and Austria's Galician province. In 1873, the German death toll from cholera was 33,156 people; Hungary lost 190,000 people in 1872–73. In 1873, cholera was also reported in Great Britain, the Netherlands, Belgium, Sweden, Norway, and France.

Cholera had settled firmly in Persia (Iran) since 1865. A major outbreak there in 1870 helped spread the disease into Turkish Kurdistan, Iraq, and Arabia. In 1871–72, cholera spread west to Egypt and east into Bukhara (in Uzbekistan) and Russian Turkistan. It resurfaced in Mecca in 1872 and entered the Sudan through its port of Suakin on the Red Sea. Syria faced a serious epidemic in 1875.

Cholera was extremely virulent in India during 1875–77 (see INDIAN CHOLERA EPIDEMIC OF 1875–77). In 1862, it struck China, affecting Peking (Beijing), Manchuria and Shanghai (untold thousands of people died). It spread from India to Indonesia in 1863–64 and again to China and Japan in 1864–65. From Thailand and Malaya in 1873 it penetrated Sumatra, Java, and Madura, while from Singapore it was carried to Borneo and the Celebes. Japan's most serious invasion occurred in 1877–79, with 158,204 cholera cases and 89,207 human deaths recorded in the last year alone. See also ZANZIBAR CHOLERA EPIDEMIC OF 1869.

Further reading: Pollitzer, *Cholera;* Marks and Beatty, *Epidemics.*

Asiatic Cholera Pandemic of 1881–96

Fifth in a series of cholera pandemics (see ASIATIC CHOLERA PANDEMIC OF 1817–23, et al.), marked by German physician Robert Koch's discovery that cholera was indeed a specific gastrointestinal infection.

The pandemic began, as had its predecessors, in India. Traveling from its endemic home in the Lower Bengal region, cholera exploded with tremendous virulence in the Punjab and Lahore region of northwest India during 1881–82, causing heavy casualties. Outbreaks occurred in Korea in 1881, in Thailand in 1882, during both these years in Mecca (Arabia), China (also in 1883), and Japan, and in the Philippines in 1882–83. From Mecca, returning Muslim pilgrims carried cholera to Damietta in Egypt's Nile

River delta. During 1883, cholera raged throughout Egypt.

Cholera erupted in Toulon, France, in April 1884, and later there were small outbreaks in Marseilles, Paris, and other cities, affecting 10,000 people all over the country. Some of the same areas were reinfected in 1885.

Italy's strict quarantine regulations were breached in 1884, with the city of Naples recording a major outbreak in August–September. Cholera plagued Italy through 1886–87 but did not cause epidemics.

Spain suffered a brief invasion of the disease in 1884, a more virulent one in 1885 (160,000 cases and about 60,000 deaths), and another minor incursion in 1890.

Cholera failed to establish itself in Great Britain thanks to timely preventive measures. Prompt diagnosis of a case on board a ship bound from Naples and Marseilles to New York, prevented its arrival in North America. However, the South American continent suffered seriously in 1886 (Argentina), 1887 (Chile), and 1888 (Argentina and Chile).

In Asia, cholera troubled China in 1888, 1890, and 1895; Japan in 1885, 1886, 1890, 1891, and 1895; Korea in 1888, 1890, 1891, and 1895; and the Philippines in 1888–89. After causing massive outbreaks in northern India during 1891, cholera raged through Afghanistan and Iran in 1892 and then entered Russia (see RUSSIAN CHOLERA EPIDEMIC OF 1892–93), where the morbidity was staggering.

Meanwhile, in 1892, the disease was prevalent in France and Germany, with the city of Hamburg suffering seriously (see HAMBURG CHOLERA EPIDEMIC OF 1892). Both countries were reinfected in 1893–94 but not in epidemic form.

South America was attacked several times in the 1890s: Brazil in 1893–95, Argentina in 1894–95, and Uruguay in 1895.

On the African continent, cholera was prevalent in 1893 (Tripolitania [western Libya], Tunisia, Algeria, Morocco, and French West Africa), 1894 (Sudan, Tripolitania, and French West Africa), 1895 (Morocco and Egypt), and 1896 (Egypt).

For a few years after that, cholera lay dormant, but it erupted again in many regions in 1899. See also FRENCH CHOLERA EPIDEMICS OF 1848–49, 1853–54, AND 1865–66; GERMAN CHOLERA EPIDEMICS OF 1830–90.

Further reading: Pollitzer, *Cholera;* Marks and Beatty, *Epidemics.*

Asiatic Cholera Pandemic of 1899–1923

Sixth in a series of cholera pandemics (see ASIATIC CHOLERA PANDEMIC OF 1881–96) that originated in India. During 1899, cholera once again broke out in northern India, causing major outbreaks in Bombay, Calcutta, and other cities in 1900. In fact, in 1900, mortality from cholera (805,698 deaths) was the highest ever recorded in India during a single year. Cholera also spread south to the former Madras Presidency (province) and lingered in the country through the ensuing decade. Meanwhile, in 1900, it invaded Afghanistan and the Persian Gulf region in the west and, in 1901, Burma (Myanmar) and Singapore in the east.

In 1902, Indian Muslim pilgrims bound from Madras to Mecca by sea, transported cholera to Jedda (Jidda) in Saudi Arabia. What followed, from the end of February 1902 in Mecca, was an explosive outbreak that killed about 4,000 pilgrims in the city. Intensive measures to prevent the disease from encroaching into Egypt failed, and it moved from Asyut (Assiut) across the rest of the country. According to one source, some 34,000 people succumbed to the epidemic here.

From Burma and Malaya, the epidemic spread in 1902 to infect China, Manchuria, Korea, Japan, and the Philippines, perhaps rekindling preexisting cholera foci in those countries.

In 1903, cholera attacked Syria via the Sinai Peninsula, Palestine, Asia Minor, the coastal areas of the Black Sea, Mesopotamia (Iraq), and Persia (Iran). During the spring of 1904, caravan traffic transported cholera through Samarkand into the Caspian Sea port of Baku, where it erupted in September 1904. Cholera continued its westward march into Transcaucasia, north via Astrakhan (see ASTRAKHAN CHOLERA EPIDEMIC OF 1823, RUSSIAN CHOLERA EPIDEMIC OF 1829–31), and then along the Volga River up to Samara (Kuibyshev). Some scholars believe it penetrated to as far east as western Siberia.

In 1905, cholera did not emerge beyond the valleys of the Ural, Don, and Volga rivers and was virtually dormant through 1906. It flared up once again in 1907 in the Volga basin and, in the following year, spread as far as St. Petersburg and some Baltic ports in the west, many Black Sea ports to the south and eastward into Transcaspia, Turkistan, and Siberia. The situation eased somewhat in 1909 and then was followed by the Russian Cholera Epidemic of 1910 (q.v.). Once that abated, the cholera situation was fairly quiet in Russia until the First World War began, when major outbreaks occurred (see RUSSIAN CHOLERA EPIDEMICS OF 1915–22).

The Americas remained free of cholera during this pandemic. A ship carrying Russian immigrants to South America infected the Atlantic islands of Madeira during a stopover in October 1910. The resulting outbreak (1,769 cases and 600 deaths), which lasted until February 1911, marked the pandemic's westernmost presence.

In 1909, cholera was introduced into the Dutch port city of Rotterdam, where it caused a minor outburst (26 cases and six deaths). Sporadic occurrences were reported from 18 other areas in the Netherlands. Elsewhere in western Europe, cholera occurred only in isolated pockets. Central and southeastern Europe were not as lucky. Cholera erupted in a small way at Apulia and Naples in Italy during 1909. During the summer of 1910, the disease was reintroduced by gypsies traveling from Russia via Brindisi. The infection quickly spread over the southern part of Italy, killing 1,400 people over a few weeks. In the following summer, most of Italy (including Sicily) was infected, but serious outbreaks occurred only in a few areas. Apparently, an importation from here caused an outbreak (733 cases) in Tunisia in 1911.

Cholera arrived in Hungary in 1909 and caused several outbreaks in 1910 and 1913. Both Hungary and Austria suffered seriously during World War I (1914–18), mainly because of importations by Russian and Serbian prisoners of war. Austrian troops introduced cholera into Prussian Silesia but without any major consequences. Again, Russian prisoners interned in Germany introduced the disease into the prison camps there, but it did not spread, except marginally, into the civilian population. The German Army, vaccinated against cholera, suffered a fairly low incidence except in the Turkey-based regiments. The Balkan countries were plagued by serious outbreaks of cholera from 1910 to 1922.

Cholera erupted frequently in Saudi Arabia during this pandemic. One of the most severe outbreaks occurred in Islam's holy city of Mecca late in 1907 (perhaps an importation from Odessa) and killed 25,000 or more in the kingdom of Hejaz during 1908. Other Arabian outbreaks were in 1909 (Hejaz), 1910 (Mecca), 1911 (Mecca), and 1912. The situation in Persia was similar; cholera was widespread in 1906, returned via the north in 1908, and was prevalent in 1911–12, 1914–19, and again in 1922–23. Turkey suffered in 1916, Mesopotamia in 1918, 1919, and 1923, and Palestine in 1918.

India was seriously affected throughout the first decade of the twentieth century, with hundreds of thousands of cholera deaths recorded in most years—1904 (189,855 deaths), 1905 (439,439 deaths), 1906 (682,649 deaths), 1907 (400,024 deaths), 1908 (579,814 deaths) and 1909 (227,842 deaths). More than half a million deaths occurred annually during 1918 and 1919 in India.

Other Southeast Asian areas, particularly Burma, Indochina, the Philippines, and Indonesia, also bore the repeated onslaught of the disease throughout the pandemic period.

Further reading: Pollitzer, *Cholera;* Marks and Beatty, *Epidemics.*

Asiatic Cholera Pandemic of 1961–75   Pandemic of so-called *el tor* cholera (paracholera) that spread in three phases over much of Southeast Asia, the Middle East, Africa, and parts of Eastern Europe.

This pandemic was caused by *Vibrio el tor*, a different strain of the *Vibrio comma (cholera vibrio),* isolated in 1905 by F. Gottslich from the bodies of six Muslim pilgrims housed at the El Tor quarantine station outside Mecca. Endemic in Sulawesi (formerly the Celebes Islands), Indonesia, it had caused several outbreaks there since the 1930s. There, in January 1961, a major cholera epidemic began in the seaport of Makassar and soon spread (aided by the movement of troops and the Chinese population) to central and northern sections of Sulawesi.

During its first phase (1961–62), most of the island territories in Southeast Asia were infected, mainly via sea routes, starting with Java (May), Sarawak (July), Kalimantan, Macao, and Hong Kong (all in August), Philippines (September), Sumatra, and Timor (November). Paracholera (as the disease was sometimes called) was also reported from Canton even before it reached Hong Kong. It is estimated that over 12,000 cases and nearly 2,000 human deaths occurred in these areas during 1961. The pandemic continued to spread even in 1962—Sabah (January), Taiwan (July), and Irian Jaya (October). There were over 13,000 cases and 1,977 deaths in 1962 in these areas.

In 1963, *Vibrio el tor* invaded the Asian mainland and reinfected all the Western Pacific rim countries except Taiwan. Malaysia was attacked in May, Korea in September, and Bangladesh in December. Also by December, Singapore, Thailand, Cambodia (by rail from Thailand), and Burma (Myanmar) were infected. Vietnam was struck in January 1964. The epidemic penetrated India in March 1964 via the port of Madras. Both here and in Calcutta (struck in April), the infection was apparently transported by sea through Indians returning from Burma. In less than a year, most of the country was engulfed.

From India, the disease traveled to Pakistan (June 1965) and then very quickly to Afghanistan (early July), Iran (mid-July), and adjoining territories of the former Soviet Union (August 21). Surprisingly, Iraq escaped the infection until August 5, 1966. The westward march of the pandemic led to panic, the introduction of strict repressive measures, and severe

disruption of international trade. Perhaps because of these measures, the pandemic was relatively quiescent between 1967 and 1969 except for the reinvasion of Malaysia and Singapore in 1968 and Hong Kong, Macao, and Korea in 1969. Laos, in Indochina, was attacked for the first time in 1969.

The following year, 1970, was one of the worst in the history of cholera. The pandemic intensified once again to infect 24 new countries in Asia (6), Africa (15), and Europe (3).

The third phase began when Soviet (Russian) authorities announced an imported outbreak caused by the *Vibrio el tor* in the city of Astrakhan on August 10, 1970. Subsequently, between August 14 and September 19, 1970, *el tor* outbreaks were reported from six Middle East countries: Lebanon (August 14), Israel (August 21), Dubai (August 27), Syria (September 2), Jordan (September 3), and Saudi Arabia (September 9). Also hit were Libya (August 23), Ukraine's port of Odessa (September 4), and Tunisia (September 19). The presence of *Vibrio el tor* in Iraq and Iran prior to the outbreak in Astrakhan, and in Egypt prior to its Middle East eruptions, is assumed. Two different serotypes (microorganisms with common antigens) of the *vibrio*—Inaba and Ogawa—were responsible for these outbreaks.

In November 1970, the pandemic (Inaba serotype) traveled from the Arabian Peninsula to Ethiopia, the French-owned Afars and Issas (Djibouti), and in December 1970 to Somalia. Meanwhile, in July 1970, Guinea-Bissau became the first West African country to be invaded—apparently by the air routes—by the Ogawa serotype. The infection spread very rapidly to Sierra Leone (September 24), Liberia (October 6), Ivory Coast (October 20), Mali and Togo (November 24), Dahomey (December 16), Upper Volta (Burkina Faso) (December 17), and Nigeria and Niger (December 27). Ghana, although infected in January 1971, did not experience cholera outbreaks until November. Istanbul, Turkey, experienced a virulent attack in October (Inaba serotype) as did Czechoslovakia.

In 1971, cholera raged in nearly all these countries and attacked new ones: Cameroon (February), Chad and Uganda (May), Mauritania (June), Algeria and Morocco (July), Senegal (August) and Angola (December). In March, Kenya and Oman became infected, as did Yemen, subsequently. Spain was invaded in July and Portugal in September—perhaps through citizens returning from North Africa. Over 100,000 new cholera cases occurred during this year. Two severe epidemics were recorded—in Indonesia (23,555 cases) and in India (51,000 cases).

In 1973–74, cholera occurred in Mozambique, Malawi, Zimbabwe, South Africa, and Tanzania (for the first time). Italy suffered an outbreak in August 1973 and Portugal between April and November 1974 and in 1975. In the east, Sri Lanka, Java, Sumatra, and some of the Philippine islands were invaded between 1973 and 1975.

Further reading: Barua and Burrows, eds., *Cholera;* Howe, *A World Geography of Human Diseases.*

Asiatic and European Influenza Pandemic of 1830–31
Series of influenza epidemics occurring mainly in Asia and Europe in 1830–31 and believed to be part of a global pandemic at the time.

The pandemic apparently began (although this remains a matter of some dispute) in China late in 1829. In October and November of that year, influenza was reported from the port city of Canton (Kwangchow or Guangzhou). Influenza also occurred in other unspecified parts of China in January (crew members of a British ship were infected on the 25th) and in September 1830. From China, the infection was transported along the shipping routes to the Philippines, where Manila was struck early in September.

Through the subsequent months, influenza may have spread south through the Philippine Islands. In January 1831, it arrived in Borneo and in Sumatra. The seaport of Grisee in Surabaya (Surabaja) province in northeastern Java (Indonesia) experienced a severe epidemic late in March. It affected the inland areas and spread to the island of Madura in mid-April. Early in June, the western sections of Java were affected, too.

The epidemic continued to move northwest, arriving in Singapore in mid-June, in Malacca at the end of June, and in Penang in mid-July (all on the Malay Peninsula). Outbreaks were reported from various Indian cities in April and December 1832, but it is not clear if they were offshoots of this pandemic or precursors of the next. Japan was also attacked by an influenza epidemic in 1831–32.

The first inkling of the pandemic's presence in Europe came from Moscow, in Russia, which reported an outbreak in November 1830. St. Petersburg was affected in January 1831. How the pandemic arrived in Europe is not definitely known. Some believe it may have traveled from China by the overland route across Siberia and the Urals or via the Central Asian republics. Once in Europe, it spread rapidly to infect the Baltic area (notably Tartu in Estonia) in February and Warsaw in March. In April, Breslau, Berlin, and East Prussia were invaded; in May, influenza reached Budapest, Prague, Vienna, Hamburg, central Germany, Denmark, Sweden, and Finland. England, Scotland, the rest of Germany, Paris and the northern part of France were infected in June. In July, influenza penetrated southern France, the Netherlands, Belgium, and the Swiss city of Geneva. It was quiescent during the summer but reappeared in Rome in mid-November and spread to Naples and Sicily in December and to Spain and Gibraltar in January 1832.

Shipping traffic carried influenza across the Atlantic into the United States. The mid-Atlantic states were apparently the first to be affected; the flu outbreaks in Philadelphia and Boston peaked during December 10–17, 1831. Influenza cases were reported from Cincinnati as early as mid-November. The disease progressed slowly south along the Atlantic coast, arriving in Georgia's Burke County in February 1832. Most of the United States had been affected by then.

Everywhere, the pandemic was characterized by a high attack rate, but the case-mortality was quite low. In Manila and Penang, for instance, the epidemic infected so many residents that normal business activities had to be suspended. In Java's Buitenzorg (Bogor) province (population 219,415), 51,588 cases and 277 deaths were reported. No doubt the morbidity rate (23.5 percent) is an understatement, but the mortality rate of 1.3 percent may be quite accurate. Morbidity (incidence of disease) was 15.5 percent and mortality 0.3 percent in the Javanese province of Surabaya (311,192 population).

The pandemic spread extensively, but mildly and erratically, throughout Europe. Ten percent were infected in Geneva, and about 75 percent in Naples. Mortality was negligible in England and estimated at about 2 percent in Glasgow, Scotland. In Boston, total mortality was 20 percent higher, undoubtedly attributable to the influenza epidemic. The disease was relatively dormant in 1832 but erupted in pandemic form in 1833 (see EUROPEAN INFLUENZA PANDEMIC OF 1833).

Further reading: Patterson, *Pandemic Influenza 1700–1900;* Beveridge, *Influenza: The Last Great Plague.*

Asiatic and European Influenza Pandemic of 1836–37
Influenza epidemics were scattered across Asia and Europe during 1836–37 and were believed by many to be interconnected. However, there is some doubt on whether or not they constituted a true pandemic (see ASIATIC AND EUROPEAN INFLUENZA PANDEMIC OF 1830–31).

Interestingly, the first intimation of the disease was from the southern hemisphere. In October 1836, influenza was reported from Sydney, Australia, and from Cape Town in South Africa. In both cities, it began to spread. In November, influenza attacked Java and Penang (in Malaya) and was also recorded in the northern Canadian territory of the Hudson's Bay Company. The latter outbreak is considered its only incursion across the Atlantic.

While influenza raged through Cape Town in November 1836, St. Petersburg in Russia was apparently infected at the same time. The following month, the infection struck many European cities, including London, Aberdeen, Stockholm, Copenhagen (and a large part of Denmark), Berlin, Hamburg, and Germany's two Baltic ports (Lübeck and Greifswald). In the early stages of influenza's movement across Europe, the Baltic area seems to have been an important disseminating center.

Within the next month, the disease had extended itself as far north as the seaport of Umea in Sweden and covered much of England, Ireland, Germany, and the Netherlands. Vienna, Paris, Bordeaux, and Geneva were also affected at the end of January 1837. Influenza erupted in Egypt and Syria in January.

In February, France, Germany's Rhineland, northern Italy, and northern Spain came under attack. British ships carried the infection to Lisbon, Portugal, early in that month. Switzerland escaped the outbreak until March, when Rome, Barcelona, and Madrid also succumbed to it. In May it was devastating Naples and, in June, Palermo and Malta. Apparently, even Iceland was hit in 1837.

Everywhere, cities were the initial focus of the influenza infection, which was then diffused to surrounding areas. During the pandemic, the most serious to strike Europe since 1781–82, morbidity (incidence of disease) was high. According to some, this pandemic may have been an offshoot of or caused by a varying strain of a previous pandemic. Perhaps the influenza outbreaks in the southern hemisphere and in southeast Asia were part of a series of unrecorded epidemics in the area during 1836 that eventually invaded Europe later in the year.

More people died during this pandemic than during the previous two pandemics. In Geneva and Copenhagen, for instance, more than 50 percent of the population was attacked by flu. Paris and Lyon suffered just as severely, while in Florence three quarters of the population fell ill. Overall mortality was unusually high in cities like London, Berlin, Hanover, Stockholm, and Glasgow.

Further reading: Patterson, *Pandemic Influenza 1700–1900*; Beveridge, *Influenza: The Last Great Plague*.

Asiatic Influenza Pandemic of 1781–82   See EUROPEAN INFLUENZA PANDEMIC OF 1781–82.

Asiatic Influenza Pandemic of 1889–90   More severe than previous influenza pandemics and certainly more widespread in its impact. It was marked by annual reappearances in the years immediately following 1890.

There is some controversy regarding the origin of this "flu" epidemic. Most accounts have traced it to Bukhara (Bokhara), capital of Uzbekistan in central Asia, and apparently it first broke out there in May 1889. Frank Clemov, a British physician, disputed this theory and placed the pandemic's source in the towns of Tcheliabinsk (Chelyabinsk) in western Siberia and Petropavlovsk in Kazakhstan in early October 1889. Regardless of which theory is accepted, there is general agreement regarding the subsequent course taken by the pandemic.

In Bukhara, the outbreak affected two thirds of the city's 80,000 to 100,000 residents and left several thousand dead. Apparently, the epidemic lingered in the city until August 1889 and perhaps would have been no more than a localized outbreak had it not been for the newly opened railway routes from the Caspian Sea across the Kara Kum (Qara Qum) desert to Bukhara and Samarkand. Built to encourage the export of carpets from these two renowned cities, the railways helped spread the epidemic to far-flung areas. In October, the city of Tomsk in Siberia reported outbreaks. Around the same time, Moscow, St. Petersburg (Leningrad), and towns along the Volga River and in the rest of European Russia were struck by the influenza's virus. Central Asian republics were invaded from the north and east in two separate waves, and the city of Kiev was infected in mid-November. By late December 1889 influenza had traveled beyond Lake Baikal to the Chita region. Stretinsk (Stretensk) was infected in January 1890 and again in August, Yakutsk in February, Vladivostok, Khabarovsk, and Sakhalin Island in June, and Blagoveshchensk in July 1890.

The Scandinavian and Central European countries were invaded in November 1889, mainly through Baltic shipping and rail traffic. Thereafter, the pandemic spread very rapidly along the highways, waterways, and rail routes, covering most of Europe by late December. The epidemic even reached Constantinople (Istanbul) by the end of the year. Great Britain was infected in mid-December, and the epidemic crossed the country with the Christmas traffic from London.

Meanwhile, across the Atlantic, New York and Boston reported influenza outbreaks in mid-December 1889, and Montreal was hit a week later. Over the next two months, the epidemic spread through much of the eastern half of the United States and established pockets of infection at San Francisco and New Orleans.

The Central and South American countries were infected in January 1890 (Mexico, Guatemala, Uruguay), February (Brazil, Argentina, and Chile), March (Peru), April (Ecuador), and October (Falkland Islands). The disease's diffusion through the

West Indies was more erratic and extended over the first six months of 1890.

In Africa, the first outbreaks were reported in January 1890 from Egypt, Morocco, Tunisia, Libya, and Cape Town in South Africa. The West African countries were struck from February to June. Zanzibar was infected in March, Botswana in April, Mozambique in July, Mauritius in August, Réunion and Malawi in September, and Ethiopia's mountainous region in November 1890.

Persia (Iran) was invaded in January 1890 by two separate waves from Russia. From here, the epidemic is believed to have traveled overland to Pakistan. Beirut was attacked via the Mediterranean late in January and Yemen in early April. The virus arrived in Colombo, the capital of Ceylon (Sri Lanka), on a ship from England and lingered in its rural areas until July. Late in February, the disease entered India's port of Bombay. The Indian railways quickly transported it to the bustling cities of Calcutta and Madras. Smaller cities such as Poona, Benares (Varanasi), and Meerut were attacked in mid-March. In June, rural Bengal was still suffering. Kashmir was invaded in December 1890.

Southeast Asia reported influenza epidemics in February 1890 (Singapore, Japan, and Hong Kong), March (Malaysia, North Borneo), April (Tientsin in northern China), July (Peking/Beijing), September (Yunnan province in China), and October (Shanghai).

In March 1890, the epidemic reached Australia and New Zealand. Otago, Wellington, Dunedin, Christ-church, Tasmania, Melbourne, Sydney, and much of southeastern Australia reported epidemics in March. Adelaide and Queensland were invaded in April and Auckland and Perth in May 1890.

During its journey across the world, the disease left few countries untouched and had a high attack rate. Like the pandemics of 1957 (see ASIAN INFLUENZA PANDEMIC OF 1957–58) and 1968 (see HONG KONG INFLUENZA PANDEMIC OF 1968), succeeding waves of this pandemic were more severe than the initial outbreak. Even after it had passed, many countries continued to suffer recurrent influenza epidemics during successive years. In some cases these caused many more deaths than the pandemic itself—mainly due to secondary pneumonia or other respiratory diseases—particularly among the elderly.

Further reading: Patterson, *Pandemic Influenza 1700–1900;* Beveridge, *Influenza: The Last Great Plague;* Henschen, *The History of Diseases.*

Astrakhan Cholera Epidemic of 1823 Offshoot of the Asiatic Cholera Pandemic of 1817–23 (q.v.), marking the westernmost limit of that pandemic.

Cholera reached the Russian port city of Astrakhan (on the Caspian Sea's Volga River delta) via vessels from Resht in northern Persia (Iran) (see PERSIAN CHOLERA EPIDEMICS OF 1821–22, SYRIAN CHOLERA EPIDEMIC OF 1822–23) and via land travelers from Tiflis (Tbilisi) in Georgia in September 1823. An official report received from Tiflis in mid-August had forewarned the Russian government of cholera's westward progress. The outbreak was brief—lasting only two months—but intense. Of the 392 cholera cases reported between September 10 and October 4, 1823, 205 were fatal. According to historian Roderick McGrew's research, these statistics are not very reliable; the reporting of such data, he believed, could not have been accurate given the vast distance from Astrakhan to the central Russian administration as well as the frequent inability of doctors to correctly diagnose cholera.

Officially, the Russian government accepted the theory of contagion and advised that cholera-infected patients be isolated and quarantined. There are conflicting reports regarding whether the local government enforced these quarantine measures or not. Nevertheless, the epidemic remained localized within the Astrakhan region and did not spread north into European territory. This has been attributed by some scholars to the severe European winter of 1823–24 rather than to any specific preventive measures undertaken by the Astrakhan administration.

The Medical Council in St. Petersburg dispatched two of its representatives to Astrakhan. By the time they arrived and confirmed the outbreak as being one of Asiatic cholera, the epidemic was beginning to subside. However, cholera's entry into Russian territory prompted the creation of a special cholera council at St. Petersburg. The council established a sound medical and administrative framework enabling it to deal with future cholera epidemics. Their recommendations were implemented when the next cholera epidemic struck in 1829–30 (see PERSIAN CHOLERA EPIDEMIC OF 1829–30).

Further reading: McGrew, *Russia and the Cholera, 1823–32.*

Astrakhan Plague of 1727–28 Epidemic of bubonic plague that invaded the Volga River port city of Astrakhan during 1727–28.

The outbreak began rather slowly and may have been caused by Russian military incursions into plague-infested Persian territory during this period. Astrakhan was an important center in the silk trade, and the infection may have been an importation from across the Central Asian steppes. It is also possible that the outbreak resulted from local foci (disease areas). The first case occurred in July 1727 when a soldier returning by ship from Gilan in Persia was found to be suffering from plague-like symptoms. Upon examination, physicians discovered buboes in his groin area, but he did not die until August 27 and no other cases were reported, so they concluded that he had died of dropsy and leg wounds.

A week later, another soldier returning from military duty in Persia and exhibiting characteristic plague symptoms died, leaving no doubt as to the cause. His remains were cremated immediately, and his companions rushed out of town. Throughout the mild winter of 1727–28, a scattered outbreak of plague continued before exploding upon Astrakhan in a big way in April 1728. By the end of the month, plague had claimed 411 victims and attacked another 315 people, who had to be isolated.

During the spring and summer of 1728, the governor of Astrakhan urged citizens to head for the suburbs and outlying areas. He ordered the evacuation of the garrison and all government offices in the city. His advice was only partially heeded and the situation deteriorated rapidly. People left stricken homes for refuge with healthy relatives, but secretly took their infected belongings with them. This defeated the very purpose of the mass evacuation and spread the infection even farther. The bodies of plague victims were secretly disposed off to escape detection by the surgeons and to enable survivors to continue living in the infected house. June (1728) was the worst month: 1,300 deaths were recorded by June 21, mostly among migrant summer laborers. On June 30, the governor finally ordered the evacuation of the entire city.

Mortality rates stabilized by early August, but the imperial government forbade any movement of people or goods from the south until June 1729. This ban aggravated the growing food crisis in Astrakhan. Overall, it is estimated that 3,000 people died during this epidemic in the city (population 20,000). Many of these were migrant workers already weakened by malnutrition. In 1738–39, Russia was struck by another epidemic of plague (see RUSSIAN PLAGUE OF 1738–39).

Further reading: Alexander, *Bubonic Plague in Early Modern Russia.*

Athens Plague of 430–429 B.C.   See PLAGUE OF ATHENS, GREAT.

Augsburg Typhus Epidemic of 1703–04   Deadly outbreak of epidemic typhus fever in the southern German town of Augsburg during the War of the Spanish Succession (1702–1714). Augsburg (located in Bavaria at the confluence of the Wertach and Lech rivers) was infected first by French and Bavarian

soldiers occupying the town in 1703, and then by the English and Imperial armies who besieged the town the following year. Annual burials rose from 900 human bodies in 1702 to 1,245 in 1703, increasing dramatically in 1704 to 3,113. These excess deaths among Augsburg's inhabitants were due mainly to typhus fever; an abrupt drop to 748 deaths in 1705 indicates the end of the epidemic.

Further reading: Prinzing, *Epidemics Resulting from Wars;* Cloudsley-Thompson, *Insects and History.*

Australian Influenza Epidemics of 1890–91   See SYDNEY INFLUENZA EPIDEMICS OF 1890–91.

Australian Influenza Epidemic of 1918–19   Epidemic that affected Australia in two waves: the first (a mild one) in late 1918, and the second (a rather more virulent visitation) in early 1919. It was part of a global pandemic of influenza (see SPANISH INFLUENZA EPIDEMIC OF 1917–19) that ravaged many countries (see INDIAN INFLUENZA EPIDEMIC OF 1918–19; INDONESIAN INFLUENZA EPIDEMIC OF 1918).

In September 1918, influenza outbreaks were reported from Sydney, Australia, in which nearly 30 percent of the population was said to be affected. In October, severe influenza and pneumonia (this often fatal) were prevalent in the southern parts of New South Wales. Later that month, the federal government introduced rigid quarantine measures for ships arriving from infected ports. These measures remained operative until May 1919 and clearly succeeded in keeping the more virulent infection at bay until early 1919, even as neighboring New Zealand suffered intensely during late 1918 (see NEW ZEALAND INFLUENZA EPIDEMIC OF 1918–19). Meanwhile, outbreaks were reported from some of the quarantined ships.

In mid-January 1919, influenza broke out at Melbourne, Australia, and spread across the province of Victoria in three waves. The first occurred in February 1919, the second in April and May, and the third in July and August. In Victoria, the highest mortality (18.7 percent) was recorded during the second wave. Overall, 3,316 people died in Victoria during the nine-month period from January 1, 1919, to September 12, 1919.

In New South Wales, the epidemic began somewhat mildly but became more virulent as it progressed. It peaked in two waves during June–August 1919, recording a mortality rate of 33.5 percent. During the same nine-month period, 5,869 deaths were registered in the province of New South Wales. The people in South Australia, Queensland, Western Australia, and Tasmania (infected in August 1919) were not as severely attacked.

Influenza broke out frequently in Australia in the years immediately following the epidemic. For instance, Sydney suffered an outbreak in February 1920. Melbourne, Adelaide, and Brisbane suffered severe influenza complicated by pneumonia in June–July 1923. Milder outbreaks were again reported in the country in 1924.

Further reading: Jordan, *Epidemic Influenza: A Survey*; Mackenzie, ed., *Viral Diseases in South-East Asia and the Western Pacific*.

Australian Murray Valley Encephalitis Epidemics

Outbreaks of a new disease called Murray Valley Encephalitis (MVE) in Australia during the twentieth century. Known also as Australian Arbo-Encephalitis, MVE hits the human central nervous system, causing high fever, rigidity of the muscles, mental confusion, and coma. Caused by an arbovirus (arthropod-borne virus), MVE is transmitted in Australia by the mosquito *Culex annulirostris* from an intermediate host such as the waterfowl to man. The disease is not spread from man to man. In fact, many infected people exhibit no outward manifestations of the disease. MVE is now known to occur only in Australia and Papua New Guinea.

The first cases were noticed in southern Australia's Murray River Valley area in the spring of 1917. During the following summer, 134 cases were reported from New South Wales, Queensland, and northern Victoria. Nearly half of those affected were children under five years of age—a comparatively younger age group than that affected by the Japanese B Encephalitis virus (see JAPANESE ENCEPHALITIS EPIDEMICS OF THE 1920S AND 1930S). Mortality was high; according to one estimate, this MVE outbreak claimed 94 lives during 1917–18. The causative virus was successfully isolated from the central nervous system of three fatal cases during this outbreak, only to be lost soon thereafter. (It was rediscovered during a 1951 epidemic of MVE in Australia.)

There was also an outbreak of MVE in 1922 and another in 1925–26. After a long hiatus, MVE resurfaced in the 1950s; the epidemic in 1951 killed 19 people. It was followed by another MVE epidemic in 1974 that led to ten deaths.

Further reading: Paul, *A History of Poliomyelitis*; Shaw, ed., *Australian Encyclopedia*.

Australian Rubella Epidemic of 1938–41

Massive and widespread outbreak of rubella (also called German measles) that first struck Australia in 1938 and lasted until 1941.

Rubella was no stranger to Australia, where there had been a number of outbreaks of the disease in different areas during the late nineteenth and early twentieth centuries—for example, in 1899, in 1917, and in 1924–25. All of them were caused by a fresh importation of the rubella virus from outside the country. Even in Australia's major cities, there did not then exist a large enough pool of susceptible persons to keep the rubella virus spreading indefinitely. Many people had immunity acquired by natural infection.

Caused by a filterable virus, rubella begins with fever, headache, sore throat, and coughing and generally produces a reddish, somewhat elevated but usually short-lived (three days) rash. It is less dangerous than measles (rubeola) and is primarily a childhood affliction. During the epidemic of 1938–41, many adults were infected, too. Morbidity statistics are not available because rubella was not declared a notifiable disease until 1953 in Australia. The epidemic peaked in the country in 1940.

This extensive epidemic was important in that it led to the discovery of the relationship between rubella and congenital malformations, such as deaf-mutism, cataracts, blindness, heart malfunction, and microcephaly. To the Australian ophthalmologist N. McAlister Gregg, goes the credit for showing that women who suffered from rubella during pregnancy (particularly in the early stages) ran the risk of giving birth to a child with congenital defects. Following this discovery in 1941, immunization against rubella was introduced for women of child-bearing age in Australia.

Further reading: *Health and Disease in Tribal Societies*; Bett, *The History and Conquest of Common Diseases*.

Australian Scarlet Fever Epidemic of 1875–76

Major epidemic of scarlet fever that extended over several provinces in southeastern Australia and caused high mortality.

Scarlet fever, a dreaded and highly infectious childhood disease, was introduced into Sydney, Australia, late in the 1830s via infected passengers arriving from England on immigrant ships. The first scarlet fever epidemic reportedly occurred in 1840–41 in the Sydney area; 69 patients were treated at the city dispensary. During the next few decades, the disease continued to plague Australia in epidemic waves (1849–50, 1858–59, 1863–64) and endemic form.

The epidemic of 1875–76 was more widespread and virulent than any of its predecessors; it also lasted longer (approximately 40 weeks in Sydney). A scarlet fever epidemic raging in England in 1874 may have been responsible for the outbreak in Australia in 1875. In Sydney, the epidemic began late in September 1875 and continued halfway through 1876. The disease, which struck in two stages, was particularly acute between November 1875 and June 1876.

During the first phase (12 weeks from early November to the end of January), 236 people (41 percent of total mortality) died. The second phase (early February to the third week of May) claimed 248 victims (43 percent of total). There was a brief reappearance late in June, but by mid-July the epidemic had subsided.

The epidemic caused more than 575 deaths (mainly children under five years of age) in Sydney alone. Unlike the city's measles outbreak in 1867, this epidemic affected children across class boundaries. Nearly one third of all deaths were due to complications of the disease. It is estimated that 8,000 to 10,000 Sydney residents suffered from scarlet fever during the epidemic. Overall, 5,000 people died in the provinces of New South Wales, Victoria, South Australia, and Tasmania.

The onset of scarlet fever is rapid; rising fever is followed by a red, sore throat and a bright red rash all over the chest and limbs. A few days later, the fever subsides and the skin starts to peel. The mere mention of the disease struck terror in the minds of people. A concerned and worried Australian populace prompted government inquiry into the origin and spread of the disease. Government preliminary reports suggested ways of coping with infectious diseases and eventually became the basis of the official policy for the management of such diseases. Some of the recommendations, regarding quarantine and fumigation, for instance, were implemented during the Sydney Smallpox Epidemic of 1881–82 (q.v.). The scarlet fever epidemic thus was an important step toward the formulation of an official public health policy in Australia.

Further reading: Curson, *Times of Crisis: Epidemics in Sydney 1788–1900;* Marks and Beatty, *Epidemics.*

Australian Smallpox Epidemic of 1788–89

First recorded epidemic of smallpox in Australia, literally decimating the aboriginal population in the Sydney area.

In 1788, months after the arrival of Britain's First Fleet, which brought white settlers into Sydney, a smallpox-like disease was observed among the aborigines in southeastern Australia. In late March or early April of 1789, the disease became more virulent and spread rapidly along the usual aboriginal routes between Botany Bay and Broken Bay and, in particular, around the Port Jackson area. Apparently, it also spread inland in some sections. It lasted between one and two months.

According to one account, the epidemic killed over half the aboriginal population in the region. Eyewitnesses have described the grisly discovery of many human corpses washed ashore at the various coves and inlets. Terrorized by this strange and unfamiliar disease, natives fled the scene, carrying the infection with them. Families routinely abandoned their sick members to die; no doubt, many perished as much from want of food as from the disease. A few of the patients were reportedly taken to Sydney for treatment, but most died without knowing what had struck them. There were so many deaths that individual burials had to be suspended and the corpses dumped on communal burial sites. Only one white settler, a crew member of the ship *Supply,* was infected. He died soon after contracting the infection early in May.

Some scholars doubt that this affliction was indeed smallpox. The rash and the heavy mortality, they argued, could also have been caused by a type of chicken pox to which the aborigines may have had no resistance. It may also have been an outbreak of native pox, a disease indigenous to the country.

Similarly, there is much speculation about the origin of this epidemic. Some have suggested that the disease was introduced into the country by members of the First Fleet, which landed at Botany Bay in mid-January 1788. Some have attributed its source to crew members of the French expedition led by La Pérouse because its ships were anchored at Botany Bay between January and March 1788. Another surmise is that the infection was brought by the *Supply,* whose crew member Joseph Jeffries died of it. Yet another theory is that some "variolous matter" imported by the First Fleet—perhaps to inoculate the settlers and aborigines—either accidentally or deliberately led to the outbreaks that killed hundreds of aborigines.

In terms of mortality, this was the most severe epidemic ever to hit the Sydney area. Its psychological impact on the aboriginal community was tremendous. Sydney's first successful smallpox inoculation was carried out in May 1804. However, the natives suffered several more such outbreaks during the century, all of which grossly depleted their numbers.

Further reading: Curson, *Times of Crisis: Epidemics in Sydney 1788–1900;* Hopkins, *Princes and Peasants: Smallpox in History.*

Austrian and Prussian Typhus Epidemics of 1805–07

Outbreaks of louse-borne typhus fever that killed thousands of soldiers and civilians following the occupation of Vienna and the Battles of Austerlitz and Jena during the Austrian and Prussian phases of the Napoleonic Wars (1803–15).

The French occupied Vienna in November 1805, with the predictable result that the city's hospitals soon became crowded with wounded French troops, among whom a severe epidemic of typhus broke out. A few weeks later, on December 2, the decisive Battle of Austerlitz took place, after which both French and

Allied wounded troops were removed to the nearby Moravian town of Brünn (Brno, the Czech Republic), where one quarter of them—12,000 men—died from typhus fever. The disease soon spread among the inhabitants of Brünn and subsequently through the surrounding regions, killing tens of thousands of civilians in Moravia, Silesia, Austria, Galicia, and Hungary.

As the French Army crossed and recrossed central Europe, its dumping places for sick and wounded soldiers grew ever larger; troops at the Battle of Jena in October 1806 would patch their wounds and return to the field rather than risk death in the disease-ridden *ambulances*. In the latter part of 1806 and the first half of 1807 Napoleon marched through Prussia. All along the military routes soldiers were left to die in overcrowded, understaffed, and grossly filthy hospitals, where typhus fever, as well as dysentery and other diseases, were rampant. As usual, typhus fever spread from the hospitals to the civilian population, killing thousands of people in Königsberg (Kaliningrad), Marienburg, Bromberg, and other places in East Prussia and along the Vistula River. See also DANZIG TYPHUS EPIDEMIC OF 1807.

Further reading: Prinzing, *Epidemics Resulting from Wars;* Quennevat, *Les vrais soldats de Napoleón.*

B

Bahamian Yellow Fever Epidemic of 1862–64 Outbreak of yellow fever in the Bahama Islands (or Bahamas). The disease had been a problem in the West Indies, where the people did not know that it was mainly transmitted by the *Aëdes aegypti* mosquito; most doctors then propounded its causation to be miasma or contagion and emphasized the significance of either local insanitary conditions or quarantine precautions respectively (both views were partly correct).

During the U.S. Civil War (1861–65), the British-owned Bahamas was an important base for blockade-running to the Confederacy (the U.S.'s Southern states). British-built, privately owned ships evaded the Union (Northern) blockade of the 3,550-mile Southern coastline to supply the Confederacy with goods of all kinds. Vessels frequently plied between the Bahamian port of Nassau and such Confederate ports as Charleston, South Carolina, and Wilmington, North Carolina. One experienced blockade runner, Thomas E. Taylor (see below), told of many yellow fever victims in Nassau, where he remembered counting 17 funeral processions passing his house one day and also burying three good friends on one day in the summer of 1864. Taylor himself contracted the disease and went to Halifax, Nova Scotia, to recover. Wilmington was also hard hit by the yellow fever epidemic, which killed about 2,500 of its 6,000 inhabitants.

Notable among the persons who died then from yellow fever was the newly consecrated first Anglican bishop in the Bahamas, the Reverend Charles Caulfield, who succumbed on September 4, 1862. The epidemic of yellow fever was the last serious one in these islands.

Further reading: Craton, *A History of the Bahamas;* Taylor, *Running the Blockade.*

Bangkok Poliomyelitis Epidemic of 1952 Severe epidemic of poliomyelitis that struck the city of Bangkok, Thailand's capital, in 1952.

The infection was most probably an importation from Singapore, where the disease had been prevalent throughout 1950 and 1951. The polio epidemic in Bangkok, believed to be Thailand's first, began in September 1952. The first reported patient was a Swiss woman who died four days after contracting the infection. The next case occurred in a pregnant Danish lady who was taken to Singapore, where she was kept in an iron lung (device for artificial respiration) until her child was born. During the period September to December 1952, 388 polio cases were reported in Bangkok city. These included cases among foreigners living in the city and native Thais. The epidemic seemed to have affected all age groups, and overall mortality was six percent.

Then the outbreak subsided, a few paralytic cases (involving weakness or paralysis of one or more muscles) were noticed but none involved the spinal column (called non-paralytic polio). Most of the milder and more common polio infections, it must be remembered, were generally not reported and sometimes not even diagnosed. These cases fall into two categories: abortive poliomyelitis (brief illness generally exhibiting one or more symptoms such as sore throat, headache, vomiting, and fever) and inapparent poliomyelitis (a silent infection that nevertheless builds antibodies against the virus strain). All three polio viruses were found in samples of the Thai population, thus indicating that the mild, non-clinical forms of polio had previously occurred in the country. See also VIETNAMESE POLIOMYELITIS EPIDEMICS OF 1958–60; TAHITIAN POLIOMYELITIS EPIDEMIC OF 1951.

Further reading: *Poliomyelitis: Papers and Discussions Presented at the Fourth International Poliomyelitis Conference;* World Health Organization, *Poliomyelitis.*

Bangladeshi Smallpox Epidemic of 1971–73 Major epidemic of smallpox among the refugees escaping a civil war in Bangladesh (called East Pakistan until December 1971).

The outbreak began in November 1971 at the Salt Lake refugee camp near the city of Calcutta in India, where thousands of refugees from neighboring Bangladesh were temporarily housed (see INDIAN-BANGLADESHI CHOLERA EPIDEMIC OF 1971). The refugees were to have been vaccinated on arrival, but with thousands more crossing over into India every day, very few actually received the vaccination. In the crowded and filthy conditions of the camps, smallpox spread very rapidly. Moreover, the initial outbreak was misdiagnosed so that no action was taken to contain it until the end of January 1972. By then, several million Bangladeshis had sought refuge in that area.

On December 16, 1971, Bangladesh became independent. Subsequently, thousands of Bangladeshis started returning home, many carrying smallpox with them. Meanwhile, the infection was also spreading very quickly in India and Pakistan. In Bangladesh, the epidemic was initially confined to three districts in the southwest—Barisal, Faridpur, and Khulna. Upon investigation, however, it was found that 27 of the country's 57 subdivisions were affected.

In March 1972, smallpox invaded Khulna, the country's third largest city. An intensive containment and eradication program was launched in Khulna on April 28. Instead of mass vaccination, it focused on immunizing high-risk groups, and the outbreaks were rapidly controlled within four to six weeks each. In the city's refugee camps, procurement of relief supplies was made contingent upon showing proof of vaccination. Eradication and surveillance efforts received monetary aid and other assistance from the World Health Organization and the United Nations Relief Organization in Dacca, the capital of Bangladesh.

According to *The Washington Post*, in the two months ending on April 11, 1972, some 7,000 people had died from smallpox in Bangladesh. The number of smallpox cases reported by India (27,407), Pakistan (7,053), and Bangladesh (10,754) during 1972 is believed to be only one tenth of those that actually occurred.

In December 1972, 1,019 smallpox cases were reported in Bangladesh. This soared to 3,919 in January 1973 and even further to 5,282 in February. Every district in the country was affected. The epidemic peaked in April before finally subsiding. Asia's last case of smallpox occurred in Bangladesh on October 16, 1975.

Further reading: Fenner et al., *Smallpox and Its Eradication*; Hopkins, *Princes and Peasants: Smallpox in History*.

Barbadian Yellow Fever Epidemic of 1647

First veritable account of yellow fever on the West Indian island of Barbados, where more than 5,000 persons perished from the "new distemper" (what the Barbadians then called the acute infection) within a few months in 1647.

The early English colonists on Barbados brought in many slaves for labor in the production of sugarcane; evidently, in the 1640s yellow fever (carried by *Aëdes aegypti* mosquitoes) arrived with blacks from West Africa aboard Dutch ships involved in the profitable slave trade. The mosquitoes, which can carry the yellow fever virus and transmit it to humans by their bites, found favorable conditions for breeding in water supplies on board ships. Once in Barbados, the insects found a suitable warm climate to further breed and transmit the infection to men, women, and children. While many black African slaves were immune to the fever, after recovering from it, many white Europeans (sailors and settlers) and native Indians on Barbados were severely attacked; within a month, nearly 80 percent of the victims perished, and the living were hardly able to bury the dead in 1647.

Called the "Barbados distemper" by Massachusetts Governor John Winthrop, who established in 1647 North America's first ship-quarantine regulations to protect his English colony from infection, yellow fever spread from Barbados to Mexico's Yucatán Peninsula, the West Indian islands of St. Kitts and Guadeloupe, and Havana, Cuba.

Further reading: Howe, *A World Geography of Human Diseases*; Wain, *A History of Preventive Medicine*.

Barbadian Yellow Fever Epidemic of 1691

Disastrous outbreak of yellow fever that killed several thousand persons on Barbados, easternmost of the Caribbean islands, during the summer of 1691. A dreaded scourge ever since the Barbadian Yellow Fever Epidemic of 1647 (q.v.), yellow fever also conferred immunity upon many older Barbadians who had survived earlier attacks of this highly fatal disease of the warm regions of America and Africa.

On the populous island (about 55,000 people), then a British colony, the mosquito-borne yellow fever virus infected and killed native Indians of all ages. It was, however, far more lethal among the fighting men of a British naval fleet stationed in Barbados and sent there to engage in battle with French forces in the West Indies during the War of the Grand Alliance (1688–97). In the summer of 1691, thousands of the British on Barbados fell victim to the infection, whose onset was sudden, with chills, fever, headache, general pains, nausea, and vomiting. Jaundice appeared between the second and fifth days, after which convulsions, coma, and death occurred in many cases. Some 3,100 men from 18 British ships perished from yellow fever, leaving an insufficient number to attack the French West Indian island of Martinique. The fleet returned to Great Britain later that year, having hardly enough men to navigate the ships into port. Crew members of a British ship that laid off Barbados during the next two years died from yellow fever daily; a total of about 600 seamen succumbed in that time.

Further reading: Cartwright, *Disease and History;* Cloudsley-Thompson, *Insects and History.*

Barcelona Yellow Fever Epidemic of 1821

Epidemic of yellow fever in the Mediterranean port of Barcelona, Spain, killing about a sixth of the city's population during the summer and fall of 1821. Because the first victims were ship's crew and dock workers, it was assumed the disease was brought to Barcelona aboard the *Gran-Turco* and other ships that had recently arrived from Cuba.

At first, most cases were confined to Barceloneta, a poor neighborhood near the harbor, and it is this initial concentration of the illness among the poor that led to accusations of neglect and suppression of the facts on the part of city officials. In fact, the epidemic offered competing political factions the opportunity to accuse each other of lack of conscience and even of having poisoned wells and distributed contaminated food. As deaths increased through August, most of Barcelona's wealthier citizens left the city.

Faced undeniably with a major epidemic—the illness had spread through the entire city and hundreds of people were dying every day—authorities closed off Barcelona and sank the contaminated ships in early September. Most of the city's high officials then withdrew to the town of Villafranca, 25 miles away (the mayor chose to stay). Doctors and pharmacists were ordered to remain, while the police and 3,000 militiamen, half of whom died, heroically attempted to prevent riots and pillaging. People without financial means who tried to find safety in the countryside encountered peasants who drove them away with gunshots, and because a cordon was placed around the city, they could not return; thus trapped, many died of thirst and starvation. The French set up a cordon of 15,000 soldiers to prevent refugees from escaping through the Pyrenees into France. Other measures taken by the French included closing their ports to ships from Catalonia and quarantining ships from all other ports in Spain. Madrid also protected itself by closing its access points and exhorting citizens to denounce any Catalonians who had fraudulently entered the city; even bull fights were suspended.

As food became scarce among Barcelona's poor, rioting and looting broke out; free soup was then made available and a subscription taken up throughout Spain to help raise money. Finally, on October 11, 1821, through the help of two businessmen who supplied the necessary funds, people were evacuated to make-shift cabins outside the city. In November the epidemic gradually declined, and with the onset of cold weather in December, finally ceased altogether. Barcelona's port was reopened on Christmas Day.

An estimated 18,000 to 20,000 people died in Barcelona from yellow fever from August through the end of the year, most of them in September and October. Other places in the surrounding region were severely affected too, including Tortosa, Tarragona, and the Balearic Islands.

Further reading: Hoffmann, *La peste a Barcelone;* Peset Reig, *Muerte en España (política y sociedad entre la peste y el cólera).*

Basel Plague of 1610–11

Severe epidemic of mainly bubonic plague that killed approximately 3,600 persons out of some 6,000 who contracted the disease in Basel, or Basle, Switzerland, in 1610 and 1611.

For more than 250 years after the Black Plague or Black Death (q.v.) of the mid-fourteenth century, European countries, cities, and towns suffered minor and major outbreaks of plague (chiefly bubonic, but also pneumonic and septicemic in form). The Swiss city of Geneva had a plague outbreak in 1528, and the Swiss town of Grindelwald endured one in 1688; plague occurred in both bubonic and pneumonic form in both of these outbreaks.

In January 1610 the city of Basel reported its first cases of bubonic plague; authorities were frightened to see about 40 percent of the population of about 15,000 inhabitants contract the disease, which is transmitted by the bite of an infective flea carrying the plague bacillus (*Yersinia pestis*). Most likely diseased rats (primary hosts of plague) traveled with merchandise into Basel, and rat fleas sought out other hosts (especially human beings) after the rats died from plague. Depending on where an infected flea bites its human victim (which is usually in the groin, armpit, or neck), painful lumps (buboes) develop in those areas; severe headaches, high fever, nausea, vomiting, and black spots on the skin, among other symptoms, accompany the buboes; and between 30 and 50 percent of those stricken will die if untreated.

During the 15-month-long epidemic in Basel, morbidity (amount of disease or sick rate) and mortality (death rate) were high, according to reliable sources. One source claimed there were 6,408 plague infections and 3,968 fatalities during the epidemic, but another source stated that those figures included infections and deaths resulting from other causes, too. Basel recovered, reporting fewer plague deaths afterward, but suffered Switzerland's last epidemic of plague in 1667–68 along with several towns in the canton of Zurich.

Further reading: Cipolla, *Fighting the Plague in Seventeenth Century Italy;* Lien-Teh, *A Treatise on Pneumonic Plague.*

Beijing Pneumonia Epidemics of 1949, 1952–53, and 1958–59

See PEKING PNEUMONIA EPIDEMICS OF 1949, 1952–53, AND 1958–59.

Bengali Smallpox Epidemic of 1769–70.

See IN-DIAN SMALLPOX EPIDEMIC OF 1769–70.

Black Assize.

See CAMBRIDGE TYPHUS EPIDEMIC OF 1522; EXETER TYPHUS EPIDEMIC OF 1586; LONDON TYPHUS EPIDEMIC OF 1750; OXFORD TYPHUS EPIDEMIC OF 1577.

Black Death (Black Plague, Bubonic Plague, Second Plague Pandemic)

Calamitious, widespread epidemic that devastated Asia and Europe in the mid-fourteenth century. This acute infectious disease, which in its earliest stages and in some places seems to have been predominantly of a pneumonic type (thus helping to account for its rapid and terrifying spread), was marked by swelling of the lymph nodes or buboes (hence known as the "bubonic" plague). It was also called the "black death" because of the black blotches, caused by subcutaneous hemorrhages, which appeared on the skin of diseased human beings near the time of death. An overwhelming infection of the blood led to rapid putrefaction in victims, who usually died within two to four days. The bubonic plague was caused by the bacillus *Pasteurella pestis (Yersinia pestis),* transmitted to persons by fleas from infected rats. The pneumonic plague, resulting as a complication of the bubonic type and as an invasion of the lungs by the bacterium, spread from person to person without the intermediary transference by fleas. Beside the black blotches on the skin, the plague showed itself in swellings in the groin or armpit and in bleeding from the lungs; it was also characterized by very high fever, delirium, and prostration in its victims.

Originating in central Asia, the disease killed an estimated 25,000,000 Chinese, Indians, and other Asians during the 15 years before it entered Constantinople (Istanbul) in 1347. From there it quickly spread to Genoa, Naples, Venice, Marseilles, and other Mediterranean ports; ships carrying Crusaders returning from the Middle East were a factor in this respect. By late 1347 the plague had hit Dalmatia (a

Croatian province on the Adriatic) and the islands of Cyprus and Sicily. Thousands of inhabitants of southern France, Spain, and Italy succumbed to the Black Plague before it reached Paris in June 1348 and London several months later. While raging in England and Ireland, the then mysterious malady spread to the Netherlands, Germany, Norway, Sweden, Denmark, and Russia, and by 1350 all of Europe (including Iceland and Greenland, according to some sources) was in the grip of the plague.

Historical estimates of the mortality directly due to the plague vary from one fourth to three fourths of the population of Europe and Asia; at least 25,000,000 Europeans died between 1347 and 1351. Half of London (some 100,000 persons) was said to have perished; two thirds of the students at Oxford University died. Four fifths of the population of Marseilles died. The Pope at Avignon, where half of the population died, consecrated the Rhône River to permit corpses to be thrown into it for Christian burial. More than a third of Italy's population perished. Villages everywhere were drastically depopulated by the plague, which extended into Egypt and Africa and continued to rage and carry off many thousands of people during the next three decades (in the early 1380s many towns and cities suffered their "fourth visitation" of the pestilence).

At the time medical and lay authorities throughout Europe sought to give rational explanations for the virulent plague, which was clearly contagious. They issued many treatises trying to explain to the public the causes, symptoms, and treatment of the disease, which was in general blamed on celestial, terrestial, and miasmatic facts as well as contagion (transference from infected persons). The plague was attributed to any and all of the following: corrupted air and water, hot and humid southerly winds, proximity of swamps, lack of purifying sunshine, excrement and other filth, putrid decomposition of dead bodies, excessive indulgence in foods (particularly fruits), God's wrath, punishment for sins, and the conjunction of stars and planets. Religious fanatics asserted that human sins had brought the dreadful pestilence; they roamed from place to place, scourging themselves in public. In places, the plague was blamed on cripples, nobles, and Jews, who were accused of poisoning the public wells and were either driven away or killed by fire or torture. There was panic everywhere, with men and women knowing no way to stop "death" except to flee from it.

The segregation of the sick was ordered in many cities, but in some the quarantine practice and stations were put into effect too late (such as in Venice and Genoa, where half the people succumbed). Various procedures of disinfection began and continued, such as the fumigating of letters and washing money with vinegar. Social confusion resulted; laborers were scarce so that many fields went unplowed; wheat was not sowed, vines not trimmed. In England, the wages paid to fieldhands nearly doubled because labor was at a premium due to the many dead. Food prices rose greatly, trade was disrupted, numerous leaders in church and government perished, and intelligent persons fostered an obsessive cult about death. The ravages of the Black Death helped bring the Hundred Years' War to a standstill; both sides (the English and French) signed a truce that was thrice renewed (1347–51); hostilities erupted again in 1355.

To many historians, the Black Death marked the end of the Middle Ages and the start of the modern age. Its devastation cleared the way for Europeans to form new social conditions, to systematize land-holding relations between owner/farmer and tenant/laborer on the basis of rent, to strike a balance between capital and labor. See also PLAGUE OF ENGLAND, GREAT; PLAGUE OF FLORENCE (BLACK VOMIT).

Further reading: Bowsky, ed., *The Black Death*; McNeill, *Plagues and Peoples*; Tuchman, *A Distant Mirror: The Calamitous 14th Century*; Ziegler, *The Black Death*; Smith, *Plague on Us.*

Black Death in the Middle East   Bubonic plague epidemics that struck various countries of the Middle East during the Black Death (q.v.) pandemic of the fourteenth century, seriously depopulating them and permanently altering their economic and social structure.

The plague disease first entered the region from southern Russia. Muslim leader Malik Ashraf (of the Jalayirid dynasty), returning to Baghdad in 1347 after an attack on Tabriz (which borders Azerbaijan, where plague was then raging), is believed to have introduced the infection. His troops laid siege to Shaykh Hasan Buzurg (town near Baghdad) but had to abort the siege, reportedly because of intense heat and shortage of provisions. In reality, the siege was lifted because plague had struck the army and penetrated even the city of Baghdad.

Early in the autumn of 1347, plague reached Alexandria in Egypt through its flourishing maritime trade with the Black Sea ports and Constantinople (Istanbul). From there, it traveled eastward to Gaza, where it caused a severe epidemic between April 10 and May 10, 1348. According to one estimate, 10,000 people died in Gaza during this outbreak, and the markets had to be shut down. The governor of Gaza himself fled and sought refuge in the village of Budda'arsh. The epidemic then traveled north along the Syrian coast and infected many cities in Syria

and Palestine—Asqalan (Ascalon), Acre (Akko), Jerusalem, Sidon, Beirut, Damascus (July 1348), Homs (Hims), and Aleppo (October 1348), to name a few. Five hundred deaths occurred in Aleppo every day at the height of the epidemic.

Sometime in 1348–49, the epidemic reached Antioch, perhaps by sea. Its residents fled north into Anatolia (Asia Minor), carrying plague with them. Very few survived the journey. Plague simultaneously arrived in the Islamic holy city of Mecca, probably with Muslim pilgrims. It was said, however, that non-believers had brought this visitation upon the city. Thousands of people, including pilgrims and regular inhabitants, died. In 1349, plague attacked Mawsil (Mosul) and reappeared in Baghdad. To the south, the country of Yemen was attacked in 1351 when King Mujahid returned from imprisonment in Cairo. The infection may have derived from the Mediterranean coast or been newly introduced from the Far East.

From eyewitness accounts, it is clear that the epidemics in Damascus and Aleppo, for instance, involved pneumonic plague as well. Many writers have described in great detail how people in the streets, their skin mottled, spat out blood and died soon thereafter. This is why the epidemic spread so rapidly. Even wild and domestic animals died by the hundreds, apparently of plague.

Medieval Muslims traditionally explained a visitation of the plague as the will of Allah or God; others categorized it as a punishment for the moral aberrations of its members. Islamic religious law forbade its members from believing in the contagion theory and from entering or fleeing the epidemic area. Some writers stressed the role of medicine in treating plague patients while others urged penance, prayer, and supplication in addition to medicine. In fact, in Damascus, public prayer meetings and rituals were held for days. Various preventive measures were suggested. Blood-letting was reportedly quite common; many believed it would relieve the patient. For the buboes (swellings of lymph glands), everything from cold water to surgery was advocated.

The governor of Damascus ordered the killing of all dogs in the city during the epidemic, perhaps because they were eating the abandoned human corpses piled up on the streets. The high cost of burial prevented many people from burying their dead. The governor then abolished burial fees so that proper burials could take place. At the city's Umayyad (Ommiad) Mosque, mass funerals became routine affairs. Mortality was particularly high in the rural areas of Palestine and Syria; many farm workers died during the sowing season, and others fled to the cities. At harvest time, few were left to gather the crops. There was no formal legislation controlling the exodus of people from villages to the cities, even though peasants were expected to return to their land within three years. With the migration or death of most inhabitants, entire rural areas became ghost-like.

Cities suffered too—economically and because of high mortality. During a severe epidemic, many fled the cities, abandoning homes and businesses to burglars and petty criminals. Tax evasion was rampant in this chaos.

The precise demographic impact of the plague pandemic on the countries of the Middle East is almost impossible to ascertain. In Damascus, at its peak in September–October 1348, the epidemic claimed more than a thousand human lives every day. Overall mortality in the city was estimated between 25 percent and nearly 38 percent. Syria lost about a third of its population (400,000 deaths) in this epidemic, which subsided after March 1349.

Further reading: Dols, *The Black Death in the Middle East;* Twigg, *The Black Death: A Biological Reappraisal.*

Blackfoot Indian Smallpox Epidemic of 1837–38

Grave epidemic of smallpox that claimed the lives of about 4,000 Blackfoot Indians, who then occupied a vast territory stretching from the Upper Missouri River area (Montana) to northern Saskatchewan.

In late summer of 1837 several passengers aboard a keelboat on the Missouri River bound for Fort McKenzie contracted smallpox. The boat also carried supplies and other goods for trade to the Blackfoot (or Blackfeet) Indians, whose name derived from their custom of dyeing their moccasins black. Earlier, in June 1837, smallpox had broken out among a Siouan Indian tribe in middle Missouri (see MANDAN INDIAN SMALLPOX EPIDEMIC OF 1837), and had spread thereafter to the Assiniboin and Crow Indian tribes, neighbors of the Blackfoot, who were skillful hunters of buffalo and not friendly to the white man and other tribes.

Before the keelboat reached Fort McKenzie, the agent in charge of the fort concluded that the goods and supplies were smallpox-contaminated, and he tried to detain the boat until cold weather set in. However, his trading clients, the Blackfoot, refused to listen to his warnings about disease and threatened to bring the boat to the fort themselves if he did not allow it to dock there as scheduled. The agent complied with the Blackfoot demands, and trade between the Indians and whites was carried out. Within ten days after the Indian traders returned to their villages, hundreds of Blackfoot fell victim to the deadly smallpox virus. By early 1838, some 4,000 of them had succumbed to the disease.

Smallpox had been transmitted again and again from the white European settlers to the Native Americans (the Indians) between 1520–24 and 1836–40, when the disease catastrophically affected Indian tribes from the eastern United States to Alaska. Some authorities contend that the reason for high mortality occurring among the North American Indians in the latter years was that the disease was transmitted to some Indian tribes who had not been exposed to smallpox for a long time. This was the case with the Blackfoot, who had evidently been infected by the virus only one other time—56 years before the 1837 smallpox outbreak. In 1781 more than half the Piegan (Pikuni) Indians—one of the three tribes of the Blackfoot nation (the Kainah and Siksika [Blackfoot proper] being the other two)—had fatally contracted the disease after raiding an infected Shoshone Indian camp; by the year 1837 most Indian survivors of that smallpox outbreak had died of other causes, thus leaving a largely susceptible, younger Indian population. The Blackfoot did not associate the disease with the white man in 1781, nor did they blame them for their infection in 1837.

Further reading: Dobyns, *Their Number Becomes Thinned: Native American Dynamics in Eastern North America;* Washburn, *The Indian in America.*

Black Plague   See BLACK DEATH.

Black Vomit   See PLAGUE OF FLORENCE (BLACK VOMIT).

Boer War Typhoid Epidemic   See BRITISH TYPHOID EPIDEMIC IN THE BOER WAR.

Bolivian Hemorrhagic Fever Epidemic of 1959–64

Epidemic caused by a previously unrecognized virus striking two distinct rural populations in the tropical prairies of eastern Bolivia, affecting over 750 persons of a total population of 4,000 to 6,000 in the endemic area. The disease, caused by the Machupo virus, one of a class of arena-viruses (i.e., sandy viruses), is spread by the rodent *Calomys callosus*, particularly by the rodent's urine. Since males in the Bolivian outbreak were twice as likely to acquire the disease as were females, it has been conjectured that victims came into contact with infected rodent urine while harvesting crops.

The first recorded case of the outbreak took place in early 1959 near San Joaquín, a village with a population of 2,500 and the capital of Mamoré province. From July through December 1960, 21 cases occurred in the small settlements around San Joaquín. From October 1960 until mid-1962, there were 107 cases with 44 deaths in Orobayaya (population

600), which lies 70 miles from San Joaquín. El Mojon, a village near Orobayaya, was also the site of deaths from the mysterious ailment before the town was abandoned and burned by panicking villagers. A total of 476 cases were recorded from the start of the epidemic through 1962. Thirty percent of these cases ended in death. In late 1962 or early 1963, cases began to occur within San Joaquín, which had previously been unaffected. There were over 260 new cases in 1964. The death rate for the 18-month period ending in mid-1964 (when the rodent vector was discovered and a successful rodent abatement program was undertaken) was 20 percent.

The incubation period for the Machupo virus is seven to 14 days. There is gradual onset of chills, fever, headache, nausea, and vomiting. In more severe cases, there is widespread hemorrhaging, with bleeding gums and blood in the vomit, urine and stool. The virus is similar to but distinct from that first noted in Argentina in 1953.

Further reading: *Harrison's Principles of Internal Medicine,* 11th ed.; MacKenzie et al., "Epidemic Hemorrhagic Fever in Bolivia"; MacKenzie, "Epidemiology of Machupo Virus Infection."

Bombay Plague of 1896–97 See INDIAN PLAGUE OF 1896–97.

Boston Smallpox Epidemic of 1666 First major smallpox epidemic to ravage Boston. Some historians believe that the disease originated in England and was transported across the Atlantic Ocean by settlers to the Massachusetts Bay Colony; others think that some American Indians introduced smallpox into Boston, for the French and Indians in Canada had been suffering from it during the last five years. In 1666 Boston had about 4,000 inhabitants.

The smallpox (variola) virus did not infect all the Bostonians who were exposed to it (because some people are inherently immune to smallpox), but a large number of citizens came down with headaches, backaches, fever, malaise, and sometimes convulsions and delirium, before showing the characteristic smallpox rash. Some of the survivors of the disease were left with pockmarked faces, and others were left blind or infertile.

Simon Bradstreet, English diarist and a founder of Cambridge (near Boston), estimated that "there dyed about 40" persons during the epidemic. John Hull, another English diarist, confirmed Bradstreet's death toll, writing that there were "several hundreds" of cases and "betwixt forty and fifty" fatalities. Hull also noted that the Boston smallpox outbreak worsened as the weather became colder and that it was "a very dying time." Hull's observations concur with modern knowledge of the smallpox virus, which prefers cool, dry weather to hot or humid weather, although epidemics have occurred during all times of the year.

Further reading: Hopkins, *Princes and Peasants: Smallpox in History;* Shurkin, *The Invisible Fire;* Winslow, *A Destroying Angel: The Conquest of Smallpox in Colonial Boston.*

Boston Smallpox Epidemic of 1677–78 Serious outbreak of smallpox that ravaged Boston in the Massachusetts Bay Colony in 1677–78.

In 1675 the American Congregational clergyman Cotton Mather predicted in one of his sermons that "very soon God will lift up his hand against Boston." The smallpox outbreak two years later seemed to fulfill his prophecy when ships from England carried the disease to Boston. The 1677–78 epidemic cost Boston many important leaders who succumbed to the disease. At the height of the outbreak on September 30, 1677, a reported 30 people died on that one day. The epidemic was much more severe than the Boston Smallpox Epidemic of 1666 (q.v.), in which a total of just 40 people reportedly died.

Boston imposed strict quarantine laws and forbade travel to surrounding areas in order to try to contain the disease. The epidemic also led to the first medical document (or pamphlet) published in America; Reverend Thomas Thacher, the first minister of Boston's Old South Church, published a broadside entitled *A brief rule to guide the common-people of New England how to order themselves and theirs in the small-pocks or measles* (1677–78), which described the disease, offered solutions for treatment and control of it, and presented a hypothesis of the causes of smallpox. The document was needed then to help calm the public and the fright evoked by the disease.

Since Thacher's publication, scientists and physicians have made great progress in understanding smallpox, which is caused by a brick-shaped virus and is spread from person to person. This variola virus prefers cool, dry weather to hot and humid weather, although epidemics have occurred at all times of the year. The strain of smallpox that affects human beings does not affect animals; thus, there must be a sufficiently large population of susceptible persons for the disease to spread. Boston in 1677 was suitable for smallpox to spread. However, the virus will not necessarily infect all persons exposed to it, for some people have an inherent immunity; the virus can survive on clothing or bedding and can be transported over distances that way.

Smallpox's incubation period is usually nine to 12 days from the time of a person's infection. Symptoms appear abruptly: headache, backache, chills, fever, nausea, and sometimes convulsions and delirium; the fever and pain intensify on the second day; in the next days, the smallpox rash appears, first in the mouth and throat before spreading to the face, upper back, chest, and then arms and legs. The rash evolves into pimples, blisters, pustules, and then scabs. Sometimes the internal organs are attacked, leading to toxemia or internal hemorrhaging; death is almost certain in these cases (in seventeenth-century Boston it certainly was). Also, large amounts of skin can be lost, leading to bacterial infections and death.

The mortality rate of infected persons was generally one in four in past centuries; survivors were often left with pockmarked faces; some were left blind or infertile; no one escaped smallpox unscathed.

Further reading: Hopkins, *Princes and Peasants: Smallpox in History*; Shurkin, *The Invisible Fire*; Winslow, *A Destroying Angel: The Conquest of Smallpox in Colonial Boston*.

Boston Smallpox Epidemic of 1702–03   Severe outbreak of smallpox in Boston in the Massachusetts Bay Colony between 1702 and 1703. About four percent of Boston's population (some 300 persons out of about 7,000) died from smallpox and scarlet fever, which had broken out at the same time (thus it was difficult to determine the number of deaths from smallpox alone).

The epidemic was so dreadful that it prompted the selectmen of the Massachusetts Bay Colony to pass an act or law that authorized the enforced quarantine of diseased people. December of 1702 was the peak of the epidemic. The famous American Congregational clergyman Cotton Mather observed at the time that "more than fourscore people, were in this black month of December, carried from this Town to their long Home." Smallpox infected three of Mather's children; he was lucky, however, because all three survived. The characteristic smallpox rash left many survivors of the disease with pockmarked faces or blindness or infertility. See also BOSTON SMALLPOX EPIDEMIC OF 1721–22.

Further reading: Winslow, *A Destroying Angel: The Conquest of Smallpox in Colonial Boston*; Duffy, *Epidemics in Colonial America*; Shurkin, *The Invisible Fire*.

Boston Smallpox Epidemic of 1721–22   Boston's worst eighteenth-century smallpox epidemic, which killed 844 of the 6,000 people infected in a population of 11,000 and during which the New World first made use of inoculation. The sixth to grip Boston since its original settlement, the smallpox epidemic occurred when enough people without immunity (not previously infected) had accumulated to sustain an epidemic. Complacency about safeguards, like Boston Harbor's island-sited quarantine hospital (established in 1717), and forgetfulness of the terrors

attending such a pestilence, left Boston vulnerable. In April 1721, the British ship *Seahorse,* carrying a crew infected with smallpox, entered Boston Harbor, bypassing the harbor hospital, and docked. Despite isolation of the sick crew members at a house by a wharf, the disease spread into the town.

The two major strains of smallpox included *variola minor* (known as alastrim) and *variola major,* the more severe variety, which usually killed 20 percent to 40 percent of those infected. Highly infectious smallpox traveled from person to person, transmitted primarily via contaminated particles from the nose or mouth, which another person inhaled. Indirect infection was possible through the bedding or clothes of the infected. No treatment, other than that for accompanying illnesses, softened the virulence of smallpox, although vaccination prevented it. Within ten to 16 days, victims developed high fever, headaches, and body aches. Some vomited and showed signs of colic or toxemia. Next, skin blemishes, from which the disease takes its name, covered the body. Rash pustules first filled with clear lymph and later with pus, after which scabs formed and then dropped off, leaving scars, pits, and spotty pigmentation. Aftereffects could include pockmarks, especially facial, and, less commonly, arthritis, encephalitis, pneumonia, myocarditis, osteomyelitis, and blindness. Smallpox immunized a survivor to any further attacks.

As the 1721–22 epidemic got under way, the selectmen set about to control the disease by flagging infected houses, locating nurses, and appointing guards. By June, Harvard University announced the closing of commencement to the public to minimize contagion. A thousand people fled Boston. Although half the adults were immune due to previous outbreaks, the young were helpless. As sickness became pervasive, terror mounted, peaking in September through November 1721. Daily death counts rose. Church bells tolled for the dead all day, day after day. Trade and business came to a standstill. Refusing to dock, sloops carrying fire wood left their cargo at Castle Island. Streets by day were empty except for mourners going to services. At night, carts collected bodies. The sick were quarantined. But Sunday church services were never restricted. North Church posted prayer requests for 222 sick on October 7 and 322 on October 14.

Religious leader Cotton Mather advocated use of variolation as described in articles by Timonius and Pylarinus published by the Royal Society. A common practice elsewhere in the eighteenth century, variolation was an inoculation that induced a minor smallpox infection. Developed in Asia and passed along as a folk remedy, variolation was introduced to Europe by European physicians resident in Asia. Lady Mary Wortley Montague, immortalized by the great poet Alexander Pope, helped popularize its use in England in 1721. Unbeknownst to the colonists, British scientists at the time established that about ten percent of those variolated were likely to die during a full-scale smallpox epidemic. Acceptance of the heathen technique demonstrated a shift from values centered on the spiritual and the afterlife to the enlightenment philosophy of improving the secular world. On June 6, 1721, Mather sent an appeal to Boston's physicians to use variolation as a preventive measure. Later, he wrote to Dr. Zabdiel Boylston, who responded by using variolation on his own son and a slave. The subsequent controversy that erupted over inoculation raised questions about the secular vs. the religious domain, as well as the safety of the patient, contagion, and the authenticity of future immunity.

The community split over variolation at a July 21 selectman's meeting, attended by Boston's physicians, officials, and many citizens. Dr. William Douglass presented evidence refuting the value of variolation and exposing its hazards. Dr. Boylston presented evidence of the seven variolations he had performed. The selectmen sided with the physicians opposing variolation. Variolation became cause for public indignation in the midst of a city already stricken with frenzied panic and a widespread, virulent disease. Many (seldom the clergy) saw variolation as an attempt to thwart God's will as the only provider for Man's present and future good. Tabloids carried charges, countercharges, and testimonials. There was an attempt on Cotton Mather's life.

By November and December 1721, the pestilence began to abate. Refugees returned to Boston. North Church numbered only 50 staying at home because of illness by December. No one died of smallpox in February or March 1722. Two died in April and one in May. At a town meeting in May, Dr. Boylston complied with the request to stop any inoculations. Many came to realize that inoculation actually worked by seeing that those inoculated survived. Thus, the edict against inoculation came to be relaxed. During the 1721–22 epidemic, inoculation had preserved the lives of 280 people. Dr. Boylston had inoculated 247 people, six of whom died.

Further reading: Duffy, *Epidemics in Colonial America*; Fenner et al., *Smallpox and Its Eradication*; Hopkins, *Princes and Peasants: Smallpox in History*; Winslow, *A Destroying Angel: The Conquest of Smallpox in Colonial Boston*.

Boston Smallpox Epidemic of 1763–64

Outbreak of smallpox that struck Boston from 1763 to 1764 and killed only 170 inhabitants out of a population of some 15,000 to 20,000 people.

Out of the first 12 or 13 cases of smallpox reported in 1763, ten or 11 persons died, according to colonial diarist James Gordon of Boston. These initial deaths led to a great panic in the town, because the inhabitants remembered the pain and suffering that earlier smallpox outbreaks had wrought (see BOSTON SMALLPOX EPIDEMIC OF 1721–22). Many Bostonians, including notable members of the government, fled across the Charles River to nearby Cambridge to escape the onslaught of this dreaded disease. In accordance with a law passed years earlier, the Boston selectmen successfully placed many of the smallpox-infected houses under quarantine.

The recent development of a smallpox inoculation changed the course of this epidemic dramatically, in comparison to some earlier Boston epidemics. Townspeople had voted to allow inoculations beginning on March 13, 1764; this process of inoculating people continued through April 20, 1764. In a letter written by colonist Benjamin Gale to Dr. John Huxham, Gale stated that only five human deaths occurred in the first 3,000 inoculations. By the end of the epidemic, nearly 5,000 inhabitants had been inoculated, and among those 5,000 there were 1,025 poor citizens of Boston (cared for by the Overseers of the Poor); this was the first epidemic instance where special provisions were made for the inoculation of the poor. The inoculations caused 46 deaths, while 124 persons out of 699 infected naturally with smallpox perished. In all, Boston had a mortality rate of less than one percent during the epidemic, which eventually spread to Cambridge. In Cambridge, 649 persons were inoculated, and only two deaths resulted. Thirty-eight natural cases of smallpox broke out in Cambridge, and just four proved fatal

Further reading: Blake, *Public Health in the Town of Boston, 1630–1822*; Duffy, *Epidemics in Colonial America*; Winslow, *A Destroying Angel: The Conquest of Smallpox in Colonial Boston*.

Brazilian Malaria Epidemic of 1938–40

Devastating outbreak of malaria that infected as many as 290,000 persons and killed at least 26,000 of them in Brazil's northeast coastal region, especially in the Jaguaribe River valley.

Earlier, in 1930–31, successive malaria outbreaks struck the seaport of Natal and the surrounding region in northeast Brazil. The *Anopheles gambiae* mosquito (the most efficient malaria vector or carrier in the world), which had never before been found outside Africa, was discovered to be responsible for the Natal epidemics. The mosquito bites a person with malaria, sucking in blood containing the Plasmodium parasite, which it transmits to a healthy person through a bite. For the next seven years the parasitic disease was allowed to brew in the Natal area because the Brazilian government was unable to destroy the mosquito vector, which managed to escape from the area on board ships and trucks traveling northwest along the coast, eventually infesting the Jaguaribe River valley more than 200 miles away and regions farther north.

During the rainy season, malarious mosquitoes bred abundantly in water wells and other stagnant water bodies in the Jaguaribe and other river valleys. The native people, who cultivated sweet potatoes in the streambeds of dry rivers (after the rainy season), were attacked by hordes of diseased mosquitoes, which swarmed among the population in the open countryside and compelled many wealthy inhabitants to flee to the cities and the poor to nearby villages (the mosquito vector does not thrive in cities).

Since 1923 the Rockefeller Foundation had been in Brazil fighting another mosquito-borne disease, yellow fever, and in mid-1938 it joined with the Brazilian government to organize a counterattack against the malaria-carrying mosquitoes. However, this campaign, headed by Dr. Fred L. Soper, was not initiated until after the 1939 rainy season, for there was no hope of checking mosquito reproduction during the wet season. Consequently, diseased mosquitoes during the rainy season moved up the river valleys. Along the Jaguaribe River, lined with houses that formed a continuous village, the vector easily jumped from one house to another, infecting the inhabitants. Fatalities were high among infants and children under five years old, whose resistance was sometimes lowered to such an extent that other diseases they acquired proved fatal (if they did not die from malaria). The use of quinine had limited effect; the most effective preventive measure in this pre-DDT period was destroying the mosquito larvae through spraying crude oil and Paris green (insecticide prepared from copper acetate and arsenic trioxide) on the surface of stagnant water, or through the age-old method of drainage.

During the 1939 dry season the Rockefeller Foundation succeeded in clearing the *Anopheles gambiae* out of one coastal village near the Jaguaribe valley, where only 6,124 malaria cases were reported in the valley during the 1940 wet season as the result of exterminating the mosquitoes with Paris green and pyrethrum sprays. By November 1940 the malarious mosquitoes had been driven from the valley. It had been the biggest battle so far in which spray-killing played a major role in combating malaria.

Further reading: Ackerknecht, *History and Geography of the Most Important Diseases;* Harrison, *Mosquitoes, Malaria and Man.*

Brazilian Plagues of 1899–1988   Outbreaks of bubonic plague affecting over 6,000 persons in Brazil's coastal cities during a 35-year period, before becoming primarily a malady endemic to rural, inland areas, particularly in the northeastern part of the country. Santos, a city lying just inland of São Paulo in southeastern Brazil, is widely said to have been the first site of bubonic plague in the Western Hemisphere, although other sources claim that the disease first appeared in Argentina in that same year.

Various theories have been put forth about the source of the Santos outbreak of plague, which is caused by the bacteria *Yersinia pestis* and is spread to man via infected fleas and rodents. A ship docked in Santos in October 1899 was reported to have large numbers of dead rats on board, and crew members were said to be infected with the disease shortly thereafter. The ship had sailed from Oporto, Portugal, a known focus of bubonic plague. Other theories regarding the source of the plague outbreak include the notion that the disease came from a contaminated rice ship originating in Rangoon that had stopped in Africa, or that plague was previously extant in Brazil or elsewhere in the Americas—possibly for centuries—without the knowledge of the public. A probable case of plague was seen in the Santos yellow fever hospital sometime prior to the sailing from Oporto. The beginning point of the epidemics, therefore, cannot be ascertained. The initial Brazilian cases were part of a worldwide pandemic of plague that began in Hong Kong in 1894 (see HONG KONG PLAGUE OF 1894).

A few months after the first cases were noted in Santos, São Paulo also became infected. Other Brazilian ports—Rio de Janeiro, Fortaleza, Pernambuco, and Rio Grande do Sul—soon became foci of the illness. In Rio de Janeiro, the capital, news of the Santos outbreak created a panic among the health authorities, who knew of plague only from medical textbooks. The first case was seen in that city on January 8, 1900. By the end of that year, 295 victims had been taken by the disease; the dead including one of the leading physicians, who died of pneumonic plague, the deadliest form of the disease. The government expeditiously founded an institute in Rio for the production of anti-plague serum. Over the next few years, due to the government's efforts at serum therapy and rodent control, bubonic plague was successfully wiped out in the capital and in Santos.

Recife, the capital of Pernambuco state, was also among the cities hard hit during the initial epidemic. Officials confirmed the presence of the disease in Recife at the end of March 1902. There were 148 deaths from plague from March through July, with the peak of the epidemic occurring in April. By October, there was only one death from plague, and it seemed as if the epidemic had passed. That was not the case, however, and 166 more persons perished from the disease in 1903. Plague continued to take an average of 17 lives per year in Recife from 1904 through 1918.

By 1934, public health measures had sharply reduced the incidence of cases and the number of deaths in major population centers, where most of the over 6,000 Brazilian cases had been reported. After that point, the disease continued to be a problem only in inland, rural areas, particularly in the northeast. There were 2,973 cases and 815 deaths from the disease in the northeastern states during the period 1935–49, out of 3,125 cases and 890 deaths throughout Brazil during that same period. From 1950 through 1963, an additional 461 cases were reported in Brazil, again, principally in the northeast. Bubonic plague has never been entirely eradicated in Brazil; there were 578 cases in 1968–69, more than in any other country in the Americas. Thirteen hundred cases were reported during the years 1970–75, more than a third of the cases occurring in 1975. Only 98 cases were reported in Brazil in 1980, and the incidence of the disease continued to decline during the eight years following. Mortality rates during recent outbreaks have been low (3%) compared to death rates for plague elsewhere, probably due to an active national surveillance system leading to early identification and treatment.

Further reading: Rail, *Plague Ecotoxicology*; Pan American Health Organization, *Plague in the Americas*; Gregg, *Plague*.

Brazilian Smallpox Epidemic of 1555–62

First smallpox (*variola major*) epidemic to strike Brazil after the Spanish conquest. In 1555 the disease struck the French Huguenot settlers at Rio de Janeiro and soon spread into the interior forest regions and then up the coast. Before the epidemic ended, it had reportedly killed half the native population of Brazil.

Contemporaries described the disease as a form of pox so loathsome and foul-smelling that none could stand the great stench. Prior to the 1500s, Brazil's Indians had lived in isolation from European diseases. They were a community that lacked immunity, and when the smallpox disease arrived, it was devastating to the population.

There was no discrimination among those the disease attacked; men, women, and children were all vulnerable. There were sometimes as many as 120 sick Indians to a hut with no one to tend them or bury the dead. With so many sick or dying, the task of making manioc flour was neglected; manioc flour was the chief food of the Indians. If anyone was lucky enough to survive the epidemic, he or she was probably faced with starvation. Many Indians offered themselves as slaves just for a free meal.

The first symptoms of smallpox are a fever and sharp back pain, after which a rash appears. It then passes through stages of papule, vesicle, and then eruptions, which dry up and leave scars or pockmarks. There is a 12-day incubation period, and it is only at the eruption stage that the disease is contagious.

The native cure was to lay the sick on beds of leaves and branches that were then laid over trenches filled with fire. It was believed that this would rid the body of poison.

Jesuit missionaries had arrived in Brazil ten years before the epidemic began; Brazil was an important foreign province to convert to Christianity. They labored nonstop in their efforts to cure and convert the Indians; they would apply leeches, wash the Indians, and pray. Neither the Indian nor the Jesuit remedies worked as the death toll rose. Some missionary villages lost as many as 30,000 Indians within three months.

The Jesuits were at a loss to explain why God was taking their flock, but attributed the disease to punishment by the Almighty. Many Indians did believe that it was some sort of divine punishment. Others realized that the Jesuits carried the disease, and they came to fear the missionaries. Indians abandoned their homes and fled to the forests in droves. By the late 1500s the coast of Brazil was almost unpopulated by Indians.

Smallpox would attack in wave after wave in the ensuing centuries, killing more Indians than any other disease; an estimated three million Indians died between 1550 and 1850 in Brazil.

Further reading: Hemming, *Red Gold: The Conquest of the Brazilian Indians, 1500–1760*; Burkholder and Johnson, *Colonial Latin America*.

Brazilian Smallpox Epidemic of 1660

Hemorrhagic smallpox outbreak that spread throughout the Jesuit missions along the banks of the Amazon river in Brazil and killed an estimated 44,000 native Indians.

The Jesuits arrived in Brazil in the 1500s determined to convert the "heathen" natives. They established ten Christian missions in Mainas, a region of Peru east of the Andes that covered some 1,500 miles along the banks of the Maranon, Huallagua, and Ucayali rivers, and also along the Amazon as far upstream as Manaus in Brazil.

The epidemic began in 1660 at Maranhão (São Luiz) on Brazil's coast. During the spring rains, the epidemic spread to Belém (Pará), where it destroyed over half the native population. It was termed "the great fire" by the Indians as the sickness swept through the region (northeast Brazil and the lower Amazon).

Smallpox utterly devastated the Indian population, sometimes taking as much as 90 percent (it has been termed one of the worst genocides in history). The native Indians had never been in contact with the disease and lacked immunity to it.

Hemorrhagic smallpox is the deadliest strain of the virus and is most always fatal. It is severely infectious, characterized by initial back pain, headache, and high fever. In three to five days, a rash develops and goes through stages of papule, vesicle, and pustule. When there is bleeding under the pustule, it is the sign of hemorrhagic smallpox.

Both Jesuits and Indians were at a loss to explain the high death toll of the Indians when only a small percentage of Portuguese and Spanish succumbed to the disease. The Jesuits blamed it on a lack of devotion by the Indians, believing it was God's punishment. Many did come to realize that they could very well be the carriers of the disease. They labored nonstop trying to cure the Indians by applying leeches, washing the sick, and praying. The Indians would lay the sick on beds made of branches and leaves, or over trenches filled with fire as a cure. Neither remedy worked; the Jesuit priests found themselves alone, surrounded by sick and dying Indians. They nursed the Indians, dug graves with their own hands, and heard confessions.

The Jesuits, filled with zeal and determination to convert the masses, would gather nomadic tribes into villages or groups. These groupings allowed the disease to spread rapidly, sometimes wiping out whole missions. Indians fleeing from the epidemic only carried it farther inland to previously unexposed populations. The missions were eventually abandoned as more disease and revolts and slave raids took their toll.

Brazil continued to suffer periodic outbursts of smallpox, and the laboring Jesuits remained powerless. In 1669, another epidemic struck, taking an estimated 22,000 Indian lives. And again in 1695, the Jesuit missions were struck by yet another wave of hemorrhagic smallpox.

The epidemics also served to precipitate animosities between the colonists and the Jesuits. The colonists had arrived in Brazil with high hopes of becoming wealthy farmers; they used the natives as slave labor, which the Jesuits were against. The colonists were frustrated by the rate at which the Indians died and blamed the pious Jesuits. A long series of rebellions took place between the colonists and the Jesuits, who were detested and were eventually expelled from Brazil in 1760.

Further reading: Hemming, *Red Gold: The Conquest of the Brazilian Indians, 1500–1760*; World Health Organization, *The Global Eradication of Smallpox*; Shurkin, *The Invisible Fire*; Hopkins, *Princes and Peasants: Smallpox in History*.

Brazilian Smallpox Epidemic of 1665–66

Epidemic of *variola major* smallpox that struck along the coast of Brazil in 1665–66.

Variola major smallpox is the severest strain of the disease and often develops into hemorrhagic smallpox. Characterized by a high fever, back pain, and a rash, smallpox is contagious only when the rash reaches the pustule stage. If there is bleeding under the pustules (pus blisters), it is hemorrhagic smallpox and most often fatal.

The epidemic broke out in the coastal town of Pernambuco (now Recife) and spread southward to Rio de Janeiro. The mortality rate was enormous; 40 to 50 persons at once would sicken and die. There were no healthy people left to aid the sick, go for medical assistance, or seek what little remedies there were.

The virus especially affected the African slave population in Brazil. Due to severe smallpox outbreaks in the last century, the native Indian population had declined so much that the demand for African slaves had become greater. As the slave trade increased, so did the risk of smallpox. The mortality rate of slaves was so high in this epidemic (1665–66) that many wealthy proprietors or landowners lost all their slaves and were reduced to poverty. With no one to work the land and plant crops, famine followed and lasted well into the 1700s.

As the disease traveled south, it lost some of its impact; yet another epidemic struck the port of Bahia (now Salvador) in 1680–84 and coincided with a three-year drought. This epidemic so ravaged the slave population that sugar production (from the sugar cane crop) was drastically reduced because of the lack of laborers.

Further reading: Hopkins, *Princes and Peasants: Smallpox in History*; Shurkin, *The Invisible Fire*.

Brazilian Smallpox Epidemic of 1878

Epidemic of smallpox (*variola major*) responsible for the deaths of at least 56,791 persons in and around Fortaleza, the capital of Céara province, in northeast Brazil. The devastation from the outbreak was swift and intense; half of the victims were felled in an eight-week period. Most of them were refugees from the *sertão*, or interior, of the province, who had crammed into Fortaleza to escape wretched drought conditions inland.

After the long, hot summer of 1877, the winter rains never arrived in the sertão. The region was essentially an agricultural one, populated by mixed race peasants referred to as sertanejos. Faced with starvation on their lands, the sertanejos abandoned the interior in droves. Four hundred thousand persons fled for the coast on foot during March 1878; some 100,000 people or as many as 150,000 perished en route. The coastal towns of Fortaleza, Arcati, Pacatuba, and Baturité swelled to many times their normal population. Fortaleza, for example, with a native population of about 25,000, is said in one account to have harbored about 65,000 persons— there had been more, but the government encouraged many to leave with free steamboat passage, and others succumbed to hunger and disease. Another account states that, at the time of the epidemic, Fortaleza housed 170,000 people, of which 110,000 were refugees. Exhausted and starving, huddled for the most part in primitive and filthy refugee camps, the surviving sertanejos greeted the variola virus.

The first smallpox cases were seen in August 1878 and are said to have come from Arcati. From August through October, 1,472 smallpox deaths were recorded in Fortaleza. The incidence of the disease then increased sharply. In the beginning of November, about 100 persons were dying per day. By the end of the month, approximately 9,800 had perished in Fortaleza alone. These figures are based on official burial records and are said to be underestimates, as many bodies were buried surreptitiously at sea or in the woods. Another report states that smallpox was in every corner of the city by November, and that 40,000 persons were stricken in that month. The epidemic peaked in December. Eight hundred forty-four deaths were recorded on December 10; approximately 14,400 victims died in Fortaleza during that month. Hemorrhagic (or black) smallpox, the most deadly course of the disease, was reported in December, and claimed the life of the provincial president's wife.

Burial of the thousands of corpses presented a problem for local officials. Gravediggers, paid in money, provisions, and liquor, were hastily recruited for the awful task of digging mass graves, with 12— sometimes as many as 25—bodies thrown in a trench together. The gruesome work went on virtually round-the-clock. The workers fainted—some died— reportedly from the unbearable stench.

Meanwhile, corpses lay in the many refugee huts until picked up by the body carriers, who kept up a daily procession to the cemeteries. Adult bodies hung suspended from poles, two or three together, while corpses of children lay in trays atop the carriers' heads. Smallpox can be transmitted via contact with corpses, but the sertanejos reportedly came to ignore the bodies, which lay in so many of the huts. There was no attempt to limit contact with those already stricken with the highly contagious disease. At Christmas of 1878, the dying were brought into the churches for confession in an eerie procession of hammocks. There was virtually no attempt to vaccinate the populace. One report indicates that fewer than 5,000 had been vaccinated in Fortaleza. The surrounding towns were hit as hard or harder than the provincial capital. In Pacatuba reportedly more than half the people were stricken. Only in the city of Baturité was there an organized vaccination program, and the death rate there was much lower than in the neighboring towns.

An organized anti-variola campaign was begun in Fortaleza in 1900. Gradually, the disease was brought under control in Céara. There was only one case in 1902 and another in 1904. Smallpox was not entirely eradicated from Brazil until World Health Organization efforts in 1971.

Further reading: Hopkins, *Princes and Peasants: Smallpox in History*; Guerra, *Osvaldo Cruz*; Smith, *Brazil, the Amazons and the Coast.*

Brazilian Smallpox Epidemic of 1905

Outbreak of smallpox in Recife, Brazil, killing about 3,800 people before moving on to Rio de Janeiro, where it left 3,600 dead. It was one of the first times that the government stepped in to take measures against a disease in Brazil.

The Brazilian state of São Paulo had started a comprehensive public health program in 1892 that required smallpox vaccinations for all its citizens. It also attempted to assist other Brazilian states in setting up vaccination programs. Despite these measures, smallpox broke out in the city of Recife; the government there then passed a bill requiring compulsory vaccination. However, an anti-vaccination campaign arose and soon escalated into riots and revolt. Powerful rural groups, mostly wealthy planters, were concerned with the cost of public health programs, and what they considered interference by the state government in their domains. The government eventually won the rich planters over to the vaccination program, arguing that potential immigrant workers would not come to a place that was disease-ridden; the planters were in danger of losing their cheap labor supply and consequently consented to have government vaccination programs set up in various cities but not in rural areas.

Smallpox was brought to Brazil by Spanish and Portuguese explorers in the 1500s; it was particularly devastating to South American Indians and others because they had lived in isolation from European diseases and lacked immunity. The microbes that cause the smallpox virus thrive in large pools of people, and South American cities, with their crowded and unsanitary conditions, were ideal for the virus to multiply and spread. Smallpox is not a disease that strikes hard and fast; instead it travels in small pockets of infection, affecting a few persons who pass it on to others, thus forming a chain; this allows the virus to hang on and travel from place to place. The first symptoms of the virus are back pain and fever, followed by a rash that develops into pustules, which erupt and then crust over and fall off, often leaving the victim scarred.

The World Health Organization's campaign against smallpox, started in 1967, succeeded in eradicating smallpox from Brazil. The last known case of smallpox in Brazil was in April 1971. The World Health Organization compiled a 1,476-page book entitled *Smallpox and Its Eradication* that details the history of smallpox throughout the world and the eventual eradication of the disease.

Further reading: Baxby, *Jenner's Smallpox Vaccine*; Shurkin, *The Invisible Fire.*

Brazilian Smallpox Epidemic of 1967–71

Epidemic in Brazil, serving as the impetus behind the World Health Organization's (WHO) Smallpox Eradication Campaign between 1967 and 1971.

In 1967, there were an estimated ten million cases of smallpox in the world. The principal areas of outbreak were India, Pakistan, Bangladesh, the Indonesian archipelago, Africa, and Brazil. In Brazil, there were a total of 33 outbreaks and 1,492 cases.

In the Brazilian coastal city of Vitória in Espírito Santo state, 51 cases of children with smallpox were reported in 1968 in the city hospital; the children had all entered the hospital for other medical reasons, and none of them had been vaccinated against smallpox; later five of the children died. Also, there were no quarantine measures set up for the patients, and there was no vaccination of staff and patrons. Because of a lack in preventive measures, hospitals in Brazil were helping spread the disease. The largest smallpox outbreak occurred in Bahia state (north of Espírito Santo) in 1969, where 507 cases were reported.

Smallpox has unique characteristics that make it an ideal candidate for complete eradication. It is an exclusively human disease, and there are no animal carriers. It is slow to travel and has a long incubation period of 12 days. This makes it possible to trace all those who had contact with an infected person and isolate them. Smallpox is highly recognizable and contagious only in the eruption stage. There is no carrier state, and the one vaccine introduced by Edward Jenner in 1796 serves in all strains of the virus.

The first signs of smallpox are back pain and fever. A rash develops that erupts into pustules, which form crusts and separate in about three weeks.

WHO set up mass vaccination sites and surveillance teams to search out cases, give vaccinations, and make reports to a central smallpox office. In 1968, 12 million vaccinations were performed, twice as many as the year before.

WHO estimates that if no cases of smallpox are reported within two years of the last known case, the area is considered free of smallpox. In 1970, programs were begun in all states of Brazil and 30 million vaccinations were performed. On April 19, 1971, the last case of smallpox was reported in Brazil.

Further reading: World Health Organization, *The Global Eradication of Smallpox*; Baxby, *Jenner's Smallpox Vaccine*; Shurkin, *The Invisible Fire.*

Brazilian Yellow Fever Epidemics of 1849–1902

See RIO DE JANEIRO YELLOW FEVER EPIDEMICS OF 1849–1902.

British Cholera Epidemic of 1832

First epidemic of Asiatic cholera in the British Isles, appearing in October 1831 when a ship from the North Sea port of Hamburg (Germany) docked at the town of Sunderland on England's northeastern coast. From Sunderland it quickly spread to Scotland, Ireland, and other parts of Britain. Londoners awaited its arrival in a state of panic and on February 6, 1832, observed a day of national fasting and penance in the hope it might be averted; a few days later London's first case of cholera was reported. Fatalities in London numbered about 5,300 persons until autumn, when the disease subsided, and 1,500 more deaths occurred the following year. Mortality from cholera for the entire country for 1831 and 1832 was an estimated 31,000.

Cholera had emerged from India early in the nineteenth century to scourge large areas of the world in four devastating pandemics (1817–23, 1826–37, 1846–63, 1865–75). The rapid spread of this genuinely global disease, second only to influenza in its extent, was made possible by the increasing use of modern methods of transportation introduced during the industrial revolution. Before this time, cholera was largely confined to India and adjacent countries.

Cholera is a water-borne disease caused by the comma-shaped bacillus *Vibrio comma*. The bacillus often will not survive the stomach juices, but when it does, it multiplies quickly in the alimentary tract and causes radical dehydration from which the victim may die in a matter of hours. The horror of cholera lay in its terrible symptoms, including incessant diarrhea and vomiting, severe muscular cramps, and prostration. Worst of all, a shrinking of the facial features and soft body tissues occurs due to the sudden loss of body fluid, and discoloration of the skin from ruptured capillaries turns the shriveled victim black and blue. Recovery can be rapid, but an individual who succumbs will be dead within one or two days from the appearance of symptoms, which begin to manifest two or three days after ingestion of *Vibrio comma*.

The story of cholera in the Western world is inseparable from the problems of nineteenth-century urbanization, sewage control, and public water supplies. Burgeoning populations outpaced the capacity of city governments to develop adequate sewage systems and to ensure clean and ample water. Impure water carries the cholera bacillus and causes most cases of it, but because the bacteria is passed in human feces, tiny particles of which can then be carried to food by unwashed hands or by flies and roaches, proximity to raw sewage and careless personal hygiene further spread the disease. Families crowded together in dirty tenements, people in coal mining districts where sanitation was particularly crude, and laundresses and nurses handling the soiled bed linen of the sick were especially at risk.

Cholera is not a carrier disease, as the bacteria normally remain in the body of a recovering patient for less than two weeks.

The threat of cholera in 1831 prompted the Royal College of Physicians to create a Central Board of Health and to produce guidelines for the establishment of England's first local boards of health. Responsibilities included setting up temporary hospitals, providing the poor with medical care, paying for funerals when necessary, cleaning sewers and slaughter-houses, closing cesspools, and fumigating private houses. These were important first steps toward a comprehensive concept of public health administration.

Cholera was initially thought to be a communicable disease, and on these grounds St. Bartholomew's Hospital in London refused to admit cholera patients. The controversy over rival theories of the origin and spread of epidemic diseases was fired by the great cholera outbreaks of the 1800s, and was finally resolved toward the end of the century with the advent of bacteriology and the discovery of the cholera-causing bacillus by German scientist Robert Koch (see BRITISH CHOLERA EPIDEMICS OF 1848–1849 AND 1853–54).

Further reading: McNeill, *Plagues and Peoples;* Marks and Beatty, *Epidemics;* Smith, *The People's Health, 1830–1910.*

British Cholera Epidemics of 1848–49 and 1853–54 Second and third visitations of Asiatic cholera

in Britain, occurring during the third global pandemic of 1846 to 1863. More severe than the first attack in 1832, the epidemic of 1848–49 claimed an estimated 54,000 to 62,000 human lives from autumn 1848 to the end of 1849. The outbreak of 1853–54 caused about 31,000 more deaths. In both cases, the disease was introduced into Britain from Hamburg, Germany.

In 1854 Dr. John Snow correctly hypothesized that cholera was waterborne. Noticing that a disproportionate number of people who used water from the Broad Street pump in central London were dying, Snow demonstrated the connection between consumption of this sewage-laden water and the incidence of cholera. He further stated that cholera entered the system by mouth, a notion that was by no means taken for granted at the time. Snow's idea challenged the centuries-old theory of miasma, which held that epidemics were caused when foul air, contaminated by rotting matter or stagnant water, attacked individuals whose weak constitutions made them susceptible to these corrupted vapors. Snow's idea that cholera was caused by the ingestion of a specific microorganism supported the rival "germ" theory. The germ theory, however, relied on contagion as the explanation for epidemics and supplied the justification for quarantine, a procedure ineffective for diseases that are not primarily contagious, including cholera. The so-called anticontagionists adopted Snow's hypothesis because, ironically, his association of cholera with contaminated water lent evidence to the miasmatic theory. Intensified awareness of the hazards of impure water resulted, but the confusion significantly impeded progress in medical research.

The Broad Street pump was closed, and deaths from cholera in that locale abruptly stopped. Authorities instituted new measures to promote public sanitation and improve water quality. But despite Snow's brilliant insights, the medical establishment largely ignored his conclusions. Thus the mystery of cholera remained, and erroneous medical theories persisted until the German scientist Robert Koch identified the cholera bacillus in 1884.

Further reading: McNeill, *Plagues and Peoples;* Marks and Beatty, *Epidemics;* Smith, *The People's Health, 1830–1910.*

British Cholera Epidemic of 1865–66 Fourth and final epidemic of Asiatic cholera in the British Isles. Part of the broader pandemic of 1863–75, the disease was first imported into England's southern port of Southampton in September 1865, probably from Egypt, and a few months later appeared in the northeastern port of Hull, brought by European immigrants on their way to the United States. This epidemic, less devastating, than those of 1832, 1848–49, and 1853–54, caused approximately 15,000 human deaths, 5,000 of which occurred in London.

Heightened awareness of the need for improved public sanitation and clean water supplies probably contributed to the containment of cholera during this visitation. But resistance to the work of English physician John Snow, who traced cholera to contaminated water in the epidemic of 1832 and correctly hypothesized the existence of microorganisms as the cause of the disease, resulted in slow adoption of truly effective prevention. Careful handling of patients' excreta, through which the cholera bacillus is passed, and boiling household water, which kills the bacteria, would have saved many lives had these simple methods been promoted by the medical profession and the central and local boards of health (see BRITISH CHOLERA EPIDEMIC OF 1832; BRITISH CHOLERA EPIDEMICS OF 1848–49 AND 1853–54).

While Europe and the United States continued to experience large-scale epidemics, England was spared from cholera after 1866, largely due to strict quarantine of ships from foreign cities, which prevented the disease from entering the country.

Further reading: Creighton, *A History of Epidemics in Britain*; Smith, *The People's Health, 1830–1910*.

British Columbian Typhoid Epidemics of 1908–13

Outbreaks of typhoid fever that killed hundreds of people, mainly in the interior Rocky Mountain valleys of British Columbia, Canada. Caused by bacteria (*Salmonella typhosa*), typhoid fever is carried by water, milk, and food (notably fish and shellfish) contaminated by human feces and urine; it can be contracted by direct contact with a diseased patient and from an asymptomatic carrier of the fever.

About 1880 typhoid-infected railway construction workers introduced the disease into British Columbia, which had become Canada's sixth province in 1871. Sporadic outbreaks occurred until 1908, when more cases erupted in the crowded, confined towns in the province's southern interior region; there sanitary conditions were poor, and sewage problems in the mountainous river valleys provided opportunities for person-to-person typhoid transmission as well as pollution of water supplies. British Columbia reported 70 human deaths from typhoid in 1908, 55 deaths in 1909, and 101 deaths in 1910. Chinese workers on the railways, as well as in the mining and lumbering industries, were forced to live on the outskirts of the towns, high up on the mountain slopes. Ironically, as outcasts they rarely caught typhoid fever during this time.

Between 1910 and 1913, however, severe typhoid outbreaks struck the construction workers on the Canadian Northern Railway in the Thompson and Fraser river valleys in southern British Columbia; several hundred people perished in the camps and towns, such as Fernie. Sewage problems in the settlements had been ignored by most authorities, despite warnings by the provincial board of health, which finally in 1912 initiated a small vaccination campaign for protection. However, very few doses of vaccine were distributed in the interior, where 67 persons out of 527 who contracted typhoid died in 1913 (all of British Columbia had 700 infections and 85 deaths that year). Because of an economic recession in the province in 1913 and the start of World War I in 1914, there was a halt to major construction and thus many transient workers left the region. Out of 206 typhoid cases in 1915, only seven were fatal. Incidence of typhoid continued to decline in the following year.

Further reading: Huckstep, *Typhoid Fever*; Roland, ed., *Health, Disease and Medicine*.

British Encephalitis Epidemic of 1919–31

Epidemic of about 12 years' duration that claimed thousands of human lives throughout England, Scotland, and Wales. The first cases reported in England occurred during the first quarter of 1918, but it was not until the following year that the outbreak reached epidemic proportions.

Encephalitis is a disease of the nervous system that manifests a variety of bizarre symptoms, both mental and physical. The main symptom of "encephalitis lethargica," the variety most prevalent in the early years of this epidemic, is constant fatigue and stupor. In another type, the patient shows acute agitation, sleeplessness, and jerking of muscles; these symptoms began appearing with frequency in 1923. Rolling of the eyes, paralysis of the eye muscles, and accelerated breathing are other common symptoms. Mental disorders include delirium and severe disorientation. The fatality rate of encephalitis is as high as 50 percent, and sometimes much higher. Although people of all ages are susceptible to encephalitis, the majority of cases are found in the 10 to 20 age group. Incidence declines with increasing age.

Encephalitis was first recognized and identified as a specific disease by an Austrian physician, Constantin von Economo, who brought it to the attention of the medical profession in 1916. Shortly thereafter the disease began appearing all over the world, and continued in epidemic form globally for the next several years. Because physicians in England had no clinical experience of the illness, it was mistaken at first for botulism.

In the five-year period 1919–23, 2,373 human deaths occurred from encephalitis in England and

Wales out of 4,380 recorded cases; from 1924 through 1929, 7,368 deaths occurred out of a recorded 13,900 cases; and in 1930 and 1931, 1,878 deaths occurred out of 1,386 recorded cases. Lack of notification explains the higher number of fatalities over cases recorded in 1930–31. To the recorded cases—as a highly fatal contagious disease, notification of encephalitis became mandatory in England and Wales on January 1, 1919—should be added many mild cases that went unrecorded.

Encephalitis was widespread in Scotland by 1923, appearing in rural as well as highly populated areas. Although significant numbers of cases were reported in Ireland, encephalitis did not become epidemic there.

Even in mild cases, death or permanent brain damage may ensue due to residua or sequelae (pathological consequences), sometimes occurring years after an initial case. Relapses also often occur. Encephalitis is a carrier disease, so that a perfectly healthy person who is infected but shows no symptoms may infect another person. Thus, isolation and other precautionary measures, in the case of carriers, are of no effect in preventing transmission of infection. Like influenza, encephalitis usually occurs mainly during the winter months.

Further reading: Ackerknecht, *History and Geography of the Most Important Diseases*; Greenwood, *Epidemics and Crowd-Diseases*; MacNalty, "Epidemic Diseases of the Central Nervous System"; Stallybrass, "Encephalitis Lethargica: Some Observations on a Recent Outbreak."

British Influenza Epidemic of 1918–19

Part of the calamitous, worldwide Spanish Influenza Epidemic of 1917–19 (q.v.), striking the British Isles between mid-1918 and early 1919.

During the first wave of what was called the "Spanish flu," which reached England in June 1918, morbidity (incidence of disease) was highest among those under 35 years old and progressively declined in older age groups; this is the typical pattern for flu. Despite fewer attacks among older people, however, and following the usual mortality pattern of influenza, most human deaths occurred in this older age group, mostly due to pneumonia triggered by the flu virus. In addition, the attack rate was highest during the first of the pandemic's three waves that hit Britain, yet mortality was lower than the succeeding two waves. In the British Isles, as elsewhere, most deaths occurred in the autumn of 1918, during the second wave. Altogether approximately 200,000 people died in England and Wales. What was extraordinarily atypical was that during the second, most lethal wave, about half of the total fatalities occurred among the younger population. Death from flu in the 20 to 40 age group in such incredibly high numbers had never happened in Britain before, and has not been experienced since. This explosion of deaths among young people is a feature of the epidemic that remains unexplained satisfactorily to this day.

Influenza causes death, in the majority of cases in a "typical" epidemic, through virulent infection, which leads to pneumonia. Perhaps ten percent of the deaths in Britain in 1918 in the autumn wave were due to a particularly severe pneumonia that would develop suddenly, killing its victims—of all ages—within 48 hours or less.

Fewer British people died in the third wave of early 1919, but again, as in the second wave, 50 percent of the deaths were among younger people. Different viral strains were probably responsible for each separate wave, explaining the variations in severity each time, although this is not certain. The duration of the second wave was only about six weeks in any given location, while the first and third waves lasted longer.

Unlike the so-called filth diseases such as typhus fever or plague, which were often largely confined to economically deprived social classes, influenza, a highly infectious disease spread through the air, attacks universally. In 1918, vaccines were undeveloped, but some inoculation with flu serum did take place. Masks were used to little effect, since viral matter could pass through the sides, and chemical sprays to "cleanse" the air were unfortunately completely useless.

Further reading: Beveridge, *Influenza: The Last Great Plague*; Henig, "Flu Pandemic"; Ryle, "Zero Grazing."

British Influenza Epidemic of 1950–51

Sudden influenza outbreak in Newcastle in the north of England and in Aberdeen and Edinburgh in Scotland during the last week of December 1950. It is probable that the virus was imported to Britain through these port cities from Scandinavia, where influenza was then circulating.

During the next six weeks (January–February 1951) the illness was reported from most places in England, Scotland, and Ireland, although in varying intensities. In Ireland, for example, influenza broke out sharply in Belfast, while Dublin was only mildly affected. The highest attack rates and mortality rates were in northern England, where the epidemic began, and in Liverpool and its surrounding area. Influenza was far more deadly in Liverpool than anywhere else in Britain—weekly death tolls in that city were as high as those during the Spanish Influenza Epidemic of 1917–19 (q.v.), one of the most lethal epidemics of any kind in history. During the six weeks of the epidemic, an estimated 50,000 fatalities occurred in England and Wales, due either directly to influenza or indirectly through secondary bacterial complications leading mostly to death from pneumonia and other respiratory sequelae. Successively since 1918, when 86 percent of deaths occurred among people under age 55, the percentage of deaths in younger age groups decreased steadily, until in 1951 those under 55 accounted for only 12 percent of deaths from flu and flu-related causes.

Virologists determined that two distinct subtypes of influenza A, the "Scandinavian" subtype and the "Liverpool" subtype, both consisting of a variety of different strains, were responsible for this epidemic.

Although the epidemic of 1950–51 was not a global pandemic, many areas of the world were affected, including South Africa, Australia, and most of Europe.

Further reading: Bradley, "Discussion: Influenza 1951"; Isaacs and Andrewes, "The Spread of Influenza"; Burnet, *Viruses and Man.*

British Influenza Epidemic of 1957–58

Outbreak in 1957 of a new antigenic subtype of the influenza A virus (the most important of three viral types), labelled H2N2 (formerly designated A2); replaced subtype H1N1 (A1), which had been the main influenza type prevailing since the Spanish Influenza Epidemic of 1917–19 (q.v.). Appearing first in China in February 1957, this so-called "Asian flu" spread, over the next several months, throughout the entire world. The H2N2 virus was much less deadly than its predecessor, H1N1, which caused at least 20,000,000 deaths worldwide, including 200,000 deaths in England and Wales, in 1918 and 1919. Nonetheless, the Asian flu of 1957 caused widespread sickness and considerable mortality.

England was hit hardest with the virus in August, September, and October, and experienced a minor second wave in December and January 1958. Although it is impossible to calculate morbidity rates for influenza, an estimated 12,000,000 people were infected in 1957 and 1958; total deaths in England for this epidemic are estimated at 16,000. The highest attack rate was among children aged 5 to 14 years, although the majority of deaths were caused by secondary virulent complications in older age groups. High attack rates among younger people, with few deaths, and lower relative morbidity but much higher mortality among older age groups, is typical for most influenza epidemics. The 1957–58 outbreak was somewhat distinctive in that during September, half the deaths attributed to flu occurred among people less than 55 years old, recalling the pattern of the 1918 epidemic (see BRITISH INFLUENZA EPIDEMIC OF 1918–19). In October of 1957 and the following winter

months, however, the pattern of deaths became more typical of most influenza outbreaks, with most deaths occurring among people over 55.

Most deaths were in people, regardless of age, with preexisting lung disease whose condition became fatal upon infection with influenza. In otherwise healthy individuals, however, a life-threatening form of pneumonia often developed; about 20 percent of deaths were due to pneumonia caused directly by influenza virus.

Of the several types of vaccine available in 1957, the one with the best demonstrable results conferred immunity in 30 percent to 60 percent of cases with reaction times from two to four weeks after inoculation. Because a different vaccine must be prepared for each new strain of influenza virus, an appropriate vaccine often cannot be prepared in time to prevent widespread infection; early detection of a new, genetically altered viral subtype is therefore crucial. In 1957, vaccination was not extensively used. See also ASIAN INFLUENZA PANDEMIC OF 1957–58.

Further reading: Beveridge, *Influenza: The Last Great Plague;* Stuart-Harris, "Influenza and Its Complications"; Stuart-Harris, "Influenza."

British Influenza Epidemic of 1968–70

Outbreak of the "Hong Kong flu," so named because the virus that developed into a global pandemic was first detected in that Chinese city, erupting in July 1968 and quickly spreading around the world. Britain reported its first serious cases in December 1968.

This viral strain was not a new subtype, but a less genetically changed variant (H3N2) of the subtype H2N2, which caused the Asian flu of 1957 (see ASIAN INFLUENZA PANDEMIC OF 1957–58). Natural immunity (immunity gained from an infection of influenza) was therefore effective to some degree in individuals who had been infected either by the first occurrence of the Asian flu in 1957 or during any of the subsequent localized epidemics involving that strain. A peculiar aspect of this pandemic was that, whereas the United States was severely affected during the first wave of 1968–69, Britain (and Europe), with similar attack rates, experienced far fewer human deaths. The second wave of 1969–70 was much more lethal.

The first wave appeared in England in late December 1968 and lasted through May 1969. The attack rate was more or less the same for all age groups, with the exception of people over 65 who experienced a lower rate. The second wave, much shorter and much more deadly, started in early December 1969; morbidity rose sharply and quickly declined toward the end of January 1970. In just eight weeks, an estimated 30,000 people died of influenza and influenza-related respiratory diseases, mostly pneumonia and bronchitis.

Because the virus in both waves comprising the epidemic of 1968–69/1969–70 was the same, the difference in duration and virulence of the two waves remains puzzling to virologists. Vaccination was not used extensively and thus could not have significantly affected relative attack rates, and the natural immunity conferred on a large segment of the British during the first wave apparently had no affect on the intensity of the second wave. See also HONG KONG INFLUENZA PANDEMIC OF 1968; RUSSIAN (RED) INFLUENZA EPIDEMIC OF 1977–78; U.S. INFLUENZA EPIDEMIC OF 1968–69.

Further reading: Beveridge, *Influenza: The Last Great Plague*; Miller, Pereira, and Clarke, "Epidemiology of the Hong Kong/68 Variant of Influenza A2 in Britain."

British Smallpox Epidemic of 1796 Widespread epidemic of smallpox that caused over 3,500 deaths in London and an estimated 35,000 deaths throughout the British Isles.

The epidemic's terrible destructiveness stands out as background to one of the momentous events in the history of medicine. This was the experimentation and propagation by Dr. Edward Jenner of vaccination, or inoculation against smallpox with cowpox virus. Having heard from his English country neighbors that people who had had cowpox—a disease often contracted by milkmaids and others working closely with cattle—never contracted smallpox, Jenner conducted experiments first on his infant son and then, seven years later in 1796, on a young boy called James Phipps. Jenner discovered that when smallpox virus was introduced into a person already inoculated with cowpox, little or no reaction to the smallpox resulted. This meant that people would not only forgo the mild attack of smallpox that always accompanied variolation, but also avoid risk of death from an unexpectedly virulent case (see LONDON SMALLPOX EPIDEMIC OF 1721). In addition, while persons inoculated with smallpox virus could infect others with smallpox, those inoculated with cowpox virus could not.

Jenner brought his findings to the attention of the world in a paper he published in 1798. The safety from smallpox that vaccination conferred and the consequent elimination of the spread of infection could have extinguished one of the most terrible diseases to ever afflict mankind. However, despite the fact that vaccination was immediately received with enthusiasm by governments throughout Europe, North and South America, India, China, and other parts of the world (more than 100,000 people were vaccinated in Britain alone by 1801), the practice

was not universally accepted until many decades later. In Britain, influential physicians as well as large numbers of common citizens resisted the procedure fiercely, and as a result deadly epidemics continued to occur in Britain throughout the nineteenth century.

Further reading: Hopkins, *Princes and Peasants: Smallpox in History*; Shurkin, *The Invisible Fire*; Smith, *The Speckled Monster*.

British Smallpox Epidemic of 1816–19 Major epidemic of smallpox that started in central England in the town of Derby in the spring of 1816 and spread during the following three years to many areas of the country, including Nottinghamshire, Staffordshire, East Anglia, and as far south as London and Canterbury. Mortality figures for this epidemic are difficult to estimate; in London, for example, the bills of mortality (formal statements) upon which historians rely for statistical information about deaths, were inadequately kept. It is clear, however, that babies and young children were the chief victims (as was normally the case until the mid-1800s, when the older population began to contract smallpox in high numbers).

Rising unemployment at this time helped increase the incidence of smallpox among the poorer population, whose numbers were forced to wander from place to place in search of work, a condition that always facilitates the spread of disease. A contemporary spoke of "the public exposure of hideous objects just recovering, loaded with scabs, at the street corners." In Ireland, a poor harvest in the fall of 1816 caused the same general vagrancy, especially in the northern towns, where smallpox spread quickly among the children of displaced peasant families. Smallpox was also widespread and highly fatal in Scotland during these years.

The epidemic of 1816–19 was the first widespread outbreak of smallpox to occur in the British Isles after the introduction by physician Edward Jenner of the preventive technique of vaccination during the British Smallpox Epidemic of 1796 (q.v.). This life-saving procedure was met with strong opposition from people who either preferred the older, but less safe, technique of variolation (see ENGLISH SMALLPOX EPIDEMIC OF 1751–53), or who rejected both treatments for various medical and religious reasons. During this epidemic the controversy about the merits of both vaccination and variolation became heated, as it would continue during subsequent epidemics throughout the rest of the nineteenth century. In the meantime, because there is no cure for smallpox, thousands of people died through resistance or inaccessibility to either preventive technique.

Further reading: Creighton, *A History of Epidemics in Britain*; Smith, *The Speckled Monster*.

British Smallpox Epidemic of 1837–40

One of the worst epidemics of smallpox ever to afflict England and Wales, which claimed nearly 42,000 lives from July 1837 (when registration of death by cause began) through December 1840; in London, 6,449 fatalities were recorded. Most deaths occurred in 1838.

This epidemic began in the west and southwest part of England, where the cities of Exeter, Bath, and Liverpool were experiencing high fatalities early in 1837. The infection spread through Wales in the winter of 1837–38, and during 1838 spread to the eastern areas of England, where deaths in the city of Norwich were especially high. In 1839 the disease subsided somewhat but surged again in 1840, concentrating mainly in the manufacturing towns of Lancashire, which continued experiencing an unusually high number of deaths from smallpox through 1841.

Once again the controversy over vaccination, or inoculation with cowpox virus, which had met with bitter opposition since its introduction in 1796 (see BRITISH SMALLPOX EPIDEMIC OF 1796), became inflamed as thousands of people throughout Britain died unnecessarily. Legislation passed in 1840 banned the less safe procedure of variolation, or inoculation with smallpox virus, and made vaccination compulsory, a law that was resented and ignored by many, and therefore unsuccessful in preventing further serious outbreaks of smallpox. Other legislation designed to enforce vaccination would be passed in following decades, as frequent outbreaks erupted and a devastating epidemic afflicted England once more in 1870–71 (see BRITISH SMALLPOX EPIDEMIC OF 1871–72). The fearful smallpox epidemic of 1837–40 coincided with a major epidemic of typhus fever, which caused approximately 28,000 deaths (see ENGLISH TYPHUS EPIDEMIC OF 1837–38).

Further reading: Creighton, *A History of Epidemics in Britain*; Smith, *The People's Health, 1830–1910*; Smith, *The Speckled Monster*.

British Smallpox Epidemic of 1871–72

Last great outbreak of smallpox in the British Isles, which caused approximately 42,000 deaths in England and Wales in two years. London's death count was about 10,000. In Scotland, the epidemic continued through 1874; approximately 6,300 people died from smallpox in this four-year period. Ireland's worst year was 1872, with about 3,250 fatalities, nearly all of which occurred in the largest towns, Dublin, Cork, and Belfast. This epidemic was part of a broad pandemic of smallpox due largely to the spread of the disease by French soldiers during the Franco-Prussian War (1870–71), and was carried to England by refugees in the autumn of 1870. However, smallpox had been endemic in England for centuries, and in the generation since the last major epidemic of 1837–40, sporadic eruptions in various part of Britain caused thousands of deaths, notably in 1848, 1851, 1852, 1858, and 1863–65.

Unlike most smallpox epidemics since 1700, where infants and young children comprised the highest number of fatalities, the epidemic of 1871–72 saw a high proportion of deaths among adolescents and adults, a change partially explained by the severe epidemic of scarlet fever in 1868–70, which claimed over 82,000 lives, mostly among the under-five population, and the fact that many people of adult age had either never been vaccinated or passed through childhood without contracting smallpox, which confers immunity to further infection. The disease also was more prevalent in cities than in small towns and rural areas, and among the poorer classes, who continued to ignore or resist vaccination for themselves and their children, despite numerous acts of Parliament that mandated compulsory vaccination. Resentment of what was viewed as interference in their private affairs and a feeling of resignation in the face of the general deprivation of their lives, in addition to inflamed rhetoric by various anti-vaccination groups, combined to strengthen their opposition to a procedure they distrusted, and made the road to universal prevention of smallpox impossible. Nonetheless, smallpox gradually declined in the following decades, a phenomenon that remains largely unexplained.

Further reading: Creighton, *A History of Epidemics in Britain*; Hopkins, *Princes and Peasants: Smallpox in History*; Smith, *The People's Health, 1830–1910*.

British Smallpox Epidemic of 1901–02

Last epidemic of smallpox (*Variola major*) to afflict the British Isles, claiming over 1,300 human lives in London and nearly 1,400 in Glasgow, the two cities with the greatest number of fatalities. Cases mounted in London in the late summer of 1901 and quickly spread through surrounding areas; by 1902, the whole of England was experiencing unusually high numbers of cases.

This epidemic, although relatively minor in comparison to previous outbreaks, is notable for being the last severe occurrence of smallpox on a widespread scale in Britain's history. At the same time it highlighted the strange, unexpected decline of the disease. Vaccination, which provides temporary immunity to smallpox, had helped reduce the spread of infection over the previous decades, but so much opposition to the practice arose among anti-vaccination groups in the last quarter of the nineteenth century that the British Parliament modified previous legislation, which had made vaccination mandatory. Thus, neglect of preventive measures against smallpox coincided with its gradual, natural disappearance from the British Isles. A few spectacular incidents occurred in the 1970s when individuals contracted the infection as a result of laboratory accidents.

A much milder, though still fatal, form of smallpox, *Variola minor*, continued to erupt in Britain, sometimes in epidemic proportions, through the 1960s.

Further reading: Hopkins, *Princes and Peasants: Smallpox in History*; Smith, *The People's Health, 1830–1910*; Smith, *The Speckled Monster*.

British Typhoid Epidemic in the Boer War Epidemic of typhoid fever in South Africa during the Great Boer War (1899–1902), striking some 77,000 British troops and killing about 13,000 of them. Hundreds of Boers, South African Dutch colonists or farmers who were fighting the British, were also affected and perished.

Typhoid fever, a communicable disease caused by the bacterium *Salmonella typhosa*, has frequently occurred among soldiers in action and thus has been called the "campaign" disease. Before the Boer War, it was a serious illness in the Napoleonic, Crimean, Spanish-American, and U.S. Civil wars (in the latter war, the Union Army alone suffered 81,360 deaths from either typhoid fever or dysentery, another waterborne disease).

Most common in tropical climates, typhoid fever is usually caused by contaminated water or food. At the time of the Boer War, filtering or boiling water were measures known to prevent contamination, and yet these procedures were not fully practiced by the British troops in South Africa. Early in the war, during a march to Bloemfontein, many thirsty British soldiers drank straight from the Modder River, whose waters were then polluted or contaminated with the infectious typhoid bacillus (the disease had been prevalent in the native villages upstream); the British Army's water filters had become clogged at the time, and the frustrated soldiers could not wait for their boiled water to cool in the hot African climate. The disease was contracted by the soldiers, some of whom spread it through direct contact with others.

Those with the illness suffered severe abdominal pain, high fever, diarrhea, and delirium, sometimes dying by the second week of their infection. Because the effectiveness of the preventive vaccine for typhoid was questionable, only 14,626 British soldiers

out of 328,244 then in South Africa were vaccinated; some 64,000 men were sent home for medical treatment. Between February 1900 and the end of 1902, the disease was contracted by 42,741 troops, 11,327 of whom died from it; during that period, 6,425 troops were killed on the battlefields of the war. All in all, about 400,000 British troops were dispatched to South Africa before the Boers capitulated to end the 32-month-long war, which brought approximately 8,000 British deaths from battle wounds and some 13,000 from typhoid fever.

Although hygienic and sanitary practices in the British military improved a great deal following the war, the substantial decline in typhoid fever was largely due to the British Army's adoption of total vaccination of all troops going abroad. Whereas in the Boer War typhoid fever was contracted at the rate of 105 per 1,000 men (with mortality [death rate] at 14.6 per 1,000), in World War I (1914–18) the disease was contracted at 2.35 per 1,000 men (with mortality at 0.139 per 1,000).

Further reading: Cartwright, *Disease and History*; McGrew, *Encyclopedia of Medical History*.

Burmese Dengue Hemorrhagic Fever Epidemics of 1970 and 1971 Two epidemics of dengue hemorrhagic fever (DHF) that began in the port city of Rangoon (Yangôn) in Burma (Myanmar) in 1970 and 1971.

Burma's first outbreak of a dengue-type fever occurred in Rangoon in 1963. This was found to be caused mainly by the chikungunya virus. Then, in 1970, Rangoon was invaded by a DHF epidemic; 1,974 cases and 87 deaths were reported. Once again, the chikungunya virus was the main culprit, but this time dengue viruses 1 and 3 were also isolated. The Burmese cities of Bassein and Moulmein were also infected during this epidemic.

In 1971, DHF returned to cause another epidemic in Rangoon, this one registering 685 cases and 34 deaths.

During the 1960s and 1970s, DHF epidemics were reported in many countries of Southeast Asia (see THAI DENGUE HEMORRHAGIC FEVER EPIDEMICS; SINGAPORE DENGUE HEMORRHAGIC FEVER EPIDEMICS), in the Western Pacific and, more recently, in the South Pacific. DHF is now known to mainly target Asian children under 14 years of age.

Further reading: Howe, ed., *A World Geography of Human Diseases*.

Burundian Meningitis Epidemic of 1992 Short, severe outbreak of cerebrospinal meningitis (CSM) that killed 215 out of 1,239 persons reported infected in the country of Burundi in east-central Africa in

August–September 1992. Although located south of Africa's so-called "meningitis belt" (sub-Sahara), Burundi had suffered periodic CSM outbreaks from 1935 to 1972 but afterward did not report this acute bacterial disease until the 1992 epidemic.

Infected, asymptomatic human carriers apparently brought the disease from western Tanzania into Burundi, where cases were first recorded on August 19, 1992. (The disease is generally spread to and from others by aerial droplet infection and is characterized by fever, headache, vomiting, and stiff neck.) Cases occurred throughout Burundi and were especially serious in the province of Ruyigi in the east, where a total of 867 cases were reported between August 19 and September 21. Although all age groups were affected in Burundi, two thirds of those stricken were under 30 years old and a fourth of all infections were children under ten years old. In some persons, onset of CSM was sudden, with acute fulminating attacks causing death within 24 hours.

More than 17 percent of those afflicted by CSM died in the Burundian epidemic; this was high considering the effective modern medications available. International medical aid was promptly called in and a vaccine was provided to Burundi's infected communities, thus curtailing the epidemic by the end of September 1992.

Further reading: Hartwig and Patterson, *Cerebrospinal Meningitis in West Africa and Sudan in the Twentieth Century*; World Health Organization, *Weekly Epidemiological Records*.

C

Cádiz Yellow Fever Epidemic of 1800 Epidemic of yellow fever that killed thousands of people in Spain's southern port city of Cádiz during the summer and fall of 1800. The first cases were reported in early August in the harbor area, which led to the assumption that the illness was imported into Cádiz on a ship from Cuba that had anchored on July 6, three of whose passengers had died of yellow fever during the crossing.

During August 1800 yellow fever spread rapidly through the entire city; by September, 200 people were dying every day. Churches could not accommodate the need for sacraments and burials, bells no longer tolled at each death—bells would be ringing all day and night—and fever victims were buried outside the city walls. Commerce came to a standstill as the port and the city gates were closed. As usual in most large-scale epidemics, the plight of the poor became urgent. Municipal authorities were able to maintain social order, principally by supplying food and medical care to the residents of the poorer *barrios*. In an attempt to clear the city of what were believed to be contaminated, disease-causing miasmas, drains were cleaned, streets and houses hosed down, resins and wood burned along the streets, and cannonshots fired in hopes of purifying the air. To ward off infection people covered their faces with cloths soused in vinegar, carried garlic in their mouths or pockets, or wore aromatic amulets.

Physicians—dozens of whom died—stood helpless in the face of this destructive fever. The ignorance of the medical profession was admitted by José María Mociño, an attending physician during the epidemic: "I cannot disguise the fact, that in effect we found ourselves in disagreement about the nosological determination of the disease, about its etiology, about its pathological nature, and as a consequence about the therapeutic, preventive, and hygienic measures it necessitates." Mociño firmly believed that miasmas caused yellow fever, and attributed its disappearance in December to cold winter winds sweeping away the "swampy emanations." Despite the fact that it was clearly noted in Cádiz that people from the Americas and Africa, who presumably had had the disease before, did not contract the fever, many medical men were adamantly opposed to the idea of immunity to it. The theory of contagion was also continually debated. Numerous investigations and studies were undertaken, yet no one had the remotest suspicion that specific mosquitoes carried the yellow fever virus. All records of the epidemic mention the unusually hot summer of 1800, a condition that allowed mosquitoes imported aboard ships from tropical climates to thrive.

As estimated 7,400 to 8,500 people, or 13 percent to 15 percent of the population, died of yellow fever from August to December in Cádiz. The disease spread to many places throughout the surrounding region, including Medina Sidonia, Jerez, and Seville. In the following few years yellow fever would terrorize most of southern Spain (see SPANISH YELLOW FEVER EPIDEMICS OF 1803–05).

Further reading: Peset-Reig, *Muerte en España*; Mociño, *Disertación de la fiebre epidémica, que padeció Cádiz*.

Cádiz Yellow Fever Epidemic of 1810 Outbreak of yellow fever striking Spain's seaport of Cádiz in mid-September 1810 during the Spanish War of Independence against France (also called the Peninsular War, of the Napoleonic Wars). French troops outside the city made the threat of yellow fever even more alarming than usual, as Cádiz faced the decimation of its small national army as well as large numbers of deaths among its citizens and the thousands of refugees it harbored from the surrounding countryside.

Fortunately the epidemic, which began late in the summer season and thus had less time to intensify and spread, did not prove as deadly as others in Cádiz had been, particularly the Cádiz Yellow Fever Epidemic of 1800 (q.v.). Bartolomé Mellado, a prominent Spanish doctor who reported the first cases of the illness to city officials and wrote a detailed account of the epidemic, counted 2,788 deaths through December 1810. It was assumed that the disease was brought to Cádiz by ships from nearby Gibraltar, where the virus had appeared several weeks earlier (see GIBRALTAR YELLOW FEVER EPIDEMICS OF 1804–28). Yellow fever continued to harass Cádiz and other cities in southern Spain during the next three years, reaching as far north along the Mediterranean coast as Murcia and Alicante.

Further reading: Cloudsley-Thompson, *Insects and History*; Peset-Reig, *Muerte en España*.

Cairo and Alexandria Diphtheria Epidemics of 1882–86

Outbreaks of diphtheria in Egypt's two most important cities; killed a total of almost 3,500 inhabitants from 1882 to 1886. At this time diphtheria cases were increasing alarmingly around the world, in both warm and cool climates.

Called "cynanche" (inflammation of the throat) by Egyptians, diphtheria and its transmission were not well understood when numerous inhabitants of Cairo and Alexandria contracted the disease, which is caused by a specific bacterium that primarily infects the tonsils, pharynx, larynx, or nose and is transmitted through droplet infection from diseased persons. During the course of the epidemics, Cairo suffered much more severely than Alexandria did, reporting more than seven times as many fatalities from diphtheria than the latter city; Cairo's population of about 374,000 people was rather larger than Alexandria's, about 231,000. Authorities then could do little to help the victims of diphtheria, who were mainly children, and in 1883 infections escalated in both cities. The contagion remained prevalent until abating about three years later, and continued to be a health problem in Cairo and Alexandria. Many years later, in 1932, diphtheria erupted severely in both places, and victims' mortality ran as high as 48 percent.

Further reading: Henschen, *The History and Geography of Diseases*; Newsholme, *The Origin and Spread of Pandemic Diphtheria*.

Calcutta Smallpox Epidemics of the 1800s

Smallpox epidemics of varying intensity that repeatedly attacked the Bengal city of Calcutta, India, during the nineteenth century.

The first epidemic, in 1832–33, claimed 2,814 victims in the city. The death toll for the second epidemic, which struck Calcutta in 1837–38, was 1,548 people. During this period, smallpox also infected the city of Lucknow to the west, where it was attributed to economy measures introduced by the government, such as shutting down the vaccine depart-

ment. Another bout of smallpox hit Calcutta during 1843–44, claiming 2,949 human lives.

The worst outbreak of the century came in 1849–50, when 6,431 deaths were reported among Calcutta's 387,398 native Indian residents—3,329 of them during the first five months of 1850. More than 32,000 residents (about one in every family) were estimated as being infected with smallpox. The city's European residents were not spared either; 76 were hospitalized and 12 deaths (mainly among soldiers and sailors) were recorded. The situation was so serious that during one specific week in 1850, the ratio of Calcutta's smallpox deaths to its population was far higher than London's overall mortality rate from smallpox for any three-month period since 1837.

Smallpox again affected Calcutta in 1857, causing 3,177 deaths. Another epidemic struck in 1865, claiming 4,923 lives. Calcutta was also infected during smallpox outbreaks in India in 1873–74 and in 1884–85; in between, the Bengal Vaccination Act of 1880 was enacted. Thereby, vaccinations were declared mandatory in the port of Calcutta and in areas under the jurisdiction of the lieutenant-governor of Bengal, for all residents and new arrivals.

Calcutta suffered a major outbreak in 1894–95, with 2,220 deaths in 1895 alone. During this visitation, eyewitnesses reported that the bedding of smallpox victims was often thrown into the streets where it was picked up by ragpickers and promptly recycled. Also, sickrooms of smallpox patients were often dark and dingy, with little air or light, and were visited by large numbers of relatives and friends. It is not surprising that the infection continued to spread.

Further reading: Hopkins, *Princes and Peasants: Smallpox in History*; Arnold, ed., *Imperial Medicine and Indigenous Societies*.

Cambridge Typhus Epidemic of 1522 (Black Assize)

First of three famous assizes (county court sessions) that took place in sixteenth-century England, at which many presiding officials, jurors, and spectators became infected with what was probably louse-borne (or "epidemic") typhus fever during Lent at the castle of Cambridge in 1522. A near-contemporary chronicler relates that at these assizes, "the justices and all the gentlemen, bailiffs and other, resorting thither, took such an infection, whether it were of the savour of the prisoners, or of the filth of the house, that many gentlemen, . . . thereof died, and almost all which were present were sore sick, and narrowly escaped with their lives." Unlike the two later Black Assizes of the 1500s (see OXFORD TYPHUS EPIDEMIC OF 1577; EXETER TYPHUS EPIDEMIC OF 1586), in which the deaths of prisoners are specifically mentioned, the presence of fever or distress among the prisoners being tried at Cambridge is not recorded, although an allusion to them as a cause of the infection is clearly made.

Until the late nineteenth century, English prisons or "gaols" were notoriously filthy and the lives of prisoners unspeakably wretched. Typhus fever was so rife among the men incarcerated in these places that it became known as "gaol fever." The human body-louse, which transmits the disease from man to man, thrives in insanitary conditions where water and soap for bathing are unavailable and people are crowded together, as in jails, ships, and tenement housing. England's three Black Assizes of the 1500s drew the attention of contemporary observers because the fever affected members of the privileged classes. Outbreaks of typhus fever in prisons were a common occurrence in England, but they were little noted until prison reform became a social issue of the 1800s.

Further reading: Creighton, *A History of Epidemics in Britain*; Zinsser, *Rats, Lice and History*.

Canadian Cholera Epidemics of 1832 and 1834

Acute outbreaks of cholera that took the lives of al least 25,000 persons in eastern Canada in 1832 and 1834.

In early 1832 authorities in Lower Canada (Quebec) initiated precautionary measures to prevent the entry of cholera-infected persons from England, Ireland, and other places (see BRITISH CHOLERA EPIDEMIC OF 1832; ASIATIC CHOLERA PANDEMIC OF 1826–37). In February 1832, a quarantine station was established on Grosse Isle in the St. Lawrence River, about 30 miles east of the city of Quebec. Cholera reportedly entered the station with Irish immigrants aboard ships as early as April 1832, but the disease remained isolated until the brig *Carricks* docked at the station on June 3. During the *Carricks'* voyage from Ireland, 45 out of 145 passengers aboard died from cholera; the sick were removed to the quarantine hospital, but no effort was made to lessen contact with them during the rest of the incubation period (from one to six days) of this communicable disease.

Another ship, the *Voyageur*, cleared quarantine on Grosse Isle on June 7 and then dropped off some suddenly sick passengers in Quebec's port before heading upriver to Montreal. Between June 8 and June 15, one Quebec hospital admitted 250 cholera cases, of which 161 were fatal. The disease then spread quickly to nearby Pointe Levi (Levis), Beauport, and other towns in Lower Canada. When the disease seemed to abate, the superintendent of Grosse Isle's quarantine station was unfortunately and prematurely ordered to discontinue the inspec-

tion of ships on June 20, but cholera-contaminated ships continued to arrive at Grosse Isle. The river port of Trois-Rivières (Three Rivers), situated between Quebec and Montreal, forbade vessels from entering and thus remained free of cholera in 1832.

When the ship *Voyageur* arrived in Montreal on June 9, 1832, one passenger had already died of cholera and another sick passenger managed to visit a soldier friend at a waterfront inn before dying. The soldier contracted the disease and infected 46 others in his garrison before he too died. In the next two weeks, there were some 800 human deaths from cholera in the Montreal area. By September, a reported 1,843 persons had died, including about 70 Indians at Caughnawage village (where 157 Indians had been attacked by cholera). Montreal was not safe from the disease until November 1832, when a total of 1,885 fatalities had been recorded in the area. The infection spread to neighboring towns in what is now southeastern Quebec province, where there were an estimated 4,000 deaths from cholera (a seventh of the population then); from this area, cholera reached New York State (see U.S. CHOLERA EPIDEMIC OF 1832).

In 1832 physicians did not know that cholera was spread by water, milk, or food contaminated by human stool or that it was caused by a bacterium (*Vibrio comma*). Patients were often subjected to ineffective methods, bloodletting, and transfusions of saline fluid. In the city of Quebec, the Hôtel-Dieu and other hospitals were quickly filled, and it was necessary to open other establishments to house the sick; tents were also erected on the nearby Plains of Abraham to accommodate the sick. A special cholera cemetery, the Champs des Morts, had also been built and was busily operating by September 15, by which time at least 3,851 deaths had been recorded from cholera in and around Quebec City, where the mortality rate was nine times that of Paris and 16 times that of London.

Upper Canada (Ontario) also suffered from the epidemic between mid-June and August 1832; either refugees from Montreal or some of the 11,000 immigrants conveyed cholera with them. Among the worst hit towns and cities were Brockville, Kingston, and Johnstown (Prescott) on the St. Lawrence River, York (Toronto) on Lake Ontario, and London near Lake Erie.

Canada then remained free of cholera for almost two years, until July 1834, when infected Irish immigrants again carried the disease into Grosse Isle and, without detection, passed through the quarantine and landed at Quebec city. There the epidemic lasted until October, killing 2,509 persons during that time. Montreal was also struck, listing 913 fatalities from cholera. Trois-Rivières also reported cases in 1834. In

Upper Canada, York and Kingston suffered the most fatalities; the village of Galt (now part of the "new" city of Cambridge), southwest of York, was nearly depopulated because of the epidemic. Some 2,500 out of York's 10,000 inhabitants became infected with cholera.

To the east, Nova Scotia and Newfoundland, both of which had escaped the disease completely in 1832, were not as fortunate in 1834, when the port city of Halifax reported many thousands of infected citizens; troops stationed at Fort Massey were seriously attacked. The cholera epidemic lasted about three months in Nova Scotia and killed 20 or more victims daily.

Further reading: Ackerknecht, *History and Geography of the Most Important Diseases;* Heagerty, *Four Centuries of Medical History in Canada;* Marks and Beatty, *Epidemics.*

Canadian Cholera Epidemic of 1849

Cholera outbreak that spread mainly in Canada East (Quebec) and Canada West (Ontario), the disease having at first entered the country through emigrants from abroad or from the neighboring United States (see U.S. CHOLERA EPIDEMIC OF 1849).

About 38,000 immigrants in 1849 passed through the Grosse Isle quarantine station on the St. Lawrence River, east of the city of Quebec—some 11,000 more than the year before. During the summer of 1849, about a fourth of the population of Grosse Isle had cholera at one time; there were 60 fatalities once within two weeks. In addition, at the start of the epidemic, immigrants lodged in houses in Quebec city died of the disease, and afterward, between mid-July and mid-August 1849, the total number of fatalities in Quebec rose to 1,185 people.

Before the disease entered Montreal, the city's board of health issued directions to the public, advising persons how to avoid contracting cholera. (It was not yet known that the disease was caused by the bacteria *Vibrio comma,* although the British scientist John Snow published in 1849 his opinion that contagious matter might come from a diseased human intestine and might enter the system in contaminated water.) Cholera cases were reported in Montreal in early June 1849, and by mid-month 45 or more fatalities were being recorded on some days. Daily fatalities were a steady 25 by mid-July. The disease became so acute in Montreal in August that there was an insufficient number of required jurors for that month's court term. At the epidemic's close in mid-October, thousands of persons had become infected with cholera in Montreal, a city of approximately 55,700 inhabitants.

Health authorities in Toronto (formerly called York) in Canada West (Ontario) attempted to prevent the disease from entering the city, after learning that it had infected the city of Kingston on Lake Ontario in late May 1849. A month later Toronto reported its first cases of cholera; when the epidemic ended in September, the mortality rate stood at about 60 percent in this city of about 30,000 people.

In 1851 Canada had limited cases of cholera except for a serious outbreak in Quebec City, where 282 human deaths occurred within a two-month period in the summer. The disease broke out in 1852 on board the ship *Advance,* sailing from New York to Quebec. A Canadian working on the ship while it was in Quebec's port contracted it and passed it to fellow workers and two sailors from the ship. Within two months (September to November), cholera had killed about 150 people in Quebec. Another cholera outbreak in 1853 was probably averted because of precautionary measures; when a cholera-infected ship from Liverpool, England, entered Quebec's port in the autumn of 1853, authorities found that 34 persons had died during the ocean voyage and five others were still sick; immediately the sick were sent back to Grosse Isle for quarantine.

Further reading: Ackerknecht, *History and Geography of the Most Important Diseases;* Heagerty, *Four Centuries of Medical History in Canada.*

Canadian Cholera Epidemic of 1854

Outbreak of cholera, a serious intestinal disease spread by polluted food and water, that claimed the lives of several thousand persons in southern and eastern parts of Canada during three months in the summer of 1854.

In mid-June 1854 at the Grosse Isle quarantine station on the St. Lawrence River, east of Quebec city, authorities unwittingly allowed immigrant passengers from a recently docked ship, which had lost 45 passengers to cholera during a transatlantic voyage, to mingle with passengers from a non-cholera-infected ship, which soon passed inspection and entered Quebec city's port. (Transmission usually occurs through ingestion of water contaminated with feces or vomitus of patients.) Nine persons from the cholera-free vessel came down with cholera about five days later and spread the infection to others in Quebec City, where a reported 724 people died from it by August 28. Earlier, some sick immigrants had gone to Montreal, where the disease soon erupted on June 22 and killed 396 persons in the following week. About 1,300 human deaths occurred in Montreal during the nine-week-long outbreak there.

In late June 1854 cholera spread also into Canada West (Ontario), first being reported in the city of Hamilton (on the west end of Lake Ontario) and two days later in Toronto and Kingston (ports also on the lake). In Toronto and Kingston, cholera deaths numbered about 25 a day during most of the following two months. Physicians sometimes ineffectively treated patients with intravenous injections of milk and blood serum during the epidemic.

To the east, in New Brunswick, infected immigrants and others aboard a ship brought the disease into the port of St. John in the summer of 1854. It spread rapidly in this crowded, unsanitary port city, where many immigrants congregated close together in housing along lanes and alleyways. Also, St. John's water supply, obtained mostly from wells, became contaminated from poorly dumped sewage. About 1,500 inhabitants of St. John and its suburb Portland perished during that summer from cholera. From St. John, the disease spread inland to New Brunswick's capital, Fredericton, and other towns, such as St. Andrew and Woodstock.

The cholera finally subsided throughout southern and eastern Canada by mid-September 1854, but it had been carried by immigrants to areas in the west, such as the rich wheatland of the Red River country of Manitoba, where there were relatively few inhabitants. That same year, at a medical conference in Ottawa, a committee of Canadian doctors drew up a memorandum to educate the public about cholera, the bacterial cause of which was not identified until about 1883 by the German physician Robert Koch.

Further reading: Ackerknecht, *History and Geography of the Most Important Diseases;* Heagerty, *Four Centuries of Medical History in Canada.*

Canadian Indian Smallpox Epidemic of 1780–82

Virulent outbreak of smallpox that killed thousands of Indians (Chippewa, Sioux, and others) in Canada between 1780 and 1782. At the close of the epidemic, it is estimated that three fifths of the Indians living in the western and northern Canadian regions had perished from this highly contagious viral disease, characterized by acute fever and a skin eruption of tiny pimples. The pockmarked faces of Indian survivors of smallpox were seen by white Europeans, who had carried the disease to the New World, for many years afterward in North America.

Both the Chippewa or Chippeway (also called Ojibwa) and the Sioux (Dakota) Indians contracted smallpox through the wearing of infected clothing they confiscated in raids on white traders and settlers. The Chippewas dominated the area from eastern Lake Huron to the Turtle Mountains in northern North Dakota in 1780, when smallpox began ravaging them. The Sioux, who had been forced westward by hostile Chippewas, inhabited the northern Great Plains and western prairies up into Canada. In 1780 smallpox broke out among Indian groups in the middle Missouri River region and spread north and west

into Canada. Living crowded together in wigwams, huts, tepees, and dugouts, with no concept of sanitation or quarantine, the Indians were severely infected, having little or no immunity to the disease (permanent immunity usually follows recovery from a first attack). Whole tribes fled to the open plains to escape the invading pestilence that blinded many and disfigured nearly all those who survived.

The variola (smallpox) virus was transmitted from the Chippewas to tribes they traded with, spreading to the Cree and other Indians in the Canadian forests. The Sioux carried it to other tribes of the plains, the Arikara, Hidatsa, and Mandan, among others, who infected other Indians to the west and to the Rocky Mountains. Villages were depopulated as whole Indian families succumbed; many men, dehydrated and unable to bear the high fever, dove into rivers and lakes to cool themselves; more men than women and children perished in some villages. Dogs and wolves feeding on the corpses of smallpox victims also died of the disease; as a result of a great loss of hair due to smallpox, the fur of the wolves became useless to traders.

At the peak of the epidemic in 1781, the Chipewyan Indians (another tribe) west of Hudson Bay were decimated. Leaving their fields untilled or their crops buried beneath the snow, the Indians who survived the outbreak remained in such a state of despair and despondency afterward that few of them had gained sufficient strength to hunt and fish by 1783. The Cree living south of Hudson Bay were struck again by smallpox in 1784 and 1838.

Further reading: Simpson, *Invisible Armies;* Heagerty, *Four Centuries of Medical History in Canada.*

Canadian Indian Smallpox Epidemic of 1837

Outbreak of smallpox that killed thousands of Assiniboin, Cree, Blackfoot, Piegan (Pikuni), and other Plains Indians inhabiting territories in the interior of Canada around the Saskatchewan, Swan, and Red rivers in 1837.

After spending the spring of 1837 hunting and killing bison (buffalo) on the plains of Saskatchewan and Manitoba, about a thousand Assiniboin and Cree Indians traveled southward to trade their furs at Fort Union, a major trading post of the American Fur Company, located in northeastern Montana on the Missouri River, near the mouth of the Yellowstone River. The Indians ignored warnings to stay away from the fort, where inhabitants had become infected with smallpox. After arriving at the fort in June 1837, a large number of Indians contracted the highly contagious viral disease, which blinded or disfigured many of them for life. Many Assiniboin and Cree fled from the fort on horses, believing they could run away from the deadly contagion, only to quickly spread the smallpox northward into the northern department of the Hudson's Bay Company, another important fur trading company. Only about 150 Indians infected at Fort Union survived, and thousands of other Indians in the areas of the Saskatchewan, Swan, and Red rivers suffered severely when the infectious virus entered their villages.

Later that summer (1837) members of a party of more than 5,000 Blackfoot and Piegan Indians contracted smallpox while trading at Fort McKenzie in the Upper Missouri Valley. Seeking to escape the dreaded infection, Canadian bands of these allied tribes fled northward and unwittingly infected the Kainah (Blood), Sarsi (Sarcee), and Atsina (Gros Ventre) tribes, all united with the Blackfoot to defend their lands. Close contact among the Indians gathered together in their usual large encampments during the summer months helped spread the smallpox virus. By November 1837, the Indian tribes in the Qu'Appelle River valley (southern Saskatchewan) were badly infected, as were a number of them living along the North Saskatchewan River in the parkland between Carlton House and Edmonton House (two trading posts of the Hudson's Bay Company).

An extensive vaccination campaign by the Hudson's Bay Company arrested the epidemic before the end of the year, so that the disease did not spread to the nearby Wood Cree Indians, who joined the Plains tribes in the parkland to hunt bison during the winter. Company fur traders estimated that some of the Canadian tribes lost up to 75 percent of their members during the epidemic. See also BLACKFOOT INDIAN SMALLPOX EPIDEMIC OF 1837–38.

Further reading: Heagerty, *Four Centuries of Medical History in Canada*; Shortt, ed., *Medicine in Canadian Society*.

Canadian Influenza Epidemic of 1890   See EUROPEAN INFLUENZA PANDEMIC OF 1889–90.

Canadian Influenza Epidemic of 1918–19   Serious outbreak of influenza that attacked at least a sixth of Canada's approximately six million citizens between July 1918 and January 1919. During the closing days of World War I, the infection spread to military troops on both sides (the Allied and Central powers) and to civilians all over the world, making its way to Canada on ships (see SPANISH INFLUENZA EPIDEMIC OF 1917–19).

In mid-July 1918 the ship *Somali* was placed in quarantine at Grosse Isle in the St. Lawrence River, east of Quebec City, when nine crew members were hospitalized there with influenza. A few days later a majority of the *Somali's* crew of 177 members was hospitalized because of flu. Though special precau-

tions were now taken at the Grosse Isle quarantine station, the infection entered the city of Quebec later that month (July). Because some patients exhibited symptoms that resembled acute pneumonic plague before they died, Quebec authorities first thought that pneumonic plague, not influenza, was beginning to spread through the country.

Farther upriver at Montreal, a military transport ship, *Nagoya*, had managed somehow to dock on July 9, 1918, with about 100 of its 160 crewmembers suffering from influenza. Precautions were then taken that kept Montreal free from the infection until September. On October 14, the medical record for that day listed 165 deaths out of 378 cases in the city; during the next three days, another 6,283 cases and 839 fatalities were reported. Montreal's Board of Health adopted strict measures to combat the disease: all public meeting places, including schools, theaters, and dancehalls, were ordered closed; the clergy were asked to reduce their church functions; stores were to be closed by 4 P.M. each day; and emergency hospitals were opened. By November 7, there had been a reported 17,252 cases and 3,028 fatalities in Montreal. However, since only the severe cases were reported, it was estimated that at least 100,000 city inhabitants had contracted influenza. (In the entire province of Quebec, 530,704 cases were recorded between July and November 1918.)

To the east along Labrador's coast, whole villages were struck by the disease, with many deaths. There was no medical and nursing service in this desolate region; in many cases, those who recovered were too weak to bury the dead victims, and dogs sometimes fed upon the bodies. New Brunswick's situation was not nearly as ghastly, reporting 1,394 fatalities during the epidemic.

About the same time that the disease hit Quebec, the province of Ontario became infected, particularly the cities of Toronto, Hamilton, St. Catharines, London, and Collingwood; a total of 300,000 cases reportedly occurred in Ontario. Fewer cases and fatalities appeared in the western provinces of Saskatchewan, Alberta, and British Columbia. Among the 61,063 Canadian troops stationed in the country, 10,506 had contracted influenza by mid-December 1918; in addition, 45,960 Canadian troops stationed overseas were infected. After January 1919 Canada suffered fewer and fewer outbreaks, and fear of influenza subsided.

Further reading: Heagerty, *Four Centuries of Medical History in Canada*; MacPhail, *History of the Canadian Forces, 1914–19*.

Canadian Measles Epidemic of 1846–47   Widespread measles (rubeola) outbreak that killed untold hundreds of Canadians—white and Indian—in the

western, interior regions of present-day Manitoba, Saskatchewan, and Alberta.

Caused by a virus spread by sneezing and coughing, and characterized by fever and reddish spots, measles first appeared in Manitoba's Red River district at the Hudson's Bay Company's Norway House (a fur-trading station) in early June 1846. Measles-carrying crewmen on the company's riverboats brought the infection to Norway House, where other boat brigades and crews soon caught it. Healthy crews and fur-traders arriving there from Manitoba's York Factory on Hudson Bay were infected, along with brigades arriving at Norway House and Cumberland House (another local trading station that became infected) from areas to the west on the Saskatchewan, Swan, and Athabasca rivers. Unwittingly, many sick men brought the disease home to their communities in the west and northwest (north and central Saskatchewan and Alberta), where the infection seemed to accelerate.

In the summer of 1846 Ojibwa (Ojibway) Indians contracted measles after trading at Norway House, and later that summer Indians dwelling around Fort Alexander in the Red River district were ravaged by the disease. By August 10, there was a report that 31 Indians living near York Factory had perished from measles. Traders and Indians from York Factory apparently carried it inland to Île-à-la Crosse in north-central Saskatchewan, where the Chipewyan Indians were severely struck by measles (and influenza) and suffered high fatalities. At that time (October 1846), inhabitants of the English River area in southwest Ontario were also suffering from the epidemic. By December, it had moved north to affect Fort Chipewyan at the western end of Lake Athabasca (northeast Alberta), where both Chipewyans and whites were victims.

The epidemic, which came to an end in early spring 1847, did not extend north into the Mackenzie River district of the Northwest Territories, probably because the Indians' usual, autumn fur-trading was completed before the arrival of riverboat crews at Fort Simpson, the principal trading post on the upper Mackenzie. Nor did the epidemic spread south into the United States. The Hudson's Bay Company was affected because the epidemic incapacitated many able-bodied men employed to bring boatloads of valuable furs to market from the Canadian wilderness.

Further reading: Shortt, ed., *Medicine in Canadian Society*; McGrew, *Encyclopedia of Medical History*.

Canadian Smallpox Epidemic, Great   Worst outbreak of smallpox among the Indians of Canada, killing thousands of them between 1755 and 1757. Infected French settlers in what is now Quebec spread the disease to the Indians, who later called 1755 the "Year of the Great Smallpox Epidemic."

The Canadian Indians first contracted smallpox about 1639 (see HURON INDIAN EPIDEMICS OF 1634–40), and the disease remained prevalent in varying degrees afterward. Some French and British soldiers arriving at Canadian ports in 1755 carried the contagious variola (smallpox) virus and infected colonists in Quebec city, Montreal, and other settlements as far westward as Niagara, New York. By October 1755 the Montagnais Indians in the Montreal area had become badly infected through contact with the whites, who also infected the Seneca and other tribes in present-day northern New York.

After the start of the French and Indian War (1756–63), waged between the British and French and each side's Indian allies, smallpox spread to Fort William Henry, at the southern end of Lake George, New York, and to Fort Edward, about 20 miles to the south (forts then held by the British). In addition, numerous Indians were smallpox-infected and thus were hindered from waging war against the British, and the French were not able to execute numerous military movements and invasions at this time because of the effects of smallpox. Furthermore, in order to enlist the aid of the Indians during the war, both the British and French came to the assistance of infected Indians and provided them with food and medicine and helped them bury their dead during the epidemic.

In midsummer of 1757 French General Louis de Montcalm led an army of some 6,000 French troops and 2,000 Indians to Fort William Henry, which was captured on August 9. Marching out of the small, unsanitary fort with the honors of war, the defeated British were treacherously beset and "butchered" by the Indians, whom Montcalm was unable to control. The Indians also plundered and looted the fort, and many contracted smallpox and died on their way home. Later, some of the Indian survivors testified in councils held at Michillimakinac, Detroit, that the British had thrown some kind of lethal medicine at them during the siege of the fort.

Scanty records of the smallpox epidemic were kept, but in 1757 the disease was reported to be raging in the French city of Quebec, which had as many as 20 to 30 burials of victims daily. Patients with smallpox admitted to the city's hospitals totaled between 2,500 and 3,000; about 520 of them perished, many of whom were Acadians (early French settlers in Canada's eastern regions, including Nova Scotia and New Brunswick).

In 1758 General Montcalm sailed to Halifax, Nova Scotia, with a number of captured, smallpox-infected British soldiers (who had been taken prisoner at Fort

William Henry). During the voyage, the prisoners all recovered, but many of the French crew died from smallpox, leaving the prisoners to help bring the ship into the port of Halifax. Later, some persons falsely interpreted this incident as Montcalm's attempt to introduce smallpox into Canada's eastern region, to undermine the British there.

Further reading: Heagerty, *Four Centuries of Medical History in Canada*; Shurkin, *The Invisible Fire*; Hopkins, *Princes and Peasants: Smallpox in History*.

Canadian Typhus Epidemic of 1847

Catastrophic epidemic of louse-borne typhus fever that claimed the lives of more than 14,000 persons, most of them emigrants from the British Isles, between May and December 1847. Britain had instituted forced deportation to get rid of "excess" population, and many of the emigrants from Ireland were weak and suffering from the Great Potato Famine (1845–48) before they left home for Canada.

Thirty vessels with some 12,500 passengers aboard arrived at the quarantine station on Grosse Isle on the St. Lawrence River, near Quebec city, in mid-May 1847. During the ocean crossing, 777 of the passengers had died from epidemic typhus, an acute rickettsial disease carried by human body lice, which thrives under dirty, crowded conditions. The quality of the food on board the ships had been poor; also, an insufficient water supply did not allow for washing, while passengers in steerage had been extremely crowded in poorly ventilated, unsanitary conditions. Some of the passengers had contracted typhus before they embarked from British ports.

At the limited facilities on Grosse Isle, healthy people were not separated from those sick with typhus, and overcrowded conditions made it impossible to clean or disinfect bedding. By June 21, 1847, there were 1,935 typhus patients at the quarantine station and 260 sick on board vessels at Grosse Isle; 199 perished from typhus during that week, including two nurses. More ships with immigrants continued to arrive; by August 27 more than 81,000 passengers had arrived at Grosse Isle that year, and 2,503 of them had died from typhus in the quarantine sheds and hospital, which had insufficient nurses and had to use jail inmates from Quebec city to help care for the sick. The quarantine station was closed on October 28, and the last vessel docked there on November 7. The disease also spread to Canadians living on Grosse Isle and killed doctors, nurses, clergy, policemen, stewards, cooks, and others; by December more than 5,400 human fatalities had occurred from the epidemic at Grosse Isle.

Earlier that year (1847), louse-borne typhus was carried by some infected immigrants to Montreal, where a triple row of wooden boats was joined together between Wind-Mill Point and Victoria Pier to hospitalize thousands of the sick. By December, more than 3,500 out of some 11,000 typhus cases admitted to Montreal Emigrant Hospital had proven fatal. Many boards of health were formed in Montreal, Ottawa, Toronto, Kingston, and other cities during the seven-month epidemic. In Toronto and Kingston hospitals, there were 8,202 cases admitted and 1,965 fatalities; Quebec city's immigrant hospital had about 2,500 cases and 1,840 deaths.

Irish, Scottish, and English immigrants also arrived at the port of St. John, New Brunswick, in May 1847, and those infected with typhus were placed in adequate facilities on Partridge Island off St. John. During June, some 5,800 immigrants arrived there on 35 ships, and nearly 200 of them died in quarantine that month. By December 1847 almost 2,000 of the 14,000 immigrants making the trip to New Brunswick had perished from epidemic typhus; 800 persons died on the ship voyage to St. John, 600 died in the quarantine hospital, and 595 in the city poor hospital.

After the 1847 epidemic, Canada's House of Assembly adopted and sent a formal appeal to Britain's Queen Victoria, protesting this kind of immigration. As a result, Canada was reimbursed for its expenditures and steps were taken to prevent a recurrence of the epidemic catastrophe.

Further reading: Heagerty, *Four Centuries of Medical History in Canada*; Horsfall, and Rivers, eds., *Viral and Rickettsial Infections of Man*.

Cape Colony and Cape Town Smallpox Epidemic of 1713

First outbreak of smallpox to ravage the Dutch-held Cape Colony and Cape Town in South Africa. By means of soiled clothing belonging to sailors and passengers who had recovered from smallpox on a voyage from eastern India, the disease was introduced to the region when their vessel moored in Cape Town's harbor, Table Bay, in early 1713; lack of quarantine regulations allowed their clothing to be sent to the slave quarters of the Dutch East India Company to be washed.

The first victims of the disease were the washerwomen, who soon spread it among the rest of the slaves. It was deadly to the native Africans, who had never built up an immunity of any kind to this highly contagious viral disease. Between May and July 1713, Cape Town's streets were almost deserted, for nearly every family, black and white, fell victim to the disfiguring "pox." European settlers often did without firewood because their slaves were far too ill with high fevers and skin sores to cut down trees. Exactly how many perished from the disease is not known, but the natives suffered much more severely than the Europeans. Entire native Hottentot villages were wiped out; among the natives who worked as slaves for the Dutch East India Company, about a fifth died. Records kept by the Europeans in 1715 revealed that their population had decreased by 14 percent since 1712.

Further reading: Burrows, *A History of Medicine in South Africa;* Gelfand and Laidler, *South Africa: Its Medical History, 1652–1898.*

Cape Colony and Cape Town Smallpox Epidemic of 1755

Outbreak of smallpox in the Dutch-ruled Cape Colony and Cape Town that killed more than 2,000 people in ten months and nearly destroyed the native Hottentot tribes. The epidemic resulted in the establishment of segregated hospital accommodations for blacks and whites in this part of South Africa.

Smallpox-infected Europeans carried the disease to the Dutch colony from eastern India in May 1755, and quickly there was alarm; in July 580 slaves and 498 Europeans fell victim to the scourge. Fearing that the sick would be concealed, the Cape authorities ordered all townspeople, under threat of severe punishment, to report all cases of smallpox. The dead were speedily buried in their contaminated clothing within 24 hours of death. A foul stench reportedly filled the air when the depth of burial was reduced; corpses were buried above corpses not yet decomposed, after existing burial grounds had filled to capacity.

Some physicians believed the disease was being spread by African slaves who lived in European households; this led to separate emergency hospitals for whites and natives. But segregation did not curb the epidemic, which by October 31, 1755, had claimed nearly 500 European lives and more than that number of slaves. Most who survived were either disfigured or blinded. The disease also spread outside the colony to the north, into the Great Namaqualand (southern Namibia), where it claimed countless more native lives, especially Hottentots (Little Namaqualand was to the south, in the Cape area). According to native reports, most of the people who lived on the land located between the Kei and Bashee rivers perished in the 1755 smallpox epidemic, which they called "gall fever."

Smallpox finally disappeared from the Cape Colony in March 1756, and on April 7 prayers and fasting were observed on a day of thanksgiving for deliverance from the pestilence.

Further reading: Burrows, *A History of Medicine in South Africa;* Gelfand and Laidler, *South Africa: Its Medical History, 1652–1898.*

Cape Colony and Cape Town Smallpox Epidemic of 1882–85

Smallpox outburst that reportedly struck at least 2,300 persons, killing 649 Bantu blacks and 51 Europeans, disfiguring nearly all and blinding many of those who survived. Afterward a law was enacted that made vaccination and notification of infectious disease mandatory in the Cape Colony and its capital, Cape Town.

During earlier outbreaks of smallpox in the colony, the natives had suffered worse symptoms and a greater number of fatalities than the white Europeans did. The disease had almost annihilated the Hottentot people by the close of the eighteenth century; it continued to visit the Cape region every seventh or tenth year. In 1840 a fourth of the population of Cape Town (which the British had taken from the Dutch in 1806) was stricken with the "pox," which apparently had been brought there by some infected Malay people.

With the outbreak of the epidemic in the British-ruled Cape Colony in May 1882, the sanitary inspector of Kimberley (home of the rich diamond mines) became fearful that the infection would spread among the mine workers; he enlisted Dr. Hans Sauer to initiate medical examinations at the Modder River, where a quarantine depot was set up (about 30 miles from Kimberley). Each person arriving there from the south was examined for smallpox, and vaccinations were given to those needing them; those who refused were placed in quarantine for six weeks. Because this procedure and the vaccinations were illegal at the time, Dr. Sauer was accused in court of assault. While carrying on his work at the Modder River, he spotted 14 smallpox cases and continued until no further cases were reported from Cape Town.

Similar controls had not been established over persons entering the Cape Colony from the north, and a group of sick Africans from what is now Mozambique nearly succeeded in entering Kimberley. Some concerned whites detained them at Felstead's Farm, where a team of physicians shortly examined them (on orders from Kimberley's civil commissioner) and stated they were not sick with smallpox. To confirm this, the Cape Colony government recalled Dr. Sauer, who diagnosed the cases as definitely being smallpox. The physicians had falsified their reports for the mining authorities, who were afraid their Bantu workers would flee if news of the disease was heard. Furthermore, many people did not want the mines closed for economic reasons, and thus they failed to report smallpox cases in the community. The epidemic escalated throughout 1884 and lasted late into 1885.

The Cape medical profession's reputation was tarnished, and Dr. Sauer became involved in questionable court proceedings and legal actions concerning libel, assault, and homicide. Nonetheless, his pressure on the government (his so-called "smallpox war") brought about passage of the Public Health Act of 1883, making vaccination and notification of all infectious diseases compulsory in the Cape area.

Further reading: Burrows, *A History of Medicine in South Africa;* Gelfand and Laidler, *South Africa: Its Medical History, 1652–1898.*

Caribbean Dengue Epidemic of 1826–28 See U.S. AND CARIBBEAN DENGUE EPIDEMIC OF 1826–28.

Caribbean Dengue Epidemics of 1963–64 and 1968–69 Outbreaks of dengue, also known as breakbone fever; more than 50,000 persons were reported infected during two separate periods. There were relatively few fatalities, and most victims fully recovered.

Caused by a mosquito-borne virus, dengue was endemic in the islands of the West Indies by the twentieth century (see U.S. AND CARIBBEAN DENGUE EPIDEMIC OF 1826–28). In 1963 a serious epidemic of dengue erupted in parts of the Greater Antilles (Cuba, Hispaniola, Puerto Rico, and Jamaica); the disease was particularly explosive that year in Puerto Rico, where 25,737 persons were infected (compared to 1,578 cases in Jamaica and 350 cases in the Dominican Republic). The following year dengue spread to the coastal Caribbean region of Venezuela, infecting 18,306 people there, and to the Lesser Antilles (Trinidad, the Leeward and Windward Islands, Barbados, and other islands), striking more than a thousand inhabitants. Both the 1963 and 1964 epidemics were caused by serotype Dengue 3 (one of the four serotypes of the dengue virus), which had been isolated from the *Aëdes aegypti* mosquito (the sole-known vector or carrier in the Americas) in the Philippines in 1956. The climatic and seasonal conditions required for the spread of dengue are favorable in the Caribbean, particularly for the breeding of the mosquito vector (also the common carrier of yellow fever). The dengue virus is transmitted not person-to-person but via the bite of a diseased mosquito.

During the epidemics, all ages and races and both sexes in the Caribbean area were affected by dengue. Those who escaped infection were immune as a result of previous infection; those stricken were attacked within a short time (three to 12 days) after the crucial mosquito bite. Their symptoms included severe frontal headaches and excruciating pains in their joints (hence "breakbone fever"), as well as a rash, chills, nausea, and prostration.

Dengue remained active in Venezuela in 1965, with 4,040 reported cases, and in the Dominican Republic,

with 527 cases. However, the morbidity (disease incidence) declined greatly in Puerto Rico (93 cases) and Jamaica (36 cases) that year. The smaller islands of the Lesser Antilles recorded a total of only eight infections in 1965. The disease seemed to leave the West Indies during the next two years and move into western Venezuela, a region not touched by the 1964 outbreak; Venezuela reported 9,080 infections in 1966–67 and a total of 35,726 infections by 1969. In 1968, Jamaica again reported a dengue epidemic that lasted to 1969 (a total of 912 cases). There were also 301 cases of dengue in the Lesser Antilles at this epidemic time. Puerto Rico, which had only three cases between 1966 and 1968, was acutely infected in 1969, with 16,665 reported cases; the serotype Dengue 2 (isolated in New Guinea in 1945) was mainly responsible for this 1969 epidemic.

The West Indies continued to be infected by dengue in the following decade; another, far more critical form of the disease, known as dengue hemorrhagic fever, was then observed in the region and has been a problem since.

Further reading: Howe, ed., *A World Geography of Diseases;* McGrew, *Encyclopedia of Medical History;* Marks and Beatty, *Epidemics.*

Cartagena Yellow Fever Epidemic of 1741 See GUAYAQUIL YELLOW FEVER EPIDEMICS OF 1740, 1743, AND 1842.

Carthaginian Plague of 396 B.C. Infectious disease, of unknown type, that afflicted the Carthaginian Army in 396 B.C. as it besieged Syracuse, a Greek city in Sicily. Taking advantage of the many deaths among his opponents, the Syracusan leader Dionysius carried out a surprise attack that destroyed the Carthaginian land and naval forces.

The symptoms listed by the Greek historian Diodorus of Sicily—inflammation and mucus in the throat; burning, pain, and fatigue throughout the body; diarrhea; pustules on the skin; and delirium—reminded Hans Zinsser (U.S. epidemiologist) of the plague described by Thucydides (see PLAGUE OF ATHENS, GREAT). Both epidemics, Zinsser thought, were caused by a severe type of smallpox that led to death on the fifth or sixth day. However, most other scholars believe smallpox did not appear in the classical world until several centuries later.

Although Diodorus says the epidemic was sent by the gods to punish the Carthaginians for looting temples, he notes other factors that helped the disease spread rapidly. Not only was the weather unusually hot and dry, but the Carthaginians were also crowded together in a marshy area that was cold at sunrise and stifling hot at midday.

The struggle for control of Sicily had brought the Carthaginians to this inhospitable place. After bringing many Greek cities in the east of Sicily under his dominion, Dionysius had set his sights on the western part of the island, long under Carthaginian sway. The Carthaginians hoped to stop this by attacking him at Syracuse. Dionysius's victory, however, pushed them back to their original territory and may have prevented them from dominating events in the eastern Mediterranean for decades to come.

Further reading: Diodorus Siculus, *The Library of History*; Bury and Meiggs, *A History of Greece*; Zinsser, *Rats, Lice and History*.

Cava Typhus Epidemic of 1083

One of the earliest observed and recorded outbreaks of typhus fever, occurring in the famous Benedictine monastery or abbey of Trinità della Cava (or La Cava) above the village of Corpo di Cava, near Salerno in southern Italy. According to old Italian accounts, "a severe fever with peticuli and parotid swellings" struck many Benedictine monks living in the monastery in August and September 1083. Medical authorities and historians were compelled to assume that the monastery (founded in 1025 by Saint Alferius) had suffered a grave typhus infection (characterized by high fever with eruption of red spots and acute headache, and transmitted especially by body lice). The disease was probably not new to Italy, for evidently in 1083 the commune of Brescia in northern Italy recorded a similar outbreak.

Further reading: Hirsch, *Handbook on Geographical and Historical Pathology*; Zinsser, *Rats, Lice and History*.

Cayuse Indian Measles Epidemic of 1847

Virulent outbreak of measles (whose medical name is rubeola) that killed hundreds of Cayuse Indians in 1847. The Cayuse tribe living in the Blue Mountains region (northeast Oregon and southeast Washington) blamed the white missionaries for introducing the highly contagious disease.

Before 1847, the Cayuse had never encountered measles, which caused a mottled rash to develop over their entire bodies. They had not developed a resistance to this Old World pathogenic virus, which was spread by coughing and sneezing. The disease had devastating effects on the Cayuse, whose own therapeutic practices of sweat baths and plunges into cold rivers and lakes (to ease the high fever and burning itching) only increased the mortality rate among the Indians.

The Cayuse were usually without life-support services, and when all members of the tribe were sick at the same time, there was no one to obtain sufficient food (protein) or to provide them with drinking water to strengthen their resistance and prevent dehydration. Dr. Marcus Whitman, who ran the mission at Waiilatpu, near present-day Walla Walla, Washington, tried to provide these services and to treat the sick Cayuse during the epidemic; he protected them against exposure, provided them with warm drinks, and in some cases tried to heal the Indians with purging and bleeding. None of Whitman's remedies helped the ailing Cayuse, who thought he had instead worsened their condition. The Indians retaliated by attacking and killing Whitman, his wife, and 12 others at the mission on November 29, 1847; the Cayuse also seized and held 53 women and children until ransomed. This led to the bloody Cayuse War (1848–55), which ended with the white settlers, aided by U.S. troops, defeating the Indians and placing them on a reservation with the Umatilla Indians.

Further reading: Dobyns, *Their Number Becomes Thinned: Native American Dynamics in Eastern North America*; Simpson, *Invisible Armies*.

Central Asian Cholera Epidemic of 1870–72

Severe epidemic of cholera that erupted in some Central Asian provinces during 1870–72, an offshoot of the Asiatic Cholera Pandemic of 1865–75 (q.v.). This serious intestinal disease (spread by polluted food and water) may have been introduced either via Persia (see PERSIAN CHOLERA EPIDEMICS OF 1866–70) or directly from India through Afghanistan or along both routes. During July and August 1869, the city of Nijni Novgorod (Gorki, Russia) hosted a large fair attended by over 200,000 merchants from Persia (Iran) and Central Asia, among other places. This may have played a major role in widespread dissemination of the disease.

Balkh was invaded by cholera in 1871; another province, Turkmenistan, was infected in mid-April 1872, and Bukhara (Bokhara) in mid-June 1872. In July, it struck the area of Kokand, northeast of Bukhara, and the city of Samarkand, where the natives and some Russian troops were infected. Meanwhile, on June 30, cholera erupted in the town of Tashkent; during the next four days, 400 cases and 273 deaths were reported. It traveled to nearby provinces and then along the Jaxartes (Syr Darya) River to the Aral Sea, infecting all the Russian fortresses en route. Tashkent (population 40,000) recorded 3,267 cases of cholera and 2,261 deaths during the course of the epidemic, which ended there on August 26, 1872. In mid-August, cholera intensified in the city of Bukhara; during the first week of September, between 1,000 and 2,000 people reportedly died each day. That epidemic subsided by mid-October.

Further reading: Macnamara, *A History of Asiatic Cholera;* Pollitzer, *Cholera.*

Ceylonese Dysentery Epidemic of 1942   See SRI LANKAN (CEYLONESE) DYSENTERY EPIDEMIC OF 1942.

Ceylonese Malaria Epidemic of 1934–35   See SRI LANKAN (CEYLONESE) MALARIA EPIDEMIC OF 1934–35.

Ceylonese Malaria Epidemic of 1968–69   See SRI LANKAN (CEYLONESE) MALARIA EPIDEMIC OF 1968–69.

Chadian Cholera Epidemic of 1971   Serious outbreak of cholera in the north-central African country of Chad, killing 2,337 out of 8,225 persons infected during five months in 1971.

The outbreak in Chad began in May 1971, following cholera's advance from West Africa eastward across Nigeria in 1970 (see WEST AFRICAN CHOLERA EPIDEMICS OF 1970–71). This bacterial disease, which is spread by contaminated food or water, traveled from Kano in northern Nigeria to Maiduguri (another town) in northeast Nigeria before entering the Lake Chad area, which became the center of cholera's diffusion into the country. In early May 1971 Chad's capital city, Fort Lamy (N'Djamena), reported cholera cases, but because of good sanitation and disease control measures, Fort Lamy suffered only 22 cases and five human deaths during a two-week epidemic there. However, the large surrounding region or district, Chari-Baguirmi, which became infected about June 1, suffered 6,203 infections of cholera, 1,939 of which were fatal, during an outbreak that lasted until mid-October 1971. The Lake Chad area recorded 897 cases and 281 human deaths during an outbreak there until August.

Survivors of the epidemic in Chari-Baguirmi unwittingly carried the disease with them when they fled to other regions in Chad. The region of Mayo-Kebbi to the south endured a 23-week-long epidemic that killed 92 out of 717 who were infected. The region of Quaddai in east Chad was briefly struck in late June, but with very few deaths. Kanem, a region northeast of Lake Chad, had a two-week epidemic in July, with 48 cases and 16 fatalities, and Tandjile, a region south of Chari-Baguirmi, had an eight-week-long outbreak, which killed only one person out of 27 infected.

Most of the cases in Chad occurred among the poor, who lived in crowded, unsanitary conditions; there was also excessive morbidity and mortality in the rural areas, where people were not protected by cholera vaccination. The 1971 epidemic lasted during the rainy season (May to October), when most people remained at home to farm. And because of poor transportation networks in central Chad, cholera did not spread into the relatively unpopulated regions, nor did it enter the northern region of Borkou-Ennedi-Tibesti.

In 1972 only the region of Chari-Baguirmi reported any cholera: a minor outbreak of five cases and one death. Chad remained cholera-free in 1973 and reported a few cases the following year and no outbreaks the year after.

Further reading: Barua and Burrows, eds., *Cholera;* Stock, *African Environment Special Report 3: Cholera in Africa.*

Chadian Meningitis Epidemic of 1937–39   Devastating epidemic in Chad (then part of French Equatorial Africa) that killed more than 6,500 persons out of at least 10,000 cases of cerebrospinal meningitis (CSM) from 1937 to 1939.

The disease CSM, caused by a bacterium infecting the human respiratory passages, flourishes in the dry African area between the Sahara Desert and the equatorial forests, in countries like Chad, Nigeria (northern region), and Upper Volta. Several minor, local outbreaks of CSM occurred in western Chad from 1932 to 1935, when the disease began to spread (enhanced by outbreaks in Sudan, to the east).

During the dry months in the first half of 1937, the disease entered Chad in the south near Fort Archambault (Sarh) on the Chari River and entered in the west near Moundou. The capital Fort Lamy (N'Djamena), Koumra, Léré, Mao (near Lake Chad), and other towns were quickly affected. In the south, the districts of Mayo-Kebbi and Chari-Baguirmi were seriously infected; also, the southern district of Logone was badly ravaged by CSM between January 15 and April 30, 1937, when 960 people perished among 1,108 infected.

The Chadian cold nights during the dry season prompted most of the inhabitants to sleep indoors in their poorly ventilated and frequently overcrowded mud houses; this ensured contagion of people mainly through sneezes and coughing (transmission by aerial droplets or mucus). Symptoms of CSM include fever, severe headache, and stiff neck; children often suffered convulsions. People then died after serious symptoms of vomiting, bleeding, and collapse. By the end of 1937 at least 1,287 persons had perished out of over 2,000 infected with CSM.

The mortality rate was even greater the following year, when the disease marched throughout the entire country, striking children and young adults the hardest in most places. In 1938, the native Sara people of southern Chad suffered acutely; over one third of the total number of deaths, 1,660, occurred in the Sara region; in the town of Doba alone, there were 1,008 human deaths recorded in the first half of 1938.

With total deaths of 3,064 among about 4,500 cases, the mortality rate was almost 70 percent; at the time it was the worst epidemic on record in Chad. According to the then inspector general of Health and Medical Services for French Equatorial Africa (a Colonel Ledentu), the fatalities would have numbered at least 5,000 persons if all the unreported cases had been counted that year.

The next year (1939) saw 2,250 cases of CSM, with 1,646 deaths. Many of the Chadian victims who recovered from the disease were left deaf or mentally incompetent. Outbreaks of CSM continued to occur annually in Chad from 1940 to 1977; except for severe occurrences in 1950 and 1951, the disease declined considerably during that period. Antibiotics and sulfanamides effectively reduced the mortality rate in the 1940s.

Further reading: Hartwig and Patterson, eds., *Disease in African History*; Waddy, "African Epidemic Cerebro-Spinal Meningitis."

Chadian Sleeping Sickness Epidemic of 1912–40

Outbreak of African sleeping sickness (trypanosomiasis), lasting almost 30 years, that wiped out a third of the Sara people living along the river banks in what is now Chad (then part of French Equatorial Africa).

The disease had been endemic in parts of West Africa for centuries before entering Chad. It had been reported in upper Niger in the 1300s, along the Guinea coast in 1721, and in Sierra Leone in 1803 and 1840. Transmitted by the bite of an infective *Glossina* (the tsetse fly), the disease advanced into the Congo River basin from 1885 to 1896, resulting in more than 500,000 human deaths there. It also broke out then on the Nile River in northern Uganda, where some 200,000 deaths were reported in recurring epidemics, and moved into southern Sudan between 1890 and 1906.

Chad first recorded sleeping sickness in 1901 along the old caravan routes, where shortly so many persons died from it that survivors in the villages were too few to bury their dead. More than 55 percent of the native populations of Fort-Lamy (N'Djamena), Moissala, Gorée, and Moundou perished during the first decade of the twentieth century.

Before the French colonized Equatorial Africa, the ethnic Sara people of southern Chad lived in separate, independent villages with little or no contact with the outside world. The Sara kept their trading activity limited to their local district, where along the river banks the tsetse fly became infested and carried the infectious parasitic agent *trypanosoma gambiense*. The sleeping sickness in Chad was the Gambian form, which differed from the Rhodesian form (more relative to East Africa); humans are the important reservoir of the former, and wild animals are the chief reservoir of the latter form.

Health conditions were very poor in Chad and French Equatorial Africa, and sleeping sickness, if it is untreated, is almost invariably fatal, although patients may remain relatively well for months to years. The Sara people often fled from their infected villages, thus spreading the disease widely along the rivers of the Chari basin within a few years. When bitten by a diseased fly, victims had rashes, malaise, lassitude, headaches, and low-grade fevers at first. Continuing off and on for two years, the disease progressed to hallucinations and behavioral and personality changes; with drowsiness during the day and insomnia at night, victims' level of consciousness progressively deteriorated until they lapsed into stupors and then death.

Some drugs became available to treat the Gambian form of sleeping sickness; from 1916 to 1918 Drs. Albert Schweitzer and Eugene Janot began fighting the disease in French Equatorial Africa with the use of the drug atoxyl; afterward they treated patients with tryparsamide. Many patients were cured, though overdoses of the drugs caused permanent blindness in some cases.

Further reading: Ackerknecht, *History and Geography of the Most Important Diseases*; Hallett, *Africa Since 1875*; Hartwig and Patterson, *Disease in African History*.

Chadian Smallpox Epidemics of 1922–32

Serious outbreaks of smallpox claiming at least 8,000 deaths among more than 40,000 infected in Chad in central Africa. According to the Sara people who inhabited the area, smallpox was endemic prior to French occupation in the late seventeenth century. French colonial health records in the first part of the 1900s, although incomplete, indicate that the disease at times was as deadly as cerebrospinal meningitis and sleeping sickness.

French records of 1922 reported a severe outbreak of smallpox in Moissala in southern Chad, but how many were infected or the number of fatalities was not recorded. Some schoolchildren (six of them died) of the Sara people contracted the disease in February and March 1924, supposedly following contact with an infected army wife stationed in Fort-Lamy (N'Djamena), Chad's capital. In 1925 the region experienced a devastating smallpox epidemic when the disease erupted in the Sara people's villages in Moyen-Chari, where about 6,000 among the 30,000 smallpox patients died. This rate of mortality represented about 20 percent of those infected and about 3.3 percent of the territory's population (about 180,000 people). In 1929 the subdivision of Pala was hit by another smallpox epidemic, but how many were affected is not known. The smallpox virus caused many to be blinded and disfigured, and it had a serious side effect on pregnant Chadian women, frequently inducing abortions.

Another local smallpox epidemic occurred in 1932 in the subdivision of N'Gaur, northeast of Fort-Lamy. However, since some measures were taken to prevent the spread of the disease, only eight people perished out of the 52 who contracted it. Those preventive measures included closing the marketplaces at Mallum and Kaludia, isolating those infected, vaccinating 6,107 persons, and preventing travelers from neighboring Nigeria and Cameroon from entering Chad. It was thought that all outbreaks of smallpox in Chad had been transmitted from Nigeria and Cameroon, where the disease was endemic during this period. Nomads constantly crossed the borders, making it easy for infection to enter Chad. Smallpox requires only a breath to blow its variola virus from one human mouth to another, making it easy to transmit the infection. Also, overland caravans on the trans-Saharan trade route, mainly traveling from Cameroon, helped spread the disease into central and northern Chad during this time. It is uncertain if smallpox was spread from Chad to other African lands.

Further reading: Hartwig and Patterson, *Diseases in African History*; Shurkin, *The Invisible Fire*.

Charles V's Army Epidemic at Metz

Outbreak of typhus fever and dysentery that struck Charles V's army as it besieged the French city of Metz in November and December of 1552. With the siege, Holy Roman Emperor Charles V made his last major attempt to conquer his long-time enemies, the French. But when disease overran his camp and forced him to discontinue the siege, he retired in defeat and soon turned over all imperial affairs to his brother, Ferdinand I.

Since the 1520s Charles V had had two rivals for control of the imperial lands, which included Spain, much of Germany, the Low Countries, and territories in Italy and central Europe. In their struggle for independence from the empire, many German princes had espoused the new Lutheranism, which Charles as a Catholic had sworn to defeat. The French—under King Francis I and then under Henry II—battled Charles in Italy and pushed eastward from northern France. Their conquest of Lorraine, the region in which Metz was located, threatened to cut the emperor off from his holdings in the Netherlands and Luxembourg. In the early 1550s Charles's enemies all seemed to be closing in on him; Henry made an alliance with some of the German princes. By besieging Metz, Charles hoped not only to wrest the city away from the French, but also to take the offensive against both his foes.

The siege, however, was ill-timed and poorly planned. The Duke of Guise, ruler of Metz, had supplemented the city's natural defenses by building extensive fortifications, sending away all noncombatants, razing structures outside the walls that might shelter the attackers, and laying in food, weapons, and other supplies. Against the advice of his sister Queen Mary of Hungary, who had learned of the duke's preparations, Charles decided not to wait until spring brought more favorable weather.

The siege began in October 1552, a month before the emperor himself joined the army in the field. Bitter cold, damp, and lack of adequate provisions soon took their toll, creating conditions ripe for epidemic disease among the imperial troops. Of the 75,000 or so soldiers and mercenaries whom Charles had assembled from his Spanish, Italian, and German subjects, more than 10,000 were said to have died in a month. Those from the south, not used to such cold weather, were more susceptible. By the beginning of January Charles reluctantly admitted defeat and raised the siege. But the epidemic was not yet over; after attacking some of the defenders of Metz, it spread throughout the surrounding countryside, becoming especially virulent in the summer of 1553.

Further reading: Armstrong, *The Emperor Charles V*; Brandi, *The Emperor Charles V*; Prinzing, *Epidemics Resulting from Wars*; Zinsser, *Rats, Lice and History*.

Charles VIII's Army Syphilis Epidemic at Naples

See FRENCH ARMY SYPHILIS EPIDEMIC OF 1494–95.

Charleston Yellow Fever Epidemic of 1699

First positively identified yellow fever epidemic that ravaged the city of Charleston, South Carolina. The outbreak began in late August of 1699 and killed between 160 and 180 city dwellers and another 10 or 11 people who resided in the country. According to a private correspondent, 125 English, 37 French, 16 Indians, and 1 Negro died of yellow fever in Charleston (first called Charles Towne) during the late summer and early fall of 1699. Since accurate population statistics of Charleston are unavailable for this time period, it is impossible to determine the exact percentage of fatalities; however, estimates range from three to seven percent.

The disease struck many government officials, including the chief justice, the receiver-general, the provost marshal, and nearly half of the assembly. The deaths of these town leaders caused much distress among the remaining officials and the townspeople; thus, confusion ensued. Government and business activity came to a near standstill until November, when the epidemic finally ended. This attack was the first of many subsequent epidemics that would plague Charleston during the eighteenth century.

Before yellow fever was identified as such in 1699, it was known as "Barbados Fever" or "black vomit." In Charleston in 1699, physicians recognized the symptoms, which were yellow-tinted skin accompanied by severe vomiting, usually black, resulting from internal hemorrhages, but they did not understand the causes of yellow fever. Doctors did understand that the disease occurred from July to November, with the most serious outbreaks during August and September; however, they believed inaccurately that yellow fever was a contagious disease.

Two hundred years later, scientists finally uncovered the origin of the disease. They found that the *Stegomyia fasciata (Aëdes aegypti)* mosquito carries yellow fever and infects humans with the disease. This explained why the disease was not contagious and why it occurred only during the summer months, as the cold winter weather killed the mosquitos that carried the disease. Thus, activity in Charleston returned to normal in November 1699 when cold weather killed the mosquitos—but only after many people had died.

Further reading: Duffy, *Epidemics in Colonial America*; Fraser, *Charleston! Charleston!*; Ramsay, *Ramsay's History of South Carolina*.

Charleston Yellow Fever Epidemic of 1706 Pestilence of yellow fever that swept through Charleston, South Carolina, in 1706. This followed the Charleston Yellow Fever Epidemic of 1699 (q.v.), which had caused mass chaos in the city. The French and Spanish armies stationed in St. Augustine, Florida, heard that the yellow fever was ravaging Charleston, and they saw the epidemic as an opportune time to attack Charleston. During the early 1700s, France, England, and Spain were constantly quarreling in both Europe and the American colonies.

The French and Spanish sent five vessels to Charleston, and on August 28, 1706, they asked English colonial Governor Nathaniel Johnson to surrender. He refused and sent the Charleston militiamen after the invading troops. Johnson had stationed the militiamen a half-mile outside the city; thus they were not infected with the yellow fever. The French and Spanish had grossly underestimated the fortifications surrounding Charleston, as well as the strength of the army and the desire of the militiamen to defend their city. In all, the French and Spanish killed only one person from Charleston, while the

yellow fever killed nearly five percent of the city's then population of about 1,300 people.

Like the earlier yellow fever epidemic of 1699, the Charleston pestilence of 1706 killed many prominent townspeople. The fever raged during August and through September and October, but when the winter cold killed the mosquitos that carried the disease, Charleston again was free of yellow fever. (Charleston was founded and first called Charles Towne by English colonists in honor of King Charles II.)

Further reading: Duffy, *Epidemics in Colonial America*; Fraser, *Charleston! Charleston!*; Ramsay, *Ramsay's History of South Carolina*.

Charleston Yellow Fever Epidemics of 1728 and 1732 Two epidemics of yellow fever that swept through Charleston, South Carolina, and brought the city to a standstill on both occasions. The epidemic of 1728 was the first appearance of yellow fever in ten years. This pestilence was described as a "Bilious Plague" because it was so widespread and also because it was so mysterious. Doctors in the early eighteenth century did not know how to treat the disease; consequently, the mortality rate was extremely high. In the early 1700s, physicians also did not know that mosquitos carried and transmitted the yellow fever. One local physician asserted that the yellow fever came from the West Indies; he was correct in realizing that the disease was imported, but he did not understand how the disease arrived in the United States. It was not until much later that scientists recognized that the *Stegomyia fasciata (Aëdes aegypti)* mosquitos that carried yellow fever must have survived on trade and slave ships and then disembarked in the port city.

In 1732, yellow fever returned to Charleston; it began in May and lasted until October. The epidemic reached its height in July when eight to 12 white men were buried daily. The city prohibited the tolling of funeral bells because there were so many funerals each day. Many of the wealthier residents fled to plantations in the countryside, hoping to escape the disease. The English colonial governor, Nathaniel Johnson, refused to abandon the city; however, his obstinacy caused him to lose his wife, a son, and three servants.

The yellow fever epidemic of 1732 killed 130 white men and many black slaves in Charleston. The yellow fever halted nearly all private and public business during the summer and fall of 1732. Business, however, was very profitable in Charleston during this era, and prosperity soon returned once the cold winter weather killed the mosquitos that carried the yellow fever. See also CHARLESTON YELLOW FEVER EPIDEMIC OF 1699, CHARLESTON YELLOW FEVER EPIDEMIC OF 1706.

Further reading: Duffy, *Epidemics in Colonial America;* Fraser, *Charleston! Charleston!;* Ramsay, *Ramsay's History of South Carolina.*

Charleston Yellow Fever Epidemics of 1792–99

Yellow fever epidemics that affected the city of Charleston, South Carolina, in the summer of 1792 and each summer from 1794 to 1799. In 1799, the fever killed 239 of Charleston's approximately 20,000 inhabitants. Yellow fever had plagued Charleston several times during the late seventeenth and eighteenth century, affecting mostly foreigners and children. The first attack occurred in 1699 and subsequent epidemics of primary importance took place in 1728, 1732, 1739, 1745, and 1748. The outbreak in 1792, however, was the first one to reach epidemic proportions since 1748.

When these epidemics occurred in Charleston, physicians did not understand what caused yellow fever. They did recognize the symptoms, which were yellow-tinted skin accompanied by severe vomiting, usually black, resulting from internal hemorrhages. Before yellow fever was identified as such in 1699, it was known as "Barbados Fever" or "black vomit." Physicians also understood that the disease occurred from July to November, with the most serious outbreaks during August and September. Doctors in Charleston believed inaccurately that yellow fever was a contagious disease; consequently, the local government imposed quarantine laws and established the first board of health in 1796. A few cases of yellow fever were reported in the countryside, but the disease never spread there. Toward the end of the eighteenth century, doctors began to realize that the disease was not contagious, as those in close contact with the yellow fever patients had not contracted the disease.

In the late nineteenth century, scientists finally uncovered the origin of the disease. They found that the *Stegomyia fasciata* (later renamed *Aëdes aegypti*) mosquito carries yellow fever and infects humans with the disease. This explained why the disease was not contagious and why it occurred only during the summer months, as the cold winter weather killed the mosquitos that carried the disease. Many recent historians and scientists believe that these mosquitos survived the voyages of slave or trade ships from Africa or South America. Thus, the mosquito link also explained why the disease was mostly contained in Charleston, as the mosquitoes' inability to fly long distances limited the spread of the disease. The fact that the port cities of Charleston, Philadelphia, and New York City faced the most severe and numerous epidemics helps support the theory that ships transported the mosquitoes to the United States.

Further reading: Duffy, *Epidemics in Colonial America;* Fraser, *Charleston! Charleston!;* Marks and Beatty, *Epidemics;* Ramsay, *Ramsay's History of South Carolina.*

Chilean Meningitis Epidemic of 1941–43
See SANTIAGO MENINGITIS EPIDEMIC OF 1941–43.

Chinese Cholera Epidemic of 1820–22
Part of the massive Asiatic Cholera Pandemic of 1817–23 (q.v.), reaching China in 1820, apparently via the sea route from Bangkok (see THAI CHOLERA EPIDEMIC OF 1820).

Some scholars say that the disease actually invaded China in 1817, taking the overland route from its birthplace in India (see INDIAN CHOLERA EPIDEMIC OF 1817–18). At any rate, it was an unfamiliar disease when it struck Canton in 1820. By all accounts it was a severe epidemic that ravaged many Chinese provinces. A contemporary chronicler identified vomiting, diarrhea, and painful tendons as the main symptoms of this new disease.

Later in 1820, cholera invaded two more ports—Wenchow (Yungkia) and Ningpo—before entering the Yangtze River valley. By 1822, cholera had covered northern China and moved into Beijing (then Peking). From Beijing, it is believed to have made its way across the Great Wall of China and then followed the caravan routes to Kyakhta (Kiachta) inside the Russian border. Parts of central and northern China reported outbreaks until 1824.

Subsequent cholera epidemics, which were frequent until 1932, traveled across China following basically the same route—starting in the south and moving north along the coast and by the inland route, and spreading to the heart of China along the Yangtze River. See also INDONESIAN CHOLERA EPIDEMIC OF 1821; JAPANESE CHOLERA EPIDEMIC OF 1822.

Further reading: Pollitzer, *Cholera;* Macnamara, *A History of Asiatic Cholera.*

Chinese Cholera Epidemic of 1932
Severe epidemic of cholera that affected many of China's provinces in 1932.

The epidemic began rather suddenly in March 1932 at Canton. From there it spread in April to Shanghai (where the mortality rate was the highest at 7.4 percent) and in May to the port of Swatow and inland to Hankow and Nanking. It moved north in June 1932 and invaded the Manchurian ports of Newchwang, Antung, and Dairen (Ta-lien) (see MANCHURIAN CHOLERA EPIDEMIC OF 1919). Massive flooding in Manchuria in August 1932 added to the miseries of the people already ravaged by cholera. Northwestern China, including the provinces of Hunan, Shensi, and Suiyuan, was attacked in July. Officially, over 100,000 cases and nearly 32,000 human deaths were reported during 1932.

The epidemic subsided in 1933 but not before the infection had been transported by boat to Japan, where it caused only minor outbreaks. Cholera once again flared up in epidemic form during 1937–39, 1942, and 1945–46.

Further reading: Pollitzer, *Cholera;* Huard and Wong, *Chinese Medicine.*

Chinese Cholera Epidemics of 1937–42

Cholera epidemics that invaded various parts of China during 1937–42.

The first outbreak began in May 1937 in eastern Kwangtung (Guangdong) province and spread west to Kwangsi (Guangxi) province by August; over 28,000 cases apparently occurred in Kwangtung and only 600 in Kwangsi. In December 1937, cholera appeared in the Yuan River basin and, by June 1938, had invaded the Tse (Tzu), Siang (Hsiang), and Yangtze River valleys. The Sino-Japanese War of 1937–45, extending into World War II, helped spread the epidemic into China's interior; nine provinces reported a total of 50,043 cases of cholera during 1938. Even Manchuria was affected. Hunan province marked the northernmost limit of the epidemic, recording 4,500 cases and 2,000 human deaths in 1938.

China had another major outbreak of cholera in 1939. According to one account, it began in June in the hilly rural areas of Nangpu Hsien district and spread to the adjoining districts in the west and northwest. The cities of Chungking (Chongqing) and Chengtu were important disseminating centers of infection. Others believe it originated in Hunan province (1,087 deaths) and spread from there to Kweichow (Guizhou) and 15 other provinces. The epidemic extended south and west across the provinces of Yunnan, Szechwan (Sichuan; 41,000 deaths), and Sikang, and north across Shensi (Shaanxi; 10,000 deaths) and Kansu (Gansu provinces). Kunming, Yunnan's capital, recorded 3,486 cases and a mortality rate of 74 percent. Central China was severely affected. During this visitation, cholera also penetrated southwestern China.

Minor outbreaks of cholera continued in 1940. However, they were restricted to the areas of southern Kiangsu (Jiangsu), Chekiang (Zhejiang), Fukien (Fujian), Kwangtung, Hunan, and northern Szechwan.

In 1941, cholera again invaded China, and this time the port cities, including Macao (1,475 cases), Hong Kong, Canton (Guangzhou), and Shanghai, suffered the most. Incidence was relatively low inland; only Hunan, Fukien, and Kwangtung reported outbreaks.

During World War II (1939–45) and following the Japanese occupation of Burma, the Malay states, and Hong Kong, cholera marched across southern China along different military routes. It arrived in Kwangtung along the Si (Hsi) River and crossed over the Burmese border to infect Yunnan and Kwangsi provinces. Between January and September 1942, 11,951 cases were reported from 19 Chinese provinces. Cholera continued to rage intermittently through October and November.

Further reading: Pollitzer, *Cholera;* Simmons et al., *Global Epidemiology.*

Chinese Cholera Epidemic of 1945–46

Most widespread of the cholera epidemics that struck China in the twentieth century (see CHINESE CHOLERA EPIDEMIC OF 1932, CHINESE CHOLERA EPIDEMICS OF 1937–42).

Early in 1945, cholera was prevalent in Kwangsi, Kweichow, and Yunnan but in a mild form. The first major outbreak of this epidemic originated in Szechwan province in May 1945—along the Yangtze River just upstream of Chungking. The following month Chungking and the surrounding area were infected. The epidemic then coursed along the Yangtze to Ichang, where it smoldered through the winter. The infection in Szechwan had meanwhile subsided by the end of the year. In September 1945, cholera broke out in Kwangtung, which was again infected in May 1946.

In February 1946, a serious outbreak of cholera threatened Japanese soldiers held in a prison camp at Hankow, China. These soldiers were later transported downstream to Nanking and Shanghai, which led to the introduction of cholera in these ports. In July 1946, the epidemic began to spread rather rapidly across the country. Within a few months, by October 1946, cholera had invaded much of China, reaching Inner Mongolia and central Manchuria to the north, Limchow to the south, and beyond Chungking to the west. This rapid transmission of the disease was facilitated by the dispersal of troops and the repatriation of prisoners following the end of World War II.

It was the worst cholera epidemic (see MANCHURIAN CHOLERA EPIDEMIC OF 1919) to hit the people of Manchuria, and the death toll was very high. It began in late June 1946 when the infection reached Liaoning in south Manchuria. From here it spread rapidly along the railway routes.

The epidemic in 1946 has been traced either to the Szechwan or to the Kwangtung cholera outbreaks of

1945. Those outbreaks resulting from the Szechwan source had a fairly low to moderate case fatality rate (ten per cent) while the Kwangtung outbreaks recorded high case fatality rates (25–30 percent).

Further reading: Pollitzer, *Cholera*.

Chinese Dengue Epidemics of 1978–80   Considered the first recorded epidemics of dengue in China since World War II, when Japanese troops had introduced the disease into the coastal areas (see JAPANESE DENGUE EPIDEMICS OF 1942–45).

The first, a large epidemic, was caused by dengue type 4 in the Foshan district of Kwangtung (Guangdong) province in southern China in 1978. A total of 22,122 cases, some of them hemorrhagic, and 14 human deaths were reported during the outbreak. The next year, dengue cases were found to be caused by dengue type 1 virus. Both these outbreaks were confined to some coastal districts near Hong Kong. The *Aedes albopictus* mosquito was the vector or carrier in both cases.

In 1980, epidemics caused by dengue type 3 were reported from a wider area in southern China. The coastal sections of Kwangtung and Kwangsi (Guangxi) provinces and Hainan Island were affected. This time, the *Aedes aegypti* mosquito was isolated as the main vector. A hemorrhagic tendency was observed in some cases.

These epidemics were part of a series of dengue epidemics that occurred in many countries of Southeast Asia and the Western Pacific during the 1970s and 1980s.

Further reading: Mackenzie, ed., *Viral Diseases in South-East Asia and the Western Pacific;* World Health Organization, *Dengue Haemorrhagic Fever.*

Chinese Hepatitis Epidemic of 1986–88   See XINJIANG (SINKIANG) HEPATITIS EPIDEMIC OF 1986–88.

Chinese Influenza Epidemic of 1918   Widespread influenza epidemic—offshoot of the Spanish Influenza Epidemic of 1917–19 (q.v.)—that spread across China in 1918.

The epidemic was preceded by the spread of influenza in March and April 1918, affecting many Chinese cities, including Beijing (Peking), Shanghai, and Tientsin, but this is not considered part of the pandemic that was then invading many countries worldwide.

According to Edwin O. Jordan (see below), the epidemic invaded Shanghai late in May 1918 and spread very rapidly along sea and river routes to infect many other Chinese ports. Canton's first case reportedly occurred on June 4; Hong Kong reported a sudden increase in the number of influenza patients (269 cases) hospitalized during that month. When the year ended, influenza had claimed 405 lives and pneumonia another 2,251 in Hong Kong alone—a dramatic increase over the previous year's figures. Influenza also raged at Chefoo (Yen-tai) during the first two weeks of June.

According to a report on July 27, 1918, nearly 50 percent of the city of Chungking's population was infected by the flu virus, which became more virulent as it spread. In September, influenza struck the river port of Hankow and, the following month, it again invaded Canton, Chefoo, Hong Kong, Changsha (Hunan province), and Shanghai. Both natives and foreigners suffered during the epidemic. Most of the deaths, particularly in the rural areas, were the result of pulmonary complications following the actual flu attack. Nine hundred deaths were reported from the port of Weihai (population 147,177), where influenza broke out in October–November 1918.

Overall, China suffered a milder attack than did India (see INDIAN INFLUENZA EPIDEMIC OF 1918–19). Influenza struck China again during the winter of 1919–20 and, more severely, in February 1924.

Further reading: Jordan, *Epidemic Influenza; Reports on Public Health and Medical Subjects.*

Chinese Plague of 1894   See HONG KONG PLAGUE OF 1894.

Chinese Plague of 1917–18   Outbreak of pneumonic plague in northern China during 1917–18.

The epidemic, which was traced to a wild rodent source in Ordos (part of Inner Mongolia), invaded the Chinese provinces of Shansi and Chahar during the winter of 1917–18. The disease also made brief inroads into the provinces of Chihli, Shantung, Anwhei, and Kiangsu. Since the outbreak was focused primarily in a sparsely populated area, it infected a relatively smaller number of people (see MANCHURIAN PLAGUE OF 1910–11; MANCHURIAN AND MONGOLIAN PLAGUES OF 1928–30). An estimated 16,000 people were struck by the disease during the epidemic, which lasted seven months. Prompt medical attention, particularly crucial during an outbreak of pneumonic plague, apparently helped control the spread of the infection. Scattered cases of plague were also reported from Hong Kong and Amoy in 1917–18.

Pneumonic plague occurs when pneumonia strikes a person suffering from bubonic plague. If left untreated, the patient is almost certain to die within the next day or two. In this form of plague, the infection is transmitted from person to person through droplets in the air. Pneumonic plague is thus ignited and fostered by the concurrent presence of bubonic plague in the community.

Following the epidemic, the Chinese government established a Central Epidemic Prevention Bureau at Peking (Beijing) in 1919. It also instituted measures aimed at preventing epidemics from entering the country. For instance, infectious diseases were to be reported to the police. Also, three quarantine hospitals were built at the port city of Hangchow.

Further reading: Pollitzer, *Plague;* Wong and Lien-teh, *History of Chinese Medicine.*

Chinese Plague of 1931–32

Chinese Plague of 1931–32   Severe epidemic of plague that invaded the neighboring Chinese provinces of Shansi and Shensi during 1931–32 (see CHINESE PLAGUE OF 1917–18; MANCHURIAN AND MONGOLIAN PLAGUES OF 1928–30).

Outbreaks of pneumonic and bubonic plague were a recurrent theme in both these provinces (largely because of their proximity to Inner Mongolia's diseased Ordos district) throughout the 1920s; some were severe and widespread, others highly localized. The epidemic of 1931–32, caused by an epizootic among domestic rats (*Rattus norvegicus,* the local species) was an intense one, by all accounts. It was a mixed outbreak that infected many previously unaffected districts and claimed an estimated 20,000 victims in the two provinces. More than 1,000 victims each were reported from the districts of Lin-hsien and Hsing-hsien in Shansi and from Han-shan, Micheh, and Suiteh in Shensi province. The Shansi outbreak was primarily bubonic, whereas the Shensi outbreak began as bubonic and, in the fall, changed to pneumonic in two districts. Thanks to preventive measures launched by the health authorities, the epidemic did not spread beyond these two provinces.

In the fall of 1932, plague reappeared, but this time only four districts—Mi-cheh, An-ting, Hsia-hsien, and Suiyuan—were infected. Several small and scattered outbreaks occurred in this area through the 1940s, but overall there had been a marked improvement in the plague situation here since the epidemic of 1931–32

Further reading: Pollitzer, *Plague;* Lien-teh et al., *Plague: A Manual for Medical and Public Health Workers.*

Cholera Pandemics

Cholera Pandemics   See ASIATIC CHOLERA PANDEMICS (various dates).

Colombian Smallpox Epidemic of 1776

Colombian Smallpox Epidemic of 1776   Severe smallpox (variola) epidemic striking the town of Socorro in north-central, present-day Colombia, causing many human deaths and havoc and helping precipitate the subsequent, fearful Comuneros' Uprising of 1781. The uprising, which was suppressed, was led by *comuneros* (citizens for democratic reforms), including Spaniards and Indians, and was against oppressive Spanish-colonial government taxation.

By 1776, smallpox was endemic in Colombia (part of New Granada, including Venezuela and Ecuador), occurring in periodic cycles with each new generation of non-immune people. When it struck Socorro in 1776, it struck one of the country's wealthiest settlements. About 6,000 persons out of a population of 33,170 perished; the majority of fatalities were from the lower classes, many of them infants. Poor parents sometimes had to leave dead infants at the door of a church in order to get a free burial during the epidemic.

At the time, the town of Socorro had also suffered several bad harvests, and thus the health and prosperity that Socorro had enjoyed was undercut. On March 16, 1781, *comuneros* rebelled against a proposed sales tax. On March 30, they rebelled angrily against the tobacco monopoly by the colonial government; tobacco was for many farmers their only cash crop. On April 30, mixed-blood Spaniards and Indians demonstrated against both the sales tax and the profitable tobacco monopoly. The common people had failed to profit economically as landowners had, but were not against the king; thus their slogan was "Long live the King; death to bad government." The Spanish government introduced the smallpox vaccination later in the 1780s, and the disease abated.

Further reading: Phelan, *The People and the King;* Hopkins, *Princes and Peasants: Smallpox in History.*

Congolese Sleeping Sickness Epidemic of 1895–1906

Congolese Sleeping Sickness Epidemic of 1895–1906   Devastating epidemic of African sleeping sickness (African trypanosomiasis) that killed about 500,000 persons in the Congo Free State (Zaire) in south-central Africa from 1895 to 1906.

Before 1895, this parasitic disease had long been endemic in the Congo River area as far upriver as Stanley Pool (Malebo Pool), a lakelike expansion of the river along the modern Zaire-Congo Republic border. Disease-carrying tsetse flies infested the rivers of the Congo region and attacked the people moving along these waterways. Earlier, in 1857, British explorer Dr. David Livingstone had asserted that the bite of the tsetse fly was responsible for transmitting sleeping sickness to some animals, but he was certain that human beings were immune to the bite. Furthermore, Livingstone's "discoverer," Henry Morton Stanley, who was economic development chief for Belgium's King Leopold II from 1878 to

1884, unwittingly contributed to the spread of the disease in the Congo's central and eastern regions, when he established trading stations; river boats carried disease-infected persons as well as flies into the developing population centers.

By 1896 the disease (then commonly known as "Negro lethargy") had claimed about 5,000 human lives in and around Lukolela on the Congo River. The mortality figures (one of the few times they were obtained) were gained through the efforts of Roger David Casement, British consular agent in the Congo Free State (1901–04), who found only 352 survivors of the disease in Lukolela in 1903. In a letter to the governor-general of the Congo state in 1904, Casement reported appalling, unsanitary conditions at Lukolela, where the sick were left untreated medically. (Casement gained fame for exposing the brutal exploitation of native labor by white traders of rubber in the Congo.)

After being bitten by diseased tsetse flies, Congolese natives complained of low-grade fever, chills, severe headaches, lesions, rashes, and insomnia; sometimes behavioral and personality changes occurred, with hallucinations and delusions. Without medical help, increased wasting and somnolence occurred until inevitable death. At this time, drug treatment was largely experimental and inadequate; therefore, the main effort of the Congo government was directed toward locating infected people and then isolating them in special hospitals (lazarets or lazarettos). In three main towns near Stanley Pool, located within a few miles of each other, thousands of natives of the Teke (Bateke) tribe fatally contracted the sleeping sickness; patients who tried to flee the area helped to spread the infection. By 1903 Leopold-ville (Kinshasa), the capital, on Stanley Pool, was reportedly left with less than 100 natives.

In 1903 King Leopold II attempted to fight the epidemic in his African colony by inviting a team from Britain's Liverpool School of Tropical Medicine to his Congo colony to study the disease. That same year in Uganda (a British protectorate), the Gambian form of sleeping sickness was isolated, and the tsetse fly was identified as the vector of the disease's infectious parasitic agent, *Trypanosoma gambiense*.

Sleeping sickness abated considerably in the Belgian Congo by 1912; four years before, the Belgian parliament had taken over the Congo Free State from King Leopold and created the Belgian Congo. By late 1920 sleeping sickness had advanced into northern Nigeria via the Congo, which was again ravaged by the disease a few years later, with mortality rates as high as 30 percent in areas. By 1939 almost every country in West Africa had been infected by the disease, in either the Gambian or the Rhodesian form.

Further reading: Ford, *The Role of Trypanosomiasis in African Ecology;* McKelvey, Jr., *Man Against Tsetse;* Marks and Beatty, *Epidemics.*

Connecticut Smallpox Epidemic of 1634   Pestilence carried by Dutch traders to the Connecticut River Indians that precipitated a catastrophic epidemic—a sequence of outbreaks over a period of about seven years—among Indians along the St. Lawrence River and Great Lakes and into eastern Canada. The Pequots (Mohawks of the Iroquois nation who had driven out the Mohicans) had invited both the English (Massachusetts Bay) and Dutch (New Netherlands) to the Connecticut River for trade. The English erected a palisaded settlement in what later became Newtown, just north of the Dutch trade center. At one point, the Dutch tried to conspire with the Indians again the Puritans, but it didn't work. Infected Dutch passed the disease to the Indians. Although there are no comprehensive statistics, multitudes of Indians died. Individual, firsthand accounts reported that many more died than lived. According to William Bradford, governor of Plymouth Plantation, 95 out of every 100 Indians died in the Connecticut River valley outbreak, while the English escaped infection. Both phenomena were construed to be divine providence. To the Puritans, God helped them in their righteous journey to follow His will, and destroyed the infidels obstructing their path. Once smallpox had virtually eliminated the Indians in the Connecticut Valley, English settlers from Dorchester plantation in Massachusetts were anxious to move there. After some contention, the Dorchester group reached an agreement with the Newtown English settlers over land rights. The new settlers founded Hartford, Wethersfield, and Windsor in Connecticut, and Springfield, Massachusetts.

Also known as variola, smallpox was a highly infectious virus that a victim either inhaled or picked up via particles contaminated by infected oral or nasal mucus. Because of their total vulnerability, Indians would have contracted the most virulent form of smallpox, although even the lesser variety (variola minor) would have proven fatal. After infection and an incubation period of about two weeks, victims would exhibit the symptoms of high fever, aches and pains, headaches, and sometimes vomiting. Later, spots appeared that became eruptions filled first with clear lymph and then pus, which would break, after which scabs would form and then fall off, causing scars, pockmarks, and spotty pigmentation. Accompanying or resulting infirmities could include blindness, heart problems, and arthritis, among many others. In the seventeenth century, God tested or punished with smallpox. To even try to find a cure would have been construed as an anathema.

Smallpox devastated populations never before exposed to the disease, killing up to 90 percent of those infected. According to an observer of Indians as late as in the nineteenth century, the disease was so lethal to them, they often died before the skin eruptions appeared. Because of their migratory habits as well as their panicked flights to escape contact with the diseased, Indians carried seeds of contagion far and wide. William Bradford, in his history *Of Plymouth Plantation 1620–1647*, vividly described how the Pequots of Connecticut suffered:

> For usually they that have this disease have them in abundance, and for want of bedding and linen and other helps they fall into a lamentable condition as they lie on their hard mats, the pox breaking and mattering and running one into another, their skin cleaving by reason thereof to the mats they lie on. When they turn them, a whole side will flay off at once as it were, and they will be all of a gore blood, most fearful to behold. And then being very sore, what with cold and other distempers, they die like rotten sheep.

The Indians were in such pitiable condition that they were unable to accomplish even rudimentary tasks. Overwhelmed with compassion despite fear of the disease, the English fed them, stoked their wood fires, and buried their dead. Bradford called it a miracle that the English escaped infection, although John Winthrop mentioned a Newtown smallpox death in a letter to his son.

Jesuits located in eastern Canada, recording that smallpox had broken out among Indians in 1634, observed that as soon as the Indians chose to serve God, they were destroyed by famine, smallpox, and war. North of Lake Ontario, the Hurons were ravaged by smallpox from 1636 to 1640 until only half the tribe remained, making them vulnerable later to destruction by the Iroquois. The ravaged Hurons blamed the smallpox epidemic on the Jesuits, whom they would have killed had it not been for the needed trade with the French. The Jesuits may have been culpable of spreading the disease as they went from person to person performing baptisms. The Iroquois later suffered great losses because of the disease. Some New World invaders came to exploit the Indians' susceptibility to smallpox as a tool against them. Even some of the most devout spiritual leaders relished and gloried in the sickness and death of Indians as God's judgment against them. See also

MASSACHUSETTS SMALLPOX EPIDEMIC OF C. 1617–19; MASSACHUSETTS SMALLPOX EPIDEMIC OF C. 1633.

Further reading: Bradford, *Of Plymouth Plantation;* Duffy, *Epidemics in Colonial America;* Hopkins, *Princes and Peasants: Smallpox in History.*

Constantine Malaria Epidemic of 1941   Explosive outbreak of malaria in the city of Constantine in northeast Algeria, killing about 7,725 persons from March to November 1941. In previous years there had been a low incidence of the infectious disease in the area, thus considerably increasing the susceptibility of the inhabitants to the pathogen's attack. Furthermore, in March 1941, after a season of abnormally heavy rainfall, there was an abundance of anopheline mosquitoes, which carry malaria's microorganism (a tiny parasitic protozoan that lives in the red blood cells of humans). The mosquitoes, which breed and thrive profusely in stagnant water (ditches, swamps, and marshes), may bite and infect healthy individuals, who come down with violent chills, nausea, high fever, and sweats and may die in a coma or delirium without prompt treatment.

A traveler from neighboring Morocco apparently carried malaria's parasite into Constantine, where an anopheline mosquito bit him, sucked in blood containing the parasite, and bit another person to infect him; this is the typical cycle of transmission. The epidemic erupted in March in Constantine, where eventually 85 percent to 90 percent of the area's estimated population of 220,000 became infected before the epidemic ended in November. While many adults were stricken, both native and European, a large number of the infections, especially the serious cases, occurred among children below school age; those children who survived were most likely damaged by the effects of the disease. The malaria also adversely affected pregnancies.

The epidemic in Constantine claimed the lives of about four percent of those stricken with malaria, despite systematic campaigns by authorities to eradicate mosquito larvae and to treat large numbers of sick people. Ways of controlling malaria had increased ever since a French Army surgeon in Algeria, Alphonse Laveran, discovered (1880) the parasite of malaria and explained the various forms the parasite may take when human blood is infected by the bite of the mosquito. The illness is still regarded as a problem in Algeria and other African countries, as well as other parts of the world.

Further reading: Boyd, *Malariology;* McGrew, *Encyclopedia of Medical History.*

Constantinople Plague of c. a.d. 746–48   Epidemic of bubonic plague that traveled through the eastern Mediterranean over a three-year period. Although chronological problems in the primary source—the late eighth-century Greek monk and chronicler Theophanes—make it difficult for exact dates to be assigned, the years A.D. 746 to 748 would be a good estimate. During the preceding 60 to 70 years the war-torn Near East had been regularly visited by epidemics. The Constantinople Plague began where so many others had—in Syria. Proceeding across northern Africa to Sicily and southern Italy, the plague then struck Greece and finally circled back eastward to Constantinople (Istanbul), where it raged for a year.

Because the epidemic followed shipping and commerce routes (as bubonic plague does), its journey is a good indication of the contacts between Mediterranean countries. Unlike other earlier epidemics in the area (see ANTONINE PLAGUE; PLAGUE OF JUSTINIAN), the Constantinople Plague did not make substantial inroads into northern and western Europe. Ties between West and East were slim because of ongoing disputes between the papacy and religious leaders in Constantinople and because of incursions by Gothic peoples, Slavs, Persians, and other easterners, which had gradually taken much of the old Roman Empire out of Byzantine control. In fact, Arab conquests of Syria and Palestine in the seventh century A.D. had severed the overland routes to Constantinople—one reason the plague had to follow a roundabout course before reaching the Byzantine capital.

When it did arrive there, the plague caused mass frenzy as well as widespread mortality. According to Theophanes, oily crosses appeared on clothing and the sacred garb of churches—presumably to mark the next victims. Those stricken with the disease had hallucinations: They imagined strange-looking people who stopped to talk to them or entered houses to kill the inhabitants. By the following spring and summer when the plague was at its height, the dead were so numerous that they could not be buried. Even dry reservoirs, vineyards, and orchards had to be used as cemeteries.

Once the plague subsided, the Byzantine ruler Constantine V repopulated his capital with large numbers of Slavs from Greece, who brought with them their Hellenized culture. While the Byzantines were enriched by the cultural influences, Constantine at the same time wanted to minimize some of the Slavs' foreign ways. He hoped to convert them to iconoclasm, the prohibition on all divine images—a cause he zealously upheld until the end of his reign.

Further reading: *The Chronicle of Theophanes;* Bury, *A History of the Later Roman Empire;* Franzius, *History of the Byzantine Empire;* Simpson, *A Treatise on Plague.*

Continental Army Smallpox Epidemic of 1776
See QUEBEC SMALLPOX EPIDEMIC OF 1776.

Copenhagen Poliomyelitis Epidemic of 1952
Largest and most intense outbreak of poliomyelitis or polio recorded in Denmark until that time, with over 3,000 cases. Overwhelmed by the high number of patients, about one third of whom had respiratory problems, the local doctors had to develop an innovative way of treating them.

A single hospital for communicable diseases served the more than one million residents of greater Copenhagen, but its 500 hospital beds were quickly filled when the epidemic hit. From late July through the end of December, about 3,000 polio patients were admitted; during the peak of the outbreak (a week in late August and early September), nearly 50 new cases arrived each day. Approximately 1,000 of them had some degree of paralysis, and in about 350 of these the bulbar centers of the brain (those next to the spinal cord) and the lower cranial nerves were affected. In addition to having trouble breathing, these patients were in danger of having their air passages obstructed by secretions because they could not cough or swallow on their own. Such a concentration of severe poliomyelitis cases was unprecedented in Europe.

Although the hospital had several respirators, the demand for them rapidly exceeded the supply. Hoping to keep patients alive when respirators were not available, the hospital's chief physician, H. C. A. Lassen, and his colleagues invented a new method. After performing a tracheotomy just below the larynx, they inserted a cuff into the trachea to close it off from secretions; using positive pressure, they then pumped air into the lungs from a rubber bag feeding into the trachea. The parts for the apparatus were inexpensive and easy to obtain. The only major requirement was for power to pump the air—and this was supplied by about 200 medical students per day who were paid modest amounts to pedal bicycles.

The new technique dramatically improved a patient's chances for survival. Until the end of August (when the device was created), 31 people needing therapy for advanced respiratory problems were admitted to the hospital, and 87 percent of them died. Of the nearly 300 similar patients treated by bag ventilation, about 60 percent lived for at least a month—that is, past the critical first few weeks of the illness, during which most polio deaths occur. In 1953 Swedish doctors used bag ventilation with similarly impressive results during a similar poliomyelitis outbreak in their country, which also featured a high percentage of severe respiratory problems.

Further reading: International Poliomyelitis Congress, *Poliomyelitis: Papers and Discussions Presented at the Third International Poliomyelitis Conference;* Lassen, "A Preliminary Report on the 1952 Epidemic of Poliomyelitis in Copenhagen"; Paul, *A History of Poliomyelitis.*

"Cough of Perinthus" Outbreak of disease recorded in the Hippocratic *Epidemics;* occurred at Perinthus (Marmaraereglisi) in northern Greece (now part of Turkey, on the Sea of Marmara) during the winter and spring of an unidentified year around 400 B.C. Either the Greek physician Hippocrates himself or a gifted member of his school wrote the detailed clinical account of the outbreak, whose first signs were a cough and, frequently, pneumonia. After about 40 days most victims had a relapse and developed one or more of the following symptoms: sore throat, angina, fits of coughing, disturbed vision, and paralysis of the soft palate or of the limbs.

The disease struck people of all ages, but in different ways: Children seemed to have more problems with seeing at night; few women got fever or pneumonia, but slave women were at greater risk of angina than were freeborn ones; men were afflicted in greater numbers, probably because they were outside the home more. People who had fever, chills, and trouble with breathing were more likely to die, while many others recovered, especially those who had problems only with swallowing.

Emile Littré, a nineteenth-century editor of Hippocrates, noted that paralysis and angina are characteristic of diphtheria. Another diagnosis suggested by some is influenza, which would account for the fever, coughing, and fatigue. As one scholar notes, few similar diseases cause short-lived, widespread outbreaks that often lead to pneumonia. No one illness, though, appears to encompass all the symptoms observed at Perinthus (a port town). Quite possibly the outbreak included several diseases, among them diphtheria, influenza syndrome (flu-like symptoms caused by related viruses), whooping cough, and deficiency disorders (notably one of vitamin A, which results in night blindness and can aggravate respiratory infections). Such diseases may have afflicted the inhabitants of Perinthus every year at about the same time; similar seasonal outbreaks have been seen in rural areas during the modern era. Mirko D. Grmek, author of *Diseases in the Ancient Greek World*, translates the passage describing the outbreak, found in Hippocrate's *Epidemics.*

Further reading: Jones's introduction to the works of Hippocrates (London, 1923); Hare, "The Antiquity of Diseases Caused by Bacteria and Viruses."

Cremona Diphtheria Epidemic of 1747–48 Severe epidemic of diphtheria that killed at least a thousand persons in the northern Italian city of Cremona in Lombardy in 1747–48. Physicians there were familiar with this acute infectious disease involving the nose and throat, for in 1618 and 1648 serious outbreaks of malignant sore throat or "angina maligna" (a common name then for the disease) had been documented in parts of Lombardy, especially Mantua.

After the start of the Cremona epidemic in 1747, physicians observed that the infection caused ulceration in the throats of victims, making deglutition (swallowing) difficult; in many of the cases, swelling of the neck was a prominent sign, and food and medicine were regurgitated through the nose. As swallowing and breathing became more difficult, many patients died of asphyxia, often within a few days after infection. Though the disease was known to be contagious since 1618 and sanitary and quarantine procedures were put into effect, the mortality rate was extremely high in Cremona, especially among children. In many instances, all the children in an infected family contracted the disease.

Some physicians in Cremona applied leeches to the sick or used scarification (slight incisions in the skin) along with alum, copper, and arsenic as acidic cauterizing substances. Others performed tracheotomies (operations of cutting into the trachea or windpipe). Dr. Martino Ghisi of Cremona, whose eight-year-old son was infected and recovered, observed that one of his patients, a six-year-old girl, had expectorated much mucus and pieces of gelatinous membrane formation prior to her death. During an autopsy Ghisi performed on another dead child, he discovered that the respiratory membrane from the larynx to the bronchi was inflamed and contained a whitish substance similar to that which had been coughed up by the six-year-old girl. In 1749 Ghisi, who recognized the paralytic phenomena associated with the disease, published what became an important, knowledgeable, early account of diphtheria.

Further reading: Andrews et al., *Diphtheria;* McGrew, *Encyclopedia of Medical History.*

Crimean War Epidemics Outbreaks of cholera, scurvy, dysentery, and typhus that struck British, French, and Russian combatants during the Crimean War (1854–56). While diplomatic misunderstandings and military inefficiency helped prolong the fighting, the troops fell victim more often to disease than to combat. During the war, however, both the British (under guidance from Florence Nightingale) and the Russians made improvements in medical care that not only lowered the number of human deaths from disease, but also inaugurated a period of army sanitary reform.

In 1853 Russia had demanded certain safeguards for Christians living in Ottoman Turkish lands, as well as the right to sail its warships through the Dardanelles Strait, then controlled by the Ottoman Empire. When the Turks refused, Russia invaded Ottoman territories in the Danube River region, and the Turks declared war. Fearing that Russia's aggression would upset what they saw as the balance of power in the East, Britain and France entered the war in 1854 on the Turkish side. Ongoing diplomatic negotiations did not halt the fighting, which was concentrated on the Russian naval base at Sevastopol in the southern Crimea, on the Black Sea. The allies began attacking the port in September 1854, but despite their land battles that autumn, they were unable to capture the base and a long siege began.

Disease was present before any shots were fired. Cholera, which struck parts of Europe, Asia, and America during 1840–63, infected a number of soldiers even before they left the southern ports of France. Cholera spread more widely when the troops disembarked in the East. Despite a lull in the winter of 1854–55, it continued to rage among British and French (as well as Russian) soldiers for the remainder of the war, eventually killing the French commander Armand J. L. de Saint-Arnaud. Both British and French soldiers contracted numerous other infectious diseases as they assembled at the Bulgarian port of Varna. Nor did conditions improve when the allied forces reached the Crimea. The lack of sanitation and of medical care fostered the transmission of disease, but so did shortages of food and medicine, since both sides had to transport supplies over great distances by land.

The winter of 1854–55 was particularly bad for the British. In November alone about 330 of them succumbed to scurvy, dysentery, typhoid, and other diseases. Throughout the entire winter nearly 50 percent of all soldiers admitted to the British hospitals died, many from gangrene that set in after they were wounded. The hospitals were astonishingly dirty: Bed linens were rarely changed, and in November only six shirts were washed in one British hospital that had some 2,000 dysentery patients.

The sufferings of the allied soldiers were publicized in reports by newspaper correspondents who, for the first time, accompanied the troops in battle. Outrage in Britain helped convince the government to send the Italian-born English nurse Florence Nightingale to the Crimea in late 1854. With never more than a few dozen nurses under her supervision at any one time, Nightingale carried out extensive reforms in hospital administration. Although they were nothing more than simple housekeeping matters—such as providing clean linen, washing patients, de-

livering adequate meals on time, and getting reliable supplies of medicine—her methods brought the British death rate down dramatically.

Scurvy had attacked the British soldiers during the first winter, for example, but not afterward, when they were eating better food. Among the French, however, the disease was rampant from the summer of 1855 on. In addition, the winter of 1855–56 brought a typhus epidemic to the French Army, killing several thousand; the British, on the other hand, were largely unaffected during that time. In fact, throughout the war, death rates in French hospitals remained consistently high and at times surpassed the worst British rates of the first winter. Information about disease among the Russian troops is less easy to come by, but they, too, were afflicted with typhus and other infectious diseases. Advances in medical care and nursing helped improve matters on the Russian side, as they had for the British Army.

The allies finally captured Sevastopol in September 1855, and a peace conference the following spring ended the war. The various diseases, however, continued to run their course. Cholera and typhus reached Russia and the Ottoman Empire, although the inhabitants of Constantinople (Istanbul) were largely spared. Because infected soldiers were quarantined and kept from returning to French soil until all threat of contagion was past, typhus never broke out among the French civilian population. In 1856 and 1857, however, local typhus epidemics occurred in Britain as the troops came home.

Further reading: Prinzing, *Epidemics Resulting from Wars;* Seton-Watson, *The Russian Empire, 1801–1917;* Smith, *Florence Nightingale: Reputation and Power;* Woodward, *The Age of Reform, 1815–1870,* 2nd ed.

Crusader Epidemic at Acre   Outbreaks of one or more diseases, including scurvy, that raged through the Crusader army as it besieged Acre (Akko, Israel) for nearly two years starting in August 1189 during the Third Crusade (1189–92). Although sickness and famine claimed more Crusader lives than battle did, still the Christians accomplished their goal when the beleaguered Muslim garrison surrendered in July 1191.

Previously a French possession, Acre had been captured by the Muslim leader Saladin in 1187, the same year in which he took Jerusalem. Two years later, alarmed by Saladin's conquests in the Middle East, Christian leaders in Europe began to mobilize for another crusade. Guy of Lusignan, a Frankish (French) leader who had lost his Syrian lands to Saladin, did not wait for allies from the west; in August 1189 he arrived at Acre to try to win back his lands. Contingents from Italy, Denmark, and other parts of Europe kept arriving to reinforce Guy's small army, which was also counting on large numbers of troops led by the English and French rulers. Despite their vows to defend the Holy Land, however, King Henry II of England and King Philip Augustus (Philip II) of France delayed in setting out for the east, as they instead continued their long-standing war with each other.

Meanwhile, the besiegers at Acre were in a stalemate. The Muslim garrison held out valiantly, while in turn the Crusaders were encircled by Saladin, who attacked them from the rear whenever they tried to storm the city. The Crusaders fell ill from various diseases, one of which killed Queen Sibylla, Guy's wife, and their two children. Symptoms described by the chronicler Geoffrey de Vinsauf make it clear that scurvy was one of the diseases in the camp. During the near-constant rain in the winter and spring of 1191, he writes, the Crusaders suffered from famine so harsh that men ate grass, bones that had already been gnawed by dogs, and even their horses, for which they could not get grain. Disease came in the wake of famine, causing swollen limbs and loss of teeth; only a few of the victims survived.

The situation brightened within a few weeks. Philip Augustus brought his troops in late April, and in early June the Crusaders rejoiced to see Richard the Lion-Hearted (now king of England after his father Henry II's death). The kings, however, quickly fell ill with a fever that caused the hair and nails to fall out—perhaps the same scurvy still among the soldiers—but both leaders recovered and rallied the troops. Richard's 25 ships, which were loaded with food, siege equipment, and booty from his recent conquest of Cyprus, resupplied the starving Crusaders and helped the French fleet blockade the harbor at Acre. After several weeks in which few provisions could get through to them, the Muslim garrison could hold out no longer. In July 1191 they surrendered and returned Acre to Christian control.

Further reading: de Vinsauf, *The Itinerary of Richard I and Others to the Holy Land;* Oldenbourg, *The Crusades;* Prinzing, *Epidemics Resulting from Wars.*

Crusader Epidemic at Adalia

Crusader Epidemic at Adalia   Epidemic in early 1148, during the Second Crusade (1147–49), wiping out thousands of infantry and pilgrims whom King Louis VII of France and his knights had left behind in Adalia (Antalya), a city on the coast of Anatolia (roughly Turkey).

The Crusade, which ended in failure, was intended to win back the Syrian city of Edessa (Urfa, Turkey), captured by the Franks in the First Crusade over 40 years before but now in Turkish possession. The king of France and the German emperor, Conrad III, each

gathered soldiers to defend the Holy Land. Conrad's army was massacred by the Seljuk Turks in October 1147, but Louis was more fortunate, managing to lead his troops to Adalia despite suffering heavy losses along the way. Using their knowledge of the terrain, the Turks had often launched surprise attacks on the Franks (French), forcing them to fight in narrow and dangerous mountain passes. Since the Turks had also overgrazed and destroyed the countryside, the Crusaders who did survive the attacks were often unable to find provisions.

The situation did not improve when the Franks reached Adalia on January 20, 1148. The Byzantines who controlled the city charged them exorbitant prices for food and supplies. When Louis decided to abandon the overland route and sail instead to Antioch, the Byzantines agreed to procure enough ships for the passage, but never made good on their promise. After waiting several weeks for the winter rains to stop, Louis and the knights boarded the few available ships; the infantry and pilgrims were supposed to march south under Byzantine escort.

But those remaining at Adalia were soon afflicted with a contagious disease. In his history of the Second Crusade, Louis's chaplain, Odo of Deuil, gives few details of the epidemic—presumably because he had already left the city with the king. After breaking out among the Crusaders, the disease soon spread to the inhabitants of the city, depopulating entire homes. The rapid spread, high mortality, and recent presence of foreign ships in the harbor suggest the possibility of bubonic plague, but more likely causes are typhoid, dysentery, and the other diseases that prey on weakened soldiers in crowded, unhealthy conditions. Whatever the disease, Odo says that several thousand of the Franks feared it so much, they preferred to leave the city and try to make their escape through the surrounding areas, which were filled with Turkish soldiers. They were unsuccessful; Turkish attacks killed most of those who did not succumb to the disease.

Further reading: Odo of Deuil, *The Journey of Louis VII to the East;* Berry, "The Second Crusade"; Grousset, *The Epic of the Crusades.*

Crusader Epidemic at Al Mansurah

Crusader Epidemic at Al Mansurah   Outbreak of scurvy, probably complicated by typhoid and other diseases, that attacked the Crusaders during the late winter and early spring of 1250. In the previous year the army led by King Louis IX of France had captured Damietta (Dumyât), an important Egyptian city in the east of the Nile River delta. Their ranks thinned by the epidemic, by military miscalculations, and by constant skirmishes with the Muslims, the Crusaders were unable to follow up their success at Damietta.

Well-organized and -financed at the start, the Seventh Crusade (1248–54) duplicated the strategy used in the Fifth Crusade over 30 years before. Hoping to strike at the Muslims by capturing their ports in Egypt, the Crusaders landed in the Nile delta and overran an abandoned Damietta in the spring of 1249. To avoid the summer Nile River floods and to wait for promised reinforcements from France, Louis kept the army at Damietta until October. A slow and cautious advance southward to Cairo then began. Continually fighting off Muslim raids, the Franks (French) picked their way through the many canals and tributaries of the delta until they reached the Muslim stronghold of Al Mansurah (El Mansûra). For six weeks the armies faced each other there, camped on opposite banks of the Nile.

Neither side made a move until Louis decided on a surprise attack after he learned of a river passage farther away. The gamble worked despite many Crusader casualties suffered in rash charges by some of their leaders; three days later, on February 11, 1250 (the first Friday of Lent), the Muslims counterattacked in a fierce battle. So many Muslims and Christians died on these two days, according to French historian Jean de Joinville (the seneschal of Champagne, who was himself wounded on February 8) that the dead bodies covered the river from one bank to the other. He claims that the stench arising from the corpses infected the survivors, none of whom recovered his health.

In fact, disease was soon raging in the Crusader camp, along with famine. The Muslims began an effective campaign to intercept Crusader supply ships, capturing about 80 of them. The Christians had little to eat during Lent except for unwholesome fish; their poor diet, Joinville wrote, undoubtedly helped cause the epidemic.

The symptoms he described—decaying flesh on the legs, skin that turned black as the ground or as an old boot, rotting gums, and bleeding from the nose—indicate scurvy, but other diseases probably afflicted the Christians as well. Joinville said that he himself had a quartan fever (recurring every fourth day) and "a rheum in my head [that] ran through my mouth and nostrils," while Louis, who bravely stayed among his army, became ill from dysentery on top of scurvy.

The epidemic dragged on until Easter, worsening to the point where barbers had to cut away flesh from the gums of victims just to allow them to eat. Finally, Louis realized that his position was impossible and ordered a retreat to Damietta. With the sick soldiers being carried on ships, the others marched on foot, but they were so weakened they surrendered to the pursuing Muslims. Led into captivity, Louis and his army won their freedom only by giving up Damietta and paying an enormous ransom.

Further reading: Jean de Joinville, *Memoirs of Saint Louis IX,* in *Chronicles of the Crusades;* Marks and Beatty, *Epidemics;* Runciman, *A History of the Crusades;* Strayer, "The Crusades of Louis IX."

Crusader Epidemic at Antioch Devastating epidemic, probably of typhoid, that struck the Crusaders in the summer of 1098 after their successful but difficult siege of Antioch. The Turkish stronghold in northern Syria was just a stop on the Crusaders' route to Jerusalem, which they wanted to recapture from the Muslims. The journey to the Holy City was postponed for months, however, partly because so many Christian soldiers fell ill during the First Crusade (1095–99).

Reaching Antioch in October 1097, the Crusaders discovered a heavily fortified city too large for them to surround completely. While the Seljuk Turks inside the city were able to bring supplies in through several gates, the starving Crusaders were forced to search 40 or 50 miles away for even the slightest bit of food. A harsh, cold, wet winter—which they had not expected—took its toll on the foreign soldiers, many of whom deserted.

Persistence paid off for the remaining soldiers when they captured the city during a surprise attack in early June. Within a few days, however, the Turkish leader Kerbogha (emir of Mosul) arrived to defend Antioch and ended up besieging the Franks (French) within the city. Without food for several weeks, too feeble even to guard the gates of the walls, the Crusaders seemed certain to perish, until the lance purportedly used in the Crucifixion was discovered. Fired by devotion to their faith, the Crusaders took the offensive on June 28 and routed Kerbogha's troops in the plain outside the city.

Although the siege was over, the sufferings of the Crusaders were not. Disease broke out in their ranks, undoubtedly fueled by the hot summer and the lack of supplies. The epidemic might have been typhoid, scurvy, malaria, or any of the other army diseases. In his history of the early Crusades, the twelfth-century churchman William of Tyre writes that the cause of the epidemic was not known, but that its lethal nature was certain. All groups of people died, including the papal legate Adhemar, bishop of Le Puy (who died on August 1), some of the Frankish princes, and especially women. (In addition to the wives, servants, and prostitutes who had accompanied the Crusaders, there were Christian women living in Antioch.) At least 30 to 40 corpses were buried each day.

As they waited for the epidemic to abate (it finally did in September), many princes took their small armies out of Antioch to escape the pestilence and busied themselves by capturing other towns nearby. Disease may have followed them: Without mentioning any symptoms, William of Tyre says that famine and sickness befell the troops at Marra, a town near Antioch. Weary of delay and hardship, the soldiers set fire to the town, hoping to prod their leader, Raymond of Toulouse (Count Raymond IV), into leaving. Raymond acquiesced to their wishes and set out for Jerusalem in January, with the other Crusader princes and troops following along.

Further reading: William of Tyre, *A History of Deeds Done Beyond the Sea*; Billings, *The Cross and the Crescent*; Runciman, "The First Crusade: Antioch to Ascalon."

Crusader Epidemic at Damietta Severe outbreak of scurvy that killed 15 to 20 percent of the Crusader army during its siege of Damietta (Dumyât, Egypt) in the winter of 1218–19 during the Fifth Crusade (1217–21). Attacking the valuable Nile delta—in the western half of the Muslim empire—was part of the Crusaders' strategy to get back Jerusalem. By gaining control of the Egyptian port cities, they hoped to force the Muslims to sue for peace and offer Jerusalem in exchange.

In spring 1218 the Crusaders encamped opposite Damietta, which was situated on the other bank of the Nile and protected by the sultan's army outside its walls. A large chain across the river and a fortified tower in midstream prevented the Crusaders from crossing and engaging the Muslim troops in battle. After three months of effort, the Crusaders captured the tower and sliced the chain in late August. Shocked at this feat, the Muslims nonetheless fought on, using sunken ships to block the river.

For several months both sides launched inconclusive attacks on the other. Then a torrential rain storm in late November, lasting three days straight, seemed to spell the ruin of the Christians. Floodwaters submerged their tents, swept away their food supplies, and cast adrift many transport ships. Similar floods and destruction in the Muslim camp kept the situation from becoming disastrous for the Crusaders. After the storm, however, disease spread through the Christian ranks. The symptoms described by the chroniclers make it possible to diagnose scurvy: swollen gums, loss of teeth, and legs that swelled up and festered as the skin turned black. According to the chroniclers, the epidemic killed either one fifth or one sixth of the Christians, including the papal legate, Robert of Courcon, whose preaching in France had won many adherents to the crusade.

At the same time, disease was rampant among the Muslim army and the inhabitants of Damietta. In addition, intrigues within his camp alarmed the sultan, who fled in panic with his troops in early February 1219, leaving Damietta undefended. Even after their heavy losses in the epidemic, the Crusaders were able to cross the Nile unopposed and lay siege to the town, which they conquered in November 1219.

Further reading: Billings, *The Cross and the Crescent*; Grousset, *The Epic of the Crusades*; Prinzing, *Epidemics Resulting from Wars*; Van Cleve, "The Fifth Crusade."

Cyprian, Plague of See PLAGUE OF CYPRIAN.

D

Dalmatian Plague of 1783–84 Infectious bubonic plague that killed more than 3,000 people in Dalmatia (region in southern Croatia, lying along the east shore of the Adriatic Sea), which was ruled by the Venetian Republic at the time of the epidemic. Though plague had retreated from most of Europe by the eighteenth century, it continued to infect regions in the Balkan Peninsula, which had close ties with the Ottoman Empire (Turkey), where the plague bacillus was prevalent in rats and fleas (disease carriers).

During a famine in Dalmatia in 1782, inhabitants fled inland to the Turkish region around Sarajevo in Bosnia. There they contracted plague and carried it with them when returning home in 1783 (it can be transmitted from person to person by airborne droplet infection). On the frontier between Dalmatia and Bosnia, militia were stationed to halt diseased Dalmatians, who were isolated in specially built huts, but plague nevertheless made its way farther into the coastal territory.

By September 1783 the territory close to the Croatian seaport of Split (Spljet or Spalato) had become plague-infected. A Venetian blockade was set up to deter the movement of infected persons into Split. Inland to the northwest, the town of Knin was gravely struck by plague in October and recorded 215 human deaths from it by February 1784. By then 320 persons living outside Split had also died, and a lazaret or lazaretto (hospital for the treatment of contagious diseases) had been established in the borough of Luzaz.

In mid-March 1784 some inhabitants of Split began dying suspiciously, with buboes (swellings in the groin). Venetian authorities soon confirmed the plague, enacted laws to close churches and synagogues, set up a camp in a remote area for the disinfection of flea-infested garments and goods, and opened another lazaret. All communication between Split and the rest of Dalmatia was cut off, but for three months plague continued to affect thousands of people in Split and the surrounding countryside; the dead were conveyed in boats to remote burying grounds. A reported 1,201 persons in Split (ten percent of its population) perished from plague, which ceased to kill victims there after June 1784.

Further reading: Howard, *Prisons and Lazarettos;* Shattuck, *Diseases of the Tropics.*

Dancing Mania (St. John's Dance, St. Vitus's Dance, Tarantism) Epidemics of hysteria that appeared in the form of dancing. Dancing mania, or epidemic chorea, was predominantly a psychic rather than physical illness. At various times and places in Western Europe, groups of people gathered in the streets and danced for hours, often calling out to saints to save them or to demons to release them from torment. For the most part, the various dancing manias were a manifestation of the fear, frustration, suspicion, and horror people felt during earlier plague years. Understandably, people responded to their disturbed feelings by attempting to do something about them, or at least by trying to find a culprit for what had happened or was happening in their lives and times. In this way, dancing mania was closely related to the flagellant movement—a cult desperate to find someone or something responsible for the Black Death (q.v.)—which spread throughout Europe in 1348. Participants in both movements attempted to divert the punishment of a great evil by chastising themselves.

Dancing mania appears to have occurred as early as the twelfth century. The barefoot Friar Johann Paulus told a story of a dancing mania that took place in a village in Saxony during that century, but the first large dancing mania did not appear in Germany until 1374. The epidemic began on the Rhine and in Flanders and moved to Cologne, Treves, Metz, and Liège. The large frenzy died out within a year, but smaller epidemics reappeared on and off for several centuries.

The most serious outbreak of dancing mania in Germany started at Aix-la-Chapelle (Aachen) in July of 1374; it was later referred to as St. John's Dance as its occurrence corresponded with St. John's Day

(June 24). The first part of the event was chronicled by Peter of Herental, a monk who seems to have witnessed several days of the manic dancing. According to him, the dancers were truly suffering from demonic possession and tried to free themselves through frantic dancing. These people formed a large group in the street and danced for hours. Some of them screamed and foamed at the mouth, calling out the names of demons and begging to be released. In later stages, some of the dancers appeared to be insensitive to pain and called out to onlookers to trample on them. There are other chronicles of the event that provide a more cynical explanation, saying that the dancing was conducted as a swindle. Possibly suspicion was aroused by the fact that most of the dancers were poor people—peasants, artisans, beggars, servants, and unmarried women. Their movements often ended in increased sexual activity, perhaps explaining why so many of the women were pregnant. In addition, some of the dancers asked the onlookers for money.

At first, the dancers did not appear to have any motive other than cleansing themselves of demonic possession. After a while, others joined the group and imitated the behavior of the original dancers. The craze then developed into an anti-clerical protest. Mobs shouted abuse at priests and blamed the clergy for not baptizing their children correctly. In a town near Herstal, Belgium, a number of dancers vowed to kill the clergy. The priests responded by exorcising as many of the dancers as possible. After many appeared to be healed, the clergy acquired a great reputation.

In 1518, an epidemic of manic dancing broke out in Strasbourg, France. It became known as St. Vitus's Dance (see STRASBOURG DANCING MANIA). Many of the participants are said to have danced themselves to death. There are several versions of exactly what happened, but the best known maintain that many of the dancers were cured after they were sent to the nearby monastery of St. Vitus where a Mass was said over them and holy water was sprinkled over them in the name of St. Vitus (a fourth-century Sicilian martyr who is invoked against many diseases and who is the patron of dancers).

By the beginning of the seventeenth century, although the dancing mania was beginning to die out in Germany, another dancing mania was at its height in Italy. From the fifteenth to seventeenth centuries, tarantism was prevalent in southern Italy. At the time, the illness was attributed to the bite of the tarantula (large, hairy spider). The illness was most likely psychic in origin and spread by sympathy, as the St. John's and St. Vitus's dances were. Those affected with tarantism fell into a state of melancholy and often wept. When they heard music, they displayed an uncontrollable impulse to dance and did so until they fell to the ground. It was believed at the time that those suffering from tarantism dispelled their melancholy through dancing and music.

Almost all the theories of the cause of manic dancing state that psychological factors were behind the craze. It is possible, however, that the dancing mania of medieval Germany, at least, had a physical cause; ergot of rye has a chemical compound that can cause hallucinations, agitation, colored vision, and increased susceptibility to external influences. The dancing mania at Aix-la-Chapelle may very well have been caused, at least initially, by rye bread that was infected with ergot.

Further reading: Cartwright, *Disease and History*; Marks and Beatty, *Epidemics*; Nohl, *The Black Death*.

Danzig Plague of 1602   See PRUSSIAN PLAGUE OF 1602.

Danzig Plague of 1709   Six-month epidemic of plague in the East Prussian port of Danzig (Gdańsk, Poland) that killed 24,533 city inhabitants and 8,066 people in the surrounding suburbs from June through December 1709.

A letter written from Danzig on October 22, 1709, describes the thievery, and appalling treatment, of the dead that was typical in times of plague:

> Great wickedness is committed by godless men who turn to robbing and stealing and secretly slip into the houses. In cases where they know that there is something worth stealing and one or two persons alive in the house, they ill-treat them or even murder them, and take possession of what they desire. The houses are searched daily, morning and evening; the dead are carried out and the sick handed over to the care of the plague doctors. It frequently happens that in a single day and night more than a hundred people are buried, of whom a few are provided with coffins [carpenters could not keep up with the demand for coffins]; but the majority are simply placed in a grave 12, 20, 30, even 50 together, piled up above one another—and I have often heard that the people are frequently not quite dead and are yet carried away by the impatient gravediggers like so many carcasses.

To help alleviate the suffering of the poor during the epidemic, Danzig's town council provided free bread, and paid two *Pestprediger* (plague-priests) to visit the sick. In addition to the miseries the plague caused directly, a thinned-out population and uncommonly heavy rains resulted in a crop failure, so that high prices and hunger, as well as more plague, which caused another 1,800 deaths, continued well into 1710.

Danzig's plague of 1709, the last large-scale epidemic the city would experience, was equal in destruction to the epidemic of 1602, which claimed nearly 19,000 victims (see PRUSSIAN PLAGUE OF 1602); another virulent outbreak, which killed 11,600 people, occurred in 1653.

Further reading: Nohl, *The Black Death;* Siegler, *Danzig, Chronik eines Jahrtausends.*

Danzig Typhus Epidemic of 1807

Unexpected outbreak of lice-borne typhus fever among French besiegers and Prussian defenders of the city of Danzig (Gdańsk, Poland) in the spring of 1807 at the time of Napoleon's campaigns in Prussia (roughly northeast Germany and northwest Poland). Encamped outside the city from March through the end of May, French General François-Joseph Lefebvre's 38,000 troops suffered high losses from typhus, while the Prussian garrison of 15,000 soldiers was so weakened from both typhus and scarcity of food that they were forced to capitulate (April 27); Lefebvre's capture of Danzig earned him the title "duc de Dantzig" in 1808. Napoleon entered Danzig on June 1, by which time the epidemic had largely run its course. Typhus fever would break out in Danzig with more deadly force during a siege of the city in 1813 (see DANZIG TYPHUS EPIDEMIC OF 1813; GERMAN TYPHUS EPIDEMICS OF 1813–14, NORTHERN AND CENTRAL).

Further reading: Prinzing, *Epidemics Resulting from Wars;* Siegler, *Danzig, Chronik eines Jahrtausends.*

Danzig Typhus Epidemic of 1813

Outbreak of epidemic typhus fever among the French garrison and civilian population of the city of Danzig (Gdańsk, Poland) during a siege from January 11 to November 29, 1813, following the return of Napoleon's army from Russia at the end of 1812 (see NAPOLEON'S ARMY EPIDEMICS IN RUSSIA). Much of the army was already suffering from typhus fever (see PRUSSIAN TYPHUS EPIDEMICS OF 1812–14); of nearly 36,000 troops and officers defending the city, approximately 25,000 were ill or weakened from wounds and exposure, unable to bear arms.

Thousands of soldiers died in Danzig under deplorable conditions during the course of the siege, according to Siegler: "As there were no hospitals, beds or remedies, many died from lack of care, and at the same time infectious diseases broke out and made great havoc. A cluster of dead men and horses was a common sight in the streets, and in a short time many thousands of the troops, as well as of the inhabitants, were carried away." Four hundred men died in January, 2,000 in February, 4,000 in March,

3,000 in April, and 2,000 in May. During February and March, 200 to 300 civilians died every week: "almost every family was in mourning, and many families were wiped out entirely." After having abated somewhat during the summer months, the epidemic broke out with renewed force near the end of the siege in November, killing 245 inhabitants in just two weeks; by this time typhus had also spread among the Prussian and Russian besiegers.

Added to the misery caused by typhus fever, troops and civilians—but not the army officers, who had hoarded food and supplies and lived comfortably throughout the siege—suffered extreme hardships from lack of food and fuel due to fire-bombing of the city's storehouses; many people during the latter part of the siege died of starvation and exposure. By the end of the siege nearly 16,000 soldiers and 5,600 civilians had died, the majority from typhus fever.

Further reading: Prinzing, *Epidemics Resulting from Wars;* Siegler, *Danzig, Chronik eines Jahrtausends.*

Delhi Hepatitis Epidemic of 1955–56

Large, explosive epidemic of viral hepatitis that attacked the city of Delhi in northern India during the winter of 1955–56. At that time, infectious hepatitis was considered endemic (existing in a region permanently) in Delhi (population 1.8 million), with about 5,000 cases reported each year.

During 1955–56, massive contamination of one of the city's main water supply sources led to its largest recorded epidemic of viral hepatitis. The source of the contamination, it was later discovered, was sewage from the Najafgarh drain that had accidentally backed up into the Wazirabad pumping-station (supplying water to many areas of Delhi) from November 10 to 16, 1955. Thousands of unsuspecting citizens were thus exposed to the infection during that period and many fell sick after an 18- to 62-day incubation period.

The resulting epidemic was brief, lasting six to seven weeks (December 1, 1955–January 20, 1956), and explosive, ending as suddenly as it had begun. The incidence was widespread and cases were reported simultaneously from far-flung areas of the city. Before any preventive measures could be implemented, the hospitals were crowded beyond capacity. Overall, some 97,000 cases were estimated to have occurred, 29,300 of them icteric (with jaundice). Seventy-three deaths were recorded in the latter group. The outbreak peaked between December 20, 1955, and January 4, 1956. Those in the 15–39-year-old category suffered the highest incidence (2.9 percent). The attack rate was slightly lower (two percent) in those above 40 years of age and even lower (1.2 percent) in those under 14 years of age. It was higher in men than in women and noticeably higher among upper income families, who presumably lacked the resistance and immunity possessed by their less fortunate neighbors. The attack rate among the cantonment troops was 50 per 1,000 for those on the Delhi waterline and 1 per 1,000 for those drinking well water. The rate among officers was twice that of the troops and four times that of the city sweepers. Pregnant women suffered a higher morbidity rate (three times as much) than other women and a significantly higher mortality (10.5 percent) than was recorded for the population as a whole (0.99 percent).

The initial or prodromal phase of the disease, characterized by gastrointestinal symptoms during this outbreak, lasted about two to three days. Generally, though, the course of the disease was relatively mild, with symptoms of weakness, anorexia, nausea, fever, pain in the upper abdomen, and a yellowing of the eyes and skin. The average incubation period of 40 days was longer than usual for hepatitis, but this has been attributed partly to the prompt treatment (since the contamination was discovered not long after it had occurred) of the water with additional alum and chlorine. Also, different strains of the hepatitis virus may have been involved, and the development of the infection may have been delayed in a partially immune population. Given the extent and intensity of the initial exposure, no secondary wave of infection was observed in the community.

Further reading: Melnick, "A Water-Borne Urban Epidemic of Hepatitis," and Viswanathan, "Certain Epidemiological Features of Infectious Hepatitis During the Delhi Epidemic, 1955–56," in Hartman et al., eds., *Hepatitis Frontiers.*

Dublin Plague of 1604–05   See IRISH PLAGUE OF 1604–05.

Dublin Plague of 1650–51   See IRISH PLAGUE OF 1650–51.

Durban Dengue Epidemic of 1926–27   Large outbreak of dengue fever that infected an estimated 50,000 persons in and around the seaport of Durban in east Natal, South Africa. This infectious tropical and sub-tropical disease, caused by a virus transmitted by the bite of the *Aëdes aegypti* mosquito, is characterized by agonizing pain in the joints (hence it is also called breakbone fever) and frequently produces a dandified manner of walking in its victim (hence it is sometimes called dandy fever).

Late in 1926 dengue (pronounced *den-gee* or *dengay*) swiftly attacked many inhabitants of Durban; it had apparently swept from the nearby coastal town of Stanger in the north to Pinetown on the main railway line to Durban, continuing south to Kelso Junction. About ten percent of Durban's population were bitten by diseased mosquitoes and, three to 12 days later, suddenly came down with fevers of 104° F or higher, severe frontal headaches, excruciating aches and pains in their limbs, and rashes. Victims' convalescence was long and difficult, often lasting for weeks or even months. Mortality is generally low in dengue epidemics, but in the Durban cases, hemorrhagic symptoms were reported in a large number of them: the dengue virus attacked the circulatory system and precipitated bleeding from the nose and mouth, causing numerous human deaths. The infection struck men, women, and children of all ages and races. Only those immune as a result of previous dengue infection seemed to escape the epidemic, which ended in early 1927. It has been shown that extensive dengue epidemics appear only in endemic communities that have been free from the disease for a considerable number of years; this was the circumstance in Durban, where the last dengue outbreak had occurred in 1897. Authorities initially thought that the virus in Durban had been carried widely by convalescents, but this theory was later overturned when it was proven that a person is infectious only as long as the fever lasts, which is seldom longer than the first three days. In addition, the disease's virus is not transmitted person-to-person; a mosquito becomes infected only when it bites an infectious person (or possibly a monkey) during the first three days of the sickness; the mosquito remains infected for life.

There are no known drugs or vaccines effective against dengue. Medical treatment usually consists of cool sponging to lower the high fever, codeine or other pain-relieving drugs, and, in the case of dengue hemorrhagic fever, blood plasma and adrenalin. The eradication of mosquitoes and their breeding places is basic to controlling the disease.

Further reading: Cluver, *Public Health in South Africa;* Scott, *A History of Tropical Medicine.*

E

Ecuadoran Plagues of 1908–88   Arrival of bubonic plague in the port city of Guayaquil aboard a ship sailing from Paita, Peru, in 1908; affecting close to 8,000 people in the Ecuadoran port before striking thousands more elsewhere in the country in sporadic, rural outbreaks. The disease, which is caused by the bacteria *Yersinia pestis* and is spread from infected rodents and their fleas to man, was first noted in Guayaquil's rat population and then spread to the populace there. The 1908 plague cases in Guayaquil drew Ecuador into the worldwide pandemic of bubonic plague that is said to have begun in Hong Kong in 1894 (see HONG KONG PLAGUE OF 1894).

In Guayaquil (whose population in 1905 was 81,650), the medical community fortunately had braced itself for an invasion of plague, having heard that other port cities in Latin America were infected. The formation of a bacteriological institute, the acquisition of the valuable Yersin serum (at the time, the only treatment for the infection) from Europe, and an active rat eradication project helped mute the epidemic. Nevertheless, the 1908 outbreak made a profound impression on the Ecuadoran leadership and has been credited with creating support for a costly public health campaign. From 1908 through 1913, many coastal cities in Guayas, where Guayaquil is located, and in Manabi, Los Rios, and El Oro provinces were affected by the spreading bubonic plague epidemic. Esmereldas province, somehow, was not involved. The disease spread from the coastal cities to Ecuador's sierra (mountains) quickly, chiefly via the railroad. All areas of the mountainous region were affected at some time during the period 1909–39, from Guaytacama, a small village near Ecuador's northern border with Colombia, to the province of Loja, on the southern border with Peru. The Loja outbreak, which occurred from 1918 to 1926, was a result of infection from across the Peruvian border rather than from the Ecuadoran railway line.

Plague started to disappear from the coastal cities in 1924, and the coast was considered plague free by 1930. In 1935, however, Guayaquil was again the site of plague, and remained so until the last case was recorded on April 14, 1939, bringing the total number of cases recorded in that city from the time of the initial outbreak in 1908 to 7,863, with 3,113 deaths. In the small villages of the sierra the disease persisted as a rural, endemic pestilence, requiring constant vigilance on the part of health authorities to prevent its spread.

Despite the eradication of plague in Guayaquil, periodic flare-ups of the disease have been reported along the coast. Infected fleas stowing away in bags of merchandise from Loja province were blamed for reintroducing plague to El Oro province, where small numbers of cases were recorded in 1939, 1940, 1950, and 1954. The island of Puna in the Gulf of Guayaquil was also the site of a small outbreak in 1954; again the disease came from Loja province. Wool exported from the island led to two more cases in Guayas province, not far from Guayaquil, in 1955. In the late 1950s and early 1960s, additional minor outbreaks in the coastal provinces were reported, the disease having spread there from Chimborazo province in the Andes, or from Loja province. The coastal city of Manta and its environs in Manabi province were hard hit between 1961 and 1963.

In Ecuador's interior, Chimborazo, Tungurahua, Canar, and Loja provinces have all been major sites of plague. In Chimborazo, the disease first appeared in 1909, affecting 1,420 persons, chiefly in towns, from 1909 to 1939. Thereafter, plague in Chimborazo became primarily a rural disease, with 365 more cases between 1940 and 1963. Mortality rates in Chimborazo were high, as high as 85.7 percent in 1946.

Tungurahua, adjacent to Chimborazo, had reported plague as early as 1926, with an epidemic affecting 100 persons in 1929. The disease was reintroduced in 1956, probably via infected guinea pigs from Chimborazo or via rail from the coast.

In Canar, just south of Chimborazo, 200 cases with high mortality were recorded in 1933. Smaller outbreaks were noted in 1945, 1951, and 1953, the latter said to be imported from Loja province.

Plague reached Loja province in 1918 in the Cazaderos-Alamor area before finally arriving at the city of Loja in 1926. The province became a major focus of the disease, particularly during the May through December dry seasons, with 2,795 cases and 887 deaths from 1926 through 1956. Another 222 cases were recorded in the province through 1963. Wild rodents from Peru have been blamed for the Loja outbreaks.

World Health Organization statistics indicate continued incidence of plague in Ecuador throughout the 1960s, with a sharp decline in the 1970s. There was a resurgence in the disease in Chimborazo in the early 1980s, with 65 cases occurring between January and April 1983. There were only three cases of plague from 1985 through 1988, all in 1985 in Loja, apparently having been spread there from across the Peruvian border. Hamsters and rabbits have been implicated in the spread of plague in Ecuador, along with the usual rat vector.

Further reading: Pan American Health Organization, *Plague in the Americas*; Pan American Health Organization, *Health Conditions in the Americas*.

Ecuadoran Yellow Fever Epidemics of 1740, 1743, and 1842   See GUAYAQUIL YELLOW FEVER EPIDEMICS OF 1740, 1743, AND 1842.

Edinburgh Plague of 1530   First of four major epidemics of bubonic plague to afflict Edinburgh and other towns of Scotland in the sixteenth century. Preceded by at least half a dozen less severe outbreaks during the first quarter of the century, especially the years 1502–05, 1512, 1519–20, and 1529, this visitation began in Edinburgh in May 1530 and lasted through the end of September. Aberdeen and probably many other places between the Firth of Forth, where Edinburgh is situated, and the Firth of Moray in the north of Scotland, were affected too.

Civic authorities in all Scottish burghs (chartered towns) had begun to issue strict regulations in time of plague, both to avert it and to deal with it once it arrived. Far harsher than their English counterparts, Scottish authorities ordered perpetual banishment, branding, and even death as punishments for disobeying certain decrees. For example, a tailor was hung in front of his own door because he both failed to notify the authorities that his wife had plague and attended church while she was ill (fortunately the rope broke and the man was given the lesser sentence of banishment from Edinburgh). A woman accused of bringing the plague to Edinburgh from the nearby town of Leith, and another of attending church and moving freely about while infected with the disease, were drowned for these crimes. These

and many other equally unfortunate men and women were victims of the erroneous belief that bubonic plague is spread through human contact, whereas it can be transmitted only through the bite of a flea. The flea, having ingested the deadly plague bacillus (*Pasteurella pestis*) from its plague-infected rat host, then regurgitates it into the bloodstream of a human being.

It is not known where the epidemic of 1530 originated, but it was almost certainly imported into Scotland from an English or foreign port. Although bubonic plague can remain endemic in a rat population, which can result in minor outbreaks in human communities from time to time, a major epidemic evidently requires the introduction of a fresh strain of *Pasteurella pestis* into a given rat population virulent enough to create a quantity of "plague-blocked" fleas sufficient to infect large numbers of human beings.

Further reading: Creighton, *A History of Epidemics in Britain*; Daiches, *Edinburgh*; Dickinson, *A New History of Scotland*; Shrewsbury, *A History of Bubonic Plague in the British Isles*.

Edinburgh Plague of 1568–69   Second serious outbreak of bubonic plague to afflict Edinburgh, Scotland, in the sixteenth century. Spanning two plague seasons, from September to December 1568 and from spring 1569 to autumn 1569, this epidemic may have claimed ten percent of Edinburgh's estimated population of 25,000.

As in prior years, strictly enforced regulations were issued to avoid and control the pestilence. Many involved procedures for maintaining the plague-sick in isolation huts outside the city gates. Officers were appointed to supervise the cleaning of infected houses and the removal of household members to the isolation site. Clothing and other items belonging to infected persons were cleaned in a special caldron from which nothing could be removed upon pain of death. Two men and two women were chosen to bury plague victims in graves that had to be seven feet deep (in contrast to plague-burials in England, where corpses were often hastily buried in very shallow graves). These measures were useless in stopping the spread of plague, which is transmitted to humans from the bite of fleas, whose natural host is the house-dwelling rat (see EDINBURGH PLAGUE OF 1530). Those persons forced to the isolation moor would in fact be safe from plague because the plague-infected rats would remain in the houses of the town; but when sent back to their homes, these unfortunate people would once again be at risk.

Although ignorant of the plague's true cause, people observed that major outbreaks seemed to be brought to a city from somewhere outside. Thus civic authorities were always alert to news of plague in other places. Accordingly, in September 1569, a certain merchant was blamed for importing the disease into the city the previous year, and ships arriving from Denmark, where plague was reported, were ordered to unload their cargo outside of Edinburgh.

The first medical work by a Scotsman (Dr. Gilbert Skeyne), and written in the vernacular, to make it accessible to the common people, appeared during this epidemic. Like most medical tracts of the period, this book was largely a reiteration of theories and advice that had been circulating for centuries, but it offered an interesting and important eyewitness account of the deplorably insanitary conditions of Edinburgh, where the custom of leaving human waste to rot in the streets caused contamination of the water supply, proliferation of disease-transmitting vermin, and other serious health hazards.

Further reading: Creighton, *A History of Epidemics in Britain*; Shrewsbury, *A History of Bubonic Plague in the British Isles*; Smout, *A History of the Scottish People, 1560–1830*.

Edinburgh Plague of 1585 Severe epidemic of bubonic plague affecting Edinburgh and many other towns of the east coast of Scotland. First appearing in July 1584 in the seaport town of Wester Wemyss, into which it was probably imported from Flanders, where it was then epidemic, the plague spread to several boroughs between the Firth of Tay and the Firth of Forth before reaching Edinburgh in May 1585, where it destroyed as much as ten percent of the population.

The civic authorities claimed the disease entered Edinburgh "by the infectioun of a woman who had beene in Sanct Johnstoun, where the plague was" and immediately issued a series of ordinances to combat the epidemic. Citizens were prohibited from sheltering travelers without permission; stray animals were slaughtered; and concealment of a case of plague was punishable by death. Fear of the disease caused the usual exodus from the city of all who were able to flee; in December the city recorded that due to desertion "the kirk [church] is now destitute of elders and deacons." The king left Edinburgh, moving from town to town as each refuge was successively invaded by the epidemic. A surgeon was appointed to care for the sick, and homeless children were sheltered at the city's expense. The customary isolation facilities were set up on the moor outside the city, and public gatherings, except for churchgoing and marketing, were prohibited.

The towns of Perth, Stirling, Falkland, St. Andrews, and Dundee also suffered from plague in 1585. After subsiding in winter, the plague appeared the next year in several scattered places. It probably visited Edinburgh once more, though less severely, in 1587.

Further reading: Creighton, *A History of Epidemics in Britain*; Shrewsbury, *A History of Bubonic Plague in the British Isles*; Smout, *A History of the Scottish People, 1560–1830*.

Edinburgh Plague of 1597 Last of four major epidemics of bubonic plague to attack Edinburgh, Scotland, and neighboring towns in the sixteenth century. This epidemic was widespread and killed many, but mortality figures are not known. Appearing in Inveresk at the end of June 1597 and probably imported to Scotland through the port of Musselburgh (near Edinburgh), the plague spread as far north as Dundee, and south to the English border. Edinburgh authorities gave considerable plague relief to the people of several afflicted towns, and took the usual measures in an effort to prevent its invasion of their own city, including posting watches at the town gates to inspect travelers for signs of exposure to plague, ordering beggars to leave the city, and isolating the sick upon the nearby moor. In September a couple was banished from Edinburgh forever for concealing the illness of their child, and in October a woman was ordered to be hanged for "conceilling of the pest and beand the caus of infection of sundry persons."

Bubonic plague in Scotland usually appeared first in port towns along the east coast, to which plague-infected rats were carried by ships coming from English and European ports. Quarantining of ships became a standard practice, which was effective only so long as the ships were barred from landing. Once docked, a ship's rats would move to shore and seek out permanent homes in the houses of the town, usually first invading the slums of the poor, whose dwellings were packed around dock areas and constructed of primitive materials ideal for the nesting of rats. If an epizootic was present among the rats, an epidemic of plague usually erupted among the human population through the agency of plague-carrying or "blocked" fleas (see EDINBURGH PLAGUE OF 1530).

Further reading: Creighton, *A History of Epidemics in Britain*; Dickinson, *A New History of Scotland*; Shrewsbury, *A History of Bubonic Plague in the British Isles*; Smout, *A History of the Scottish People, 1560–1830*.

Edinburgh Plague of 1604–07 See SCOTTISH PLAGUE OF 1600–1608.

Edinburgh Plague of 1644–46 See SCOTTISH PLAGUE OF 1644–48.

Egyptian Cholera Epidemic of 1883 Serious outbreak of cholera causing the death of more than

58,500 persons, mainly in the populous areas of upper Egypt. An important aspect of this one-year-long epidemic was the discovery made by German bacteriologist Robert Koch in 1883 in Egypt of the microorganism or bacterium that is the cause of the acute infection of cholera: *Vibrio comma* (or *cholera vibrio*).

The disease cholera appeared for the first time in Egypt in 1831, when Egypt's khedive (viceroy), Mehemet Ali, asked consuls of the European powers to use the city of Alexandria as an outpost to provide health assistance for the Egyptian people. Thereafter this Egyptian city became an epidemiological laboratory for Western European scientists.

At the time Mecca (the Islamic holy city in western Saudi Arabia) was the most notorious diffusion center for the spread of cholera, which broke out epidemically there 33 times between 1830 and 1912. Cholera was frequently introduced into the Alexandria-Cairo area by Muslim pilgrims returning from Mecca and spread up the Nile into upper Egypt and sometimes into the Sudan. Libya, Tunisia, Algeria, and Morocco were also infected via Egypt by cholera epidemics originating in Mecca. Various transportation routes and commercial centers were principally responsible for the spread of cholera, which was carried about by Mediterranean ships that called at North African ports.

British scientists had been studying the disease in India for some time when, in 1846–47, the English physician John Snow concluded that cholera was not carried by bad air or by direct contact. He saw intractable diarrhea, unwashed hands, and shared food as leading factors responsible for spreading the disease. In addition, Snow determined that cholera-contaminated excrement, by permeating the ground and getting into public wells, was mixing with water used for drinking and cooking; diseased discharge also ran along channels and sewers into rivers from which entire towns were sometimes supplied with water. Diarrhea, acute spasmodic vomiting, and painful cramps are symptoms of cholera. A person's face becomes drawn, his extremities cold and withered; blood pressure falls, and the pulse becomes faint. With the increase in dehydration, the patient can become stuporous and comatose and may die of shock. Without treatment, death can occur swiftly, sometimes without any warning; the disease usually runs its course in two to seven days.

With the fresh outbreak of cholera in Egypt in 1883, leading French and German bacteriologists were dispatched to Alexandria to study the disease in depth and determine its cause. The French chose the experimental method of investigation by administering the cholera-contaminated dejecta (waste) to animals. The method failed to reproduce the disease in animals. One of the members of the French group (named Thullier) caught the disease at Alexandria and died before he was able to return to France.

Robert Koch, German physician and bacteriologist, had prepared a paper in Berlin in March 1882, announcing his discovery of the tubercle bacillus, the bacterium that is the cause of tuberculosis. Dr. Koch, who headed the German group in Egypt in 1883, performed autopsies on ten cholera victims within two to three hours after their deaths. His microscopic discovery was the short, curved, comma-shaped bacillus, which, after reaching the human intestine, causes the disease.

Shortly after Koch's discovery of the *Vibrio comma*, the epidemic in Egypt came to an end. To continue his research, the German government sent him to the Medical College in Calcutta, India, where he succeeded in confirming his preliminary findings in Egypt, by performing additional autopsies as well as other tests on cholera-contaminated stools, vomit, and water. While his views were not completely accepted, his continued research, especially after the Hamburg Cholera Epidemic of 1892 (q.v.), wherein he used peptone water as an enriched medium for cultivation of the microorganism, led to new tests being devised, differentiating the specific germ of true cholera from other vibrios (rigid, motile, comma-shaped bacteria).

The *Vibrio comma* enters the human body via the mouth, usually in contaminated food or water, causing an infection in the mucous membrane lining the lumen of the small intestine. Unwashed hands or uncooked fruits and vegetables as well as sewage-contaminated water systems are the prime ways to spread cholera.

Dr. Koch's findings paved the way for the extensive study of water purification and sewage disposal. The germ theory of cholera introduced new methods for guarding against the disease, including the implementation of chemical disinfectants and heat to kill the bacillus. Further, ways for more careful handling of the sick were employed to guard against passing cholera to others. By 1893 a vaccine against the disease had been developed.

In Egypt, compulsory inoculation against cholera was instituted in 1913. While no epidemic of cholera has occurred in the country since, this is more likely attributable to safer sewage disposal and purer water supplies than to the vaccine. In recent years, it has been proven that current standard vaccines have not been effective in altering the transmission of cholera. Intensive studies continue toward developing an effective vaccine, but at present, clinical hygiene provides the only certain protection against cholera.

Further reading: De, *Cholera, Its Pathology and Pathogenesis; Oxford Textbook of Medicine;* Rosenberg, *The Cholera Years;* Stock, *African Environment Special Report 3: Cholera in Africa.*

Egyptian Cholera Epidemic of 1902

Serious outbreak of cholera that killed thousands of people in Egypt in the summer of 1902. Cholera occurs when sanitation is frequently inadequate and is spread by polluted water and food. It chiefly affects a person's small intestine.

Accounts of the 1902 epidemic in Egypt differ considerably. One account attributes it to an Egyptian Muslim returning from a pilgrimage to Islam's holy city of Mecca in western Saudi Arabia (the disease was often prevalent in Mecca, where some 4,000 people had died of it earlier in 1902). The Egyptian pilgrim brought a can containing holy water and poured it into his village's well, not realizing it was cholera-polluted; he had hoped to bring something sacred (not cholera) from Mecca to his neighbors, who had not been able to make the pilgrimage themselves. Instead, according to this account, a cholera epidemic erupted that allegedly took the lives of some 42,000 people.

Another account points to an infected well for touching off the epidemic, but differs on how the well became contaminated. Some returning Muslim pilgrims, who had contracted cholera at Mecca, developed symptoms (like diarrhea and cramps) while journeying home at Tor, a town on the east coast of the Gulf of Suez. Upon their return to Moucha, Egypt, these cholera-stricken Egyptians soon urinated in latrines close to the village's public well, located near the mosque in the center of Moucha. The well became contaminated, and water taken from it carried the disease to the village's first victims of the epidemic, in August 1902. During the next two months, according to this account, approximately 35,000 people in Egypt became infected with cholera (14,801 became ill during the first four weeks of the epidemic; 9,466 fell victim the fifth week; and morbidity dropped rapidly after 6,388 cases were recorded during the sixth week); thus purportedly there were only from 3,500 to 5,000 human deaths. Yet another source reported 31,540 deaths from the cholera, which had spread into Syria by early October.

Further reading: Gallagher, *Diseases that Plague Modern Man;* Scott, *A History of Tropical Medicine.*

Egyptian Cholera Epidemic of 1947

Catastrophic outbreak of cholera in Egypt, causing the death of more than 20,000 people, more than half of those infected with the disease, in less than three months.

Since 1923 the number of cholera cases had declined worldwide, while the disease continued to rage throughout the Indian subcontinent in periodic outbreaks. Prior to 1947, cholera had made its way into Egypt with groups of pilgrims returning from Mecca, resulting in major outbreaks that frequently began in Egypt's Alexandria-Cairo area. However, the cholera disease that entered Egypt in September 1947 is thought to have occurred as a result of the movement of British military personnel from India. Although Egypt was a sovereign independent state after 1922, British troops remained stationed there until 1952. On September 18, 1947, the first recorded cholera cases occurred in the Egyptian village of El Korein, the home of many workers employed at a nearby British military base. Unwashed hands, uncooked fruits and vegetables, and sewage-contaminated water supplies can easily spread cholera, which chiefly affects the human small intestine or digestive tract.

Thousands of traders from all over Egypt were attending a major date fair in the vicinity of El Korein at the same time that the first outbreak occurred. Many of the traders contracted cholera either directly from other infected traders or from eating contaminated dates. In a few days the disease was running rampant throughout the Nile River Delta; smaller outbreaks were also reported along the Nile as far as the town of Qinā. In less than three months, 32,978 people were sick with severe diarrhea and vomiting; death, mainly from dehydration, came swiftly to 20,474 infected persons by early December 1947.

After German bacteriologist Robert Koch identified the cholera bacillus while working in Egypt and India in 1883, methods for guarding against the dreaded disease were instituted in the two countries. Chemical disinfectants were used, as well as heat to kill the bacillus; also, those infected were carefully handled to prevent contagion of others. After 1913, when compulsory inoculation of a cholera vaccine was instituted, Egypt was generally free of cholera until 1947. The swift conveyance of this acute disease in 1947 did not allow for precautionary measures; also control measures were not instituted before this serious cholera epidemic (the worst outside of the Indian subcontinent since 1923) ended abruptly soon after the last case was recorded on December 5, 1947; it is not known if the epidemic moved out of Egypt.

Further reading: Ackerknecht, *History and Geography of the Most Important Diseases;* Stock, *African Environment Special Report 3: Cholera in Africa.*

Egyptian Diphtheria Epidemics of 1882–86

See CAIRO AND ALEXANDRIA DIPHTHERIA EPIDEMICS OF 1882–86.

Egyptian Malaria Epidemic of 1942–44   Serious epidemic of malaria infecting almost a million people in Egypt and killing as many as 200,000.

The mosquito *Anopheles gambiae*, a carrier of the protozoon responsible for the transmission of malaria to humans, traveled from Sudan down the Nile River to Egypt, where it had never been recorded prior to 1942 (tropical Africa is the natural home of the vector). The Nile River village of Abu Simbel reported the first outbreak of malaria, and government investigators found almost all of the village's 3,500 inhabitants infected at the end of April 1942. By then, malaria had spread about 4,300 miles into Egypt, especially along the Nile.

At that time (1942), much of the country had conditions suitable for malaria to spread: good breeding grounds (swamps and other stagnant water bodies) for mosquitoes, a human population that had never built up an immunity, and a population whose disease resistance had been weakened by undernourishment during World War II. Food shortages and overcrowding were among the hardships in British-occupied Egypt. Increased wartime ship traffic on the Nile helped the migration of the mosquito *gambiae* from the Sudan.

In 1942 Dr. Fred L. Soper, who had successfully fought a malaria outbreak in Brazil in 1938–40 and was a member of the Rockefeller Foundation, was assigned to the U.S. Typhus Commission in Cairo; he saw the seriousness of the epidemic and suggested a plan to the British and Egyptian authorities for immediate eradication: to spray 150 tons of the insecticide Paris green on potential mosquito-breeding places. But the authorities limited the insecticide to certain mosquito-occupied areas, and the epidemic was not halted.

By the closing months of 1943, government officials became convinced their eradication methods were futile and decided to employ Soper's program; within six months after systematically and simultaneously spraying all mosquito-breeding areas with Paris green, the epidemic ended in Egypt.

Further reading: Burnet and White, *Natural History of Infectious Disease;* Harrison, *Mosquitoes, Malaria and Man.*

Egyptian Plague of 1347–49   Catastrophic outbreak of plague in Egypt that killed hundreds and sometimes thousands of people daily during the early years of the Black Death (q.v.).

The dreaded plague entered the country through Alexandria, its chief port, with Italian merchants on ships coming from Constantinople (Istanbul); the ships carried rats infested with diseased fleas. In Alexandria, some 100 to 200 persons reportedly died each day in the first weeks of the epidemic. The mortality increased in the city as the temperatures increased, as many as 750 human deaths apparently occurring on particular days. Most of these deaths were from pneumonic plague, the most serious and highly infectious form. By the spring of 1348, human fatalities on some days evidently reached a thousand in Alexandria, where about 100,000 persons lived prior to the plague's devastation; the city would not again reach that number of inhabitants until the sixteenth century.

The important Egyptian port of Damietta was crippled by the plague epidemic, which brought its fishing trade to a standstill. The death toll in Damietta and other Nile Delta villages was large; at Bilbais, human bodies were piled in mosques, and shops and roads were littered with decaying cadavers. Plague moved up the Nile to Cairo, where human deaths averaged about 300 daily until the end of 1348. Many deaths were from septicemic plague, which infects the blood. Death was severe in Cairo, where some sources said 7,000 or more perished on some days in the late spring of 1348 and the early fall of 1349. At times there was a shortage of coffins in the city, and no shrouds were available in which to bury the dead.

From Cairo, the plague moved southward and eastward, reaching Aswan along the upper Nile by February 1349. Egyptians also helped spread the "Black Death" by land and sea to other regions in North Africa, such as Tunisia and Libya. See also BLACK DEATH IN THE MIDDLE EAST.

Further reading: Gottfried, *The Black Death;* Ziegler, *The Black Death.*

Egyptian Plague of 1834–35   Serious epidemic of mainly bubonic plague that killed at least 30,000 persons in Egypt over a period of about nine months.

In Egypt's northern port of Alexandria in July 1834, many of the workers in the cotton stores and in the harbor area came down with plague. Some British sailors who helped load bales of cotton onto England-bound ships contracted the disease also. Shortly, lazarets or lazarettos (hospitals for the treatment of contagious disease) were set up to isolate plague patients, as the epidemic continued to spread in Alexandria and then inland to Cairo on the Nile River. Some villages were hard hit; others were not infected by plague; in Cairo, a number of physicians died of it (some of them had never touched a diseased patient).

At the time it was still unknown that the plague bacillus can infect fleas that carry it to humans from infected rodents (often rats). Because for centuries plague had broken out in port cities after the arrival of infected ships, most doctors believed there was a direct connection between the disease and the exchange of goods. Doctors did not yet know that plague-ridden fleas are able to survive from six weeks up to a year after lodging in clothes, rags, carpets, and other goods, such as cotton. The contagion theory had long been popular among physicians and influenced them to use quarantine and other precautionary measures during plague outbreaks. However, French physician Antoine B. Clot, called Clot-Bey, who was then chief surgeon to Egypt's khedive or viceroy (Mehemet Ali), discounted the contagion theory and instead said that germs infecting the atmosphere were responsible for plague (the ancient miasmatic hypothesis). To prove this, he and his colleagues visited many cases of plague (in all stages of infection) in Cairo and conducted 100 postmortem examinations without taking special precautions, resulting in no ill effects. Clot-Bey inoculated himself with the blood of a plague patient and developed no symptoms at all, although the patient died. Other experiments were performed with serum from carbuncles and with clothing from plague patients; in some tests, there were no ill effects, but others resulted in plague deaths of physicians and others. (Plague pneumonia can be transmitted person to person by droplet infection, the coughing into the air of droplets from patients.)

Following the close of the epidemic in the spring of 1835, the medical authorities in Egypt concluded that about 33 percent of the plague-infected perished—mostly from the bubonic form, but also from the pneumonic and septicemic forms in some cases. During the next five years, numerous medical publications in Europe related this Egyptian epidemic, and the writings of Clot-Bey influenced students of epidemiology for the next 50 years; the medical profession in Egypt was split into two conflicting camps: miasma versus contagion.

Further reading: Gregg, *Plague: An Ancient Disease in the Twentieth Century;* Hirst, *The Conquest of Plague.*

Egyptian Poliomyelitis Epidemic of 1940–41
See NEW ZEALAND TROOPS POLIOMYELITIS EPIDEMIC OF 1940–41.

Egyptian Relapsing Fever Epidemic of 1944–46
Outbreak of louse-borne relapsing fever in Egypt, killing a reported 3,295 persons out of 128,541 infected. Relapsing fever, also called "recurrent fever," is characterized by headache, chills, and high fever. A sick person will apparently recover after a few days and then shortly become ill again; this pattern will continue if the infection is untreated.

This systemic spirochetal disease entered northern Egypt from the Libyan desert area to the west in the fall of 1944. Workers in Egypt's province of Beni Suef contracted the infection, which is transmitted by lice and ticks, and helped spread it southward into the province of Asyût (Assiout or Assiut). At the time (1944) Egypt's public health services were grossly inadequate, and typhus fever and malaria were afflicting thousands; consequently, conditions were also favorable for epidemic relapsing fever to occur.

In 1945 the epidemic moved rapidly from Asyût southward along the Nile River areas to Qina (Qena) province and eventually throughout the rest of Upper Egypt to Aswan province (southern Egypt on a map). To the north, the disease traveled from Beni Suef to the provinces of Minya, Fayum (Faiyum), and Giza—all bordering the Nile—subsequently penetrating the cities of Cairo, Alexandria, and Gharbiya, as well as the Suez Canal ports.

The epidemic ignited in 1946, with morbidity (incidence of disease) increasing progressively during the first three months of the year (some 44,000 persons were infected). Then the worst month came—April—with 35,430 cases of relapsing fever recorded. May was almost as bad, and afterward the epidemic declined due to help from the British and Americans, who supplied Egypt with DDT and other materials to combat the disease. In previous outbreaks of typhus in Egypt, DDT had been an effective method of delousing the population, but in 1946 many people, especially women in relapsing fever areas, refused to go to the DDT dusting stations; others refused to report the infection out of fear of being taken to special hospitals or to isolation camps. Thus the epidemic had increased during that period. Finally Egypt's Ministry of Health, assisted by volunteers from elite women's groups and the Muslim Brotherhood, was able to move into stricken regions to help delouse the sick in their homes and to inject acutely sick patients with Salvarsan (used for the treatment of relapsing fever, syphilis, and other spirochetal diseases) to prevent death from myocarditis. As a result, the epidemic came to an end in September 1946. Other methods for control of relapsing fever and other diseases were later introduced in Egypt, and since then no major relapsing fever epidemics have occurred in the country.

Further reading: Gallagher, *Egypt's Other Wars: Epidemics and the Politics of Public Health;* Simmons et al., *Global Epidemiology: A Geography of Disease and Sanitation.*

Egyptian Rift Valley Fever Epidemic of 1977
Severe epidemic of Rift Valley fever (RVF) that infected about 18,000 persons (killing 598 of them) in Egypt during the latter part of 1977.

In October 1977 Rift Valley fever, an arthropod-borne viral disease, broke out unexpectedly among the inhabitants in the lower region of the Nile River valley and Delta area; it paralleled a massive epizootic among the animal population of the region. This was the first time that RVF was known to have occurred north of sub-Sahara Africa. How the disease entered Egypt is not known for sure, but most likely the RVF virus entered Egypt by way of Sudan, where RVF epizootics had occurred in 1973 and 1976, being brought into the country with a large number of Sudanese camels (which Egypt imports annually). Studies have concluded that the arthropod vectors of RVF in Egypt were several species of mosquitoes (*Aëdes caballus*, *Aëdes circumluteolus*, and *Aëdes theileri*), which live on camels, sheep, or cattle; RVF is transmitted through the bite of an infective mosquito or by handling infective material of animal origin during necropsy and butchering. The RVF virus also may have come into Egypt with human beings or arthropods in air travel or with migratory birds and their ectoparasites.

Persons of all ages became infected in Egypt. They first complained of fever, malaise with an initial rigor, severe headache, and lower back myalgia (and occasionally nausea and vomiting). Their sudden fevers lasted four to seven days; complete recovery came within two weeks. Some patients developed encephalitis or ocular and hemorrhagic-like complications. The mortality rate ranged from a low of 0.2 percent among the military to 3.3 percent of the general population, to a high of 14 percent among those hospitalized. Official reports indicate that there were some 18,000 persons infected between October and December 1977; however, total infections may well have exceeded 200,000, according to other sources.

The RVF virus was first isolated in sheep and people during an epizootic in western Kenya's Rift Valley (hence the disease's name) in 1930. During the next 20 years limited RVF outbreaks occurred in several regions in East and South Africa. In terms of morbidity and mortality, the 1977 epidemic in Egypt is considered the largest and most serious outbreak of RVF among human beings and animals. In 1978 RVF broke out again in Egypt and spread to the Sinai area, infecting United Nations soldiers there. The importance of the RVF virus as a human pathogen (disease-producing microorganism) was realized as a result of these outbreaks.

Further reading: Hoeprich, ed., *Infectious Diseases*; Klingberg, ed., *Rift Valley Fever*.

Egyptian Typhus Epidemic of 1940–45 Widespread epidemic of louse-borne typhus fever in Egypt that infected more than 110,000 persons and killed as many as 20,000.

At the beginning of World War II, thousands of transient migrant workers were employed on large estates in the provinces of Beheira and Gharbîya in Lower Egypt. They lived in filthy, crowded conditions, under which epidemic typhus thrives along with the human body louse (*Pediculus humanus*) that carries this fatal rickettsial disease. Most of the lice-infested workers came from the provinces of Minûfiya and Daqahlîya in the Nile River delta of Lower Egypt, where typhus had been prevalent for the past 20 years.

Infection of louse-borne typhus occurs by the contaminative method, not by the bite of a louse; it can arise from crushed body lice or from feces of infected lice. Clothing, bedding, or dust containing dry, infected lice feces may remain contaminated for months. The mode of transmission of the infection is through a skin abrasion or by way of the conjunctiva or through the mucous membrane of the nasal passages or mouth.

The migrant workers brought the disease into the Egyptian cities of Cairo and Alexandria, and typhus incidence in these two cities increased from 16 cases per 100,000 people in 1941 to 125 per 100,000 in 1942. Between January 1943 and August 1944 Cairo reported 7,156 cases and 1,359 human deaths; most of the sick were men between 16 and 25 years old, but males between the ages of 41 and 48 suffered the highest rate of mortality (almost 50 percent); and more than twice as many men than women were infected. Cairo's most severe outbreaks occurred in the months of April and May 1943. The epidemic reached its peak in Egypt in 1943, when 40,188 cases were recorded, with 8,252 fatalities; it had spread into Upper Egypt as far as the province of Asyût (Assiut) by then.

By 1944 relapsing fever (another louse-borne disease) had swept into Egypt from Libya, and by 1946 it had killed 2,367 Egyptians and others. But the mortality rate was much lower than that for the typhus epidemic (about 20 percent). If DDT powder, a newly available insecticide, had been used to control lice infestation, the incidence of typhus would undoubtedly have been greatly reduced. When DDT was used in 1947 and 1948, typhus cases dropped to 173 and 325 respectively. Inoculations with a cox-type vaccine had also proven effective in reducing the duration of the fever and the number of deaths.

Further reading: Horsfall and Rivers, eds., *Viral and Rickettsial Infections of Man*; Simmons et al., *Global Epidemiology: A Geography of Disease and Sanitation*.

Encephalitis Lethargica (von Economo's Disease) Epidemic of 1915–26 Pandemic of an unusual form of encephalitis that was first observed in small outbreaks in Rumania and France in 1915. The disease then swept over the world, reaching Australia in 1917, North Africa in 1919, the United States in 1918–19, and parts of South America in 1919–20. Peaking during the winter of 1919–20, when tens of thousands of cases occurred in Europe alone, the epidemic then slowed dramatically; since 1926 only a very few, sporadic cases of the disease have been noted. The pandemic remains a medical mystery. Years after the disease essentially disappeared, scientists still do not know why it spread so widely before coming to a halt, or even what caused it.

In 1917, the symptoms of encephalitis lethargica were described by Constantin von Economo, a brain anatomist in Austria who first recognized it as a specific clinical entity and coined a term for it. In Vienna during the winter of 1916–17 he saw 11 cases (six of which were fatal) that did not fit any diagnosis of which he was aware. The early acute symptoms—headaches and malaise, often with fever—would be followed by somnolence and usually delirium. Patients could be awakened fairly easily, could even walk and follow instructions, but would lapse back into sleepiness if left alone. Paralysis could strike the extremities and cause rigidity and abnormal movements, but more frequently the ocular nerves were affected; in many patients the eyelids drooped considerably.

The nature and severity of the symptoms, and the course of the illness, varied significantly from patient to patient. The disease could last for weeks or for months, until the person died (as happened in an estimated 25 percent of all worldwide cases) or recovered completely (another 25 percent).

About half or more of all patients, however, seemed to be entirely free of the disease, only to be troubled by a return of symptoms from several months to five years later. In some people, the latency period lasted as long as 15 to 20 years. In children the aftereffects included personality and psychiatric disorders, such as abnormal agitation. More troubling still was postencephalitic parkinsonism, which was marked by rigidity, spasms, and fits in which the eyes rolled upward before the patient fell down. Other people could remain locked for decades in a state of suspended animation.

The exact number of people afflicted by the disease cannot be calculated; because the mildest symptoms resembled those of other illnesses, such as the common cold or influenza, many cases of encephalitis lethargica were undoubtedly not recognized as such. In London, for instance, where the disease appeared early in 1918, it was first mistaken for botulism. Because in some respects the disease resembled other diseases, von Economo investigated many possibilities in trying to determine the cause of the Vienna outbreak. Soon, he had ruled out food poisoning,

typhus, and tuberculosis. Influenza seemed a more likely candidate, especially since in many countries encephalitis lethargica coincided with the Spanish Influenza Epidemic of 1917–19 (q.v.). However, as von Economo himself pointed out, the first appearances of the disease he described came months before Vienna was struck by influenza. In searching for the etiologic agent, von Economo autopsied several of his patients and discovered lesions of the brain stem that were close to the areas affected in severe cases of poliomyelitis. He therefore concluded that the disease was the result of an entirely new virus. No such virus was ever isolated, however, nor were any antibodies to such a virus found, and the cause of encephalitis lethargica remains unknown.

The disease may have been around for centuries before von Economo observed it. When he surveyed the medical literature from the sixteenth century on, he turned up a number of reports of "sleeping sickness," "comatose fever," or "lethargic fever." Although the accounts were often too sketchy to permit accurate diagnosis, von Economo maintained that at least two of them represented outbreaks of the disease he studied in Vienna. In Tübingen, Germany, in 1712, many cases of sleepiness and noticeable central nervous system disorders were noted, while a wave of influenza in northern Italy in the early 1890s was followed by widespread somnolence, called "nona." After manifesting itself sporadically, encephalitis may have suddenly taken on epidemic form, but the reasons for its dramatic appearance and equally abrupt disappearance have never been determined.

Further reading: Von Economo's account of the Vienna outbreak is translated in Wilkins and Brody's "Encephalitis Lethargica"; Booss and Esiri, *Viral Encephalitis*; Debré, "Lethargic Encephalitis or von Economo's Disease."

English Pestilence of A.D. 664   See YELLOW PLAGUE OF A.D. 664.

English Plague of 1348–50   See PLAGUE OF ENGLAND, GREAT.

English Plagues of the 1400s   Periodic, uncertain epidemics of bubonic plague. Identification of the disease is difficult due to the absence of clinical descriptions in the unfortunately small number of surviving narrative chronicles and official town documents. The historian's task is further hindered by the medieval custom of lumping different diseases with similar symptoms under one catchall label (fever, for example), and the almost generic type of phraseology used by chroniclers. For example, we see the observation "So great pestilence had not been seen for many years," in reference to an epidemic in 1407, used in slightly varied ways in other documents throughout the century; a mortality figure of 30,000, which cannot have been consistently accurate, is also repeatedly used. Therefore, a reliable assessment of plague or other epidemics during the fifteenth century is not possible.

Further, there is much controversy among medical historians about the ebb and flow of plague in the black house-rat, a necessary condition for the presence of bubonic (and probably pneumonic) plague in human communities (see PLAGUE OF ENGLAND, GREAT). Because bubonic plague occurs mainly in the summer and autumn, historians point to unusually high mortality during these months (as indicated by parish burial records) as evidence of plague. However, several other diseases, such as typhoid fever and dysentery, are also most common in hot weather, so the recording of a "gret pestylens" or "gret mortalytie" that subsides in winter does not alone constitute sufficient proof to label a particular fifteenth-century outbreak as plague. The presence of plague in various localities at different times throughout the century is very possible and even quite likely, but this cannot be stated with certainty. What is evident beyond doubt is that many local and more widespread outbreaks of infectious disease occurred throughout the century.

A severe pestilence of some kind broke out in many parts of England, including Bristol and London, between 1405 and 1407. There were many outbreaks in the 1430s, and the famine years of 1438–39 were especially cruel. The period from about 1447 to 1454 saw several outbreaks of disease, especially in Oxford, Norwich, and London and its contiguous districts. The year 1464 is reported by an anonymous author in *A Short English Chronicle* as a year of great drought followed by "a grete pestilence through the realm," which apparently continued well into 1465 and erupted in 1466 and 1467 in London. These are just a few of the more notable national epidemics described, as was the custom, as pestilence or plague, but which offer the historian little clue as to what they actually were. A somewhat more certain incidence of bubonic plague occurred in London and other parts of England, notably Norwich, during the two summers and autumns of 1478 and 1479. Hull was scourged by disease in 1472 and 1476, and quite probably by bubonic plague in 1478.

Plague—that is, disease in general—was thought to be caused by corrupted air, or "miasma," which entered the body through open pores. Medical treatises (composed by continental Europeans, not Englishmen) advised minimal bathing, exercise, and

sexual intercourse, all activities believed to open the pores. Instructions on bloodletting were included in some medical works, and recipes made up of everyday kitchen ingredients were widely used. King Edward IV had a special plague remedy consisting of marigolds, various herbs, and "a lytell suger of candy" if the concoction was too bitter. The idea of corrupted air was put forward by well-educated men and was the prevailing theory for many centuries. In an age that could rely only on superficial observation, it was a sound guess: No one could have suspected that microscopic organisms were responsible for deadly sickness. It was the belief that miasmic air caused pestilence that caused Parliament either to prorogue many of its sessions or remove itself from London to outlying areas so many times in the second half of the century, to avoid the "corrupt and infected airs" of Westminster, where Parliament was housed. Individuals who could afford to do so regularly fled the towns where pestilence was present. The famous Paston Letters of the mid-1400s—correspondence between members of a prosperous Norfolk family—contain many references to pestilence and paint a very vivid picture of how defenseless people felt in the face of sickness.

In the minds of many medieval people, miasmic atmosphere was caused by the astrological conjunctions of the planets, which in turn were determined by the workings of God. Penance and confession was advocated by many writers as the surest way to appease God and thus avoid disease; moderate personal habits were considered extremely important too. Avoidance of physicians who, with some exception, were widely distrusted both for their frequently demonstrated ignorance and their corruption, was advised as well. See also LONDON PLAGUE OF 1499–1500.

Further reading: Creighton, *A History of Epidemics in Britain*; Gottfried, *Epidemic Disease in Fifteenth Century England*; Mullet, *The Bubonic Plague and England*; Shrewsbury, *A History of Bubonic Plague in the British Isles*; Slack, *The Impact of Plague in Tudor and Stuart England*.

English Plagues of the 1500s   Many isolated outbreaks of what presumably was bubonic plague in many parts of England. This period (1500s) is interesting for several reasons. First, the epidemiological character of bubonic plague, which was difficult to trace in earlier times due to a lack of statistical data, becomes clearer starting in 1538, when parishes begin to record marriages, baptisms, and deaths. Burial records—although they seldom noted the alleged cause of death—allow the historian to assess seasonal mortality and thereby to make informed guesses at the type of disease involved in a given epidemic.

Those records showing high death figures for the summer and fall, especially if supported by other evidence, can reasonably be assumed to have been bubonic plague, as the rat-fleas, which transmit the disease to humans from their plague-infected rodent hosts, are active only in warm weather. (Other diseases occur mainly in warm weather too, so caution must be used when labeling a given epidemic as plague if conclusive evidence is lacking.) It becomes apparent that, unlike other infectious diseases that usually affect widespread areas at once, plague often erupts in a given locality and spreads no farther or, if it does, travels only slowly and haphazardly to its next locale.

The human disease of plague is first of all dependent upon the rat disease, which must be present in the rat population of a given city or village. In order for bubonic plague to spread, plague-carrying rat-fleas or infected rats must be passively transported, embedded in clothing or in merchandise as people and goods move from place to place. Plague was often introduced into seaports and river ports by rats coming ashore from ships that had brought them from plague-infected places. It is possible that some rats actively traveled about and settled in new habitats. Burial records tell us that, especially in the early part of the century and throughout the 1520s, later 1530s, 1540s, and later 1550s, one town or another in England experienced an outbreak, severe or slight, of plague.

London was afflicted by what was probably plague at least a dozen times in the years preceding the institution of parochial record-keeping, after which the identification of bubonic plague becomes certain. In 1543 London was severely stricken by an epidemic that was probably plague, and again in 1547, 1548, and 1549. Other important local outbreaks throughout England during this time include Shrewsbury in 1536; Chester and parts of Devonshire in 1537; York and Hull in 1538; Bristol, Dover, Rye, and the north of England in 1544; Portsmouth in 1545; parts of Northamptonshire, Devonshire, and Wiltshire in 1546; Cornwall in 1547; Lincoln in 1549; Bristol in 1551. Many towns of the Thames Valley experienced plague in 1520 and 1536. Cambridge was afflicted many times during these decades, particularly in 1513 and the late 1520s.

It is during this period that civil authorities became more and more active in their efforts to control disease. Their policies reflected the current beliefs about the spread of disease, and because these policies were devised for all and any diseases, they also reveal that one disease was still largely undifferentiated from another. In 1518 Londoners exposed to plague (which may have meant bubonic plague specifically or another pestilence) were ordered to stay at home and to carry a white rod four feet long if they must go out; infected houses were closed up and marked with bundles of straw for 40 days. In 1535, in response to a disease that probably was not plague, garbage was ordered to be carted away regularly, a wise regulation for general hygiene and effective in abating some infectious diseases, but of little importance in combating plague. To help avoid contagion—again, of use for some diseases but not for plague—public events were canceled, court terms adjourned, and even attendance at church was discouraged because of the crowding involved.

London's severe mortality in 1543 prompted additional measures, including the airing of clothing worn by infected persons, the destruction of dogs, which were believed to spread disease, and the burial of plague victims in deeper graves to prevent corruption of the air from their decaying bodies. Social conscience was demonstrated in an order to provide care for sick individuals turned out of households, a measure that appeared with increasing frequency throughout the later 1500s.

Among the many medical tracts and sermons concerning the "horryble Plague of the Pestilence," perhaps the most popular, which saw about 15 editions between 1539 and 1580, was *The Myrour or Glasse of Helth necessary and nedefull for every person to loke in that wyll kepe theyr body from the sekenes of the pestylence.* Although these works provided much-needed comfort and hope, they contained the same ineffectual kitchen remedies, theories of corrupted airs, and ideas about divine and cosmological causes that had been current for centuries and would continue to be so until the advent of modern medical science. See also LONDON PLAGUE OF 1563; LONDON PLAGUE OF 1578; LONDON PLAGUE OF 1593.

Further reading: Mullet, *The Bubonic Plague and England*; Shrewsbury, *A History of Bubonic Plague in the British Isles*; Slack, *The Impact of Plague in Tudor and Stuart England*.

English Smallpox Epidemic of 1751–53

Most extensive and fatal outbreak of smallpox in England until that time. This nationwide epidemic began in London in December 1751, where it caused more than 3,500 deaths in the following year. By the spring of 1752 the disease began to spread to many areas of England. The severity of the outbreak is exemplified by the town of Chelmsford, where 95 people died out of 290 cases in a nine-month period beginning in July 1752.

The epidemic of 1751–53 was the turning point in the progress of the practice of variolation (inoculation with smallpox virus) in England. Before this time, although it had been demonstrated beyond doubt that variolation conferred immunity, the procedure was carried out on a very small scale. But with the threat of death and disfiguration by smallpox everywhere, people became more receptive to the idea, and general inoculations were carried out in many towns throughout England during these years.

It was also during this epidemic that attention was focused on the greatest problem with variolation, the fact that smallpox is highly infectious, and anyone who had been inoculated with the virus could spread it easily to others, if precautions were not taken. For example, inhabitants of many towns resented the arrival of country people for inoculation; they believed the countryfolk contributed to the spread of the disease and prolonged the epidemic. Controversies such as this set the stage for the breakthrough in smallpox prevention, vaccination (first attempted by Edward Jenner in 1796). In the meantime, the dangerous preparatory methods employed by many physicians, including bleeding, purging, and even near-starvation, were dramatically modified by the English surgeon Robert Sutton, who was active starting in the 1750s. Sutton further minimized the risk of serious illness and death by making smaller incisions in the patient and carefully selecting the viral matter. These safer practices were further developed by Sutton's son Daniel, who was instrumental in popularizing variolation and thus protecting many thousands of people from the dreaded disease. Endorsement of the procedure was given by Britain's College of Physicians in 1755, largely in acknowledgment of its success during the tragic epidemic of 1751–53.

Further reading: Hopkins, *Princes and Peasants: Smallpox in History*; Shurkin, *The Invisible Fire*; Smith, *The Speckled Monster*.

English Smallpox Epidemic of 1825–26

Second major outbreak of smallpox to afflict England in the nineteenth century (see BRITISH SMALLPOX EPIDEMIC OF 1816–19). Unfortunately, few official records about the epidemic exist, so estimates of its extent or number of cases and the deaths it incurred are based on private observations, which attest to its severity in many towns and cities throughout England, from Newcastle in the north to Canterbury in the south. London was severely affected as well. A physician at the London Smallpox Hospital observed that nearly as many patients were admitted in 1825 as in the worst outbreaks of the eighteenth century, and more than in the epidemic of just a few years before. The poorer population suffered most during this epidemic, as was increasingly the case throughout the 19th century, as cities became crowded with

underprivileged people who largely shunned preventive treatments, in contrast to the wealthier classes who routinely vaccinated their children.

Both vaccination, or inoculation with cowpox virus, introduced 30 years before, and variolation (inoculation with smallpox virus), which had been known in England for a century, were practiced widely at this time. But resistance to one or both procedures (which would continue until the decline of the disease at the end of the century) caused many people to die who otherwise could have been protected by one or the other of these simple preventive techniques.

Further reading: Creighton, *A History of Epidemics in Britain*; Smith, *The Speckled Monster*.

English Sweating Sickness (English Sweat) Epidemics

Contagious disease possibly introduced into England by French soldiers recruited by King Henry VII for his army around the time of the battle at Bosworth Field (ending the Wars of the Roses) in August 1485; subsequent outbreaks or epidemics occurred in 1507–08, 1516–17, 1529, and 1551. The English sweat is noteworthy for peculiar characteristics that make it distinctly different from many other fifteenth- and sixteenth-century contagious diseases, especially the curious fact that its history—unlike that of epidemics such as typhus, influenza, and smallpox, which have persisted into modern times—was relatively brief, and it disappeared permanently from England with its last occurrence in 1551. Thus, the English sweat was never cured or successfully controlled; it merely vanished.

Another outstanding characteristic, particularly surprising and frightening to the affluent citizenry, was the incidence of the sweat among their numbers; unlike the poor, whose crowded conditions and lack of hygiene routinely made them victims of bubonic plague and other contagious diseases, the wealthy normally escaped the more deadly epidemics. The most famous victim of the sweat was Cardinal Thomas Wolsey of England, who contracted it three times in 1517 but survived. Others of high social position who were affected included aldermen and two lord mayors of London, both dying within a week in the epidemic of 1485. It was during this first outbreak that the royal court issued a decree prohibiting persons from appearing at court except on official business, which indicates the awareness among the privileged that they were as susceptible to this deadly sickness as were the common people.

The third unusual characteristic of the sweat—in addition to its abrupt disappearance and its incidence among the rich—was the violence and rapidity with which it struck and killed its victims. A papal nuncio (envoy) visiting London in 1517 observed that "the attack lasted about twenty-four hours"; another witness wrote that "There were some dancing in the court at nine o'clock that were dead at eleven."

The sweat was so-called because those attacked perspired profusely from head to foot. Symptoms included, as described in a tract written by Dr. John Caius during the fourth and last outbreak of 1551, pains in the back, shoulder, arms, legs, and head, as well as "grief" in the stomach and liver, and "passion" in the heart. A doctor writing during the first outbreak of 1485 described how the sweat came "with a grete swetying and stynkying, with redness of the face and of all the body, and a contynual thurst, with a great hete and hedache because of the fumes and venoms."

Although the sweat resembled influenza and scarlet fever as well as plague, medical historians have been unable to definitively characterize the sickness or to identify it with other diseases current in England during the 65 years of its incidence (there were efforts to label it a lesser form of plague, for example). English sweating sickness was, and remains, an unsolved puzzle in the history of human disease.

In response to the first appearance of sweating sickness in 1485, a medical work referred to as the "little book" (a shortening of its long title) was published. Written a century earlier by a papal physician called Johannes Jacobi for use in curing plague in France, it had a wide readership in England and was reissued throughout the 1500s as a guide to the prevention and cure of disease generally. The publication of the "little book"—the first medical work ever printed in England—in response to the first outbreak of sweating sickness suggests how frightened people were of a disease that stood out in alarming contrast to plague and other forms of pestilence, which, although deadly, were evidently considered endemic and therefore usually elicited no more than routine if sorrowful acceptance.

Dr. John Caius's work of 1551, *A Boke, or counseill against the disease commonly called the Sweate, or sweatying sicknesse*, stated that the disease was caused by infection, impure spirits in corrupt bodies, evil qualities in the air, and "by the nature and site of the soil and region." His remedies included eating meats and sweet malt, and abstaining from wine.

Historians do not agree on the magnitude or relative destructiveness of English sweating sickness. Outbreaks occurred simultaneously with plague in both 1517 and 1551, and perhaps in 1485, and because record-keeping was sporadic and incomplete (and many records have not survived) it is difficult to tell how many people died from any given cause. It can be said with some certainty that the sweats of 1485 and 1507 each killed 10,000 persons throughout England. Records indicate that the sweat of 1551 was particularly severe in Devon and Essex, but it is difficult to calculate reliable figures. The effect on overall mortality from sweating sickness, except in the smallest English villages, was almost certainly relatively minor.

The 1529 epidemic (which was the severest of the sweat in England) appeared in Hamburg and other German cities, moving north into Scandinavia and east into Poland, Lithuania, and Russia. Later the Netherlands was hit, but the disease never spread to Spain and Italy. In Germany, the sick were wrongly put to bed at once, covered with warm featherbeds (thick mattresses) to sweat agonizingly, and consequently died. Angry German Catholics claimed that the sweat was just recompense for Martin Luther's Protestant heresies. See EUROPEAN SWEATING SICKNESS EPIDEMICS, NORTHERN.

Further reading: Gottfried, *Epidemic Disease in Fifteenth Century England*; McNeill, *Plagues and Peoples*; Mullet, *The Bubonic Plague and England*; Slack, *The Impact of Plague in Tudor and Stuart England*; Smith, *Plague on Us*.

English Typhus Epidemic of 1816–19

First major outbreak of epidemic, louse-borne typhus fever in England during the nineteenth century. Following a severe winter in 1814–15, an economic depression starting in 1815, and a bad harvest in 1816, this three-year visitation of typhus fever was widespread throughout the British Isles, affecting many areas of England, Scotland, and Ireland. The poorer classes were especially vulnerable to illness during these years due to unemployment and the scarcity of food.

It is not known how many cases and fatalities occurred in England during this epidemic, due to faulty record-keeping and the confusion of typhus with other types of fever, such as relapsing fever and typhoid fever. Nonetheless, a measure of the severity of the outbreak can be gauged by the observation of the apothecary of a London workhouse that, whereas he normally attended an average of 150 cases of fever each year, in 1817 the number jumped to about 600, a fourfold increase.

Epidemic typhus fever, transmitted from person to person by infected lice, thrives in conditions of poverty, overcrowding, and filth, and is therefore a disease found principally among the poor. The appalling environment in which large numbers of English working-class people lived throughout the nineteenth century invited many types of infectious disease. Although awareness of the need for public health programs began taking hold in the 1840s,

England would experience two more major outbreaks of epidemic typhus fever, as well as many other diseases, in the decades to come (see ENGLISH TYPHUS EPIDEMIC OF 1837–38, ENGLISH TYPHUS EPIDEMIC OF 1847–48).

Further reading: Creighton, *A History of Epidemics in Britain;* Woods and Woodward, eds., *Urban Disease and Mortality in Nineteenth-Century England.*

English Typhus Epidemic of 1837–38   Severe outbreak of epidemic typhus fever that spread throughout the British Isles and caused approximately 28,000 human deaths in England and Wales in the 18-month period from July 1837 through December 1838. London suffered more than 6,000 fatalities during this period. Although these figures include deaths from other types of fever, most notably typhoid, the majority were caused by typhus.

In London the epidemic declined rapidly in 1839, but continued for the next few years to cause high mortality in other areas of England, especially the industrial towns in the north. The English author Elizabeth Gaskell wrote compelling descriptions of the suffering of poverty-stricken typhus victims during this epidemic in her novel *Mary Barton,* set in the northern manufacturing city of Manchester.

The distress of the poor during this widespread epidemic alerted many people to the deplorable conditions of filth and overcrowding in which the underprivileged classes lived, conditions that encouraged the spread of typhus fever and other so-called filth diseases such as typhoid and cholera. Acutely aware of the disproportionate numbers of typhus deaths among the poor, the great public health reformer Edwin Chadwick produced a ground-breaking study entitled *Report on the Sanitary Condition of the Labouring Population of Great Britain* (1842), which documented the urgent need for improved living conditions and medical care for the poor.

Although Chadwick's efforts made an immediate impact, eradication of the conditions that helped spread infectious disease was only very gradually achieved. Another devastating outbreak of epidemic typhus fever occurred just ten years later (see ENGLISH TYPHUS EPIDEMIC OF 1847–48).

Further reading: Creighton, *A History of Epidemics in Britain;* Wohl, *Endangered Lives: Public Health in Victorian Britain;* Lewis, *Edwin Chadwick and the Public Health Movement, 1832–1854.*

English Typhus Epidemic of 1847–48   Extensive and highly fatal outbreak of epidemic typhus fever that caused more than 30,000 human deaths in England and Wales in 1847 alone. Of relatively short duration, the epidemic markedly declined by the summer of 1848. London, with about 3,000 fatal cases, was less seriously affected than the northern half of England, where the northwest counties of Lancashire and Cheshire suffered most.

The widespread incidence of typhus during this epidemic was to a large extent caused by an influx of Irish immigrants escaping famine in Ireland (see IRISH TYPHUS AND DYSENTERY EPIDEMIC OF 1846–50). They entered England mostly through the northwestern port of Liverpool, where sheds had to be built to accommodate the sick, and floating lazarettos, or quarantine stations, held many more.

Because it is transmitted by lice, epidemic typhus fever is engendered and sustained in unsanitary and crowded living conditions. The deplorable environments of working-class neighborhoods in nineteenth-century English cities therefore made the proliferation of typhus fever inevitable. Incidence of the disease in various parts of England, including London, was already high in 1846; the addition of large numbers of poverty-stricken Irish, many of whom were already infected with typhus, significantly contributed to mortality during this epidemic.

The "Irish fever" of 1847–48 was the last major outbreak of epidemic typhus fever in the British Isles.

Further reading: Creighton, *A History of Epidemics in Britain;* Frazer, *History of English Public Health, 1834–1939.*

Ethiopian Cholera Epidemic of 1889–1902   Serious epidemic of the communicable Asiatic cholera disease that lingered for 13 years in southern and eastern Ethiopia, causing much suffering and high mortality. Due to European occupation of parts of the country, in addition to new territories won by Menelik II, the newly crowned Ethiopian emperor, no established authority existed to control the disease. As a result, there are no records available to indicate the exact number of persons who contracted cholera nor the total number of fatalities that occurred during the three years. Many first-hand accounts reported by numerous Europeans in the country at the time stress the suffering from the effects of the epidemic.

Following the Italo-Ethiopian War of 1887–89 and civil strife, extensive crop failure brought famine to Ethiopia in 1889. Later that year, the first outbreak of cholera occurred in Eritrea, a plateau area located on the western coast of the Red Sea. Imported from the east by Muslim pilgrims returning from Mecca, the disease ran rampant until 1890 in the Eritrean region, taken over and colonized in March of that year by Italian forces. In the town of Asmara, so many victims were left on the streets that the Italian troops resorted to burning the corpses where they had fallen. The second outbreak was reported along the Setit River in 1891. By 1892 most of the people in southern and eastern Ethiopia were afflicted with severe diarrhea and vomiting, with the sick often dying from dehydration the same day the disease was contracted.

Caused by the *Vibrio comma* bacterium, Asiatic cholera is commonly spread by contaminated water. Few survived cholera in Adowa, Gondar, Ankobar, and Harar, the four main towns of nineteenth-century Ethiopia, all unsanitary with filthy streets full of offal, human excreta, and dead animals. In the town of Sheik Husein, where the Somali inhabitants buried their dead around the edge of the pond in which they drank, four fifths of the population died from the disease. In Dabarwa in 1889, a smallpox epidemic had struck down the population; when cholera struck the diminished number of survivors, the town was decimated almost completely.

Later a clearer understanding of the rate of mortality was known, when the epidemic traveled southeast to the British Somali ports, where records were maintained of its onslaught. The seaport of Bulhar suffered the worst effects, with 686 fatalities occurring among the 826 who contracted cholera; in Zeila, there were 277 deaths out of the 369 stricken; and in Berbera, while only 13 persons contracted the disease, 11 deaths occurred.

Further reading: Ackerknecht, *History and Geography of the Most Important Diseases*; Pankhurst, *Economic History of Ethiopia: 1800–1935*.

Ethiopian Influenza Epidemic of 1918–19   Offshoot of the worldwide Spanish Influenza Epidemic of 1917–19 (q.v.), killing more than 12,000 persons in less than a year. This influenza epidemic in Ethiopia was commonly referred to as the "Hedar basheta," because of the mounting fatalities in the month of Hedar (which began on November 10, 1918).

In April 1918 mild cases of flu first appeared in Ethiopia's western provinces and in the capital city, Addis Ababa, where an epidemic (at first misdiagnosed by some as typhus or smallpox) was raging by July. By late August the flu had seriously attacked Ras (Prince) Tafari, who had recently (1917) been named regent and heir apparent to the throne (from 1930 to 1974 he reigned as Emperor Haile Selassie I of Ethiopia). Fatalities were high, with many dying within two or three days after contracting the "mysterious" disease. Many people, including the head of the Ethiopian Orthodox Church, began to flee from Addis Ababa to the surrounding mountainous re-

gions, and a shortage of gravediggers resulted in the interring of many dead victims in shallow holes only six inches under the ground's surface.

A second, more virulent wave of influenza hit Ethiopia in October 1918; it entered from Somalia via the Gulf of Aden and was soon recognized as the Spanish flu already infecting about half the world. From the Aden Gulf coast, the disease moved inland to Dire Dawa, Harar, and Addis Ababa. The large Ethiopian Orthodox and Muslim populations were undoubtedly affected, but fatalities for these groups were unrecorded, in contrast to the many deaths recorded by the Roman Catholic Church in Dire Dawa and Addis Ababa. Many foreign diplomats in Addis Ababa, including at least 60 members of the Italian legation, died from influenza in November 1918. The infection, which some Ethiopians speculated was caused by the use of poison gas in World War I, killed young and old, male and female, rich and poor, making no distinction; a large number of deaths resulted from complications that led to pneumonia.

Two of the eight practicing physicians in Addis Ababa died during the first stage of the epidemic; another fled the city, and another preferred to treat only white Europeans. Native Ethiopians thus had limited medical treatment and were also handicapped by the lack of medical supplies (due to the closure of the pharmacies by October 1918); furthermore, Addis Ababa had only one hospital. Alcohol was substituted for medicine; leaves of eucalyptus trees, boiled in water, served as a disinfectant; and the eating of garlic, reputed to have prophylatic powers, was encouraged. Business came to a standstill, and there was administrative chaos in Addis Ababa until the end of 1918, when the epidemic abated there.

To the north, the Italian colony of Eritrea on the Red Sea sustained a mild flu epidemic until February 1919, along with the northern Ethiopian provinces of Tigre and Welo. Mortality from the disease in these places was far less than it was in Ethiopia's southwestern and western regions bordering the Sudan. By late February, the epidemic had waned in all of the country.

Further reading: Pankhurst, *An Introduction to the Medical History of Ethiopia*.

Ethiopian Malaria Epidemic of 1958   Catastrophic malaria outbreak that infected an estimated 3,500,000 persons in Ethiopia and killed approximately 175,000 of them in the latter half of 1958. The epidemic, which occurred mainly in the country's central and northern highland provinces, resulted from the increased breeding of the *Anopheles gambiae* mosquito (main vector of the parasitic disease from person to person in 1958) due to excessive rainfall and higher temperatures and humidity than normal. This prolonged mosquitoes' lives, allowing them to diffuse over a much greater area than usual.

At the end of the rainy season in late June 1958, malaria began appearing among inhabitants of Shoa (Shewa), Gojjam (Gojam), and other highland provinces (where people lived at altitudes of 6,000 feet and above). Ethiopia's capital of Addis Ababa was severely infected, as were other highland cities and towns, such as Jimma (Jima), Soddo (Sodo), and Lekemt. In some places, the mortality rate of those infected was 25 percent, particularly in Shoa and Gojjam, where populations had suffered from harvest failures and famine in 1957.

Because of limited hospital services, only a small number of malaria cases were able to receive clinical care. In ten hospitals where records were made, many more patients were admitted than in the past; in the hospital at Debre Zeyt in Shoa, there were 4,094 cases in 1958, in comparison with an average of only 948 annual cases previously. In Debre Tabor's hospital, 2,780 malaria patients were admitted in 1958, compared with an average of 126 cases in yearly outbreaks before. In parts of the upper Blue Nile river valley in western Ethiopia (near Sudan), fatalities were so high in October that there were not enough healthy persons to care for the sick, and the unattended crops were eaten and destroyed by wildlife.

Few cases occurred in malaria's endemic regions in Ethiopia (the lower elevations), where the disease is not a direct threat to life due to the considerable immunity built up by the inhabitants as a result of regular outbreaks of the disease. As in most malaria epidemics, children were particularly affected in 1958, with those infected between the age of birth and two years old having a mortality rate as high as 50 percent. Numerous infected children who survived were damaged by malaria parasites remaining in their blood, making them susceptible to other infections. Ethiopia's overall morbidity rate exceeded 15 percent for the 1958 epidemic, which ended about mid-December. The disease spread into neighboring northern Somalia with returning nomads who crossed the border into Ethiopia's Haud region to graze their animals during the rainy season.

Further reading: Colbourne, *Malaria in Africa*; Prothero, *Migrants and Malaria*.

Ethiopian Smallpox Epidemics of 1886–98

Serious outbreaks of smallpox that killed a major portion of those infected in what is now Ethiopia (Abyssinia) in northeast Africa.

After the first recorded smallpox outbreak in Ethiopia in 1768, the disease erupted epidemically seven times prior to 1886, when it severely struck Adowa (Aduwa, Adwa), a major town in Tigre province in northern Ethiopia. Out of Adowa's population of about 7,000 people, there were some 500 deaths, 300 of children under age 14. Most of the Ethiopian smallpox victims were disfigured with pockmarks and scars (a common effect of the virulent virus on most infected Africans). From Adowa, the epidemic moved eastward into the regions of Gojam and Amhara and southward into the province of Shoa (Shewa). Smallpox completely decimated the population of Arusi, a town in central Ethiopia. The western part of Eritrea (a region along the Red Sea) was so badly struck that the Mansa Bet Abraha tribe living there lost about 700 people and later referred to 1886 as "the year of smallpox" in their language. The disease was also especially severe in the eastern Ethiopian city of Harar, where it was prevalent during the next 12 years.

Fatalities from smallpox were particularly high during a great famine (the result of a serious epidemic of cattle disease) from 1889 to 1891. In addition, smallpox was spread during the war the Ethiopians were waging on their western borders against the Mahdists (a fanatical Muslim sect) in the Sudan. Ethiopia's new emperor, Menelik II, saw some 3,000 men out of his army of about 20,000 die from smallpox and other diseases during their march south from Tigre to Shoa in late 1889 and early 1890. During this period of famine, war, and disease, Italian forces advanced into Eritrea to establish a colony there.

Unhealthy conditions led to an even higher incidence of smallpox in Ethiopia, especially in the larger towns, and preventive measures were established, such as closing the road from Addis Ababa to Ankober and preventing trade caravans from entering major cities during an epidemic in 1892. Other measures of prevention were harsher, such as the removal of smallpox victims from their houses and leaving them to die from exposure to sun, rain, and cold, or to be devoured by hyenas. The burning of victims' clothing and houses was another common practice. Superstitions also played a considerable role in prevention; in Tigre, no males were allowed anywhere near a smallpox patient, for it was believed that all interactions (including sexual intercourse) while God was angry with them would increase illness (itself a judgment from God). At the time, doctors inoculated with the smallpox virus (variolation), which was an often compulsory method of fighting the disease in Ethiopia, and a considerable number of human deaths occurred because of this practice.

Smallpox continued to ravage the country, notably during the Italo-Ethiopian War of 1895–96 (won by the Ethiopians), until 1898, when an effective mass vaccination program was initiated that eliminated much of the disease in the country. The last major outbreak occurred in 1904.

Further reading: Pankhurst, *Economic History of Ethiopia: 1800–1935;* Hopkins, *Princes and Peasants: Smallpox in History.*

Ethiopian Typhus Epidemic of 1876

Outbreak of louse-borne typhus fever that killed at least 5,000 soldiers and civilians between August and October 1876 in northern Ethiopia during the Ethiopian-Egyptian War of 1875–77 (won by the Ethiopians).

Carried by human body lice and thriving under unhygienic, crowded conditions, epidemic typhus first broke out in early August 1876 among invading Egyptian troops moving inland from Massawa (Mitsiwa), an Ethiopian port on the Red Sea. By August 9 the Egyptian commander reported that 160 of his troops had been hospitalized with typhus; four to six of his men were dying of this contagious, rickettsial infection every day. About 50 miles away, allied Sudanese troops who were stationed near Asmara (Asmera) soon became infected, and by September 2 typhus had claimed the lives of 47 out of 282 Sudanese hospitalized at their base. As a result, the Sudanese troops moved northward to another base, where they unwittingly infected healthy Arab soldiers whom the Egyptians had hoped to send as replacements for the sick Sudanese. Typhus soon spread from there to another Egyptian base, infecting some 200 troops there. By late September a special camp at Massawa had been established to isolate the sick, but the epidemic worsened and did not wane until late October, by which time about 2,000 Egyptian, Sudanese, and Arab soldiers had died of typhus.

The disease spread to Ethiopians in Tigre province, particularly the inhabitants of Adowa (Aduwa, Adwa), about 75 miles south of Asmara. Evidently two thirds of Adowa's population perished from typhus. A local observer of the epidemic attributed it to a famine that was linked to miasma (poisonous air) produced by "thousands" of Egyptian corpses left unburied; others concluded that the epidemic resulted from miasma from corpses of livestock that had died of cattle plague. These faulty conclusions were reached before the body louse was discovered to be typhus's mode of transmission. Though the disease commonly occurs during famines and wartime, it is transmitted from person to person by the contaminative method, initiated when a louse becomes infected after biting a typhus patient. Ethiopian civilian fatalities were reportedly more than double the number that occurred among the invading troops. Without effective antibiotics and DDT to delouse populations, Ethiopia remained typhus-afflicted throughout the rest of the century.

Further reading: Cloudsley-Thompson, *Insects and History;* Pankhurst, *An Introduction to the Medical History of Ethiopia.*

Ethiopian Yellow Fever Epidemic of 1960–62

Outbreak of yellow fever that infected about 100,000 inhabitants of Ethiopia, in East Africa. The number of notified human deaths was 5,000 during the epidemic, but some authorities have suggested there probably were at least 30,000 deaths. Very little information about the epidemic was available until the 1970s, when some important facts emerged.

In 1940 a severe yellow fever epidemic broke out in the Nuba Mountains of southern Sudan (see SUDANESE YELLOW FEVER EPIDEMIC OF 1940), but the disease did not enter Ethiopia to the east. Because the fever's virus had never previously spread to Ethiopia from Sudan, numerous authorities and others thought there was some particular biological barrier to the eastward spread of the disease. However, in 1959 yellow fever did enter Ethiopia from the Kurmuk area on the Sudanese-Ethiopian border, and 98 Ethiopians died of it that year. The *Aëdes aegypti* mosquito transmitted the lethal virus, and the Ethiopian inhabitants of the Didesa River valley were severely struck by the disease in 1960. The *Aëdes* mosquitoes, which transmit the virus to human beings by their bite, bred abundantly after much rainfall and infested crab holes, coconut shells, fallen leaves, wells, and puddles. The epidemic, which raged for almost two years in Ethiopia, was sustained by a man-to-mosquito-to-man cycle and especially afflicted those living in towns and cities. (Ethiopia then had a total population of about one million people.)

All age groups and both sexes were infected by yellow fever; there were, however, more fatalities among adults than children and a large number of mild, unrecognized cases. After the epidemic, yellow fever was eradicated by anti-mosquito measures and inoculation with a vaccine. If vaccination had been administered after the outbreak of yellow fever in 1959, many have thought the subsequent epidemic disaster could have been averted; an efficient vaccine would have been able to produce mass immunity rapidly to diminish the chance of an accelerated introduction of the lethal virus into Ethiopia's populous areas, where the mosquito-vector may have been present.

Further reading: Bedson et al., eds., *Virus and Rickettsial Diseases of Man;* Howe, *A World Geography of Human Diseases.*

European Diphtheria Epidemic of the Late 1850s

Epidemic of diphtheria that began in Europe between 1855 and 1858 and soon spread to every part of the world, including North America, Africa, Asia, and Australia. Some of the earliest cases were found in Britain, where outbreaks of a fatal throat disease occurred in Cornwall, Lincolnshire, and Kent in late 1855 through 1856. By 1857 British health officials recognized the disease as diphtheria (though they occasionally still confused it with scarlatina), and included it for the first time among the classified causes of death when they published statistics for 1855. In that year the death rate for diphtheria was 20 per million throughout Britain, but by 1859 (the height of the epidemic) it had climbed to 517. Certain towns in Lincolnshire and Cornwall reported about 1,000 cases each, but people died from the disease in every county in Britain and Wales.

Britain's experience was not unique. From there the disease spread northward into Scotland; countries as far away as India and China were affected by the epidemic, and even in Australia many people succumbed beginning in late 1858. In Sweden thousands of children fell ill and died from the disease; the high child mortality rates stood in stark contrast to those of the preceding five decades, during which widespread vaccination had practically wiped out smallpox, a leading killer of the young.

In other countries as well as in Sweden, diphtheria claimed many more victims among children than among adults. The bacteria that cause the disease must therefore have been common enough for adults to develop immunity to it, even though severe diphtheria epidemics had occurred only in Norway, Denmark, and France (see TOURS DIPHTHERIA EPIDEMIC OF 1818–20) in the previous 50 or so years. Nevertheless, because of the pandemic of the late 1850s, diphtheria became endemic in all civilized countries in the temperate zones, where it continued to strike many people for decades to come.

The pandemic had a beneficial effect as well. By bringing the disease to the attention of researchers, it gave them an incentive to try to uncover the pathology and etiology of diphtheria, to produce false membranes in experimental animals, and to inoculate humans with diphtheritic material. These efforts were to succeed later in the century.

Further reading: Burnet and White, *Natural History of Infectious Disease;* Creighton, *A History of Epidemics in Britain;* Rosen, "Acute Communicable Diseases."

European Influenza Epidemics of 1708–09, 1712, 1729–30, and 1732–33

Series of influenza outbreaks during the early eighteenth century that appear to have moved westward through Europe and even overseas, causing widespread illness but relatively few deaths.

During the first half of the eighteenth century, the influenza virus had not yet been discovered. Influenza was thought to be the result of a poison or miasma in the air that was influenced and spread by winds, temperature changes, and barometric pressure fluctuations. Cities were commonly the centers of the disease, which was slowly transported into the countryside and other cities by travel and trade. Symptoms of influenza included coughing and sneezing, sore throat, chills, headaches, fever, aches and pains, and exhaustion. Treatments during this time focused on eliminating the "poison" and balancing the body again. Most physicians prescribed a simple cure of adequate bed rest and increased fluid intake. There were also reports of some more extreme attempts to rid the body of the disease through purges, bleeding, sweating, vomiting, and urination.

The first of these European "flu" outbreaks occurred in Rome in December 1708. It moved into northern Italy in January and February 1709, into France and Belgium (then a part of France) in March, into Berlin, Prussia, in April, and north into Denmark during the summer. Most of Germany, the northwestern Balkans, and Ireland were also affected by influenza in 1708–09, but the epidemic does not appear to have reached Norway, Sweden, the Iberian Peninsula, or England.

The next major outbreak of influenza in Europe began in Jena, Germany, in April 1712 and spread throughout the summer. The disease reached Copenhagen, Thuringia, and Saxony by early June and Holstein by July, then advanced into Bavaria and Holland in August, Württemberg in September, and northern Italy in December. This epidemic was much more severe than that of 1708–09 but not as extensive. It seems to have subsided by the end of the year and did not reach France, Spain, England, or Eastern Europe.

In 1729–30 another serious epidemic of influenza broke out in Europe and possibly gave rise to one in the Americas a short while later. Two major outbreaks were reported in April 1729 in Moscow and in the Caspian Sea town of Astrakhan, almost 800 miles away. The disease appeared to be restricted to this area but in early fall was reported in Sweden, Vienna, and upper Silesia. From there the influenza continued to spread, reaching Hungary, Poland, Germany, England, and Dublin, Ireland, by November 1729. In December it appeared in Scotland, in Switzerland, and in Paris, where monasteries were forced to cancel services due to the number of monks stricken with the illness. The disease then spread into northern Italy in January 1730, Rome and the

Papal States in February, and southern Italy and Spain in March. That month, Iceland was also affected and experienced its first epidemic of influenza.

This influenza epidemic of 1729–30 is thought to have spread throughout the world, apparently reaching the North American coast of New England in October 1732. The disease had already appeared in Newfoundland, Jamaica, Mexico, Barbados, and Peru, and in December 1732 was also reported on the French island of Bourbon (Réunion) in the Indian Ocean.

It is still uncertain whether or not this 1732–33 pandemic truly originated in Russia in the spring and spread westward by land, or if it arose in Sweden in the fall and moved south to Poland and Germany and west to England by sea. Most likely, the Russian epidemic of April 1729 gave rise to a few isolated cases in Sweden and Eastern Europe, which then blossomed and spread west and south during the fall because of cooler and drier weather, more time spent indoors in close quarters, and growing trade. How the disease reached pandemic proportions in the Americas in 1732 is more difficult to determine. It is possible that the influenza spread by European-American trade across the Atlantic Ocean, although technically this should have brought about an American outbreak by fall 1731 rather than in 1732. Western Europe was coming down with the disease during 1730 and ship sailing time to America was several weeks. Another possibility is simply that the American epidemic of influenza arose independently.

At any rate, in Europe during this time influenza flared up once again and caused a concurrent epidemic in 1732–33. The outbreak is believed to have spread in November and December 1732 from the already stricken Russia deep into Poland, central Germany, Alsace (France), Basel (Switzerland), and Edinburgh, Scotland. In January of the following year influenza broke out in London, Dublin, Paris, and Flanders, as well as in northern Italy. It also spread through southern England, where even the horses and dogs were reported ill with fevers and coughs. The outbreak of influenza continued into southern Spain and southern Italy during early spring.

Both the 1729–30 and 1732–33 influenza epidemics resulted in widespread illness and high morbidity but comparatively few human deaths. The disease affected all ages and both sexes. Those it killed were mostly infants, the elderly, and people with chronic diseases or respiratory problems.

Further reading: Patterson, *Pandemic Influenza, 1700–1900*; Hirsch, *Handbook on Geographical and Historical Pathology*.

European Influenza Epidemics of 1742–43 and 1762   Two relatively brief epidemics of influenza in Western Europe that caused widespread illness but few human deaths. (*Influenza* is the Italian word for "influence," which Italians had used to refer to the influence they believed the stars or astrological bodies brought to bear on an epidemic in Italy in 1504. The term [although heard of in England earlier] was first used in Britain in 1743 to describe the same illness, formerly referred to as a fever or a "catarrh.")

In January and February of 1742 an outbreak of influenza occurred in Germany that may or may not have contributed to an October outbreak in Switzerland and northern Italy. Whatever the case, the influenza began a slow move south into the rest of Italy. It hit Milan in November, Rome in January 1743, and Naples and Sicily in February. Meanwhile, the disease was also moving north, attacking Paris in February 1743, Belgium and the Netherlands in March, and southern England in April. At this time the epidemic contained itself. It had spread very slowly, restricting itself to parts of Western Europe, and causing only a temporary, if widespread illness.

Two decades later, a similar epidemic occurred. It began near the end of the Seven Years' War (1756–63), making movement of the military a likely factor in its dissemination. In February 1762 an influenza outbreak appeared in Breslau, Silesia (Wroclaw, Poland). From there the disease spread into Vienna, Hungary, and Denmark in March. It attacked Germany, England, Scotland, and northern Italy in April, Ireland in May, and Lille and Strasbourg, France, in June. It then moved into southern France, apparently missing Paris altogether.

This 1762 epidemic of influenza was widespread but did not appear to be very severe. Mobidity (incidence of disease) was high but mortality (loss of life) was low, with the exception of the Breslau outbreak. The epidemic clearly followed an east-to-west diffusion pattern and moved from cities to towns to villages. It subsided before reaching southern Italy, Scandinavia, or the Iberian Peninsula.

Further reading: Patterson, *Pandemic Influenza, 1700–1900*.

European Influenza Pandemic of 1781–82   Major outbreak of influenza, its origin still a subject of much scholarly debate. One of the most widespread of the early influenza epidemics, it attacked China, India, Europe, and North America and was as significant in the history of the disease as was the Asiatic Influenza Pandemic of 1889–90 (q.v.) and the Spanish Influenza Epidemic of 1917–19 (q.v.).

The pandemic was heralded by several outbreaks of the disease on different continents, but scholars doubt that these outbreaks were directly connected with the pandemic. Influenza apparently raged in France and Italy during January–March 1780. In September 1780, outbreaks were reported from the Canton region in southeast China and from Bengal and the Coromandel Coast in eastern India. During the winter of 1780–81, influenza was reported from the Russian empire and, in the spring of 1781, from the United States.

While the controversy about the original birthplace of the pandemic continues among scholars, many now agree that it must have begun in China in the fall of 1781 and spread westward from this focus. Some suggest that the pandemic may have originated in the easternmost reaches of the Russian empire and fanned out east and west from there. It is interesting to note that while many of the European countries referred to it as the Russian affliction, Russians themselves called it the Chinese catarrh. Others place its birthplace in India or the East Indies. Regardless of which theory is preferred, it is clear that the pandemic affected thousands of people in far-flung countries.

British physicians have recorded an influenza epidemic at Nagapattinam in southern India (not far from the region where the 1780 outbreak had occurred) in November 1781. Around the same time, in October–November 1781, influenza outbreaks were reported from the Malaysian-Indonesian region. Outbreaks also occurred in Japan in 1781.

It is believed that the infection traveled from China to Tobolsk (a Siberian city) and then across the Ural Mountains, invading Moscow and Kazan in December 1781. St. Petersburg was invaded in January 1782. At the height of the epidemic, it is reported that 30,000 persons fell ill in the city every day. From here, the epidemic took one of two routes. One wave moved along the Baltic Sea in February, infecting Tallinn, Riga, and Tilsit (Sovetsk) before entering Poland. Another offshoot of the epidemic traveled along Germany's Baltic coast in March, causing severe outbreaks in northern Germany in April. In the same month, the cities of Miskolc in Hungary, Copenhagen in Denmark, and Stockholm in Sweden were struck. The following month, Austria, Prague in Bohemia, and western Germany suffered outbreaks.

The influenza wave, which eventually invaded the southern Scandinavian region, apparently arrived in Newcastle-upon-Tyne in northern England late in April 1782. This point is disputed by some scholars, who say that the epidemic arrived in the British Isles through London, which, with its environs, was infected in mid-May. According to their account, the disease struck Newcastle and Edinburgh in Scotland toward the end of May. Throughout June, the influenza spread rapidly from its London focus across most of England and Scotland, even reaching Dublin in Ireland. Reportedly, there was a noticeable rise in London's death rate in June 1782.

Also in June 1782, most of France, present-day Belgium and the Netherlands, and southwestern Germany (three quarters of the city of Munich's population was attacked) were invaded. In July, the epidemic covered southern France and northern Italy, Spain, Portugal, and southern Italy (two thirds of Rome's residents fell ill) were affected during August and September. Even parts of the Ottoman Empire suffered from influenza late in 1782, but details are sketchy.

The pandemic spread as far and as rapidly as the transportation system allowed. While it was not as severe as the epidemic of 1917–19, the overall morbidity was very high in many European countries. The case mortality rates, however, were generally low. Those who died during the outbreaks were mainly the elderly and those suffering from respiratory ailments.

Further reading: Pyle, *The Diffusion of Influenza;* Patterson, *Pandemic Influenza, 1700–1900.*

European Influenza Pandemic of 1788–89   Widespread outbreak of influenza in Europe and America, characterized by high morbidity (incidence of disease), low mortality (loss of life), and a distinct diffusion path.

In March 1788 influenza was reported in two Russian cities, St. Petersburg on the Baltic Sea and Kherson on the Black Sea. By April the disease had appeared in Vienna, Warsaw, and Hungary, as well as in Eskilstuna, Sweden. From there it spread into Copenhagen in May, into Munich and London in June, and into the areas surrounding London in July. By August it had hit Scotland and Paris, by September the north of France, and by October Geneva and northern Italy.

One year later the influenza virus appeared to have reached America as well. Outbreaks were reported in Georgia; Norfolk, Virginia; Philadelphia; and New York City in September 1789. One month later influenza struck Hartford, Connecticut, and continued into Boston in November and into Nova Scotia, Canada, in December. The disease also moved westward, apparently affecting several Indian tribes; one especially severe attack appears to have occurred on New York's Niagara frontier. During this time the disease was spreading southward into the Carribbean as well. It hit the islands of Jamaica, Martinique, St. Eustatius, St. Kitts, and Dominica in October, and

Grenada in November. Its mobility among these islands is believed to have been a result of shipping and trade in the area.

There were some reports that outbreaks of influenza reached South America that winter, but these are unsubstantiated. The disease did flair up again in the northeastern United States during 1790 and again in the spring of 1791. The first American outbreak was most likely a continuation of the European epidemic, caused and spread by transatlantic shipping into American ports. Subsequent outbreaks seem to have been the result of the virus mutating during its transit up and down the coast, allowing people to be infected more than once.

This influenza epidemic of 1788–89 was so widespread that it has been referred to as a pandemic. Although morbidity was rather high (50 percent was reported in Munich and several other European cities), the outbreak was not exceptionally severe. The disease affected all people, regardless of age, sex, or socioeconomic status, but it seems to have incurred few deaths. Outbreaks caused illness and inconvenience, usually lasting no longer than six weeks. The few fatalities that did occur affected those who were elderly or chronically ill.

The diffusion pattern of this influenza epidemic was similar to that of 1732. It began in Russia and moved westward across Europe, partly due to Czar Peter the Great's eighteenth-century attempt to bring Russia out of isolation and into political and economic contact with the West. A new Russian capital of St. Petersburg and increased activity on the Baltic Sea facilitated the spread not only of trade but of disease as well. Thus the path of influenza was able to follow that of commerce, from east to west and from city into countryside.

Further reading: Patterson, *Pandemic Influenza, 1700–1900*; Hirsch, *Handbook on Geographical and Historical Pathology*.

European Influenza Pandemic of 1830–31 See ASIATIC AND EUROPEAN INFLUENZA PANDEMIC OF 1830–31.

European Influenza Pandemic of 1833 Pandemic that remained concentrated in Europe, causing higher morbidity and mortality than the Asiatic and European Influenza Pandemic of 1830–31 (q.v.). Some scholars consider it part of the earlier pandemic but others, including K. David Patterson (see below), believe it to be separate.

The pandemic apparently originated in Russia, where influenza was prevalent in cities as far apart as Perm in the Urals and St. Petersburg on the Baltic during January 1832. Clearly, the infection must have spread within this area since late in 1832. The city of Riga in Latvia was infected in February, as were the cities of Tallinn in Estonia, Memel (Klaipeda) in Lithuania, and Odessa in Russia, as well as the eastern part of Galicia (now western Ukraine).

In March, influenza arrived in East Prussia, Poland, Bohemia, Helsingor (Denmark), Berlin, and Constantinople. The epidemic struck Hungary, Vienna and eastern Austria, Saxony, Denmark, the British Isles, and the French cities of Paris and Bordeaux in April. In May, it was striking western Germany, Stockholm, western Austria, areas of northern Italy, and Serbia. In the same month, influenza also traveled from Constantinople (Istanbul) to Smyrna (Izmir, Turkey), Syria, and Cairo and Alexandria in Egypt.

During June 1833, it moved north from the Netherlands and Belgium to Uppsala in Sweden while extending itself farther in northern Italy. Switzerland escaped infection until September, while Naples and Sicily were struck in November. Spain and Portugal seem to have escaped the pandemic altogether.

In Europe, the attack rate was higher than during the 1830–31 pandemic. According to eyewitness accounts, morbidity was high in the cities of Stockholm (25 percent), Memel or Klaipeda (80 percent), Königsberg or Kaliningrad (a third of the population), Edinburgh (50 percent), London (80 percent) and Paris (80 percent). Thousands fell ill in Berlin, St. Petersburg, Austria, and Bohemia.

More people died than in the previous pandemic but case-mortality was low. Breslau (Wroclaw, Poland), Vienna, Copenhagen, Prague, Königsberg, and Edinburgh recorded a dramatic increase in mortality. London reported heaviest mortality between mid-April and mid-May. All over England, the epidemic claimed twice as many human lives in February 1833 compared to the normal figures for the month. See also ASIATIC AND EUROPEAN INFLUENZA PANDEMIC OF 1836–37.

Further reading: Patterson, *Pandemic Influenza 1700–1900*; Beveridge, *Influenza: the Last Great Plague*.

European Influenza Pandemic of 1836–37 See ASIATIC AND EUROPEAN INFLUENZA PANDEMIC OF 1836–37.

European Influenza Pandemic of 1847–48 Widespread outbreaks of influenza mainly in western Europe and the Mediterranean region (see ASIATIC AND EUROPEAN INFLUENZA PANDEMIC OF 1836–37).

Scholars are not agreed on whether it was a major epidemic or truly pandemic in nature. Most agree that it probably originated in Russia, where influenza raged in Moscow and Yaroslav during January–February 1847. In March, influenza invaded St. Petersburg, where the morbidity was very high; two thirds of its residents became ill. Although its westward march was arrested there, unlike in previous pandemics, it may have spread south to present-day Turkey sometime in the spring and summer. Along with Russia and southern France, Turkey became one of the epicenters of the pandemic.

Late in August 1847, Constantinople (Istanbul) was attacked by the flu virus. From there, it spread to Alexandria in Egypt (October), southern France (early in October), and Malta (mid-October). In southern France, the infection spread rapidly to envelop Lyons and, later in October, Nice, Rennes (in Brittany), and northwestern Italy. During November, the disease coursed through France, Britain, the Netherlands, Belgium, northern Germany, Denmark (infection continuing there through January 1848), and Bohemia. Athens, Greece, was invaded in mid-November, perhaps via the Ottoman Empire (Turkey).

In December, the epidemic penetrated farther into Britain, spread to western Germany, and caused outbreaks in Algiers and Geneva (Switzerland). Madrid and Barcelona in Spain escaped infection until the very end of December, while Liège (Belgium), Naples (Italy), and Munich (Germany) remained untouched until January 1848. Influenza did not strike Berne (Switzerland) until mid-February. Surprisingly, despite the winter season, the epidemic just faded away.

The pandemic's geographical spread was quite unusual. Sweden remained unaffected, as did eastern Europe and the rest of Russia. Influenza was concentrated in western and southern Europe (its spread aided by the new railways) and northern Africa. An outbreak of the disease in the West Indies in October–November 1848 has been linked to the pandemic. According to William Beveridge (see below), influenza also invaded North America and Brazil at this time. August Hirsch, in his *Handbook on Geographical and Historical Pathology*, mentions an epidemic that occurred in Hawaii in January 1848 as being part of the pandemic.

There was considerable morbidity during the pandemic of 1847–48. For instance, it attacked between a quarter to a half of all Parisians. In London, 1,253 deaths were ascribed to influenza through December 1847, according to the city's new system of recording deaths (which replaced the antiquated bills of mortality), and 659 fatalities for the first few months of 1848. The death count for the rest of England was 12,844; including London, it was 14,756. Influenza

was particularly intense in Geneva, where one in every three residents took ill and elderly residents became victims in large numbers.

Clearly the pandemic was not as infectious as some of its predecessors had been and, therefore, did not spread as extensively. David Patterson has argued, on the basis of available evidence, that its pandemic status "seems unjustified."

Further reading: Patterson, *Pandemic Influenza, 1700–1900*; Beveridge, *Influenza: the Last Great Plague*; Smith, *Beyond the Microscope*.

European Influenza Pandemic of 1889–90

First truly global and extensively documented pandemic of influenza in Europe and elsewhere (see ASIATIC INFLUENZA PANDEMIC OF 1889–90).

Since the mid-1800s Britain and Western Europe had been experiencing an unprecedented growth in urbanization and industrialization as a result of the Industrial Revolution. Technology and transportation were moving ahead rapidly, linking cities and countrysides. Better roads, canals, and above all the new railroad system were making easier not only long distance trade in Europe, the Americas, Africa, and Asia, but also the movement of disease.

During this time, another new development was having an effect on the reporting and documentation of disease. In the mid-1800s a number of public health agencies were set up by governments in Europe as well as in the United States, Egypt, and Latin America. These new agencies were for the first time taking censuses, publishing studies of disease, and keeping track of information and statistics that monitored public health.

Medicine as a whole had also improved by the late 1800s. Not only had the number of doctors and medical journals increased, but also breakthroughs like Robert Koch's germ theory were promoting a much more scientific approach to disease and medicine. The germ theory, along with the visible spread of influenza along the new communication and trade routes, caused many younger doctors to spurn the older miasmatic theories of disease along with their dated remedies of bleeding and purging. Instead, they recognized that influenza was contagious, and even tried to isolate the microorganism that caused it. Their entire approach to the disease had become quantitative and exact.

The influenza pandemic of 1889–90 was itself quite unexpected. Aside from a few scattered outbreaks, influenza had not appeared since the late 1840s (see EUROPEAN INFLUENZA PANDEMIC OF 1847–48). In the late 1880s, however, Russia began experiencing a number of severe outbreaks in most provinces and especially along the Baltic coast. From central Russia to Siberia to the Black Sea, influenza was attacking at rates of over ten cases per 10,000 people.

The influenza pandemic that developed in late 1889 and spread globally seems to have begun in eastern Russia and spread outward from there. The outbreak originated in Tiumen, Siberia, in mid-October and moved rapidly by rail, horse, foot, and river. Influenza struck towns on the Volga River in late October and reached Astrakhan on the Caspian Sea in mid-November. It spread along the Ural River and into the central Asian republics in December 1889 and January 1890. It did not, however, make it all the way across Siberia and eastern Russia into Asia by land routes, due to the harsh, sparsely populated, frozen, and mountainous terrain. Asia was for the most part infected by oceanic trade several months later.

The disease was meanwhile moving toward Europe. By mid-November it had struck St. Petersburg and Moscow, western Russia, the Ukraine, and the Baltic. From there it spread by Baltic shipping and the European railroad into Stockholm, Copenhagen, Danzig (Gdansk), Warsaw, and Berlin in late November and early December. By the end of the month influenza had attacked Sweden, Germany, Switzerland, Austria, Belgium, the Netherlands, and France, and was moving south into Italy and the Balkans, west into Spain and Portugal, and north into Great Britain. By the end of January the entire European continent and the British Isles had been hit by the influenza epidemic.

The spread of influenza showed a typical pattern, this time more definitively documented by the new public health records. Urbanization, transportation, and accessibility routes were quite important to the transmission of the disease. Influenza spread like wildfire between major cities, while small towns and rural areas were normally hit one to two months after an outbreak in the nearest city. Extremely isolated areas (like northern Sweden, Iceland, some Alpine villages, and the Scottish Hebrides) were attacked a few months, rather than weeks, later.

From Europe, the pandemic spread to the Americas. Boston, New York, and Montreal were hit in mid-to-late-December. Canadian Manitoba, Virginia, South Carolina, and the American midwest experienced outbreaks in early January. By February influenza had attacked Nova Scotia, Saskatchewan, Newfoundland, and Louisiana, and was spreading into the coastal areas of Mexico, Guatemala, Uruguay, Brazil, and Chile. It reached the Peruvian and Ecuadoran coasts in March and April of 1890 and moved among the islands in the West Indies in a random fashion throughout the first few months of that year.

In Africa the disease was progressing in a similar manner. Influenza hit the North African coast in January and February 1890 and proceeded down the Nile in the northeastern part of the continent. At the same time it had found its way to the southern tip at Cape Town, South Africa, from where it spread rapidly northward by train and road. The western coast of Africa was hit in the early months of 1890 as well; influenza struck the British West African colonies of Gambia and Sierra Leone in February, German Togo and Cameroon in March, and the British Gold Coast (Ghana) in April. French Senegal was not hit until June. Although there is little information about influenza transmission into central Africa, it is assumed that the disease eventually made its way inland as a result of trade along the Niger and Senegal rivers. In eastern Africa, the only definitive reports place influenza in Zanzibar in March, in Portuguese Mozambique in July, and in the Ethiopian highlands in November. The Indian Ocean islands of Mauritius and Réunion experienced influenza outbreaks in August and September of 1890.

In Asia the epidemic moved southward by land routes in January 1890, from Russia into Persia (Iran), then on into present-day Pakistan. The rest of the continent was infected mainly by the shipping trade. Influenza struck the Mediterranean and Arabian Sea coasts of the Middle East during the early months of the year. It hit Ceylon (Sri Lanka) in early February, and Bombay, India, in late February, and then swept inland by rail. Japan and Hong Kong experienced outbreaks in February, while mainland China escaped the epidemic until July, when the influenza began its move inland up the Yangtze River. Singapore, Malaya, and British North Borneo were infected in March, while Shanghai was apparently not affected until October.

In the South Pacific, Australia and New Zealand experienced their first outbreaks in March, most likely caused by a ship from San Francisco. From the port cities and towns, influenza then proceeded inland throughout the summer.

The European Influenza Pandemic of 1889–90 caused high morbidity, according to those cities and towns that recorded data on the outbreaks. London gives a morbidity estimate of 25 percent, while that for Rome is 50 percent. For the most part, morbidity rates of one third to one half are thought to be accurate. Influenza struck all persons, regardless of age, sex, or socioeconomic status. Children and the elderly were, however, less susceptible to the disease, perhaps because they were less exposed to the general public.

Influenza outbreaks were rather short. About two weeks after the first cases in an area, a significant rise in incidence would occur for about another two weeks. The outbreak would then decline over two more weeks, having lasted between one month and six weeks. Mortality estimates can also be drawn from the available data. Although death rates varied from country to country, between urban and rural areas, and between age groups, an overall mortality rate can be estimated at about 0.75 to 1 death per 1,000 persons (or 270,000 to 360,000 deaths) for Europe. This was a significant death toll, larger than that caused by any other disease in the nineteenth century. Data for the rest of the world is sparse, but a similar rate can be assumed.

Although the influenza outbreaks in most countries subsided after several weeks or months, subsequent flareups did occur for a number of years. It is assumed that the original virus mutated slightly, causing new "waves" in many cities and towns. These recurrences were much less serious, striking fewer people but typically causing higher mortality than the first epidemic. They confined themselves to a small area and lasted longer. Prior infection seems to have offered up to 50 percent immunity against a recurrence. See also SPANISH INFLUENZA EPIDEMIC OF 1917–19.

Further reading: Patterson, *Pandemic Influenza, 1700–1900*; Burnet and Clarke, *Influenza*; Beveridge, *Influenza: The Last Great Plague*.

European Influenza Pandemic of 1917–19

See SPANISH INFLUENZA EPIDEMIC OF 1917–19.

European Malaria Epidemic of 1678–82

Outbreak of malarial fever that extended over a large part of Europe, killing untold thousands of people between 1678 and 1682. The infectious disease, caused by a parasitic protozoan that spends part of its life cycle in the blood of human beings (to whom it is usually transmitted by a particular mosquito), had appeared now and then in some European areas since 1557–58 (the first known European epidemic of malaria).

Throughout the 1600s, the British Isles suffered serious outbreaks of "ague," what the English then called malaria, which may have been brought home by returning soldiers and sailors from overseas duty in malarious regions of Africa, the Caribbean, and India. The London area recorded 5,237 human deaths from malarial fever in 1665, and in 1677 there were sporadic cases of ague throughout the English countryside. The following spring the disease erupted far more seriously and struck a large part of the population in the summer and fall (which was extremely hot and dry). People of all ages and socioeconomic classes were infected. Patients became exhausted to death with recurring episodes of malaria; many died

from malarial complications, such as anginas, "peripneumonies," and pleurisies. The city of London reported many fatalities from the fever in the summers of 1678 and 1679. England's King Charles II contracted malaria at Windsor in August 1679 and was cured by treatment with Peruvian bark powder (a crude quinine derivative from the cinchona tree) administered by Robert Talbor (or Tabor), an apothecary apprentice who later was appointed physician to the king and knighted. Malaria continued to attack English men and women of all classes. London recorded 1,347 deaths from it between August 10 and November 2, 1680; country parish registers sometimes indicate that the number of burials for death from malaria far exceeded the number of baptisms during the epidemic years.

Much of modern Belgium and Holland was severely attacked by the disease, which the Dutch called "febris epidemica" or "morbus epidemicus" at the time. In the hot, dry fall of 1678, numerous inhabitants of the Dutch city of Leiden (Leyden) suffered from symptoms similar to those noted in English victims: shaking chills, head and back pain, sweating, insomnia, and tiredness. In Leiden, weekly human deaths from malaria were as high as 150 (the epidemic's usual mortality count was about 20 fatalities each week). A large number of Flemish inhabitants in Belgian towns and cities contracted the disease, which also affected France's King Louis XIV in Flanders in 1680 (Louis was at war against the Dutch, English, and Germans).

Robert Talbor, who came to France from England in 1679 to treat members of the French aristocracy stricken with malaria, cured Louis XIV's eldest son (the dauphin) and other members of the royal family. For his services, Talbor received 2,000 louis d'or (French gold coins) and a generous annual pension from the king. Malaria became endemic in parts of France, including Paris; especially hard hit were Alsace and Lorraine, bordering Germany, which also endured malarial outbreaks at this time, along with Austria and Hungary (detailed information is meager). Some of the same regions were visited by malaria epidemics in 1718–22, 1748–50, 1770–72, and 1779–83.

Further reading: Bruce-Chwatt, *The Rise and Fall of Malaria in Europe*; Creighton, *A History of Epidemics in Britain*.

European Malaria Epidemics of 1805–12 and 1823–27

Local outbreaks of malaria preceded by and combined with devastating pandemics that swept over a great part of Europe, claiming many thousands of human lives in cities and rural areas.

Southern regions of France suffered heavily from epidemic malaria, which was especially deadly in the Garonne River valley and the port city of Bordeaux in the early part of the nineteenth century. At the time the parasite (plasmodium in human blood) causing malaria was not known, nor had the female anopheline mosquito, which transmits the infectious disease through its bite, been identified yet. France's southern regions had natural swamps and artificial ponds and stagnant water bodies—all good breeding places for the malaria-carrying mosquitoes. Along with malaria outbreaks in the Garonne Valley, epidemics also occurred during the digging of a canal from Arles on the Rhône River to Port-de-Bouc on the Mediterranean and in the vicinity of Marseilles and Fos. Quinine (a very bitter alkaloid) was then used in the treatment of malaria (it had been used in most of Europe since 1640). In 1800 Napoleon ordered 150 quintals of a quinine derivative—a crude powder from the bark of Peru's cinchona tree—which he distributed to 42 French cities where the malarial fever was most severe; Marseilles received about 1,100 pounds of powder. Despite the use of *quinquina* (what the French called the powder drug), malaria attacked many with recurrent cycles of shaking chills, fever, and sweats; some 3,000 people in the Landes region in southwestern France died from the parasitic disease in 1805.

Other areas known for endemic malaria included the Netherlands provinces of Friesland and Zeeland (particularly its low-lying islands), as well as the country's coastal areas; they were among the most malarious regions in Europe. The disease was most fatal in Holland (and Zeeland) during the months of September and October. In the town of Middelburg, Zeeland's capital, 534 persons died from malaria between 1802 and 1812.

Epidemic malaria devastated the British on Walcheren Island in the North Sea (in Zeeland province) during the Napoleonic Wars (1803–15). After failing to seize Antwerp in late summer 1809, the British left a garrison of about 15,000 soldiers on Walcheren, which they had seized from the Dutch. Thousands of these non-immune British troops—in this endemic malaria region—were stricken with the disease between September and November 1809; more than 4,000 of them died.

Malaria was also endemic in Ostfriesland (East Friesland), on the North Sea coast of Germany. In 1810 more than a quarter of Ostfriesland's population contracted *wechselfieber*, what the Germans called malaria.

During the construction of the St. Martin's Canal outside of Paris, France, in 1811, malaria broke out in various suburbs such as La Villette and Pantin. It is likely that some of the canal workers (former French soldiers) had carried the disease home with them from Germany and (later) from Russia, from where they retreated in defeat in late 1812. During the following ten years, the disease remained confined to its habitual endemic regions, with noticeable outbreaks in Middelburg (Zeeland) and Holland.

Another extensive malaria pandemic began in Europe around 1823. The French region of Alsace, along the Rhine border with Germany, reported an incidence of the disease that was as high as 23 percent of the hospital patients in Strasbourg, Alsace's chief city. Many French (and British and Russian) expeditionary soldiers contracted malaria in Greece in 1821 while they helped the Greeks launch their struggle for independence against Ottoman Turkish rule; the soldiers carried the fever home. Russians in western Siberia suffered a serious epidemic with high mortality in 1824. At the Baltic seaport of Königsberg (Kaliningrad, Russia), where conditions are temperately favorable for malaria, an epidemic erupted in 1825 that lasted until 1833; it was of a severity rarely seen in so high a latitude (epidemic malaria no longer occurs in many temperate zone countries).

Violent storms ravaged Germany's North Sea coastal communities in 1825, followed by an unusually hot summer in 1826 when a grave malaria epidemic struck the area; more than 10,000 persons became ill, and many perished. The North Sea also overflowed into Holland, and malaria broke out in numerous Dutch coastal areas in the summer of 1826. The city of Groningen in the northeast Netherlands recorded some 8,000 diseased persons (3,000 of them died) out of a population of about 30,000; Amsterdam, to the south, had about 2,400 human deaths from malaria in 1826. Little is known about exact fatalities from malaria in Belgium (then ruled by Holland and other European countries), but the Belgian coastal areas were infected, along with Denmark's coastal communities, in 1826–27.

Malaria was still very active in Greece in 1828, when in only a few months it killed 450 members of a French expeditionary corps in the seaport of Navarino (Pylos) in the Peloponnesus, despite the recent availability of a new, more refined cinchona bark powder for treatment of patients. Though most European countries had fewer outbreaks, Denmark's Baltic Sea island of Lolland (Laaland) suffered suddenly and seriously from malaria in 1830; more than 20,000 people were infected in Lolland's county of Maribo alone, and there was a high mortality there and in neighboring counties. Malaria did not return to epidemic proportions or prevalence in Europe until the years 1845–49, 1855–60, and 1866–72, when the disease struck many parts not only of Europe (many mentioned above) but also of India and North America.

Further reading: Bruce-Chwatt, *The Rise and Fall of Malaria in Europe*; Russell, *Malaria*; Russell, *Man's Mastery of Malaria*.

European Smallpox Pandemic of 1870–75 Devastating epidemic triggered by war. Up to this time smallpox cases in Europe had been gradually declining in number and severity because of the introduction of vaccines, both voluntary and compulsory, in several countries. At the outbreak of the Franco-Prussian War in July 1870, southern Germany required all infants to be vaccinated, but in the northern part of the country and in France such vaccination was not mandated. Germany had very few cases overall. In France smallpox had been festering silently, and the death rate due to the disease had increased about sevenfold since the middle 1860s. In Holland and Belgium it was already epidemic. War preparations, troop movements, and the migration of Parisian citizens out of their city exacerbated the previously isolated smallpox outbreaks in France. The disease began to spread rapidly, killing between 60,000 and 90,000 people in France in 1870 and 1871. It reached northern Germany in the fall of 1870, through the 373,000 French soldiers who were captured and sent to Prussian prison camps. Because of the adoption of the clothes and belongings of dead French soldiers by German civilians, the disease spread farther. Although most severe in northern Germany because of its lack of stringent vaccine requirements, the entire country was hard hit and between 1871 and 1872 reported 162,000 deaths. The disease was not so prevalent among the German soldiers themselves, due to mandatory army revaccinations every seven years. Thus, of the 8,463 (out of 800,000 soldiers in the army) who caught smallpox, only 459, or less than 6 percent, died. In the French Army, on the other hand, out of one million soldiers 125,000 were infected and 23,470 (almost 19 percent) died.

This smallpox epidemic was not limited to France and Germany. It spread throughout the continent, running especially rampant in Belgium, Holland, and Austria, which had no compulsory vaccination laws. It spread as well to the Americas (in Philadelphia alone over 2,000 died in 1871), the West Indies, and Africa. The year 1871 had one of the worst mortality rates everywhere. In Belgium 21,315 persons died; in England 23,126; and in Holland 12,476. The majority of these deaths were of children under ten years of age. After 1871 the disease spread farther south into Switzerland, Austria, and Italy as French soldiers retreated out of Germany.

The smallpox pandemic of 1870–75 is estimated to have killed at least 500,000 Europeans. The differences in severity of outbreaks and in mortality rates between countries with and without compulsory vaccination became clear and led to a major revamping of health care policy. England, for example, passed the Vaccination Act of 1871, in order to enforce its earlier Vaccination Acts of 1840, 1853, and 1867 by allowing prosecution of violators. In Germany a Vaccination Act of 1874 was passed, which forced all children to be vaccinated by age two and then again at age 12. These new laws succeeded in essentially eradicating the disease in Germany and in substantially reducing the number of cases in England, which was still divided over the legality and effectiveness of compulsory vaccination. The continuing debate between those who attributed the disease to atmospheric conditions or to an unsanitary environment ("anticontagionists") and those who believed viruses to be responsible for smallpox prevented the acceptance by the English public of vaccination as effectual protection. This public uncertainty and opposition eventually rendered the British Vaccination Acts ineffectual and allowed smallpox to persist in England and to spread once more to Italy, Spain, Austria, France, and Russia.

Further reading: Hopkins, *Princes and Peasants: Smallpox in History*; Rolleston, *The Smallpox Pandemic of 1870–74*.

European Sweating Sickness Epidemics, Northern Invasion into Europe of the mysterious and deadly "English Sweat," which appeared first in the German port city of Hamburg on July 25, 1529, possibly imported by ship from England, where an epidemic had erupted in London two months before. Until this time, the English Sweating Sickness had been confined to the British Isles, where it had appeared in 1485, 1507–08, and 1516–17. During the fall of 1529 the infection spread through Prussia, Germany, Switzerland, and Austria. One thousand to 2,000 people died from the sweat in Hamburg in the first few weeks; in Vienna, it caused havoc among Ottoman Turkish troops who were besieging the city; in the Bavarian town of Augsburg, it reportedly attacked 15,000 people in the first five days; and in Marburg, it caused religious reformers Martin Luther and Huldreich Zwingli to interrupt their meeting during the Council of the Reformation. The sweat also appeared in Scandinavia and the Low Countries. In Amsterdam, it supposedly broke suddenly from a mist, killed 500 mostly young and robust people in five days, and just as suddenly vanished. It seldom stayed in one locality more than 14 days, and its virulence varied greatly from place to place. By the beginning of December 1529 the disease had run its course; it would never again be seen in continental Europe.

The arrival of the English Sweat in Germany spread panic comparable to that caused by the plague. It was a frightening disease, killing its victims usually within 24 hours. Symptoms included chills, tremors, fever, heart palpitations, weakness, and profuse sweating, which was frequently treated with a rigorous heating regime wherein the patient lay in a blazing hot, air-tight room, heaped in blankets and furs. Like the Black Death (q.v.) and later the Spanish Influenza Epidemic of 1917–19 (q.v.), the victims of the English Sweat were mostly healthy young adults, a phenomenon that heightened its terror. No explanation of its origin, its sudden appearance in 1485, its initial confinement to England, or its incursion into Europe in 1529, has ever been found. (It would erupt once again, exclusively in England, in 1551.) See also ENGLISH SWEATING SICKNESS (ENGLISH SWEAT) EPIDEMICS.

Further reading: Hansen, *Geschichte der Epidemien bei Menschen und Tieren im Norden;* Marks and Beatty, *Epidemics;* Zinsser, *Rats, Lice and History.*

European Typhus Epidemic of 1566   See MAXIMILIAN II'S ARMY TYPHUS EPIDEMIC.

European Typhus Epidemics of 1805–07 and 1812–14, Central   See AUSTRIAN AND PRUSSIAN TYPHUS EPIDEMICS OF 1805–07; FRENCH TYPHUS EPIDEMICS OF 1813–14; GERMAN TYPHUS EPIDEMICS OF 1813–14, NORTHERN AND CENTRAL; GERMAN TYPHUS EPIDEMICS OF 1813–14, SOUTHERN; NAPOLEON'S ARMY EPIDEMICS IN RUSSIA.

Exeter Typhus Epidemic of 1586 (Black Assize)

Severe and sudden outbreak of typhus fever at the assize (county court session) held at Exeter, England, on March 18, 1586. The similarity of the circumstances to the Black Assize at Oxford nine years before was noted by the chamberlain of Exeter: This outbreak "was not much unlike to the sickenesse that of late yeares happened at an assise holden at Oxford" (see OXFORD TYPHUS EPIDEMIC OF 1577).

At Exeter, 11 of the 12 jurors died of typhus. Many of the courtroom spectators and officials were infected, and it was reported that the fever quickly spread into the surrounding English countryside. Ill and undernourished prisoners from a captured Portuguese ship were tried at the assize, many of whom died, and it is believed that the fever may have originated among these men in their crowded and filthy prison quarters. Since epidemic typhus is transmitted from man to man by the human body-louse, which thrives under such conditions, this is a likely supposition. But because little importance was attached to personal cleanliness until the nineteenth century, and lice were therefore common pests, the epidemic at Exeter could have been engendered by any louse-ridden person in the courtroom.

Further reading: Creighton, *A History of Epidemics in Britain;* Zinsser, *Rats, Lice and History.*

F

Faeroe Islands Measles Epidemic of 1846 Outbreak of measles that was the subject of a classic epidemiological study by Peter Ludwig Panum, a Danish physician who visited 52 villages on the Faeroe or Faroe Islands and treated about 1,000 patients himself. Because it came 65 years after the last previous measles case on the islands, the 1846 epidemic struck a largely nonimmune population. More than 6,000 of the 7,782 inhabitants came down with the disease.

Communicable diseases of many kinds were rare in the Faeroes, a group of 17 isolated islands lying between the Shetlands and Iceland. Panum thought that tuberculosis and syphilis were almost nonexistent, and he found no evidence of smallpox or scarlet fever in recent memory. The Faeroese people were less fortunate in other ways, however. The Danish government was too concerned with its own financial troubles to do much to alleviate widespread poverty and improve unhygienic conditions on the islands, which were under its control. As a result, other diseases—such as rheumatism, bronchitis, and skin problems—were quite common, as Panum observed.

Largely free from infectious disease but living in poverty, famine, and squalor, the Faeroese population was highly susceptible to a virus introduced from the outside. On March 28, 1846, a local carpenter returned home with measles, which he had caught when visiting several friends in Copenhagen. Despite the isolation of many individual villages, the disease traveled rapidly throughout the islands. The frequent fish kills, in which many men from different villages gathered together to hunt whales and various fish, were a prime opportunity for the disease to spread. By interviewing victims and tracing the chronology of events that triggered local outbreaks, Panum confirmed what had been known for centuries: Measles is spread through direct human contact. He also supplied conclusive evidence of the permanent immunity that measles confers on its survivors. In talking with 98 elderly people who had had the disease in 1781

(the date of the last epidemic) or earlier, he found that not a single one succumbed in 1846.

Although the epidemic struck over 75 percent of the Faeroese people, it did not slow the growth rate of the population. For centuries prior to 1800 no more than 5,000 people lived on the islands at any time; in the mid-1830s, however, over 7,000 lived there, and the number increased to more than 8,000 by 1850. Nor did the epidemic halt the social, economic, and political progress taking place on the islands. In the 1830s and 1840s the Faeroese, often led by their Danish administrators, had begun to make fishing and agriculture more productive, to fight for the abolition of the state-controlled trade monopoly, to establish schools and libraries, and to seek representation in the new Danish legislature. The attempts at reform continued in the aftermath of the epidemic, and many reached fulfillment in the following decade.

Further reading: Panum, *Observations Made During the Epidemic of Measles on the Faroe Islands in the Year 1846;* Winslow, *The Conquest of Epidemic Disease;* Jones, *Denmark: A Modern History;* West, *Faroe: The Emergence of a Nation.*

Fiji Islands Dengue Epidemics of 1971–73 and 1975 Epidemics of varying intensity that marked the return of the dengue-fever virus to the Fiji Islands after a long absence. Dengue epidemics were also reported from many other South Pacific islands in the 1970s.

The first epidemic began in March 1971 when Fiji's extremely susceptible population was struck by the dengue type 2 virus. (Tahiti was also attacked at the same time.) The epidemic in Fiji climaxed in July when 740 dengue cases were reported. By April 1972, 3,111 cases had been recorded, and, although the incidence declined noticeably after that, cases continued to be reported until 1973. Apparently, 43 percent of young adult urban dwellers were infected. A few hemorrhagic cases were observed at Fiji's Suva Hospital, but dengue did not cause any human deaths.

The dengue epidemic of 1975 was more explosive. It was part of a series of dengue outbreaks caused by the dengue type 1 virus, which occurred across the South Pacific. Early in 1974, the virus invaded the Marshall Islands. Thereafter, Nauru (mid-1974), the Gilbert and Ellice Islands (Kiribati and Tuvalu) (late 1974), the New Hebrides and the Fiji Islands (both in January 1975), Tonga, French Polynesia, and the Samoan Islands (all three groups in mid-1975) were infected by dengue fever in quick succession.

In Fiji, the epidemic began early in January 1975 in the capital, Suva, when a dengue-like illness developed among people attending a religious retreat. Laboratory analysis of these and other cases, which had been reported from elsewhere in the city, revealed the culprit as the dengue type 1 virus, which had last visited Fiji in 1944–45. The outbreak spread very rapidly until mid-March and then slowly tapered off by mid-June. Elsewhere on Viti Levu (Fiji's largest island), the epidemic lasted until late July. On some of the other island groups, the epidemic got off to a slow start but accelerated after mid-March.

By July 1975, 16,203 confirmed dengue cases had occurred all over the country. It must be remembered that not everyone who was ill sought treatment nor were all the diagnosed cases reported to the authorities. The numbers, therefore, do not accurately convey the extent of the epidemic. Among these cases, the highest incidence occurred in the 10- and 29-year-old age groups, with the 20- to 29-year-olds suffering the most. Children below ten suffered the least. Overall, males were affected at a slightly higher rate than females. More than 12 deaths were reported from the Suva area between February and April; at least six of them were caused by hemorrhagic complications and shock. It is estimated that hemorrhagic manifestations—60 percent to 70 percent involving superficial bleeding—occurred in one out of every ten patients.

In Fiji, the *Aedes aegypti* (the yellow fever mosquito) was soon discovered to be the primary vector, but the *Aedes rotumae* (only on Rotuma Island), *Aedes polynesiensis*, and *Aedes pseudoscuttellaris* may also have been involved, although in a minimal way. Once the disease was diagnosed, the authorities promptly initiated mosquito control procedures. Most of the Suva region and all the larger villages on Viti Levu were aerially sprayed, although half the population had already been infected. Workers were trained to identify and destroy mosquito breeding sites. The Fijian government began seeking to continually improve basic health care facilities at the village level.

After a brief interruption, dengue fever again flared up in Fiji during 1980–81.

Further reading: Reed et al., "Type 1 Dengue with Hemorrhagic Disease in Fiji: Epidemiologic Findings; Mackenzie, ed., *Viral Diseases in South-East Asia and the Western Pacific.*

Fiji Islands Epidemics of the Late 1700s and Early 1800s

Several epidemics resulting from Fiji's initial contacts with Europeans and the outside world; Fiji is an island group in the southwest Pacific Ocean. The first epidemic struck Fiji in 1791–92, not long after the arrival of a European ship. It was described as a prolonged illness, with patients suffering from headache, over-powering thirst, lack of appetite, stuffy nose, and congestion/constriction of the chest. Reportedly, the disease carried off entire villages in Fiji. A period of famine followed this outbreak.

Eleven years later, in 1802–03, dysentery struck the Fiji Islands; again, the outbreak was linked to the arrival of a European ship. Native records indicate that it was a very severe epidemic with devastating mortality, far exceeding that of the Fiji Islands Measles Epidemic of 1875 (q.v.).

Fiji was visited by another epidemic in 1819—again, following the visit of two American ships. The disease, which the natives called *vudi coro*, spread through the country, but the mortality was low.

In 1839, an epidemic of severe influenza broke out in Fiji. It apparently spread through most of the villages, killing many people.

Further reading: McArthur, *Island Populations of the Pacific;* Swedlund and Armelagos, eds., *Disease in Populations in Transition.*

Fiji Islands Measles Epidemics of 1875, 1903, and 1911

Three epidemics of measles that ripped through the Fiji Islands in the southwest Pacific Ocean (part of Melanesia).

The first epidemic, also the most devastating, was part of a massive outbreak of measles that began in South Africa in 1872 and spread to the tiny island of Mauritius in 1873–74 and to southern Australia in 1874. The infection was transported from Sydney to the Fiji Islands (annexed by Britain on October 10, 1874) by the British cruiser *H.M.S. Dido* early in 1875. Measles had broken out on board the cruiser, and many highly contagious passengers were later allowed ashore. Among those disembarking were Ratu Timothe (son of Thakombau, Fiji's leading chief) and his manservant, who are credited with having introduced measles into the Fijian archipelago (some 300 islands, one third of them inhabited).

They were welcomed at Levuka, the ancient capital, by a large gathering of natives representing almost every province in the country. Following a period of festivities, the representatives returned to their respective districts, taking the infection with them. During the next four months, measles spread quickly and with terrible virulence over the entire archipelago.

In this extremely susceptible population (estimated at about 150,000), the attack rate was almost 100 percent. It is estimated that more than 40,000 islanders (20 to 25 percent of Fiji's population) died during this outbreak, which subsided only after almost everyone had been infected. An eyewitness account describes many islanders as literally terrorized to death. Given its virulence and the suddenness of its onset, and the fact that they had no previous experience with the disease, most of the people did not know how to deal with it. In some cases, entire communities were attacked, leaving no one to attend to basic needs or even to bury the dead. Many died while trying to rid themselves of the fever by submerging their bodies in the sea over extended periods. Varying mortality rates were recorded on different islands, but everywhere the very young and the elderly succumbed in large numbers. The high mortality caused a severe shortage of labor in the sugar plantations. To fulfill that demand, indentured laborers were imported from India, the first batch arriving in 1879.

Fiji was invaded by measles again in 1903. Since most of the population had acquired immunity in the previous epidemic, this outbreak mainly struck young people below 28 years of age. It claimed 1,800 victims.

The island of Rotuma, which was annexed and joined to the Fiji Islands by Britain in 1881, was attacked by a measles epidemic in 1911, even as the national census was in progress. Perhaps the most deadly epidemic suffered by that island, it killed 326 people (15 percent mortality) by the middle of that year, reducing the island's population to 1,900.

Further reading: McArthur, *Island Populations of the Pacific*; Cartwright, *Disease and History*.

Fiji Islands Ross River Fever Epidemic of 1979
See SOUTHWEST PACIFIC ROSS RIVER FEVER EPIDEMICS OF 1979–80.

Finnish Ergotism Epidemics of the 1800s
Outbreaks of ergotism recorded almost annually from 1836 to 1871, with the worst epidemics occurring in 1840–44 and in 1862–63. Throughout the nineteenth century, when Finland was an autonomous and largely isolated state in the Russian empire, its economy was based almost exclusively on agriculture to meet the country's food needs. Rye was the grain most suited to the cold climate, but also the one most readily infected by ergot. Unlike their counterparts

in Germany, most Finnish farmers did not know of improved methods of draining the land and cleaning the grain that would have reduced rye's inherent tendency toward ergot infection.

The ergotism outbreaks in nineteenth-century Finland were all of the convulsive type, in which the alkaloids (nitrogen compounds) produced by the ergot fungus interfere with neurochemical balance and cause hallucinations, tremors, and other symptoms of central nervous system dysfunction. According to A. R. Spoof, whose 1872 study *Om Forgiftningar med Secale cornutum* collected the data on these epidemics, two of them were especially widespread. In 1840 in many places in Finland, an eighth of the harvested grain had ergot, while in one area over half the grain samples were infected.

The second severe outbreak, in 1862–63, coincided with a disastrous famine, during which starving people ate any grain they had, even if it was ergotized. No area of the country was immune: At least 1,400 cases were recorded, with mortality ranging from 2.7 percent to 22.7 percent, depending on the district. Because infants and young children ate a greater amount of food in proportion to their body weight than adults did, they were especially vulnerable. In 1862, for example, 56 percent of the ergotism victims were under ten years old. The ergot epidemics and famines of the 1860s (which came to be known as "the hungry sixties") made many Finns dream of a better life across the Atlantic. The first wave of Finnish emigrants left for the United States and Canada, many of them lured by agents for overseas companies, who first began to recruit in Finland during those difficult years.

Further reading: Barger, *Ergot and Ergotism*; Matossian, *Poisons of the Past*; Singleton, *A Short History of Finland*.

Florence Dysentery Epidemic of 1425
Outbreak of acute dysentery that occurred independently of plague in Florence, Italy. Called "pondi" by the Florentines, this severe diarrheal infection that affects the colon (large intestine) struck several hundred children and adults between June and October. Florence's hot and dry summer months were ideal for the spread of the disease, which is transmitted by contaminated feces (via flies) and by infected water, fruit, and vegetables.

In sections of the city where poor sanitation and malnutrition were prevalent, children were the most vulnerable to pondi, which attacked decreasing numbers of victims with increasing age. Adults suffered the same gripping or cramping gut pain but were usually able to prevent the severe dehydration that quickly killed infected young children. Five adults and 115 children reportedly perished from pondi before the epidemic came to an end in late October. The Italian city of Milan also experienced a similar dysentery outbreak in 1425.

Further reading: Carmichael, *Plague and the Poor in Renaissance Florence*; Cloudsley-Thompson, *Insects and History*.

Florence Plague of 1348   See PLAGUE OF FLORENCE (BLACK VOMIT).

Florence Plague of 1417   See PLAGUE OF FLORENCE IN 1417.

Florence Plague of 1430   Outburst of mainly bubonic plague in the Italian city-state of Florence, where more than 2,250 persons died from the highly infectious, bacillary disease (see PLAGUE OF FLORENCE IN 1417).

In early January 1430 Florentines of all ages contracted the plague, which was transmitted from rats to humans by the bite of infective fleas. (The black commensal rat, the common host for plague, lives in close proximity with human urban populations.) Children in Florence began to die in greater numbers from bubonic and pneumonic plague than adults as the epidemic advanced into the spring and summer. Between mid-June and September about 84 percent of the children who contracted plague perished. The epidemic ended after October, and the following year the disease claimed relatively few victims and was not a serious health concern until mid-century.

Further reading: Carmichael, *Plague and the Poor in Renaissance Florence*; Hirst, *The Conquest of Plague*.

Florence Plague of 1630–33   See PLAGUE OF FLORENCE IN 1630–33.

Frankish Plagues of the Sixth Century A.D.   Repeated outbreaks of bubonic plague that swept over the Frankish kingdom (France), especially its southern and central areas. The sixth-century Frankish historian Gregory of Tours recorded several instances of *lues inguinaria* or *morbus inguinarius*—a plague or malady of the groin. In referring to an epidemic in Auvergne in 571, Gregory described a wound similar to a snakebite that appeared in the armpit or groin; those afflicted died two or three days later, often after becoming delirious. To most scholars the wounds or lesions are clearly plague buboes (swellings).

Further support for that diagnosis comes from the location of many outbreaks: Mediterranean ports or places northward along the Rhône River. Although the various Frankish rulers neglected economic administration as they battled for political power, a certain amount of foreign trade continued in Gaul (roughly, France). Port cities would have been prime targets for the black rats that carried the plague. Gregory even says that a ship from Spain brought the disease to the city of Marseilles in A.D. 588. Although at first only those families that had bought goods from the ship were affected (all eight members of one household died), the plague spread throughout the city after a while.

Gregory's first recorded instance of the plague comes about 40 years earlier than the one at Marseilles. In the late A.D. 540s the plague raged in the province of Arles, while in A.D. 571 it killed many in the cities of Lyons, Bourges, Chalon, and Dijon as well as in the province of Auvergne. Appearances of the plague then became more frequent: in A.D. 582 at Narbonne; two years later at Albi, where the majority of the people died; in A.D. 588 at Marseilles, which was attacked by the disease several times in subsequent years; and in A.D. 590 in Viviers and Avignon, at the same time that bubonic plague was raging in Rome (see ROMAN PLAGUE OF A.D. 590).

Against the continual onslaughts of plague the Frankish people had little defense. When the disease hit Marseilles in A.D. 588, King Guntram advised the inhabitants to eat nothing but barley bread and water, but many popular methods to deal with the outbreaks were less rational. Prayers, vigils, and processions—all of which Gregory mentions—were used, undoubtedly to counteract the many portents people claimed to see before the epidemics struck. See also PLAGUE OF JUSTINIAN.

Further reading: Gregory of Tours, *The History of the Franks*; Thompson, *Economic and Social History of the Middle Ages*; Scherman, *The Birth of France*.

Frankish Smallpox Epidemic of A.D. 580   Epidemic described by the sixth-century Frankish historian Gregory of Tours, the symptoms of which included fever, vomiting, severe backaches, and pains in the head and neck. Although Gregory used the term dysentery, his account suggests smallpox as a more likely, though not definite, diagnosis.

Some victims imagined they had boils inside their bodies—a notion Gregory does not consider foolish, since sufferers often broke out in tumors. If the tumors burst and discharged their pus, patients were cured; many tried herbal drinks in hopes of recovering. Children were not as fortunate as adults; when the epidemic began in August of A.D. 580, it attacked children first of all, often killing them. The example of Frankish King Chilperic I, who survived a bout with the disease only to lose his two young sons to it, was typical. Chastened by their tragedy, Chilperic and his queen Fredegund put an end to their onerous taxation of the kingdom by burning the tax rolls.

Other references to smallpox-like diseases in Europe at about the same time help support the claim that smallpox may have reached France by the late sixth century. Sigbent von Gemblours described a "pestilential illness with pustules and blisters" in A.D. 541 in France, while Bishop Marius of Avenches (in Switzerland) recorded a similar disease there in A.D. 570. Finally, Greek soldiers who fought outside Mecca in A.D. 569–70 are known to have carried home a disease that could have been measles or smallpox.

Further reading: Gregory of Tours, *The History of the Franks*; Hopkins, *Princes and Peasants: Smallpox in History*; Scherman, *The Birth of France*.

Frederick Barbarossa's Army Epidemic Severe outbreak of infectious disease, probably malaria, that nearly wiped out the army of the Holy Roman Emperor Frederick Barbarossa (Frederick I) just days after its conquest of Rome in 1167. The epidemic turned his political and military victory into a stunning defeat. At the time, the Roman Catholic Church was split by schism, with two rival claimants to the papal throne: Alexander III, who had the support of many bishops and kings in Europe, and Frederick's candidate, Paschal III. Having a sympathetic pope was important to Frederick, who wanted to bring Italy and the papal lands under his own control, away from an increasingly independent papacy.

In the summer of 1167 the emperor decided to march on Rome and capture Alexander. Meeting little opposition, his German troops took the city in about a week, although in the upheaval Alexander managed to escape. When Frederick installed Paschal as pope in St. Peter's, the imperial strategy seemed to have triumphed. Frederick's luck changed on August 1, the first night of a violent storm that lasted for several days and caused the sewers to overflow in the streets. On August 2 an epidemic struck the German camp with such virulence that in four days Frederick (who himself was taken ill) ordered his army to retreat into northern Italy.

Claiming that the victims suffered from fever, chills, headaches, pain in the limbs and abdomen, and delirium, U.S. bacteriologist Hans Zinsser (1878–1940) suggested that the epidemic may have been typhus. A more plausible diagnosis is malaria, always a threat at the height of the Roman summer. Whatever its nature, the disease continued to thin the imperial ranks even as they retreated. Almost the entire army died, from generals to common soldiers, as did many of Frederick's advisors and

bishops. The emperor's opponents in Lombardy—already chafing under Frederick's attempts to subdue them—took the opportunity to form an alliance; his hopes of securing northern Italy were effectively ended for years to come.

Further reading: Baldwin, *Alexander III and the Twelfth Century*; Munz, *Frederick Barbarossa*; Pacaut, *Frederick Barbarossa*; Zinsser, *Rats, Lice and History*.

Frederick William II's Army Dysentery Epidemic of 1792 See PRUSSIAN ARMY DYSENTERY EPIDEMIC OF 1792.

French Army Epidemics in Russia See NAPOLEON'S ARMY EPIDEMICS IN RUSSIA.

French Army Epidemics of 1798–1801 See NAPOLEON'S ARMY EPIDEMICS IN THE NEAR EAST.

French Army Epidemics of 1854–56 See CRIMEAN WAR EPIDEMICS.

French Army Syphilis Epidemic of 1494–95 First appearance of syphilis (Morbus Gallicus, or the "French Disease") in Europe, occurring at Naples, first among Spanish soldiers who were then aiding that city and who apparently had been with Christopher Columbus on his first trip to the New World.

In the fall of 1494, King Charles VIII of France invaded Italy to claim his rights to the throne of Naples. His troops were from many different countries and included mercenaries of French, Spanish, German, Swiss, English, Hungarian, and Polish origin. At the time of his invasion, Italy was weak and unable to fully resist his troops. As a result, the march to Naples (and subsequent siege) was more a march of debauchery than a military campaign. There were many female camp followers, and the troops had plenty of time to socialize with them. It was common at that time to exchange women between opposing camps, and so it was not long before the syphilis spread to both armies, especially after the French troops occupied Naples in 1495.

Charles's troops were devastated by the disease. Their numbers were depleted, and those who did manage to survive were weakened and disfigured by the disease. In the spring of 1495, his army retreated from Italy. The troops returned to their own countries, carrying the disease with them. Scholars have traced the spread of syphilis at that time to the scattering of Charles's troops. The new disease appeared in France and Germany in 1495; in Switzerland later in 1495; in Holland and Greece in 1496; in England and Scotland in 1497; and in Hungary, Russia, and Poland in 1499. The disease spread not only through Europe, but to all parts of the world that the Europeans came in contact with. The Portuguese carried it to Africa and the Orient, and the disease appeared in India in 1498.

Syphilis was immediately recognized as a new disease, but it was not defined until 35 years later. The term syphilis was first introduced by Italian physician Girolamo Fracastoro in 1530, but it was not used for a long time. Instead, the disease was blamed on those thought to be responsible for it. The Italians called it the "Spanish" or "French Disease"; the French called it the "Italian" or "Neapolitan Disease"; the English called it the "French Disease"; the Russians called it the "Polish Disease"; and the Arabs called it the "Disease of the Christians."

The Spanish did not have one particular name for it but attributed its origin to Native Americans. They were most likely correct. There is still disagreement among scholars over whether syphilis existed in Europe before the return of the first expedition of Columbus from the Americas. Diseases closely related to syphilis did exist in Europe before the return of Columbus. While it is possible that the epidemic in Naples was caused by spontaneous mutation of a spirochete (bacterium) that was already present, it is much more likely that the disease was introduced to Europe by men who had been on the voyage with Columbus. Experts have studied the bones of Native Americans and found evidence of syphilis. Columbus and his crew had a great deal of sexual contact with the native Indian population, a detail that was omitted from Columbus's report to Queen Isabella of Spain. When his crew returned from the 1492–93 voyage, many joined the march to Naples with Charles VIII. Unfortunately, they were probably already infected with the disease.

There are other reasons why the syphilis epidemic in Naples was believed to be a new disease. It was unlike other genital diseases in that it caused skin eruptions all over the body. In addition, the symptoms were quite severe: high fever, intense headache, bone and joint pains, and symptoms that were similar to smallpox. The disease was often fatal. In fact, Charles VIII supposedly died of syphilis at the age of 27 in 1498.

Syphilis gained a lot of attention and was recognized as a sexually transmitted illness almost right away. In 1496, the Parliament of Paris decreed that all people infected with the disease should leave the city within 24 hours. In 1496–97, defensive measures against it were attempted at Nürnberg, Germany; in April of 1497, the town council of Aberdeen, Scotland, ordered all prostitutes to stop practicing their trade. Six months later, the Scottish Privy Council decreed that all inhabitants of Edinburgh with syphilis were to be banished to the island of Inchkeith near Leith.

Further reading: Bollet, *Plagues and Poxes;* Fleming, "Syphilis Through the Ages"; Pusey, *The History and Epidemiology of Syphilis.*

French Army Typhus Epidemic of 1528

Epidemic of typhus fever that thwarted the French siege of Naples during the Second Italian War between Charles V (Holy Roman Emperor) and Francis I (King of France); a part of the prolonged Habsburg-Valois conflict for control of Italy.

In 1528 French General Odet de Lautrec invaded Naples; his strong army of some 28,000 men encircled the largely undisciplined Imperial (Holy Roman) army, which had been reduced by illness (partly typhus) to less than 11,000 men. The siege seemed already won, but Lautrec's men were attacked by epidemic typhus (the disease, transmitted by the human body louse, had earlier broken out in upper Italy and spread to lower Italy). The men were staying in crowded, marshy camps and, as is common in times of war, were unable to keep clean. Typhus fever, which is a disease of dirt caused by an organism called *Rickettsia prowazeki,* spread quickly among the men. Within 30 days, more than half of the army had died, including Lautrec and Count Pedro Navarro (Spanish military engineer). There are some records that estimate only 4,000 of the original 28,000 French soldiers remained; also, some estimate twice as many non-belligerents perished from typhus.

The French siege was ruined, and those who survived the fever retreated. On the way, they were chased and killed by forces led by the Prince of Orange (Philibert de Chalon), in the service of Charles V. Thus, the French Army was wiped out.

Further reading: Bollet, *Plagues and Poxes;* Cartwright, *Disease and History;* Prinzing, *Epidemics Resulting From Wars.*

French Cholera Epidemic of 1832–33

First of several deadly epidemics of cholera that ravaged France in the nineteenth century. Part of a worldwide pandemic that started in India in 1826, cholera advanced relentlessly westward across Eastern Europe in the early 1830s, as France and other countries helplessly awaited its arrival (see ASIATIC CHOLERA PANDEMIC OF 1826–37). Having no experience with cholera, a disease new to Europe, French health officials were sent to already-stricken foreign cities to study preventive measures and medical treatments. Although most members of the medical establishment did not endorse the idea of contagion, the government's Council of Health insisted on quarantine measures. Accordingly, border guards were set up in August 1831 to stop infected people and goods from entering the country. When cholera appeared six months later, these measures were abandoned.

In Paris the disease came to public notice on March 29, 1832, during carnival festivities, when masked dancers revealed faces suddenly turned blue from acute dehydration and shriveling of the skin; dozens were carted off to a quick death and hasty burial, many still in their costumes. The speed with which these ghoulish symptoms overtook the victims, who often died within hours, caused immediate and widespread panic. Passers-by were lynched in Paris for carrying harmless powders, merchants accused of poisoning their wine, strangers suspected of introducing the illness into fountains and wells. The sporadic and unexpected course the disease seemed to take was disconcerting as well. One section of a neighborhood would be ravaged while another remained untouched, or one side of a street would be stricken and the other spared. (This phenomenon was noticed in England by John Snow, who correctly postulated a theory of waterborne microbes; see BRITISH CHOLERA EPIDEMICS OF 1848–49 AND 1853–54.) Those who supported the theory of contagion were hard-pressed to explain these haphazard appearances in terms of direct transmission from one infected person to another, while anticontagionists felt that cholera's checkered progress corroborated their belief that contaminated air (miasma) engenders and diffuses disease. Despite the debates about cholera's origins, most medical discussion focused on treatment. Two prominent Parisian physicians, François Broussais and François Magendie, advocated opposite approaches, both widely used. Broussais believed cholera overstimulated the body and prescribed ice, cold drinks, enemas mixed with opium, and the traditional leeches and bleeding, while Magendie used hot air baths, hot water bottles, and camphorated alcohol to stimulate the system. These approaches and others were completely useless. Many physicians openly acknowledged their failure to understand and treat the disease; others adamantly insisted on their success. Desperation for relief led enterprising French charlatans to advertise miraculous cures in newspapers and billboards. As in times of plague, people who could afford to do so fled the cities and towns to escape infection; 120,000 left Paris almost at once; 10,000 left Marseilles in January 1833.

France's country people had always resisted professional medical help as harmful and intrusive, and their distrust of doctors and the upper classes in general merely intensified during the cholera epidemic; many believed that government authorities paid doctors to deliberately infect them. On the other hand, attending physicians considered most peasants hopelessly addicted to an unclean, intemperate life that made them especially predisposed to cholera and other diseases.

Unlike childhood diseases such as smallpox and measles, which were considered a sad but inevitable fact of life, or influenza, which was fatal mostly to the elderly, cholera killed as many healthy young adults as people of other age groups, a characteristic it shared with plague. An estimated 100,000 people died from cholera in France during the 1832–33 epidemic. With its harrowing symptoms, high case-mortality rate of 25 percent to 50 percent, and likelihood of killing people in the prime of life, cholera caused more terror than any disease in European history except plague.

Further reading: Ackerknecht, *History and Geography of the Most Important Diseases*; Ackerman, *Health Care in the Parisian Countryside, 1800–1914*; Delumeau and Lequin, *Les malheurs des temps*.

French Cholera Epidemics of 1848–49, 1853–54, and 1865–66

Destructive and widespread outbreaks of cholera that ravaged France following the country's first experience of the disease in 1832 (see FRENCH CHOLERA EPIDEMIC OF 1832–33). In the epidemic of 1848–49 cholera appeared first in Marseilles and in northern France and the English Channel ports; it then spread to Paris and to the west and southwest regions. In 1853–54, Paris and Normandy were hit especially hard; and in the somewhat milder but deadly attack of 1865, France's Mediterranean shoreline, areas in the north, and Normandy and Brittany were most affected. Approximately 150,000 people died in each of the first two epidemics.

No advances in medical or etiological understanding of cholera had been made since the first onslaught of the disease in 1832. "Let us confess our ignorance about cholera if we want to be sincere" wrote a French hospital physician during the epidemic of 1849. A worldwide scourge appearing almost without interruption throughout the nineteenth century, it was not until the German researcher Robert Koch discovered the causative bacillus in 1883 that the nature of cholera and how to prevent it, if not treat it, was revealed. Prior to this discovery, alleviation of symptoms understandably continued to be the major focus of medical care, in addition to calming the hysteria that the threat of cholera often induced. French health authorities emphasized improvement of hygiene and general living conditions. Excessive eating, drinking, and indulgence in sensual pleasures was believed to predispose a person to cholera and other diseases, and avoidance of intemperate habits was accordingly advised. Peasants continued to resist the care of professional physicians, preferring instead their own home remedies and the advice of midwives.

Cholera again erupted in France, less seriously, in 1873, 1884, 1892, and 1910–11. See also ASIATIC CHOLERA PANDEMIC OF 1846–63.

Further reading: Ackerknecht, *History and Geography of the Most Important Diseases*; Ackerman, *Health Care in the Parisian Countryside, 1800–1914*; Delumeau and Lequin, *Les malheurs des temps*.

French Diphtheria Epidemic of 1818–21   See TOURS DIPHTHERIA EPIDEMIC OF 1818–21.

French Dysentery Epidemic of 1738–42   Period of severe outbreaks of dysentery in northern and western districts of France. Dysentery became widespread in Brittany in 1738, and in the autumn of 1740 the region experienced a deadly epidemic affecting mostly children; an even greater outbreak in Brittany the following year claimed over 30,000 human lives. In Anjou, an epidemic in the summer of 1742 was especially fatal among children. The urban population experienced a lower case-mortality rate than the rural peasantry, probably due to the somewhat cleaner environment of town and city dwellings.

Dysentery is an infectious disease transmitted by bits of feces contaminated by the causative bacteria. Its spread was thus facilitated by the primitive living conditions of the countryside, especially in economically depressed provinces such as Brittany and Anjou. Exposed dunghills in farmyards, lack of personal cleanliness, crowding of families in farmyards, lack of personal cleanliness, crowding of families in small rooms and often in one bed, ensured the rapid transmission of dysentery. Food shortages, drought conditions, and vagrancy due to unemployment contributed to the spread of the disease during these years in France and elsewhere in western Europe.

Further reading: Delumeau and Lequin, *Les malheurs des temps*; Post, *Food Shortages, Climatic Variability, and Epidemic Disease in Preindustrial Europe*.

French Dysentery Epidemic of 1779   Deadly epidemic of dysentery that killed an estimated 175,000 people throughout France, principally in the western provinces, during the summer and fall of 1779. Rural areas were much more seriously affected than towns and cities, basically because the appalling living conditions of the peasantry facilitated the spread of the disease (see FRENCH DYSENTERY EPIDEMIC OF 1738–42).

A doctor assigned to poor parishes in the province of Maine observed that most of the ill lay on straw, many out of doors, so sick "they were forced to stay in their mire," while fear of contagion drove neighbors and even parents away from the sick.

Another physician working near St. Malo in Brittany noted the resistance to help and the breaking of social and family cohesiveness that was so common among the rural poor: "the obstinacy of the peasant, his reluctance to take any kind of medicine, his fondness for drinking wine and spirits as soon as he is sick, the impossibility of a good administration of aid for their great misery and the dreadful spread of this scourge which smothers all feelings of humanity and gratitude, even filial love, are the main causes of this mortality." Distribution of food by civic authorities and relief from taxes helped alleviate some of the misery endured by the poor during the epidemic.

The main treatments applied by doctors and surgeons to cure dysentery were bleeding, purging, and emetics, methods that had been used for centuries for almost every type of illness. It is understandable that country people were resistant to these mostly useless and frequently harmful procedures. When doctors restricted their advice to a strictly controlled diet, which they often prescribed for their least ill patients, the proportion of successfully treated cases of dysentery increased significantly.

Both doctors quoted above attributed the spread of dysentery to "corrupted air" and "lethal miasmas," referring to the reigning theory that diseases were caused by infective air contaminated by filth or stagnant water.

Further reading: Delumeau and Lequin, *Les malheurs des temps*.

French Dysentery Epidemic of 1792   See PRUSSIAN ARMY DYSENTERY EPIDEMIC OF 1792.

French Influenza Epidemic of 1740   Uncommonly severe and fatal epidemic of influenza and other respiratory diseases in the early months of 1740; especially widespread in France's western provinces of Normandy, Brittany, and Anjou. The bitterly cold and protracted winter of 1739–40 was cited in parish records throughout the region for causing these pulmonary illnesses, which mostly struck adults and the elderly. Many parishes recorded twice or three times the usual number of burials from February through May, particularly in Anjou.

In Paris, the hospital Hôtel-Dieu, which primarily serviced the city's destitute, recorded a 35 percent increase in deaths from the previous year—7,894 for 1740, over 5,837 for 1739, mostly attributed to respiratory ailments. By comparison, deaths for the entire city rose only 14 percent, reflecting the disproportionate number of fatalities among the poor. Although people of all economic strata were affected by the epidemic, higher mortality in the poorer population was experienced everywhere. Families crowded in small, often inadequately heated rooms and sharing just one or two beds, were much more susceptible to contagious infection than people living in more spacious and effectively warmed quarters, especially during long periods of unusually harsh weather.

This acute respiratory epidemic coincided with equally destructive epidemics of dysentery and typhus fever affecting the same region of France (see FRENCH DYSENTERY EPIDEMIC OF 1738–42; FRENCH TYPHUS AND TYPHOID EPIDEMICS OF 1740–42).

Further reading: Delumeau and Lequin, *Les malheurs des temps*; Post, *Food Shortages, Climatic Variability, and Epidemic Disease in Preindustrial Europe*.

French Miliary Fever Epidemics of the 1800s

Outbreaks of miliary fever that occurred more or less continuously in France during the nineteenth century but appeared in epidemic form only occasionally. Profuse sweating is the main symptom of miliary fever (the French name is *suette miliaire*), hence its presumed association with the English Sweating Sickness Epidemics and the Picardy Sweat (qq.v.); but this connection is by no means certain. High fever usually occurs only in severe or fatal cases, along with delirium, convulsions, and loss of breath. The other characterizing symptom of miliary fever is a rash with small blisters, which led doctors to confuse the disease with measles and scarlet fever, especially since miliary fever often occurred immediately before or during outbreaks of these two diseases. Age incidence helped in diagnosis: Whereas measles is a children's disease, miliary fever attacked mainly adults.

Curiously, miliary fever appeared far more often in rural than urban areas. The first notable outbreak in the nineteenth century occurred in 1821. In 1831–32 it accompanied France's first outbreaks of cholera, and it was very widespread in 1841–42 in the southwest, where it affected some 30,000 people. In 1850 epidemics occurred in departments near the German and Swiss borders, and in 1860 in the French province of Burgundy. In March 1887 it broke out in Montmorillon in western France, and spread quickly through the surrounding area; the mortality rate during this epidemic ranged from nine to 25 percent depending on the locality. The last significant outbreak occurred in 1926.

Miliary fever was mostly confined to France, although it did appear in Belgium, Germany, Switzerland, northern Italy, Austria, and some Slavic states.

Further reading: Ackerman, *Health Care in the Parisian Countryside, 1800–1914*; Keller, *Die Letzte Grosse Epidemie von Suette Miliare*.

French Plagues of 1450–1520

Period in France during which outbreaks of plague appeared less of-

ten and were of somewhat milder intensity than previously experienced or would be experienced in following decades. This period marked the end of the Hundred Years' War with England and the beginning of a demographic rise and general reconstruction of areas that had been decimated not only by incessant battles on French soil but also by merciless pillaging, food shortages, and natural disasters.

Nonetheless, plague erupted many times throughout this era, starting with its spread in 1452–53 during the final military campaigns of the war. The worst years were 1464, 1478–84 (with over 100 recorded outbreaks), 1494, 1502, and 1514–19. These outbreaks were not necessarily seriously destructive or of long duration; evidence from tombstones indicates that plague had become far less deadly, and French annalists almost certainly exaggerated their accounts, perhaps allowing memories of past visitations and fear of future ones to color their assessment of contemporary experience. Other diseases, especially measles, smallpox, and syphilis, seem to have been more fatal and prevalent, although reports of syphilis may also have been exaggerated. Reports of plague on occasion certainly included, or referred entirely to, other diseases, since plague *(la peste)* was a general term for malady, as well as designating bubonic or pneumonic plague specifically.

Whereas during the Black Death (q.v.) in 1350 Jews and lepers were accused of engendering plague, starting around 1450 people began to believe that sorcerers and sorceresses conjured the disease. Trials of suspected individuals were conducted throughout France, and many men and women were put to death for alleged activities with magic. Some of these trials were just: Gilles de Rais (Retz), a companion of Joan of Arc, was executed in Nantes (1440) for sacrificing children in magic rituals.

France was slow to institute preventive measures against plague. From the mid-1400s, measures that had already been in force for decades in other places, particularly Italy, slowly began to be adopted by French towns. Brignoles, in Provence, was the first (1451) to inspect travelers and deny them entry if they had come from a town with plague. In 1464 the town began to expel persons suspected of being sick; and in 1494—the first town in France to do so— Brignoles authorities required a "bill of health" from travelers, a verification from towns they had passed through that that locality was free of plague. Lille prohibited the sale of furniture (1471) and of clothes (1484) that had belonged to plague victims, and Orléans was the first town in France, in 1482, to "disinfect" houses of plague victims and goods originating in places thought to be infected with plague. Towns also began recruiting surgeons and hiring men called *corbeaux* or "crows" (because they wore bird-like masks and had a somewhat sinister aspect) to carry and bury corpses. Hospitals, the first of which opened in Bourge-en-Bresse in 1472, were set up for the isolation of plague victims. By 1520, many towns were appointing special "plague captains" or "plague bureaus" charged with ensuring that the town's anti-plague regulations were carried out.

France would see a recrudescence of plague, war, famine, and social dislocation during the next 120 years.

Further reading: Biraben, *Les hommes et la peste en France;* Delumeau and Lequin, *Les malheurs des temps.*

French Plagues of 1520–1600 Eight decades of frequent and virulent outbreaks of bubonic plague in France, accompanied by food shortages and famines, flooding, harsh weather conditions, peasant uprisings, and religious wars (1562–98). Reports of plague from many localities indicate its widespread prevalence during these years. In 1521–23, 86 French accounts of plague are recorded; for 1563 and 1564, 66 accounts; and from 1580–88, 253 accounts; 1524–35, 1544–47, and 1596–98 were also periods when plague was especially active. These visitations of plague were often devastating. At Paris in 1522, the chronicler Versoris recounted that he lost his wife and 11 other household members; that more than 40 people were buried in one day in the cemetery of Saints-Innocents, where normally 30 people buried in two or three months was considered a high number; and that the poorest were most affected, one depressed quarter, Petits-Champs, having been "cleaned out" of its poor. "In short," Versoris concluded, "this year could . . . be called the great mortality, which was not only in the city of Paris, but throughout the realm of France."

Many cities began recording plague deaths and other statistical information during this period. Paris, in the epidemic of 1580, designated "quarteniers" to record facts in assigned quarters of the city and report their findings to town officials. Angers, in 1584, kept a list of hospitalized plague patients as well as fatal cases; Bordeaux maintained a list of dead in 1585; and Dijon, in 1585, recorded the number of residents who fled the town during the epidemic.

As epidemics flared with more and more frequency throughout France, town councils began to establish bureaus of health or special health "captains" to enforce plague regulations, who often in turn hired armed men to ensure obedience and maintain civic order. Force was nearly always required to contain the social unrest that inevitably arose from appearances of plague, as angry crowds looking for a way to vent their fear attacked lepers, sorcerers, pilgrims, travelers, and Jews, accusing them of generating epidemics and pillaging houses emptied of their in-

habitants due to plague. Such was the havoc plague epidemics caused that terrible physical punishments and even death were ordered for whose who disregarded the rules. Throughout the sixteenth century towns began conducting burials at night and prohibiting funeral services to avoid instilling more panic in their already disquieted inhabitants.

Soldiers were often hired by municipal authorities or regional governors to guard towns whose residents had fled for safety. Other times, when towns had little money, a "garde bourgeoise" made up of well-to-do citizens would be formed. When inhabitants refused to serve, as at Limoges in 1563 and Cordes in 1564, city magistrates would be forced to guard their deserted towns themselves. Towns also employed men called *corbeaux*, or "crows," to carry plague victims and bury the dead. Considered infectious, they had to carry a sign or wear special costumes, typically a black cloak and a beak-like mask, to warn off others, and they were isolated in separate, out-of-the-way quarters. Doctors, surgeons, and nurses (male and female) were hired by municipalities to advise them on anti-plague policies and to tend the sick. Often, doctors and surgeons would be willing to offer counsel only, and towns found themselves paying high prices for the services of attending physicians. Monks and nuns frequently served as nurses, their dedication usually precluding the need for special inducements by town authorities.

Food shortages added to the misery of plague; at Beaujeu in 1573 "the people died like flies," the poor "eating grass like animals." Wealthier citizens, as at Fougères in 1582, fled their towns to avoid both starvation and plague, leaving indigent plague victims behind, often shut up in isolation hospitals with little means of nourishment and no medical care. Frequently the reverse happened. The cities of Angers in 1583 and Apt in 1587 banished their poor, and when reports of plague in neighboring towns reached Lyon in 1580, beggars and vagabonds were ordered to leave the city "under pain of whipping." But many cities were more charitable to their poor during times of plague, providing them free shelter, food, and medical care.

France would suffer even more dramatically from plague in the seventeenth century (see FRENCH PLAGUES OF 1625–40).

Further reading: Biraben, *Les hommes et la peste en France;* Canard, *Les pestes en Beaujolais, Forez, Jarez, Lyonnais du XIVème au XVIIIème siècle;* Delumeau and Lequin, *Les malheurs des temps.*

French Plagues of 1625–40 Fifteen-year period of the deadliest and most numerous outbreaks of plague that France had experienced since the Black Death (q.v.) of the mid-fourteenth century. Serious fiscal problems resulting in peasant revolts and government repression, severe food shortages, random killing and pillaging by soldiers, and virulent outbreaks of other diseases accompanied the miseries caused by plague.

Plague appeared only sporadically during the first quarter of the seventeenth century, but accelerated dramatically starting in 1625. More than 200 separate reports were recorded for 1628–30, and the yearly average for the ten-year period 1631 through 1640 was approximately 28 outbreaks, according to contemporary records. Many French towns had to make new cemeteries or bury plague corpses in surrounding fields or private gardens to accommodate the abnormally high numbers of deceased. The worst large-scale epidemic was suffered by the city of Lyon in 1628.

By this time most anti-plague regulations and precautionary measures had been long established (see FRENCH PLAGUES OF 1520–1600; FRENCH PLAGUES OF 1450–1520). What was new to the period was a more generous treatment of the poor, who accounted for the highest proportion of plague victims. Municipal authorities allocated more funds than ever before for their care, building isolation hospitals (sometimes no more than a small, rudimentary shelter), feeding them, and hiring physicians, nurses, and other attendants. The poor of Chalon-sur-Saône, either sick with plague or suspected of being so, were fed and cared for at town expense from 1628 through 1633, and Bar-le-Duc in 1634 issued free medicines at apothecary shops. Orphans were cared for by towns or religious houses; at Amiens Capuchin monks took in 3,000 children orphaned by the epidemic of 1635–36. But the reverse was also true: Residents who could afford to do so, and often doctors and priests as well, sought safety in the countryside or other towns, leaving the sick to meet their fate. At Saint-Rambert in 1631 "half the inhabitants left with their families, at the expense of the poor who are in huts, infected by or suspected of having the contagion and ready to die of hunger," while at Feurs in the same year, "the officials and notables of the town were obliged to see all the doctors, apothecaries, surgeons and those who had the means to live in the country retreat and abandon the place."

The expense of plague epidemics was enormous. The city of Angers, for example, dispensed 100,000 *livres* (old French monetary unit) to implement its plague regulations and care for 8,000 sick during its epidemic of 1626–27. Salaries for doctors, "plague consultants," guards to watch town gates, police for maintaining civic order, men to carry and bury the dead, and other employees of town health bureaus, as well as money for food, medicine, and construction of isolation lodgings, were paid for through taxes, which citizens often bitterly protested, heavy borrowing from financiers or great lords, and some private contributions.

Purification of air was then considered effective in combating plague, and highly respected specialists who practiced *parfumage* or *aériement* were hired by towns to disinfect houses, articles of clothing, and individuals suspected of being infected with plague—many of whom, at Lyon in 1629, lost consciousness from the strong doses of "sweet perfume" they received. Many towns, such as Foncouvette in 1630, Corces in 1631, and Bourg-en-Bresse in 1636, paid young boys and girls to be shut up in newly fumigated houses, usually for 40 days, to test the efficacy of these disinfections. Other means of purifying the air included bonfires and the firing of cannons and firearms, whose powder was considered an excellent disinfectant, as was tobacco, which people used in abundance for this purpose. Towns also cleaned their roads and thoroughfares in the hopes of warding off infection, an action unfortunately taken only during times of plague; cleanliness, although of little use in arresting plague, would have helped reduce typhus fever and other "filth" diseases.

In the face of these devastating epidemics people sought consolation in their religious faith. Parish priests led supplicatory processions, and in virtually every town visited by plague, statues, altars, and chapels to the Virgin Mary were built in the hopes of winning mercy. But expressions of pessimism and resignation to what was considered God's will, found in many journals and chronicles, show that faith did little to ease the fear and desolation most people felt.

With the exception of one significant resurgence in 1650–53 and another that was less widespread in 1668–69, plague was relatively quiet in France until the great disaster at Marseilles in 1720–22 (see PLAGUE OF MARSEILLES).

Further reading: Biraben, *Les hommes et la peste en France;* Canard, *Les pestes en Beaujolais, Forez, Jarez, Lyonnais du XIVème au XVIIIème siècle;* Delumeau and Lequin, *Les malheurs des temps.*

French Plague of 1720–22   See PLAGUE OF MARSEILLES.

French Polynesian Measles Epidemic of 1854

First recorded outbreak of measles in Tahiti, Mooréa, and other of the western islands of French Polynesia (the Society Islands) in the South Pacific in 1854.

Measles was introduced into Tahiti in April or May 1854 by an American ship en route from New Castle in New South Wales, Australia, to San Francisco. Like most virgin-soil epidemics (see FIJI ISLANDS MEASLES

EPIDEMICS OF 1875, 1903, AND 1911; TONGAN AND SA-MOAN MEASLES EPIDEMICS OF 1893), its effect was devastating on the island communities. Mortality was highest in the south and west of the island of Tahiti, with Darling's trading station recording close to 100 human deaths and Davies's trading station much the same. Given the scattered communities along Tahiti's eastern coast, the death rate was believed to be quite high except along the northeast corner.

The epidemic spread to the neighboring island of Mooréa, where nearly one tenth of the population apparently perished. By the time the epidemic had subsided on Tahiti in September 1854, it is estimated that between 700 and 800 people had died. According to one account, this included people of all ages but mainly boys and men. This latter fact has been disputed and is not believed to be accurate in the light of subsequent census counts. The generally accepted mortality rate for this epidemic is ten percent. Nearly 20 percent of all marriages were brought to an abrupt end by this epidemic.

The epidemic also attacked the islands of Huahine (35 deaths), Maiao (five or six deaths), Raiatéa and Tahaa (60 deaths; three percent mortality), and Borabora and Maupiti (deaths were mainly among the older people).

Further reading: McArthur, *Island Populations of the Pacific.*

French Polynesian Measles Epidemic of 1950–51
Measles epidemic that began in Tahiti late in 1950 and spread to some of the surrounding South Pacific islands in French Polynesia.

The disease was introduced into Tahiti by sailors returning home from the Fiji Islands. Tahiti had been free from measles for 22 years so that when this epidemic began in December 1950, amid a highly susceptible population, it spread very rapidly. Nearly 90 percent of the cases occurred, as might be expected, among those under 22 years of age who had no previous exposure to the disease.

The epidemic was particularly devastating early in January 1951 when a large number of cases were reported. Authorities state that, over the following two to three months, the epidemic spread to other islands in the Society, Tuamotu, Austral, and the Marquesas groups. Around the same time, Tahiti was also struck by an epidemic of poliomyelitis (1951), which also spread just as rapidly through the island. The measles outbreak apparently ended by September 1951.

In Tahiti and its dependencies, most of the deaths in 1951 occurred in those under 25 years of age. Elsewhere, many older people died during the outbreak, leading to the hypothesis that the previous measles outbreak on some of the islands may have occurred more than 22 years ago. It is estimated that the crude death rate for the year increased by about 50 percent because of the epidemic.

Measles needs a constantly growing pool of susceptible individuals for endemicity, which the relatively small populations of these Pacific island groups could not then provide. Therefore, once the epidemic had run its course the disease disappeared until the next epidemic struck in 1960. See also FRENCH POLYNESIAN MEASLES EPIDEMIC OF 1854; TAHITIAN POLIOMYELITIS EPIDEMIC OF 1951.

Further reading: McArthur, *Island Populations of the Pacific;* Howe, *A World Geography of Human Diseases.*

French Polynesian Smallpox Epidemic of 1841
See TAHITIAN SMALLPOX EPIDEMIC OF 1841.

French Smallpox Epidemic of 1870–71   See EUROPEAN SMALLPOX PANDEMIC OF 1870–75.

French Sweating Sickness Epidemic   See PICARDY SWEAT.

French Typhus Epidemics of 1813–14   Outbreaks of lice-borne typhus fever carried by French troops to many places in northeastern France on their return march from battles in Germany in 1813 and after engagements with Allied armies in the first part of 1814, during the final stages of the Napoleonic Wars. Epidemics erupted in the provinces of Alsace, Lorraine, Champagne, and Burgundy as soldiers passing through these areas sought refuge on their homeward journey.

The scene described by a resident of Pont-à-Mousson was common:

> Who will ever forget those hundreds of wagons filled with unhappy wounded men . . . and packed in with them were sick men suffering from dysentery, typhus fever, etc. . . . . Those unfortunate men piteously begged only for a place in a hospital already filled with dying men, only to receive in reply a forced refusal, and so they were under the cruel necessity of going further to die, with the result that they infected all the towns and villages along their route, wherever they were granted a generous hospitality.

In mid-November 1813, 5,000 sick soldiers were sent to the town of Metz. Despite efforts to contain the disease, typhus spread quickly—60 soldiers died per day. Convalescing men quartered in civilian houses infected their hosts, while people working as sick-attendants brought typhus home to their families. Large numbers of people from the surrounding area pouring into Metz before the approaching German Army in January 1814 extended the epidemic, and over the next few months 30,000 more sick and weakened soldiers arrived in the city, several thousand of whom died from typhus. By April 1814, nearly 7,800 soldiers and 1,300 civilians had died in Metz, mainly from typhus fever. Strasbourg (or Strassburg), which was spared at first through successful isolation measures, lost many citizens to typhus fever during a siege in the early part of 1814. Paris was also attacked by typhus, although not as catastrophically as other places; from the latter part of February through June, 2,559 soldiers died in the city's hospitals. Civilian deaths rose by about 5,000 in 1814, perhaps 2,000 of them caused by typhus fever. Soldiers whom Parisian hospitals could not accommodate were taken by boat to towns along the Seine and Loire rivers, including Rouen and Tours, where typhus killed hundreds of men and hospital employees. See also MAINZ TYPHUS EPIDEMIC OF 1813–14.

Further reading: Prinzing, *Epidemics Resulting from Wars;* Connelly, *Blundering to Glory: Napoleon's Military Campaigns.*

French Typhus and Typhoid Epidemics of 1740–42   Exceptionally virulent wave of both typhus and typhoid fevers affecting principally the northwest region of France. In the rural areas of Brittany and Anjou, typhus caused an estimated 55,000 human deaths. Destitution and undernutrition resulting from years of economic stagnation and exceptionally harsh weather ensured that typhus fever, a lice-borne disease whose spread is accelerated by vagrancy and lack of personal hygiene, would infect large numbers of the region's peasant population.

During the winter of 1741–42, typhus erupted in the French eastern province of Lorraine, particularly in prisons, where conditions were especially conducive to the growth and spread of lice. Outbreaks of illness whose clinical descriptions suggest typhoid fever (and in some cases malaria as well) were also reported during this period from towns in Normandy, Auvergne, and other places. Deadly epidemics of dysentery and influenza added to the miseries of much of northwestern France during these years of excessive hardship (see FRENCH DYSENTERY EPIDEMIC OF 1738–42; FRENCH INFLUENZA EPIDEMIC OF 1740).

Further reading: Delumeau and Lequin, *Les malheurs des temps;* Post, *Food Shortages, Climatic Variability, and Epidemic Disease in Preindustrial Europe.*

G

Gdansk Typhus Epidemics See DANZIG TYPHUS EPIDEMICS OF 1709, 1807 AND 1813.

Genoa Typhus Epidemic of 1799–1800 See ITALIAN TYPHUS EPIDEMICS OF 1796–1800.

German, Austrian, and Swiss Plagues of the 1500s Period in which outbreaks of plague occurred with frequency throughout most regions of Germany, Austria, and Switzerland.

In northern Germany, some of the more serious epidemics of plague occurred in Hamburg in 1537, 1547, and 1564; in Lübeck in 1543, 1548 (16,000 deaths), and 1564 (17,000 deaths); and in Rostock in 1564 (10,000 deaths). Both 1564 and 1565 were plague years for most of northern Germany (and most of western Europe): "There was a dreadful death from plague everywhere in towns and in the countryside." Plague again struck most places in northern Germany in 1596, 1597, and 1598, including the cities of Hamburg, Lübeck, Bremen, Rostock, Lüneburg, Hanover, and Magdeburg. The miseries of plague were multiplied by a widespread famine throughout the region in 1597.

In Bavaria plague was widespread in 1552 and again in 1562 and 1563. In Nuremberg in 1562 the plague prevented Carnival festivities from taking place, and Regensburg recorded major epidemics in 1520 (3,000 victims) and in 1562 (2,000 victims). The city of Augsburg experienced some 20 outbreaks of plague throughout the century in which nearly 60,000 people died.

Plague was especially persistent during the sixteenth century in Switzerland, particularly in the cities of Basel and Geneva. Most outbreaks in Austria took place in the 1520s, 1560s and 1570s.

It became more and more common during this period for people of high social and professional rank—people with positions in royal households, government officials, lawyers and judges, and members of universities—to leave their cities when plague broke out and move temporarily to other places. In

1527, for example, the University at Tübingen sent its several departments to various localities far removed from the town. German religious reformer Martin Luther admonished the public to ask themselves if fleeing the plague did not mean neglecting one's Christian duty toward one's neighbor, and when the faculty of Wittenburg University withdrew to Jena in 1527, Luther, who was a faculty member, not only stayed behind but also took plague patients into his home.

Further reading: Biraben, *Les hommes et la peste en France;* Hansen, *Geschichte der Epidemien bei Menschen und Tieren im Norden;* Sudhoff and Sticker, *Zur historischen Biologie der Krankheitsreger.*

German, Austrian, and Swiss Plagues of 1663–68 and 1675–83 Two final periods of widespread outbreaks of plague in Germany, Austria, and Switzerland before the disease's disappearance from western Europe in the early eighteenth century. The worst years for western Germany were 1665 and 1666, when Cologne (Köln), Düsseldorf, Münster, Bonn, Koblenz, Mannheim, Mainz, Frankfurt, and other towns in the Rhine River region were sites of major epidemics. Both 1663 and 1664 were malignant plague years for Hamburg; a report from July 23, 1664, states that the plague there had gotten "very out of hand."

In Switzerland, 1667 and 1668 were the most serious plague years, particularly for Basel; a *Pestkonferenz* (plague meeting) was sponsored by Zürich in the town of Bremgarten to which officials from neighboring places were invited to discuss how they might prevent the plague from spreading from Basel, where the disease was rampant, to their cities. Many towns in Bavaria, including Bamberg, Nuremberg, Regensburg, and Ingolstadt, reported plague in 1679, and the cities of Leipzig, Dresden, Erfurt, Magdeburg, Halle, and other smaller cities in eastern Germany experienced outbreaks from 1679 to 1683. Plague was present in Austria from 1675, especially in Vienna, which in 1679 experienced its worst plague epidemic (see PLAGUE OF VIENNA, GREAT), and erupted in many parts of Bohemia and Silesia from 1677 to 1680. Many towns and villages during these years commemorated the end of a plague epidemic by holding a festival on the anniversary of its disappearance.

This period was preceded by 25 years of relative absence of plague from most places in Germany, Austria, and Switzerland, and with the exception of sporadic, localized outbreaks over the next 30 years, was the last time plague appeared in epidemic form over extended areas in these countries.

Further reading: Biraben, *Les hommes et la peste en France;* Hansen, *Geschichte der Epidemien bei Menschen und Tieren im Norden;* Treichler, *Die Staatliche Pestprophylaxe im alten Zürich und diesbezügliche Vereinbarungen.*

German Cholera Epidemics of 1830–90 Sixty-year period in which outbreaks of cholera occurred at varying intervals in many areas throughout Germany. The disease first reached Germany in 1831 as part of the second worldwide pandemic of Asiatic cholera that had begun in India in 1826 (see ASIATIC CHOLERA PANDEMIC OF 1826–37). German authorities attempted to prevent the disease from crossing their borders as they watched the deadly infection make its way westward from Russia through East Prussia and Poland during the spring of 1831. Large sums were spent, to no avail, in setting up military cordons, inspection offices, and quarantine buildings; ships were stopped at river and sea ports, travelers were questioned at train stations; packages, letters, and money crossing town borders were checked and fumigated. Residents along the Baltic and North Sea coasts helped troops watch for ships coming from foreign cities.

Cholera's first appearance in Germany was in Berlin in August 1831. Hamburg's first case was reported on October 8, and an outbreak occurred again the following summer. Nearby Lübeck, also a northern port city, was attacked in the summer of 1832. Cholera again broke out in many areas of Germany, especially the north, from 1848 to 1850, from 1853 to 1859, in 1866 and 1867, and in 1871. These periods roughly coincided with epidemics in other European countries. Although these outbreaks were serious and claimed thousands of lives, they were minor in comparison with the disastrous Hamburg Cholera Epidemic of 1892 (q.v.).

The approach of cholera caused unprecedented panic among nineteenth-century Europeans. An acute enteric disease that can kill within hours, cholera is characterized by the sudden onset of violent symptoms, which include abdominal pains, vomiting, and a profuse diarrhea that rapidly dehydrates the victim and causes the skin to shrivel and turn blue or black. The case-mortality rate is often more than 50 percent in untreated patients, and until the twentieth century, medical treatments were more or less useless in any case.

Further reading: Ackerknecht, *History and Geography of the Most Important Diseases;* Evans, *Death in Hamburg;* Hansen, *Geschichte der Epidemien bei Menschen und Tieren im Norden.*

German Epidemics of 1618–48 See THIRTY YEARS' WAR EPIDEMICS.

German Plagues of 1462–65 Terrible outbreaks of plague that killed thousands of people in widely distant cities in Germany from 1462 to 1465. In the Bavarian town of Regensburg, the black plague arrived and killed 6,300 people in 1462. The town council fled for safety, meanwhile agreeing with the regional cathedral authorities that Regensburg's citizens should hold a great propitiatory procession (presumably to save the people left behind). The next year also brought a great scourge that lasted about eight months and claimed 2,500 lives; much was made of the fact that 16 monks died in the Convent of St. Emmeran in one month's time. Other places in Bavaria afflicted by plague during these years included the cities of Nuremberg, Munich, and Augsburg.

Accounts from the northern port city of Hamburg assert that an explosive affliction struck Germany, that it originated in the Rhineland region, and that medical assistance did not help. Conditions in the Baltic seaport of Rostock were particularly dismal; parents wrapped their dead childrens' bodies in coarse cloth as did children their dead parents' bodies. Coffins were not used. Corpses were carted away at night to any churchyard, where they were cast into large pits already loaded with corpses.

Plague reports for 1462–65 also survive from the towns of Magdeburg, Erfurt, and Merseburg and other places in central and eastern Germany.

Further reading: Hansen, *Geschichte der Epidemien bei Menschen und Tieren im Norden;* Schöppler, *Die Geschichte der Pest zu Regensburg.*

German Smallpox Epidemic of 1871 See EUROPEAN SMALLPOX PANDEMIC OF 1870–75.

German Sweating Sickness Epidemics of 1529 See EUROPEAN SWEATING SICKNESS EPIDEMICS, NORTHERN.

German Typhus and Dysentery Epidemics of 1757–63 Period of localized epidemics of typhus fever, spread primarily through troop movements in Germany and Silesia (the western region of present-day Poland) during the Seven Years' War (1757–63).

In contrast to the War of the Austrian Succession (1740–48) when thousands of troops moved continually throughout Germany and parts of Eastern Europe, spreading typhus and other "camp fevers" over wide areas (see GERMAN TYPHUS, TYPHOID, AND DYSENTERY EPIDEMICS OF 1741–43), armies during the Seven Years' War were smaller and moved from place to place quickly, leaving less time to infect large numbers of civilians. Nonetheless, typhus fever and dysentery, which inevitably arose in armies where crowding and lack of hygiene facilitated their spread, claimed far more lives than fighting.

Towns in Silesia were infected by Austrian and Prussian troops in 1758, particularly Breslau, where 9,000 soldiers and camp followers died that year, as well as 9,000 townspeople, mostly from typhus. Schweidnitz and Landshut in Bavaria also suffered epidemics of typhus in 1758. Many places in northern Germany, which was not involved in the war, were infected in 1757, including Dresden, where annual burials doubled. In 1760 Dresden was again infected, this time by invading troops, causing an increase in yearly burials of 75 percent. Eisenach suffered many deaths from typhus both in its military hospitals and among its civilian population.

Further reading: Prinzing, *Epidemics Resulting from Wars*; Cloudsley-Thompson, *Insects and History*.

German Typhus Epidemic of 1734

Virulent outbreaks of epidemic typhus fever among army troops and civilian populations over widespread areas of Germany during the War of the Polish Succession (1733–38). Polish armies moving through Silesia (present-day southern Poland), Prussia, and the shores of the Baltic Sea in 1734 spread the disease throughout those regions, and in the west, French and German soldiers stationed on either side of the Rhine River in the fall of the same year brought typhus to many towns in the area, including Heidelberg, Heilbron, and Germerscheim. Thousands of soldiers and civilians died from typhus.

Further reading: Prinzing, *Epidemics Resulting from Wars*; Cloudsley-Thompson, *Insects and History*.

German Typhus Epidemics of 1813–14, Northern and Central

Destructive epidemics of lice-borne typhus fever disseminated through Germany by infected soldiers following battles at Leipzig and other places near the Elbe River between Napoleon's army and Allied forces in 1813 (see NAPOLEON'S ARMY EPIDEMICS IN RUSSIA).

After his defeat in Russia, Napoleon gathered a new army of 500,000 recruits that, even before the decisive Battle of Leipzig in October 1813, had lost an estimated 219,000 men to disease, compared with 105,000 directly to war casualties. Lice-ridden men crowded together in barracks, hospitals and private homes spread typhus among themselves, hospital workers, and civilians who were forced to give them shelter. Allied forces pursuing French troops after Napoleon's defeat were well aware of the danger of contracting typhus fever: As the fever-ridden French army retreated, it infected local villagers along the way. Soldiers, dead or dying, littered the roadways, and pursuing allied soldiers refused to rest or sleep in the same spots once occupied by dying soldiers and corpses.

Dozens of towns in Saxony became infected with typhus fever. According to a pastor in Dresden, after the Battle of Bautzen in May 1813, homeowners were compelled to quarter as many as two, three, or four hundred soldiers, many of whom suffered from wounds, scurvy, and infectious disease (mostly typhus), because the hospitals were overcrowded and could not accommodate them. Entire families perished from sickness and wagons carrying the dead were often heard along the streets.

Typhus deaths among residents increased even further after the Battle of Dresden on August 26 and a siege of the city from mid-October to mid-November. More than 21,000 soldiers died in Dresden in 1813. In the city of Leipzig, 80,000 French soldiers died of wounds and diseases, mostly typhus fever, after the battles of Dresden and Leipzig, while civilian deaths rose to 1,528 in November and December 1813, compared to 200 deaths in the same months the following year. Typhus was epidemic throughout most of Brandenburg. Deaths from typhus among Berlin's civil population increased 400 percent in March, April and May of 1813 and again rose sharply from November 1813 through February 1814. Typhus afflicted many places along the Elbe River, including Magdeburg, Wittenberg, and particularly Torgau (see TORGAU TYPHUS AND DYSENTERY EPIDEMIC OF 1813). South of Leipzig, troops spread typhus through Weissenfels, Altenburg, Wittenberg, Jena, Weimar, and other places. Erfurt hosted nearly 20,000 sick and wounded French and Prussian soldiers in 1813, thousands of whom civilians were forced to quarter; Prussian forces then besieged Erfurt, which accelerated the diffusion of typhus among those trapped within the city.

Battles in the region of the Main and Rhine rivers resulted in further dissemination of typhus fever. French, German, and Russian soldiers poured into Frankfurt, filling its hospitals and civilian houses. Civilian deaths from typhus rose dramatically in Hanau, Wiesbaden, Koblenz, Limburg, and many other towns and villages in the Rhineland.

Typhus was active in many places in the north of Germany at this time, but not as a result of French troops retreating after the battles fought in and around Leipzig, who passed mainly through the central, western, and southern provinces. In Hamburg, an epidemic raged through the city during a siege in early 1814, spreading first through military hospitals and then to the civilian population: In the garrison, 60 or 70 (at one time as many as 100) died every day between the start of February and the end of March. At the beginning of the siege the garrison numbered some 25,000 or 30,000 men. By the end of March, at least 10,700 bodies had been interred by the town moat, with about 8,200 people dead from typhus fever and some 2,500 from wounds. Civilian fatalities were also high, since residents were forced to house typhus patients that the overflowing hospitals could not accommodate. Surviving troops and refugees spread typhus through the surrounding area, including the towns of Altona and Lübeck. Epidemics broke out in Kiel and parts of the province of Mecklenberg during the first part of 1814.

Typhus fever in Germany abated through the spring of 1814 as Napoleon's retreating troops gradually reached France. Between 200,000 and 300,000 civilians died in Germany from typhus in 1813 and 1814, including the southern regions (see GERMAN TYPHUS EPIDEMICS OF 1813–14, SOUTHERN).

Further reading: Brett-James, *Europe against Napoleon: The Leipzig Campaign;* Prinzing, *Epidemics Resulting from Wars;* Cloudsley-Thompson, *Insects and History.*

German Typhus Epidemics of 1813–14, Southern

Epidemics of typhus fever throughout the southern regions of Germany disseminated by French and Russian troops after Napoleon's campaign in Russia (see NAPOLEON'S ARMY EPIDEMICS IN RUSSIA).

In the latter part of 1812 and first few months of 1813, French soldiers returning from Russia perished in the thousands from disease, lack of food, and exposure during the long westward march through Poland, Prussia, and eastern Germany. By the time the survivors reached southern Germany, their numbers had so decreased that typhus fever could be controlled through isolation. Authorities in Bavarian border towns, for example, inspected troops for typhus, sending infected men to barracks and lazarets (lazarettes) outside the towns. These precautionary measures, which were possible only because of the relatively small numbers of troops involved, prevented the disease from spreading through the civilian population of Bavaria, although military hospitals in Bayreuth, Plassenburg, Altdorf, and especially Bamberg were crowded with typhus patients.

The civilian population of southern Germany thus remained largely free of typhus until November 1813, when troops and prisoners passing through the area after battles near Hanau and Leipzig spread the infec-

tion almost everywhere. The isolation enforcement that had been so effective the previous spring in Bavaria was useless in the face of these enormous groups of men: Typhus-carrying French soldiers and troops, marching through the country from Saxony and Würtzburg to Bohemia, spread the fever to the citizenry in cities and rural areas. Many soldiers died in agony from the fever: thousands perished in hospitals. Case-fatality rates were especially high in towns in Upper Franconia and in Würzburg. Among the worst hit towns of Bavaria were Bamberg, where 20 patients a day died in the miliary hospital and whose residents also suffered severely; Regensburg, where townspeople were infected by residents serving French prisoners; and Ingolstadt, where 2,000 prisoners died. Württemburg was thoroughly infected with typhus, as were towns in Baden, which were forced to host thousands of sick prisoners transported there from France.

Freiburg's 9,000 residents accommodated 210,000 troops: In the garrison lazaret and university hospital in December 1813, there were more than 1,200 sick troops crowded into room space normally holding only 500 patients. Most suffered from typhus or diarrhea. Because of lack of clean linen and clothes, they were forced to remain lying on sacks of straw in their filthy uniforms. Many dead bodies were loaded onto large carts and driven away for burial each morning. The fever also contaminated civilians and wiped out whole families. The epidemic there continued through February 1814. Karlsruhe and many smaller towns in Baden, towns in the Rhineland including Worms and Kreuznach, as well as Darmstadt and other places south of the Main River suffered severe outbreaks due to the presence of infected French prisoners and passing troops.

Because of lack of hospital space and an effort to contain the disease, troops sick with typhus fever were put on boats at Trier and other places along the Moselle and Saar rivers; dead soldiers were simply thrown overboard, and many boats were left to float without a helmsman and with no way to procure food.

As this phase of the Napoleonic Wars came to a close, troop movements through Germany gradually ceased, with a consequent abatement of typhus fever through the early summer of 1814.

Further reading: Brett-James, *Europe against Napoleon: The Leipzig Campaign;* Prinzing, *Epidemics Resulting from Wars.*

German Typhus, Typhoid, and Dysentery Epidemics of 1741–43

Period of unusually high numbers of deaths throughout southern and western Germany caused mostly by epidemic typhus fever and other "camp fevers" carried to many localities by army troops involved in the War of the Austrian

Succession (1740–48). Historically associated with times of war and deprivation, typhus, the deadliest of the camp fevers, is transmitted by infected human body lice, which thrive wherever human beings are crowded together and deprived of means to bathe and otherwise rid themselves of vermin; typhoid and dysentery are bacterial diseases also facilitated by substandard living conditions.

Austrian troops moving across Bavaria and French troops garrisoned in various Bavarian towns brought typhus and the other camp fevers to many places, including Nuremberg, Augsberg, Landsberg, Passau, Ingolstadt, and Amberg. Both French and Austrian troops in the eastern regions of Bohemia and Silesia (part of present-day Poland) spread typhus and dysentery throughout those regions. Hanau and its surrounding villages along the Main River hosting English and Austrian troops after the Battle of Denningen in 1743 were severely infected with typhus and dysentery; a hospital set up near Hanau for British soldiers was rife with typhus, which infected most if not all the patients and killed nearly half of them. Dysentery was brought by army troops to Koblenz, Mainz, and Giessen.

Many towns in Thuringia and Hesse-Homburg in central Germany also experienced epidemics of typhus in 1740 and 1741, although they were not affected by the war. Outbreaks had occurred in some of these areas since 1737.

Further reading: Post, *Food Shortages, Climatic Variability, and Epidemic Disease in Preindustrial Europe*; Prinzing, *Epidemics Resulting from Wars*.

Ghanian Malaria Epidemic of 1952–54

Outbreak of malaria that struck nearly 77,000 inhabitants (killing about 4,250) in the populous southern coastal regions of present-day Ghana in West Africa between 1952 and 1954. The fatality rate was thus over five percent for the three-year epidemic.

The British colony known as the Gold Coast (which became the independent state of Ghana in 1957) recorded its first human deaths from malaria in 1920. This communicable disease caused by a parasitic protozoan and transmitted to persons by the bite of an infective female anopheline mosquito did not become a major problem until the mid-1940s. The southern tropical areas of Ghana, especially the swamps and other stagnant water bodies, were ideal for the anopheline mosquitoes to breed and spread the tiny parasite. In 1952 Ghanian officials reported about 28,000 malaria infections and almost 24,000 the following year, mainly in and around the seaport cities of Sekondi, Cape Coast, and Accra (the capital).

Malaria became the number one menace in Ghana, where many of the deaths occurred among children under the age of three. The aftermath of this unpleas-

ant infection (which brings violent chills, high fever, aching, nausea, and vomiting) is severe, for the illness stifles physical and mental growth and depresses fertility. In 1954 more than 24,000 Ghanians perished from it. Afterward the gradual use of DDT spray eliminated many mosquitoes and greatly reduced the case incidence of malaria, which remains a problem at times in parts of the country.

Further reading: Hartwig and Patterson, *Disease in African History*; Scott, *Epidemic Disease in Ghana*.

Ghanian Meningitis Epidemics of 1945–49

Serious outbreaks of cerebrospinal meningitis (CSM) that occurred annually between January and April in Ghana's northern region, where about 34,000 people contracted the acute bacterial disease and at least 3,200 died from it between 1945 and 1949.

In 1906 present-day Ghana (then known as the Gold Coast of West Africa) suffered a severe CSM epidemic that left some 20,000 people dead in less than five months. Afterward CSM remained limited to the savanna (grassland) of the north, where a major epidemic began in January 1945 at the start of the dry season. As usual, cold weather forced native groups to sleep indoors in crowded, poorly ventilated houses, where they were more susceptible to infection. Infection was from aerial droplets and discharges from the sneezes and coughs of infected persons. By May almost 10,000 CSM cases had been reported in Ghana's northwest districts of Lawra, Wa, and West Gonja. Within two to five days after contracting the disease, patients suffered blinding headaches, fever, dizziness, delirium, and stiff neck pain that lasted one to three weeks. Even with sulfa drugs administered to the sick in hospitals and special emergency camps in the bush, some 1,000 persons died by the time that outbreak ended in early June.

After that devastating epidemic in 1945, CSM continued its unpredictable state in Ghana with two moderate outbreaks: 1946 saw some 700 CSM cases and 1947 had almost 1,300 cases. In 1948 another major epidemic afflicted an estimated 11,000 Ghanians, especially in the Kusasi district, where around Bawku alone 5,700 people were stricken. Another serious epidemic of CSM occurred in some of the country's northern districts, where a total of some 10,000 cases were reported. In both 1948 and 1949, sulfa drugs and improved living conditions helped keep the mortality rate to about ten percent.

Further reading: Patterson, *Health in Colonial Ghana*; Scott, *Epidemic Disease in Ghana*.

Ghanian Plague of 1908

Outbreak of bubonic and pneumonic plague in the eastern and central regions of present-day Ghana during ten months in 1908, killing reportedly 300 of the 344 who became infected.

Plague entered Ghana (then the British colony known as the Gold Coast) in January 1908 through shipping at its port city and capital Accra. Upset by the alarmingly rapid spread of the then unidentified, highly infectious disease and its high mortality rate, medical authorities in the Gold Coast requested that burials of victims not take place until postmortem examinations were made. Plague was then diagnosed, and tests on the area's dead rats soon confirmed the existence of the plague bacillus *Yersinia pestis (Pasteurella pestis),* which is usually transmitted by diseased rat fleas to human beings.

In February 1908 British professor W. J. Simpson, a leading authority on plague, arrived in Ghana, where he set up a sanitary cordon extending from Nungwa (north of Accra) to the interior districts of Nsawam and Teimang; no one was allowed to pass into the area without a valid certificate of vaccination. More than 16,000 persons in Accra were inoculated against plague (using a method introduced into India by bacteriologist Waldemar Haffkine in 1897). And an intense rodent eradication program began. These measures eventually brought the epidemic to an end in October. See also ASHANTI PLAGUE OF 1924–25.

Further reading: Scott, *Epidemic Disease in Ghana;* Scott, *A History of Tropical Medicine.*

Ghanian Plague of 1924–25   See ASHANTI PLAGUE OF 1924–25.

Ghanian Sleeping Sickness Epidemic of 1936–41
Serious outbreak of African sleeping sickness (trypanosomiasis) that killed more than a thousand persons out of a reported 34,651 who became infected in Ghana (includes part of the former Gold Coast). The popular belief was that Ghana had been struck by an outbreak that had started in the Congo (Zaire) about 1912 and then moved gradually westward through Cameroon, northern Nigeria, Dahomey (Benin), and Togo to finally reach Ghana by 1930. The development of the Gambian type of sleeping sickness (in which humans are an important reservoir of the infectious agent, *Trypanosoma gambiense,* a hemoflagellate) increased the disease to epidemic proportions in northern Ghana, particularly in Gambaga, Walewale, Nakpanduri, Bawku, and Tamale, in 1936.

Transmitted by the bite of an infective tsetse fly *(Glossina),* the disease caused fever, headache, lymph node enlargement, anemia, somnolence, and rash, among other symptoms noticed in the sick Ghanians. Human beings and tsetse flies congregated near water sources (rivers and lakes) were the foci for the epidemic. Ghana's wetter southern regions were also affected in 1936, when cases were reported in Sunyani, Kumasi, Dunkwa, and Mpraeso (the latter two towns in the forest belt saw an increasing number of infections among Europeans). Cases of sleeping sickness were relatively few in the capital of Accra and other coastal towns during the epidemic.

By 1937 the acute disease was a serious health menace and the so-called Trypanosomiasis Campaign was established in the northern town of Gambaga; in some districts the epidemic was controlled, in others it was continually spreading in the countryside. Destruction of tsetse fly habitats was certainly difficult at first, for they were sometimes located in sacred religious groves beside the only water supplies of native villages. Eventually a major campaign involving the hand-catching of flies and the digging up of tsetse pupae proved beneficial. Patients received intravenous tryparsamide with some success, but case incidence in Ghana increased in 1938 (5,611 cases) and in 1939 (6,826 cases). In some northern villages, such as Tumu, the infection rate was as high as 16 percent of the inhabitants in 1939.

The epidemic gradually declined during the next two years until the local health authorities had informed many people about measures to protect them against biting tsetse flies. Sleeping sickness waned in Ghana during the next decades.

Further reading: Hartwig and Patterson, *Disease in African History;* Scott, *Epidemic Disease in Ghana.*

Ghanian Smallpox Epidemic of 1945–47   Grave epidemic of smallpox that killed 608 persons out of 3,196 reported infected in the West African country of Ghana (a part of the Gold Coast) from 1945 to 1947.

Before smallpox was eradicated in Africa in the 1970s, the largest recorded upsurge in smallpox cases occurred there in the years following the end of World War II (1939–45). This upsurge was supposedly fueled by military movements associated with the war and by the European powers' relative neglect of disease control measures in the African colonies. Some 99,000 cases of smallpox were reported throughout Africa in 1944 and 1945; Ghana (then under British control) reported 143 cases and 38 deaths from smallpox in 1944. In 1945 the disease infected 702 persons in Ghana, mainly in the north and Volta region. Although adults were immune because of previous smallpox infection, all age groups contracted the dreaded "pox," which is one of the most communicable of all diseases. The transmission of smallpox requires only a human breath to blow the variola or smallpox virus from one mouth to another. And smallpox can be carried by articles touched by a victim, by persons who visit a patient, and even by a diseased corpse. Death commonly occurs between the eighth and fifteenth day after contracting the disease (if untreated) and results from overwhelming toxemia or hemorrhaging. In 1945 there were 128 fatalities from smallpox in Ghana—a mortality rate of more than 18 percent.

The natives of Ghana had suffered from smallpox since the late fifteenth century, and a common method for treatment after the eighteenth century was variolation (vaccination with the smallpox virus), which was also responsible for helping spread the disease. Annual notifications of smallpox cases began in Ghana in 1901; serious outbreaks occurred in the country, with mortality rates between ten percent and 50 percent reported. By 1937 the glycerinated lymph vaccine used against smallpox had been replaced by a much more stable "dried" vaccine, which proved to be more effective and reduced the danger of the disease, which became almost unknown in urban areas.

In 1946 there were 616,000 smallpox vaccinations administered in Ghana, whose population then was about five million people; that year saw 1,646 infections with 311 fatalities from the disease. With about the same number of vaccinations in 1947, Ghana had 848 or 852 cases, most of which occurred (as in 1946) in the north and Volta region and the most serious in the east along the southern part of the Ghana-Togo border and in the Keta and Ho districts, with the disease spreading to the Akwapim ridge, thus threatening Accra, Ghana's capital. In 1947 there were 169 deaths from smallpox, including 56 in the district of Bawku and 79 in the nearby districts of Navrongo and Zuarungu in northeastern Ghana.

More than a million and a half smallpox vaccinations were performed in Ghana in 1948, and the fatality rate was considerably lower among the 1,262 cases recorded. When a moderate smallpox outbreak occurred along the southern part of the Ghana-Togo border in 1948, a vaccination campaign was undertaken jointly by the health authorities of both countries. As a result of the global smallpox eradication campaign that began in 1967 with the aid of the World Health Organization, Ghana and other West African regions were almost completely free of the disease by 1970.

Further reading: Hartwig and Patterson, *Disease in African History;* Scott, *Epidemic Disease in Ghana.*

Ghanian Tuberculosis Epidemic of 1942–44

Outbreak of tuberculosis (TB) that killed more than 3,200 persons in urban centers of southern Ghana (the Gold Coast) in West Africa. A chronic bacterial infection involving the lungs, bones, and other body organs, TB is spread through air droplets, mainly by inhalation of tubercle bacilli coughed up by infected persons.

In Ghana, TB began to reach epidemic proportions in 1942 during World War II, when the country's population continued to grow fast along the southern coastal region, especially in the two largest cities, Accra (the capital) and Sekondi. All forms of this wasting disease killed a reported 1,062 persons in 1942; the high incidence of infection was primarily due to many people's intimate contact with infected persons. In 1943 there were 1,094 human deaths from TB (a mortality rate of 264 per 100,000 persons), and in 1944 there were 1,048 deaths in the coastal area and cities. That same year the potent antibiotic streptomycin was discovered to combat the tubercle bacillus (*Mycobacterium tuberculosis*). Using streptomycin and other drugs, TB was gradually brought under control, and fatalities dropped to 944 in 1945 and declined with effective antibiotic therapy to 179 in 1957. Since then, the TB contagion has remained a problem that Ghanian health authorities have seen reemerge in patients with AIDS (acquired immunodeficiency syndrome). See also AFRICAN AIDS EPIDEMIC.

Further reading: Hartwig and Patterson, *Disease in African History;* Scott, *Epidemic Disease in Ghana.*

Ghanian Yellow Fever Epidemic of 1926

Outbreak of yellow fever that struck about a thousand inhabitants of the small town of Asamankese in what is now southern Ghana (then part of the British-controlled Gold Coast). It was the first large epidemic of yellow fever wholly among black natives ever observed in West Africa; as a result, a Yellow Fever Commission (established in 1925 in nearby Accra, Ghana's capital) closely studied the epidemic and concluded that the *Aëdes aegypti* mosquito was the vector for the disease in the region.

In May 1926 the natives of Asamankese began to be afflicted by yellow fever, but they concealed the infection from the medical authorities. The approximately 5,000 black inhabitants of Asamankese, located inland about 50 miles northwest of Accra on the coast, were very skeptical about the role of mosquitoes in spreading diseases and resented the medical authorities' enforcement of a quarantine and insect larval control—which they called "white man's humbug." The black village chief insisted that the gods were scourging his people and they must be appeased; he preferred his own methods of combating the disease and, after several human deaths, enlisted the services of an expensive "juju man" (fetishist) from Togo, bordering Ghana on the east, to free his village from the "curse." When the juju man's son and the chief's sister died from the infection, the juju man lost all his credibility, and

Ghana's recently established Yellow Fever Commission was permitted to examine the chief's stricken people.

Medical officials then isolated all victims and their contacts, and larvae and adult mosquitoes were sprayed with various fumigants and chemicals, and quarantines were enforced in Asamankese. When the epidemic came to an end in September 1926, at least 150 black Africans had died from the disease. The authorities were embarrassed that yellow fever on this scale had gone undetected for so long so close to Accra. At the time there was some question whether blacks were vulnerable to the disease, one of whose main symptoms is jaundice, which is harder to detect in blacks; furthermore, there was some doubt whether yellow fever made blacks very ill if they did contract it. The commission invalidated these questions.

Further reading: Williams, *The Plague Killers;* Patterson, *Health in Colonial Ghana.*

Gibraltar Yellow Fever Epidemics of 1804–28

Five outbreaks of yellow fever, varying in severity, which occurred in the British colony of Gibraltar between 1804 and 1828. The outbreak of 1804, part of a widespread epidemic that affected most of the surrounding Spanish province of Andalusia, killed 1,082 British garrison soldiers and others during the usual summer and fall yellow fever season; in comparison, just 91 people had died from all causes in Gibraltar during the previous two years. Less deadly outbreaks, also coincidental with epidemics in adjacent regions, occurred in 1810, 1812, and 1814; the Cadiz Yellow Fever Epidemic of 1810 (q.v.) was assumed to have been brought to that port city directly from Gibraltar.

Yellow fever struck Gibraltar once again with great intensity in 1828. According to official records, 1,183 people died, whereas a private observer counted 1,631 deaths. Such discrepancies between public and private statistics were common during epidemics, reflecting a common tendency of governments to underplay the severity of outbreaks of disease. The epidemic of 1828 occasioned a great debate between contagionists, who believed yellow fever was transmitted from person to person, and anti-contagionists, who believed that all diseases were caused by environmental factors, particularly infectious miasmas. Although data collected from direct observation and detailed questionnaires seemed to deny the contagionist view, the fact that particular mosquitoes transmit the yellow fever virus—and not infectious air—would not be discovered until the turn of the century.

Further reading: Coleman, *Yellow Fever in the North;* Peset Reig, *Muerte en España.*

Gilbert and Ellice Islands Measles Epidemics of 1890 and 1936

Two epidemics of measles (rubeola) that ripped through parts of the British colony of Gilbert and Ellice Islands (now the Pacific island nations of Kiribati and Tuvalu, respectively).

The first epidemic struck the northern and central islands (atolls) of the Gilbert group in 1890. Butaritari (Makin), northernmost among them, was severely affected. Almost 1,000 human deaths occurred on 11 of the islands during this measles epidemic, whose course was complicated by dysentery. About 500 of the fatalities occurred on the island of Tabiteuea, which was left with only 4,000 residents.

In 1936, measles was unexpectedly reintroduced into the Gilbert Islands from Fiji to the south and quickly became epidemic. By all accounts, it was a severe outbreak. One source reported 14,282 cases and some 100 deaths in a population of approximately 27,000 persons. Another estimated the casualties at 400 to 500. The epidemic reportedly spread to the Ellice Islands as well.

Further reading: Carroll, ed., *Pacific Atoll Populations;* Simmons et al., *Global Epidemiology.*

Granada Typhus Epidemic of 1489

Earliest recorded serious typhus fever epidemic in Europe. During the siege of Granada in southern Spain, when the Spanish Christian forces of King Ferdinand V and Queen Isabella I were fighting to take it from the Moors (Spanish Muslims), an outbreak of typhus occurred in the Spanish Army. The soldiers suffering from the disease developed red spots on their chests, backs, and arms, according to reports.

The Spanish Army was formally surveyed at the start of 1490: About 20,000 men were listed as missing, including 3,000 killed by the Moors. The generals calculated some 17,000 soldiers had died of typhus. At the time, physicians thought that the disease was contagious and caused by the plague. Some even believed that it originated from unburied corpses; others said that it was introduced by Spanish soldiers who came from the island of Cyprus, where the fever was then prevalent. Some writers who observed the epidemic decided that the disease was new and had come to Europe from somewhere in the East.

The exact origin of typhus fever remains obscure, although it is possible that it did begin in the East and spread to Europe with infected rats aboard ships. Typhus is a disease of dirt, tending to thrive under dirty, crowded conditions; it is caused by *Rickettsia*, a microorganism that lives in certain ticks and lice. The disease most likely was transferred from infected rats to lice, which transmitted it to human beings in 1489.

The Spanish soldiers who came from Cyprus had fought with the Venetians against the Ottoman

Turks, who may have carried typhus to the Spaniards as well as to the Saracen Arabs in the East. Thus the disease was contracted by King Ferdinand V's soldiers.

Typhus fever has always been a dangerous enemy for armies during wartime, when sanitary conditions are poor, dirt accumulates, and soldiers have a hard time keeping clean; when they are exposed to infected lice, the disease becomes a menace.

Further reading: Sigerist, *Civilization and Disease*; Zinsser, *Rats, Lice and History*; Crawfurd, *Plague and Pestilence in Literature and Art*.

Great Plague of Athens   See PLAGUE OF ATHENS, GREAT.

Great Plague of Iceland   See PLAGUE OF ICELAND, GREAT.

Great Plague of London   See PLAGUE OF LONDON, GREAT.

Great Plague of Milan   See ITALIAN PLAGUES OF 1629–31.

Great Plague of Vienna   See PLAGUE OF VIENNA, GREAT.

Greenlandic Smallpox Epidemic of 1733–34   Severe epidemic that killed perhaps several thousand native Greenlanders soon after their first contact in centuries with western Europeans. Around 1430 repeated attacks of smallpox had wiped out a European settlement on Greenland, cutting the island off from the rest of the world for about 300 years. In 1721, however, Hans Egede and some fellow Danes established a year-round trading colony and mission at Godthab (Nuuk), on the west coast of southern Greenland. Despite the withdrawal of commercial backing, the threatened loss of Danish government subsidies, disease and hardship, and conflicts with other European missionaries, the Danish settlement endured, but the Greenlanders it affected paid a terrible price. With no immunity from smallpox, which had swept over Europe with greater and greater intensity from the mid-1500s on, the Greenlanders quickly succumbed when the disease arrived on their island.

Several natives who traveled to Denmark in 1728 caught smallpox and died there the following spring. Nonetheless, six other Greenlanders sailed to Copenhagen in 1731, but only one of them—a young boy named Carl—lived to return in the spring of 1733. The smallpox he brought with him spread as he visited friends and relatives around Godthab. According to the diaries and letters of Egede and other Europeans, the first victim died on August 27, 1733, while Carl (who had appeared to be recovering) fell ill again and died on September 4. Unfamiliar with infectious disease, the Greenlanders took no care to prevent transmission, and the "noxious and wasting scab and itching" (which Egede correctly suspected was smallpox) soon infected hundreds of people. The epidemic was raging on the islands off Godthab by November; throughout the winter and into the spring it claimed the lives of almost everyone within a radius of about 15 to 20 miles around the Danish settlement. Those who did not immediately fall ill often fled, many of them to Godthab, carrying the infection to the houses in which they sought refuge.

There were undoubtedly many more than the 70 deaths noted in the colony's official records, but a precise mortality figure cannot be calculated. The native settlements were widely scattered, and their people usually took flight at the first sign of the illness. Reports by missionaries and traders, however, give some hint of the devastation. On one island, for example, missionaries found only four children still alive, one of whom had smallpox scabs over her body; their father had died after burying all the other inhabitants.

Around the end of April 1734, the epidemic began to wane. The resulting depopulation, however, disrupted hunting and fishing activities for some time to come, making it difficult for the surviving Greenlanders to feed themselves, let alone provide items for trade with the Europeans. See also ICELANDIC SMALLPOX EPIDEMIC OF 1707–09.

Further reading: Gad, *History of Greenland*; Hopkins, *Princes and Peasants: Smallpox in History*; Rink, *Danish Greenland: Its People and Products*.

Green Monkey Disease in Germany   See MARBURG VIRUS EPIDEMIC OF 1967.

Gros Ventre Indian Smallpox Epidemic of 1869   Outbreak of smallpox that killed about 800 Gros Ventre Indians living in northern Montana territory in the United States in 1869. The Gros Ventres ("Big Bellies" in French), also named the Atsina Indians, had probably suffered from an earlier smallpox outbreak that struck other Prairie or Plains Indian tribes in 1860–67.

In 1869 several crewmembers aboard the U.S. river steamer *Utah*, traveling on the Milk River in northern Montana, became infected with smallpox. One of them died and was buried along the banks of the river, and subsequently a group of Gros Ventres uncovered the dead body, taking the man's contaminated clothing and thus becoming infected with smallpox. (The highly contagious virus can easily live in clothing or bedding, as well as be directly transmitted from person to person through respiratory discharges.) The infected Gros Ventres carried the variola virus upriver to their camps in the Fort Belknap region; soon most of the tribe there became infected and spread the disease to others.

Placing their dead in trees, as was the custom of the Gros Ventres, helped spread the smallpox infection to white traders, who stole the corpses' contaminated robes and skins and sold them to others. In this way, the disease spread farther into the territory, where more than half of the Gros Ventre tribe (totaling about 1,500 members) succumbed to the disease; many of the survivors were blinded or disfigured (notably with pockmarked faces).

Further reading: Hopkins, *Princes and Peasants: Smallpox in History;* Studt, et al., *Medicine in the Intermountain West.*

Guam Encephalitis Epidemic of 1947–48

Outbreak of Japanese B Encephalitis (JBE) on the Pacific island of Guam, occurring concurrently with the Guam Mumps Epidemic of 1947–48 (q.v.).

Guam's first recorded epidemic of JBE began in early December 1947 when the first official case was reported in a 22-month-old child. Within weeks, several more cases were reported, including some in people suffering from mumps. Natives diagnosed with JBE were admitted to the Guam Memorial Hospital under the observation of medical officers of the United States Navy. Americans (civilians and the military) with JBE were hospitalized at the American Navy Hospital. Some of the cases observed during the early stages of the epidemic were of an extremely serious nature, with high temperature, disorientation, coma, and convulsions. A few of the patients never recovered.

During the epidemic, 54 cases (0.65 per 1,000 population) were reported—46 among native Guamanians (including 15 children age one to four, and ten youths between 15 and 19) and the rest among civilian/military nonresidents. More males than females were infected and most of the cases occurred in the southern part of the island. The 54 cases included cases of encephalitis from JBE (16), JBE and/or mumps (15), mumps (17) and unknown etiology (6). Pure mumps encephalitis persisted through March 1948, but all other cases generally peaked early in January and subsided by early February 1948. Both epidemics peaked simultaneously. The last case of JBE was admitted to the hospital on April 6, 1948.

The warmer than normal temperatures and higher humidity during this period (December 1947–February 1948) may have been contributing factors in the spread of JBE, a mosquito-borne (*Culex annulirostris* was considered the possible vector) viral infection. Unknown in Guam or anywhere this far south in the tropics until this outbreak, JBE was probably introduced from an endemic/epidemic zone. Its course on Guam was no doubt complicated by the simultaneous activity of the mumps virus. However, JBE subsequently disappeared from the island. Later in 1948, Guam was attacked by a large epidemic of measles, during which several deaths occurred from postmeasles encephalitis.

Further reading: Hammon et al., "Epidemiologic Studies of Concurrent 'Virgin' Epidemics of Japanese B Encephalitis"; Horsfall and Tamm, eds., *Viral and Rickettsial Infections of Man.*

Guam Mumps Epidemic of 1947–48

Outbreak of mumps (infectious parotitis) on the island of Guam, an unincorporated territory of the United States.

Guam, southernmost and largest island of the Marianas archipelago in the western Pacific Ocean, was an important military base occupied by both Americans and Japanese during World War II. Mumps had apparently not been reported from the northern part of the island for almost six to eight years and from the southern area since 1930. During 1947, several stray cases of mumps occurred among natives, perhaps as a result of importations by the families of postwar American military personnel. In November 1947, however, the incidence increased dramatically, and within one month it was obvious that an epidemic was in progress.

Statistics compiled during the epidemic reveal, even in their incomplete state, an outbreak of great intensity. By the time it subsided in April 1948, a total of 1,647 people had been infected in a total resident population of 24,717 (this does not include the military, its dependents and contractors). The average attack rate was 66.6 per 1,000 people. Reports from one village indicated an attack rate there of 192.5 per 1,000 people. The American military had 82 cases of mumps in its midst, an attack rate of 2.5 per 1,000. Figures are not available for any other group. Only half of the mumps cases that occurred in Guam during this period were actually reported. Many people suffered from both mumps and Japanese B encephalitis, and it is not clear whether their numbers were included in the official statistics.

Mumps, an acute communicable disease mainly of childhood and young adulthood, is caused by a virus of the *Paramyxovirus* family. Historically, the virus has been known to cause outbreaks among large gatherings of people (military barracks, schools, and other institutions).

Further reading: Evans, ed., *Viral Infections of Humans;* Hammon et al., "Epidemiologic Studies of Concurrent 'Virgin' Epidemics of Japanese B Encephalitis and of Mumps on Guana."

Guatemalan Dysentery Epidemic of 1969–70

Severe epidemic of bacillary dysentery (shigellosis) that killed approximately 12,000 people in Guatemala in Central America. The name shigellosis derives from the Japanese bacteriologist Kiyoshi Shiga, who discovered in 1898 the disease's infectious agent, the bacteria *Shigella dysenteriae* (or *Shigella shigae*), which is found chiefly in tropical and subtropical areas.

After an absence of about 50 years, epidemic bacillary dysentery unexpectedly reappeared in Guatemalan towns and cities in the fall of 1969. Throughout the dry season (November–May), thousands of inhabitants became infected, with symptoms of high fever, vomiting, abdominal cramps, diarrhea, and sometimes blood, mucus, or pus in the stool. Although the dysentery epidemic peaked in April 1970 and the rainy season began a month later, the disease continued to be serious because of increased contamination of water supplies; infected water, fruit, and vegetables, as well as contaminated feces, commonly transmit the disease, which primarily affects the colon (large intestine). About 130,000 Guatemalan people had contracted it by the end of the epidemic in late 1970.

Along with contaminated water as a prime factor in the spread of the disease in Guatemala, malnutrition was a primary factor in the high mortality rate, which was particularly high among the very young and the elderly. Many of the stricken children under four years old suffered convulsions; dehydration and poisoning by bacterial toxins were so extreme that profound shock resulted in many of the fatalities among the young.

In Guatemala's estimated population of 4,717,000 (in 1968), dysentery's mortality rate in 18 infected communities increased from 39 deaths per 100,000 people (in 1968) to 170 deaths per 100,000 (early in the epidemic in 1969). At the close of the epidemic, the mortality rate for the entire country was estimated to be 250 per 100,000; this number varied from 334 per 100,000 in the lowlands to 190 per 100,000 in the highlands. Because the *Shigella dysenteriae* were resistant to multiple drugs and mistakes were made in diagnosis and appropriate antimicrobic therapy, the case fatality rate was ten percent to 15 percent among those hospitalized because of acute illness; in untreated patients in villages, the case fatality rate was 8.4 percent.

There were a few isolated dysentery cases among tourists from the United States, but no secondary diffusion occurred when they returned home. In late 1969 and 1970 the disease spread from Guatemala into Mexico to the north and into El Salvador to the south, resulting in serious outbreaks in both countries during these years. In U.S. states bordering Mexico and in Los Angeles's Mexican-American sections, there was a sharp increase in dysentery cases at this time; however, because of disease control and information, U.S. outbreaks were kept localized.

Further reading: Evans and Brachman, eds., *Bacterial Infections of Humans*; Hoeprich, ed., *Infectious Diseases*.

Guayaquil Plagues

See ECUADORAN PLAGUES OF 1908–88.

Guayaquil Yellow Fever Epidemics of 1740, 1743, and 1842

Severe outbreaks of yellow fever (a viral infection transmitted by the bite of the *Aëdes aegypti* mosquito) that claimed thousands of human lives in the Pacific port city of Guayaquil, Ecuador. Located in tropical coastal lowlands, the city has a hotter and more humid climate than the rest of Ecuador and is an ideal breeding habitat for the mosquito that carries the yellow fever virus, which destroys liver cells (causing jaundice, or yellowing of the skin, hence the name of the disease).

In mid-1740 Spanish trading vessels from Santo Domingo (the Dominican Republic) evidently carried yellow fever to Guayaquil, another Spanish colony; Santo Domingo was fighting an epidemic at the time and would later be ravaged by the fever in the 1790s (see HAITIAN YELLOW FEVER EPIDEMIC OF 1794–98). The highly domesticated *Aëdes* mosquitoes easily lived, bred, and multiplied in water casks aboard ships, as well as in small pools or ponds of stagnant water in Guayaquil. That summer (1740) Spanish settlers and troops and native Indians were attacked by the disease in large numbers, and mortality was apparently very high during the epidemic, which remained localized at Guayaquil, ended in early winter, and did not affect the people of Quito, Ecuador's largest city, in the mountains.

Far to the north, in 1741 yellow fever attacked a British expedition of 12,000 troops under Admiral Edward Vernon, which was vainly attempting to seize the strongly fortified Spanish port city of Cartagena, on Colombia's Caribbean coast, where the disease killed 8,431 of the British.

Guayaquil was once again struck by the fever in the summer of 1743 (most likely it was imported from Santo Domingo, which was fighting a similar epidemic then). Since much of the adult population in Guayaquil had developed immunity (recovery from a yellow fever attack brings lifelong immunity), case incidence and fatalities were greatest among new arrivals in the city. Although the disease remained endemic, the next grave yellow fever epidemic at Guayaquil did not occur until 100 years later, in 1842, when the virus reportedly arrived with travelers from New Orleans by way of Panama. See also HISPANIOLA YELLOW FEVER EPIDEMIC OF 1495–96.

Further reading: Scott, *A History of Tropical Medicine;* Cook and Lovell, eds., *Secret Judgments of God: Old World Disease in Colonial Spanish America.*

Guinean Smallpox Epidemic of 1967

Outburst of smallpox (variola) in the West African republic of Guinea from January through April 1967. Most of the 1,529 persons reported infected were under age 15 and lived in small villages in Guinea's southwest region, near the northern districts of neighboring Sierra Leone. (Guinea and Sierra Leone had the two highest variola attack rates in the world at the time.)

Smallpox was most likely introduced into Guinea by Islamic invaders after the eighth century; thereafter periodic outbreaks were reported in the region, which became the colony of French Guinea in 1893. Between 1926 and 1966, there were more than 434,000 smallpox infections and over 64,000 deaths from the disease, with the most suffering during Guinea's dry season (November–March). The 1967 epidemic in Guinea caused 103 deaths, a mortality rate of 12.6 percent.

Despite the beginning of the West and Central African Smallpox Eradication and Measles Control Program in December 1967, another outburst of smallpox occurred in Guinea that continued until late April 1968, when the rainy season began. In that four-month epidemic episode, 330 persons contracted smallpox and 23 of them perished from its effects (high fever, prostration, and bleeding into the skin). A mass vaccination program had been initiated that proved successful; only 16 smallpox cases and no deaths were reported from late 1968 to January 1969; no cases occurred between 1970 and 1976 in Guinea, whose National Smallpox Eradication Program virtually eliminated the disease.

Further reading: Breman et al., "Smallpox in the Republic of Guinea, West Africa"; Shurkin, *The Invisible Fire.*

H

Haitian Smallpox Epidemics See HISPANIOLA SMALLPOX EPIDEMICS OF 1507 AND 1518.

Haitian Yellow Fever Epidemic of 1495–96 See HISPANIOLA YELLOW FEVER EPIDEMIC OF 1495–96.

Haitian Yellow Fever Epidemic of 1794–98 Outbreak of yellow fever that occurred during the British occupation of Haiti (then called Saint-Domingue) during the French Revolutionary Wars. An influx of non-immune persons into infected ports would frequently cause epidemics.

In 1793 a ship from West Africa evidently introduced yellow fever to the island of Grenada in the West Indies. From there, the epidemic disease spread to Jamaica and Martinique, where fever-ridden troops carried it north to Santo Domingo (Saint-Domingue). French refugees brought the disease north to Philadelphia (see PHILADELPHIA YELLOW FEVER EPIDEMIC OF 1793). In June 1794 infected soldiers from Martinique arrived at Port-au-Prince, Haiti, to reinforce the British forces that had captured this chief seaport from the French. Summertime was the sickly season in Port-au-Prince, and by September 1794 about 650 British soldiers had died of yellow fever without ever seeing battle against the French. The town's swampy ground, overcrowdedness, and open domestic water containers helped perpetuate the disease. Also, insurgents in the mountains cut off the fresh-water supply to Port-au-Prince, forcing the British to drink from contaminated containers. By the end of June 1794, two fifths of the British soldiers were dead, and by November, some 1,000 soldiers were buried at Port-au-Prince—victims of yellow fever.

The disease continued to devastate the British stationed in Haiti. Out of about 4,000 additional soldiers sent there in 1795, only 1,800 lived to see the next year. In 1796 about 13,000 more soldiers arrived, of whom some 1,300 perished from the fever in May and June alone. It did not take long for new troops to be struck down by the disease; men who felt fine in the morning could be dead by night; soldiers would drown in their own bloody vomit, and some were driven fatally mad. Sometimes the gravediggers could not keep pace and had to bury as many as five human bodies in a single grave.

With no known cure for the disease, medical treatments at the time ranged from the practical use of lemonade to combat dehydration, to the bizarre practice of dousing unsuspecting patients with buckets of cold water. The popular practice of bloodletting was also used to fight "yellow jack" or "black vomit fever."

As the pace of the military campaign increased in Haiti and camps were set up in the mountains, the disease seemed to slow down as overcrowded quarters were reduced for the British, who evacuated the island of Hispaniola in 1797 because of the increasing cost of men and weapons.

Further reading: Geggus, *Slavery, War and Revolution: Occupation of St. Domingue.*

Haitian Yellow Fever Epidemic of 1802 Epidemic of yellow fever that broke out among the French troops stationed in Haiti (then called Saint-Domingue), killing an estimated 40,000 men between May 1802 and January of 1803. (Haiti was sometimes called San or Santo Domingo, the name also given to the Dominican Republic.)

In 1802, Napoleon sent some 25,000 French soldiers to the French colony of Saint-Domingue to overthrow the rule of the native black patriot, François Dominique Toussaint L'Ouverture, who had earlier led a successful rebellion and became the virtual ruler of Hispaniola (Haiti and the Dominican Republic). The troops under the command of Napoleon's brother-in-law, Charles Victor Leclerc, were successful at first yet they encountered unexpected problems from yellow fever.

The fever is often fatal, but if one survives it, he or she is immune for life. In mid-May 1802, yellow fever broke out in the major ports of Haiti, Le Cap (Cap Haitien) and Port-au-Prince; the summer months brought an epidemic of unparalleled fierceness. By the first week of June, some 3,000 French soldiers were dead. Leclerc, in despair, saw his army crumbling and no way to control the black rebels and sent urgent dispatches to Napoleon, pleading for more men.

Haiti's fever season usually ended around the autumn equinox in September, but there was no abatement in 1802 as the fever raged on; 4,000 more men died in September.

The French naval fleet in Haiti fared no better. Yellow fever, often called "yellow jack" by seamen, was the most feared of diseases and could sweep through a whole crew, leaving an empty ship in a harbor. Some 5,000 French sailors succumbed to yellow fever in the summer of 1802. Also, approximately 100 to 120 French soldiers died each day; Leclerc estimated that 29,000 men had died by midsummer of that year. All but two of Leclerc's corps commanders perished, and soon Leclerc himself fell victim to the disease. Battling it for 11 days, he died still pleading to Napoleon to send more men.

The disease continued into January 1803; the death toll mounted. The French eventually received more men and weapons and overcame the rebels. However, when war broke out between Britain and France in 1803, the British aided the Haitian rebels, and the French finally were forced to evacuate Haiti in late 1803. Of the approximately 50,000 men Napoleon sent to Haiti, only a few thousand lived to see France again.

Further reading: Marks and Beatty, *Epidemics;* Harrison, *Mosquitoes, Malaria and Man;* Stoddard, *The French Revolution in San Domingo.*

Hamburg Cholera Epidemic of 1892

Devastating epidemic of Asiatic cholera that terrorized the North Sea port city of Hamburg, Germany, in the summer of 1892. Cholera had erupted at various intervals in Europe since 1831, but not until the great epidemic at Hamburg did people die from cholera in such large numbers, an average of 140 per day. In just two months, from mid-August to mid-September, cholera killed 8,594 people (only 12 more deaths occurred from September 20 to November 12, when the epidemic ended). Of 16,956 reported cases, 8,605 people died, reflecting a case-mortality rate of about 50 percent, an extraordinarily high percentage for most diseases. Hamburg's population was approximately 66,000; over 13 percent died.

Hamburg's officials delayed announcing the presence of cholera even though they had ample evidence, which meant that simple precautionary instructions, such as boiling water and avoiding un-washed fruit, were publicized too late. Tragically, German bacteriologist Robert Koch's discovery in 1883 of the cause of cholera—a water-borne bacillus—did not help the citizens of Hamburg in 1892. Although thoroughly aware of Koch's studies—Koch himself was ordered to Hamburg by the Prussian minister of health to confirm the outbreak—only afterward did authorities acknowledge that the areas of the city through which cholera had raged corresponded to areas supplied with unfiltered water from the Elbe River. Mortality was highest near the harbor and along the river and canals. The fact that the suburb of Altona, which had installed a new water purification system a few years before, reported far fewer cases of cholera than Hamburg, provided more evidence to those who resisted Koch's assertion that cholera bacilli were carried in water (they denied they had unsanitary water). On Koch's advice, truckloads of fresh water were distributed to working-class neighborhoods, boiling stations were set up, and disinfection squads sent round to infected houses. Koch also recommended closing of schools and banning of public meetings, and insisted on a massive publicity campaign to help Hamburg's citizens understand and implement preventive measures.

Hamburg was the only city in western Europe to suffer so dramatically from cholera in 1892.

Further reading: Ackerknecht, *History and Geography of the Most Important Diseases;* Evans, *Death in Hamburg.*

Havana Yellow Fever Epidemic of 1761–62

Outbreak of yellow fever that decimated the British forces besieging Havana, Cuba, during the Seven Years' War (1756–63).

A viral disease transmitted to humans by the bite of the *Aëdes aegypti* mosquito, yellow fever was endemic in Cuba for a time after outbreaks there in 1620 (the first known), 1649 (a major one), and 1655. Afterward the disease caused only mild concern to the Spanish and natives on the island, until 1761, when it virulently entered Havana (Spain's chief naval port in the New World) apparently via Veracruz, Mexico. Thousands of inhabitants were infected and perished from yellow fever, which causes high fever, vomiting, bleeding, and jaundice. Those who recovered from the infection gained lasting immunity and were not affected in 1762 when yellow fever struck the alien British forces (led by the Second Earl of Albemarle and aided by colonial Americans) who were then attacking Havana. After bloody fighting, the British occupied the port city for about 11 months before restoring it to Spain in exchange for land in Florida. Out of 15,000 British men, about 3,000 sailors and 5,000 soldiers died from yellow fever in and around Havana, from where British ships carried the disease to Philadelphia.

That same year (1762) the inhabitants of the small coastal town of Cayenne in French Guiana also suffered from yellow fever (for the first time, reportedly); there were thousands of infections among the non-immune native population, which also endured outbreaks of the fever in 1763 and 1764 and later in 1791. Yellow fever was a barrier to colonization of French Guiana, while Havana prospered and grew in spite of the disease. In fact, Cuba became an endemic-epidemic focus of yellow fever until 1900, when William C. Gorgas, American pioneer in public health measures, succeeded in checking the disease in Cuba through mosquito control. See also HAVANA YELLOW FEVER EPIDEMIC OF 1899–1900.

Further reading: Cloudsley-Thompson, *Insects and History*; Scott, *A History of Tropical Medicine*.

Havana Yellow Fever Epidemic of 1899–1900
Debilitating epidemic of yellow fever in Havana, Cuba, breaking out after U.S. troops occupied this port city following the Cuban War of Independence (1895–98) and the Spanish-American War (1898).

U.S. Army doctor William C. Gorgas, appointed chief sanitary officer of American-occupied Havana, set about cleaning up the city; he and other experts believed that dirt and decay helped cause yellow fever, endemic to Cuba for many years. By the summer of 1900, Havana was cleaned up, but the yellow fever epidemic had grown worse, with a reported 1,400 cases at the time. An army commission, headed by Dr. Walter Reed, was sent to Havana to study the disease; Reed and Gorgas had followed the work of Dr. Carlos J. Finley, a Cuban physician who earlier hypothesized (1881) that yellow fever was transmitted by the *Stegomyia fasciata* (later *Aëdes aegypti*) mosquito, but had been unable to prove it. Reed and his associates (Dr. James Carroll, Dr. Jesse W. Lazear, and Dr. Aristides Agramonte) set out to prove Finlay's theory. They thought there was a period of incubation while the deadly parasite developed; dramatically, Carroll and Lazear allowed infected mosquitoes to bite them. Both doctors contracted the disease, but only Carroll survived, with his health seriously impaired. Lazear died five days later in a wild delirium that required two men to hold him down. (Their martyrdom was dramatized in a play, *Yellowjack* [1928], by American playwright Sidney Coe Howard.)

In October 1900 the commission reported to the American Public Health Association that "the mosquito acts as the intermediate host for the parasite of yellow fever." Later Reed and Carroll showed that the disease was due to a filterable virus, by injecting non-immune persons with filtered serum from yellow fever patients. This was the first time a specific human disease was shown to be caused by a filterable virus. Reed and his associates also proved that the fever (though definitely transmissible) was not contagious (that is, transferred by contact); they demonstrated this fact by having four volunteers sleep in a one-room shack for 20 nights, wearing the soiled pajamas of fever patients and using beds soiled with patients' vomit; no one contracted the disease.

Under the direction of Gorgas, sanitary squads destroyed the breeding grounds of mosquitoes in Havana, draining, oiling, and screening-over all water ditches in the city. As a result, there were only 37 known cases of yellow fever in 1901, and by the summer of 1902, there were no cases. Gorgas would later go to Panama to fight yellow fever successfully, which allowed the Panama Canal to be built. See PANAMANIAN YELLOW FEVER EPIDEMICS OF 1880–1904.

Further reading: McCullough, *The Path Between the Seas*; Gorgas and Hendrick, *William Crawford Gorgas: His Life and Work*; Williams, *The Plague Killers*.

Hawaiian Plague of 1899–1900
Epidemic of plague that killed 61 of 71 people infected, beginning with Hawaiian Asians, between November 1899 and March 1900, as part of the third plague pandemic reaching toward the New World (see PLAGUE PANDEMIC, THIRD).

In November 1899, two ships from Hong Kong carried bubonic plague victims into Honolulu. One of the ships, the S.S. *Nippon Maru*, arrived with two human corpses and rats infected with plague. Hawaii first discovered it had plague when a Dr. George Herbert treated the first fatally ill patient in December; shortly thereafter, four Chinese (three clinically diagnosed) died of the disease. Because the plague first took root among Hawaiian orientals, Honolulu's Chinatown was quarantined and searched for more plague victims. Despite the lifting of the quarantine and pronouncements that the plague was gone, the disease persisted, killing 36 of 44 patients within the next month (January 1900).

The bacillus *Yersinia pestis (Pasteurella pestis)* causes bubonic plague. This bacterium becomes a threat to human beings only when it becomes epizootic among nearby rats or rodents. Among 200 kinds of flea (not the human flea), the rat flea *Xenopsylla cheopis* is plague's most common carrier. People with plague experience stupor, high fever and chills, headaches, and most important, very large, lymphatic swellings under the arms, in the neck, or in the groin. Untreated, the disease can kill 60 percent to 90 percent of its victims within five days. Modern antidotes for the disease include tetracyclines, streptomycin, and chloraphenicals.

The epidemic continued to rage in Hawaii in 1900, despite a major fire in Honolulu that destroyed the homes and possessions of many Chinese; the fire began when the fire department's burning of a plague-contaminated house went out of control in Chinatown. More than 5,000 people were left homeless and without possessions. Rats were thought to be plague carriers, which was evidenced in folklore among oriental Hawaiians, and burning houses was thought to kill them. As new cases appeared regularly in Oahu and later in the other Hawaiian islands, Asians were the first victims. Ships brought the plague infection again and again to the islands. See also SAN FRANCISCO PLAGUE OF 1900–04; SAN FRANCISCO PLAGUE OF 1907–09.

Further reading: Ackerknecht, *History and Geography of the Most Important Diseases*; Gregg, *Plague: An Ancient Disease in the Twentieth Century*.

Hawaiian Smallpox Epidemic of 1853

Devastating outbreak of smallpox that ripped through the Hawaiian Islands and forced the authorities to consider the need for more hospitals and a sound public health policy.

The disease was introduced into Hawaii by an American merchant ship, the *Charles Mallory*, which had set sail from San Francisco and arrived at Honolulu harbor on February 10, 1853, displaying a yellow flag indicating a serious infection on board. The ship was therefore berthed in isolation on a reef at Kalihi. One of the passengers had smallpox. Other disembarking passengers were vaccinated and quarantined at Waikiki. Richard Armstrong, Hawaii's minister of public instruction, launched a hastily arranged vaccination campaign, and Gerrit Judd, former medical missionary, was ordered to select sites for quarantine stations and a pest hospital. When the period of quarantine ended late in March, no new cases had been reported, the smallpox patient was recovering, and the ship had left. However, other trading ships arrived regularly from California where smallpox was then rampant.

In May 1853, the disease reappeared. Two native women were stricken; their homes and the adjacent properties were cordoned off to allow infected clothing and their grass huts to be burnt. A three-man Royal Commission on Health, responsible for vaccination, hospitals, and warning and inspection of arriving ships, was established.

Smallpox spread rapidly while doctors were still preparing a vaccine. Cases were reported from most of Honolulu's districts, and June 15, 1853, was declared a national day of mourning, prayer, and fasting. The various missions—Catholic, Protestant, and Mormon—tried to alleviate the suffering by offering food, medical care, compassion, and religious rites. Nevertheless, 114 cases and 41 deaths were reported by June 18, and double that number a week later. The epidemic was at its worst in July–August with the island of Oahu alone recording more than 4,000 cases and 1,500 deaths, mainly in the Honolulu area. The outbreak subsided in the city of Honolulu during October but continued in the rural areas. Despite heroic efforts, smallpox engulfed the islands of Kauai, Maui, and Hawaii, killing at least 450 people there. The islands of Niihau, Molokai, and Lanai remained protected because of their remoteness, stricter quarantine, and better vaccine quality.

It was so explosive overall that during an eight-month period about eight percent of Hawaii's population died of the disease. When the epidemic ended late in January 1854, the official figure was 6,405 cases and 2,485 deaths. According to eyewitness accounts, this is an underestimation. Another source cites 9,082 cases and 5,748 deaths, apparently a more realistic figure.

Normal life in Honolulu was severely disrupted; hundreds of people left the city for the rural areas and even the outer islands, despite the ban on doing so. The infected among them thus spread smallpox as they fled. The affected homes were marked by yellow flags. The natives, who had openly despised Western medical treatment, were most susceptible to the disease; very few of the white settlers were infected. Even at the height of the epidemic, many natives refused vaccination. In Honolulu, vaccination acceptance was greater, but the vaccine was not of uniform quality and did not always protect. Many families nursed their patients at home and buried the dead under the dirt floors of their huts; elsewhere, patients were abandoned and left to die alone. The streets were littered with corpses. At the Kakaako pest hospital, 40 to 50 people died every day during the peak of the epidemic.

Some people felt the government was apathetic and did not do enough; they wanted to burn all the infected homes, improve the vaccine quality, and designate volunteer leaders to oversee preventive measures in every district. Judd and Armstrong were attacked for their lack of leadership and for allowing the disease to spread. Judd was subsequently forced to resign his post in the king's ministry.

The intensity of this epidemic led the Hawaiian legislature to make vaccination mandatory for both residents and visitors alike in 1854. The vaccination campaign was apparently quite effective on the island of Maui, mainly because of the leadership provided by Reverend Dr. Dwight Baldwin, a medical missionary from Lahaina.

Further reading: Daws, *Shoal of Time: A History of the Hawaiian Islands;* Kuykendall and Day, *Hawaii: A History.*

Henry IV's Army Epidemics of 1081–83

Various epidemic diseases—probably malaria, typhoid, and dysentery—that combined with the summer heat to force the German Army away from Rome. Four times, beginning in 1081, the Holy Roman Emperor Henry IV marched on the city during his bitter but inconclusive power struggle with Pope Gregory VII.

Pope and emperor had been battling for years before Henry first besieged Rome. Gregory's reform plan, which included subordinating all secular power to that of the Roman Catholic Church, threatened Henry's attempts to control Germany. Defying Gregory's orders, the emperor insisted on retaining the right to invest German bishops—to appoint them and give them their official insignia. The bishops supported Henry since they feared excessive papal control, while the pope found allies among many German nobles who wanted independence from monarchical authority. The conflict came to a head in 1080, when Gregory backed the new emperor chosen by the nobles and excommunicated Henry for the second time. Henry then put forth the anti-pope Clement III and led his army to Rome, hoping to force Gregory to back down.

The repeated sieges of Rome did not succeed, as Gregory refused to give in to Henry's demands or to budge from the heavily fortified Castel Sant' Angelo. In early July of 1081 Henry moved his army to Tuscany; he ordered a similar retreat to the countryside after Easter of 1082, following another ineffective attack. In both cases heat and disease drove the imperial army back.

A six-month siege the next year was more successful, since Henry captured a section of Rome on the northern bank of the Tiber River and even occupied St. Peter's itself. Once again, though, the emperor withdrew in June, leaving a garrison on the riverbank. When he returned late in 1083, after negotiations with Gregory had failed, he discovered that disease had wiped out the entire garrison.

Although scanty details do not allow us to pinpoint the nature of the epidemics, we can assume that typhoid and dysentery—the usual scourges of armies—were rife. The timing of Henry's retreats, coming before the long, hot Roman summers set in, suggests that malaria also menaced his troops, as it did other German armies in Italy (see FREDERICK BARBAROSSA'S ARMY EPIDEMIC).

Further reading: Gregorovius, *History of the City of Rome in the Middle Ages;* Maehl, *Germany in Western Civilization;* Prescott, *Lords of Italy;* Prinzing, *Epidemics Resulting from Wars.*

Hispaniola Smallpox Epidemic of 1507

First recorded epidemic of smallpox to strike Latin America, with the disease brought from Europe by Spanish explorers to the West Indian island of Hispaniola (Haiti and the Dominican Republic). Black slaves from West Africa may also have carried smallpox to the island, where it subsequently spread to Cuba and elsewhere in the region in the 1500s (see HISPANIOLA SMALLPOX EPIDEMIC OF 1518).

Smallpox was particularly devastating in the New World because the natives there had lived in isolation from the disease and lacked immunity. When smallpox invaded the natives on Hispaniola, it killed all but the most resilient. This first epidemic in 1507 was so disastrous that whole tribes were reportedly extinguished. At the time, both the Spanish and the Indians were at a loss to explain the high death toll of the natives. Many believed it was God's punishment.

The epidemic of 1507 eventually died out, but it served as an example of the devastation from disease that was to spread throughout Latin America. Smallpox would strike again and again in epidemic form until it was finally eradicated in 1971. Some believed that the smallpox virus brought the worst killing to strike the New World, particularly in Hispaniola.

Further reading: Cartwright, *Disease and History;* Hopkins, *Princes and Peasants; Smallpox in History.*

Hispaniola Smallpox Epidemic of 1518

Epidemic of smallpox that originated among African slaves in the silver mines of Hispaniola (Haiti and the Dominican Republic). The disease spread to Cuba and then to Puerto Rico, where it killed over half the native population in 1519.

In 1510, the Spanish king (Ferdinand V) had officially sanctioned use of slaves in the silver mines. By 1517, as many as 4,000 black slaves were being imported annually from West Africa. When smallpox struck, it spread rapidly due to the close living quarters of the slaves and natives. By May of 1519, up to one third of the Indians of Hispaniola had died from smallpox. The population of this West Indian island, estimated to be about 300,000 persons in 1492, had reportedly fallen to less than 1,000 by 1541.

The contagious smallpox disease was called the "great leprosy" by the Indians, who were virtually defenseless against it. Those who did not perish from the smallpox virus soon succumbed to starvation because there was no one left to harvest the crops. So many died that it was impossible to bury them all, and huts were pulled down over the dead in an attempt to stifle the stench of the disease.

From Hispaniola, the disease soon spread to the densely populated mainland of Central America. It spread to Cuba in 1518 and soon after to Mexico (see MEXICAN SMALLPOX EPIDEMIC OF 1520–21); evidently a black African slave carried the smallpox virus to Mexico. Also called "the Great Fire" by Mexican Indians, smallpox helped assure Spanish conquistador Hernando Cortés's victory over the Aztec Empire.

Further reading: Hopkins, *Princes and Peasants: Smallpox in History*; Cowley, "The Great Disease Migration."

Hispaniola Yellow Fever Epidemic of 1495–96

First recorded outbreak of yellow fever in the New World, claiming many native and Spanish lives on the island of Hispaniola (Haiti and the Dominican Republic). The viral infection, believed by some to have originated in Africa, was evidently brought to the Caribbean by Spanish explorer Christopher Columbus and his men during their voyages from Spain. This theory is disputed by some epidemiologists and others who believe the disease was endemic in parts of Latin America before Columbus arrived in the late fifteenth century.

The fever's virus is transmitted by the bite of the *Aëdes aegypti* mosquito; a human victim suffers from high fever, acute headache, back and leg pain, and sometimes vomiting of black bile. The virus establishes itself in non-immune persons and is frequently epidemic. In the past, sailing ships (like Spanish galleons) were ideal breeding places for the *Aëdes* mosquito and carried and spread the disease (called "yellow jack" by English sailors) easily, and it was known to wipe out whole crews.

On Hispaniola in 1495, Columbus and his men sought to "pacify" the natives (actually to take prisoners for slaves) and waged war against them. The Spanish subdued the Indians of Caonabo during a battle (called Vega Real) in the northern part of the island, but suffered severely afterward, along with numerous Indians, from an epidemic of yellow fever. The fever extended into the next year, encouraging Columbus to shift his headquarters from the northern coast of Hispaniola (and the now ruined settlement of Isabella) to a healthier location.

In 1502 Nicolás de Ovando arrived at the settlement of Santo Domingo (founded in 1496, on the southern coast of eastern Hispaniola) with about 2,500 colonists, most of whom soon perished from the yellow fever (which acquired its name from the yellowish tint extending over the victim's body). Ovando, appointed governor of Spanish possessions in America, carried on the extermination of natives, replacing them with West African blacks brought in

as slaves. In 1508 a five-ship Spanish expedition led by Diego de Nicueza sailed from Santo Domingo. During the voyage, about 600 of the 700 men on board reportedly died from yellow fever, which continued to attack Hispaniola in periodic waves well into the nineteenth century. Not until 1936 was a vaccine developed to combat yellow fever; it was discovered by South African–born U.S. physician and bacteriologist Max Theiler.

Further reading: Cloudsley-Thompson, *Insects and History*; McNeill, *Plagues and Peoples*; Bassett, "Yellow Fever."

Hong Kong Influenza Pandemic of 1968

Global pandemic that, like its predecessor (see ASIAN INFLUENZA PANDEMIC OF 1957–58), originated either in Kweichow or Yunnan province on the Chinese mainland and spread throughout the world within a year.

The virus was first isolated in Hong Kong in July 1968 and identified there as a new strain (H3N2) of the influenza A virus. In southeast China, the outbreak was reportedly accompanied by respiratory complications. From Hong Kong, where 15 percent of the population was affected, the virus moved to Singapore and to the Philippines, causing influenza epidemics in both countries. The southeast Asian mainland was also invaded. Although the virus reached Japan in July, there were no epidemics until October—and they were caused by two different strains of the virus.

By October 1968, the virus had crossed the Pacific Ocean (perhaps with American troops returning home from Vietnam) and landed in California, where it caused a small outbreak. It also moved south to Australia and west (via the Middle East) to Europe through the shipping and overland routes. The resulting epidemics were particularly severe in the United States in November–December 1968 and in Britain in 1969. In some European countries, the epidemics raged until April 1970.

Children under five years of age were hit the hardest by this pandemic, as were adults in the 45–64-years-old age group. In Great Britain, complications such as bronchitis and pneumonia contributed significantly to the high mortality figures in 1970 (see BRITISH INFLUENZA EPIDEMIC OF 1968–70). The epidemics subsided in 1970–71, only to resurface briefly in 1971–72.

Further reading: Beveridge, *Influenza: the Last Great Plague*; Pyle, *The Diffusion of Influenza*; Stuart-Harris et al., *Influenza: The Viruses and the Disease*.

Hong Kong Plague of 1894 (Chinese Plague of 1894)

Major bubonic plague epidemic—part of the Third Plague Pandemic (q.v.)—spurred international research leading to the discovery of the plague bacillus and to an understanding of its mode of dissemination. It originated in China's Yunnan province (where it had been endemic since 1866) in 1892 and spread to Canton in March 1894, killing 60,000 people in the city within a few weeks. From here to Hong Kong (just across the water), the infection spread rapidly with the constant boat traffic between the two cities. The epidemic, which by then had affected Kwantung province, peaked in Canton in May. Two months and 100,000 lives later, the epidemic eventually left Hong Kong. Plague continued to be endemic in Hong Kong until 1929.

Later in 1894 the Chinese island of Amoy was affected. The port of Newchwang in south Manchuria (see MANCHURIAN PLAGUE OF 1910–11) was invaded in 1899, and Foochow (capital of Fukien) was hit in 1901. The invasion of Amoy and Foochow led to the rapid spread of the disease throughout Fukien province. Meanwhile, the infection was also carried through shipping to Formosa (now Taiwan) and Bombay (see INDIAN PLAGUE OF 1896–97) in 1896 and to San Francisco, Glasgow, and Sydney in 1900. Scattered outbreaks were experienced in all of the world's major ports but most of these were easily contained.

Terrified that the dreaded disease would blow out of proportion, international research teams were dispatched to Hong Kong. Within a few weeks of their arrival, Swiss-born bacteriologist Alexander Yersin and Shibasaburo Kitasato, a Japanese researcher, independently discovered the plague bacillus, *Pasteurella pestis* (now *Yersinia pestis*). Subsequently, researchers working at other locations established the role of the flea in transmitting the virus from rodents to humans.

Further reading: Pollitzer, *Plague*; McNeill, *Plagues and People*; Marks and Beatty, *Epidemics*.

Houston Encephalitis Epidemic of 1964   Largest of several St. Louis encephalitis (SLE) flare-ups that broke out across the United States in the summer of 1964. The Houston epidemic's extent exceeded that of the 1954 Rio Grande Valley, Texas, and 1962 Tampa Bay, Florida, outbreaks, but not that of the 1933 epidemic in St. Louis, Missouri. By August 1964, a Houston health officer recognized that over the summer an encephalitis epidemic had been underway because 60 human deaths due to nervous system infections had occurred. Lab testing confirmed the St. Louis virus, which had never penetrated Houston before. State and federal agencies organized a strategy for assessing and controlling the disease. Each hospital reported cases of encephalitis, aseptic meningitis, and

meningoencephalitis. Doctors were to report all outside cases. During the epidemic, from the 243 cases, 27 people died. The 15-week epidemic was thought to have begun June 27, peaked on August 29, and occurred last on October 3.

The mosquito *culex quinque fasciatus* transmits the malady, although birds, especially sparrows and pigeons, and other animals participate in the infectious spread. Houston is flat; bayous stagnated by sewage breed the mosquito that carries the disease. Because of the concentration of stagnant pools and ditches in central Houston, cases were more numerous there in 1964.

Encephalitic symptoms include slurred speech, tremor, stupor, focal paralysis, ataxia, extreme tiredness, and disorientation. All occur only in the most severe cases. The seriousness of the disease increases with the victim's age. Although often fatal, the virus spreads slowly. The illness often incapacitates survivors, like those in asylums dating from a 1916–20 outbreak. The St. Louis encephalitis virus was isolated in St. Louis (thence the name) by Dr. Ralph W. Muckenfuss in 1933.

Further reading: Ackerknecht, *History and Geography of the Most Important Diseases*; Lord et al., "Virological Studies of Avian Hosts in the Houston Epidemic"; Luby et al., "The Epidemiology of St. Louis Encephalitis in Houston."

Hungarian Typhus Epidemic of 1542.   See JOACHIM'S ARMY TYPHUS EPIDEMIC OF 1542.

Hungarian Typhus Epidemic of 1566–68   See MAXIMILIAN II'S ARMY EPIDEMIC.

Huron Indian Epidemics of 1634–40   Repeated outbreaks of European-transmitted diseases that reduced the North American Huron Indian tribe to about 9,000 people, less than half its total population prior to 1634. The swift succession of epidemics from 1634 until 1640 was apparently connected with the increase in European settlements along the eastern seaboard of North America.

The first disease of white European origin, identified as a form of measles, was most likely introduced to eastern Canada by crewmembers aboard a French ship arriving at the seaport of Quebec on the St. Lawrence River in 1634. The measles-like disease first broke out among the Montagnais, a nomadic Indian people who were living around Quebec that summer (1634). Sick Indians had high fever, followed by a rash, and sometimes impaired vision and blindness; diarrhea often occurred at the end of the infection. The sickness that occurred among the French inhabitants there was much milder. The disease quickly spread from Quebec, moving into the Ottawa River valley, where it infected another nomadic Indian tribe, the Algonquin (Algonkin), in the river's northern tributaries. Members of the Montagnais and Algonquin tribes died from the disease in large numbers.

Many Huron Indians—a tribe of four confederated bands of Iroquoian-speaking Indians who called themselves the *Wendat* and whom the French named the *Huron*—came down with the same sickness after engaging in trade with the French at Trois-Rivières (Three Rivers) in southern Quebec in July 1634. Upon their embarking to return home (to the region west of Quebec), the Hurons were certain that their trading partners (the French) were responsible for their sickness and consequently refused to allow Frenchmen to board their canoes. Many infected Hurons carried the disease to their villages, where many others were stricken during the late summer and autumn of 1634—so many, in fact, that the harvesting of their crops was seriously hampered. A great many Huron Indians were ill during the winter, and there were numerous fatalities but not as many as the Montagnais and Algonquin Indians suffered.

In the autumn of 1636, another disease (thought to be influenza) broke out in epidemic proportions among the Huron in the St. Lawrence Valley and inland. At the Indian village of Ihonatiria, four out of six French missionary priests contracted the disease but recovered from high fevers and cramps. Among the Hurons at Ihonatiria and Ossossane (another Indian village), the disease remained severe, with high mortality, between September and December 1636; the supposed influenza declined in the spring of 1637 in both these villages. The epidemic followed a similar pattern in some other Huron villages, such as Onnentsati and Andiatae; however, it flared up in these places in the spring (1637) and fatalities increased, due most likely to the scarcity of food then. The Nipissing Indian tribe, wintering in Huron country at this time, also suffered fatalities: about 70 of them died from the disease (ten percent of their tribe). The Nipissing carried the infection into northern Ontario, where many deaths of Indian hunters occurred from the disease.

In the summer of 1637, another disease epidemic attacked the whole Huron Indian confederacy. The Susquehannock Indian tribe, suffering from an unidentified infection in February 1637, may have transmitted the disease (possibly scarlet fever) northward and inland from the St. Lawrence River area to Huron country, where many Indians perished from the disease within two days. No Frenchmen at Trois-Rivières or in Huron lands contracted this disease, making it likely that it was a European childhood disease that most French were already immune to. Hurons were stricken on their way to and from Trois-Rivières, while traveling up and down the St. Lawrence and Ottawa rivers. This epidemic ended in the autumn of 1637 after killing many more Hurons than the supposed flu epidemic of 1636.

A smallpox outbreak struck the St. Lawrence Valley in the summer of 1639; the disease was thought to have been carried to the region by a group of Kichesipirini Indians who were returning home from visiting the Abenaki (Abnaki) Indians in upper New England. Mortality was again high among the Algonquin. Huron traders returning home from Trois-Rivières spread smallpox to others in their villages, where the disease lingered throughout the winter of 1639–40 and killed several thousand Hurons, including about 460 children under age seven. The Hurons angrily blamed the Jesuit missionaries for spreading the smallpox through baptisms and sometimes attacked them; the Jesuits unwittingly may have helped spread the disease by their constant moving about in the area. Exact numbers for morbidity and mortality for any of the four above-mentioned epidemics were not tabulated, but French missionaries seeking to convert the Indians to Christianity documented the effects of each of the epidemics.

Further reading: Dobyns, *Their Number Becomes Thinned: Native American Dynamics in Eastern North America;* Trigger, *The Children of Aataentsic: A History of the Huron People to 1660.*

Icelandic Plague of 1402–04 See PLAGUE OF ICE-
LAND, GREAT.

Icelandic Plague of 1494–95 Devastating epidemic of bubonic plague comparable in its effects to
the Great Plague of nearly a century before (see
PLAGUE OF ICELAND, GREAT). As the previous epidemic had done, the later plague depopulated whole
areas; the numerous dead had to be buried in mass
graves. The plague seems to have spared only one
region of the island—the West Fjords, which was
somewhat isolated. From there people later migrated
to take over the many vacant farms left in the north.

A legend about the plague offers a possible account
of its arrival in the country as well as an example of
Icelandic folklore. According to the legend, a blue
cloth that had come to Hvalfjord brought the plague,
which emerged first in the guise of a bird and then
as smoke or mist. Since blue could also mean "dark"
and suggest sorrow or evil, the cloth probably sym-
bolizes the destructiveness of the epidemic. The bird
can be taken to represent the plague, which flew
over the land, while smoke or vapors were often
thought to be causes of disease.

The legend may also be a metaphor for the plague's
arrival from the outside world—in this case from an
English trading ship that had docked at Hvalfjord.
Because Iceland had few natural resources and even
less industry, it was almost completely reliant on
foreigners to bring goods and to connect the island
with larger markets. Since the early decades of the
fifteenth century, both English and German merchants had visited Iceland frequently, sometimes
with dozens of ships each year. While these ships
brought the grain, timber, sugar, and other products
so needed by the Icelanders, they also carried more
unwelcome cargo—plague.

Further reading: Gerrard, *The Icelandic Heritage*; Gjerset,
History of Iceland; Hastrup, *Nature and Policy in Iceland*.

Icelandic Smallpox Epidemic of 1707–09 Epidemic of smallpox that killed about 15,000 people, or
approximately one third of Iceland's population of
50,000, which had been counted in the country's first
census in 1703. Another census, done in 1729, noted
much lower numbers of servants per household, a
decrease that probably reflected the population decline of 20 years before. Iceland did not again reach
50,000 people until the early nineteenth century.

The 1707–09 epidemic (the "Great Pox") was the
most devastating of a series of outbreaks that had
swept the island many times since the 1200s, attacking people of all ages. An isolated, rural country
with a small and scattered population, Iceland was
repeatedly afflicted by diseases brought from the
outside world. (Iceland was under Danish rule from
1380 to 1918.)

Abysmal living conditions also made Icelanders
more susceptible to sickness in general. Most of them
were poor farmers who lived in dark, crowded
houses filled with smoke but never with sunlight
and fresh air. On a tour of the island in the early
1700s, a Danish commissioner saw many people who
had scurvy, tuberculosis, and other diseases. Nor
could Icelanders benefit from competent medical
care: The first state physician was not appointed
until 1760.

Despite the lack of medical knowledge, Icelanders
realized that exposure to smallpox could confer immunity. In recording the epidemic of 1430, an annal-
ist notes that it killed those who had not gotten the
disease during an earlier outbreak. In 1821 smallpox
vaccination was mandated in Iceland, and the series
of epidemics, which had lasted nearly 500 years,
finally came to an end.

Further reading: Gerrard, *The Icelandic Heritage*; Hastrup,
Nature and Policy in Iceland; Magnusson, *Northern Sphinx:
Iceland and the Icelanders from the Settlement to the Present*.

Indian-Bangladeshi Cholera Epidemic of 1971
Major epidemic of cholera among refugees fleeing
from a civil war in Bangladesh (known as East Pakistan until December 1971) into the neighboring Indian state of West Bengal.

The first major outbreak was reported by officials of the West Bengal state government on April 22, 1971; they said that 300 cholera cases had been discovered in the towns of Basirhat and Hasnabad. By then, an estimated 500,000 refugees had already sought shelter in West Bengal. Given the crowded and unsanitary conditions in the makeshift refugee camps, it did not take long for the epidemic to spread. According to government sources, at least 9,500 refugees had been hospitalized and 1,250 killed by the end of May 1971. On June 5, sources in Calcutta reported the death of 8,000 more in the epidemic. In a statement issued at its headquarters in Geneva, Switzerland, the World Health Organization put the death toll at 3,000 people. Overall, an estimated 51,000 cholera cases were reported.

On May 31, 1971, the government of India made a formal plea for international aid in coping not only with this massive disaster but also with the other problems created by the steady influx of refugees. The Indian parliament also met in a special session to discuss emergency measures for dealing with the cholera.

In early June, a health officer in West Bengal's Nadia district said that cholera was also raging across the border in Bangladesh, where the medical facilities had already collapsed under the strain. To prevent more cholera victims from crossing over from Bangladesh into Nadia, the security forces sealed the border.

Moreover, severely overburdened facilities were stretched even further by an ongoing smallpox epidemic (see BANGLADESHI SMALLPOX EPIDEMIC OF 1971–73). While many countries in the world were then experiencing cholera outbreaks caused by the *el tor* biotype of the *cholera vibrio*, a study of this epidemic revealed that it was caused by both the classical and *el tor* biotypes (see ASIATIC CHOLERA PANDEMIC OF 1961–75). Inexplicably, the epidemic did not spread farther west into the rest of India.

Further reading: *Facts-On-File Yearbook* (1971).

Indian and Burmese Sprue Epidemic of 1943–45

Outbreak of sprue among troops stationed in the India-Burma theater during the last phase of World War II. Sprue (also known as psilosis), common in this theater of operations during the war, is a disease that disrupts the body's normal digestive processes and leads to an excessive fat content in the stools. It slows down or interferes with the absorption of salt, calcium, and vitamins, which eventually leads to malnutrition and macrocytic anemia in the later stages. An infective agent, perhaps viral, is responsible for the initial phase of this deficiency disease. Sprue has a seasonal incidence, peaking in June

with the arrival of the monsoon rains, and a short incubation period. Chronic tropical sprue is marked by secondary complications and chiefly attacks adults.

More than 3,000 cases of sprue, some of them quite mild, occurred in the India-Burma theater. Among the Indian troops, the milder cases were diagnosed as para-sprue. However, the mild and severe cases were basically similar and could not always be differentiated. The Standing Medical Board in Pune, India, apparently declared as invalid more than 1,000 soldiers suffering from the disease—an indication certainly that severe cases also occurred in the area. A well-regulated diet is a crucial element in the treatment of sprue.

Further reading: Cope, ed., *History of the Second World War: Medicine and Pathology; Fourth International Congresses on Tropical Medicine and Malaria.*

Indian Cholera Epidemic of 1781–83

Series of cholera outbreaks of varying intensity that began along the east coast of India.

Cholera had been endemic along India's Coromandel coast at least since the 1770s. The first major outbreak of this epidemic occurred in March 1781 in Ganjam district, northeast of what is now the state of Tamil Nadu (formerly Madras province), when a unit of 5,000 British soldiers traveling from Bengal through this region was viciously attacked by cholera. Within a few days 1,143 men had been admitted to the hospital; a few hundred never recovered. Colonel Pearse, the British troop commander, described the symptoms of cholera with great accuracy but did not refer to it by name; he called it a "pestilential disorder."

Calcutta was the site of the next virulent outbreak. Within a fortnight, cholera had claimed many casualties among the local population before finally subsiding in the region.

In October 1782, British troops arriving in the city of Madras to report for duty were struck by cholera. Over 50 of them died within the first three days. By the end of the first month, more than 1,000 cases of cholera were reported among the soldiers. Earlier that year, in March, epidemic cholera had erupted in Trincomalee, Ceylon (Sri Lanka). Throughout 1782, the disease raged with terrible ferocity along India's eastern coast.

The disease next flared up in April 1783 in central India and at Hardwar in northern Uttar Pradesh (then the United Provinces); Hardwar is a famous Hindu pilgrimage site on the bank of the Ganges River where pilgrims congregate in thousands. Over an eight-day period, the epidemic swept through the town, killing approximately 20,000 pilgrims.

Simultaneously, the Maratha armies (British allies) fighting Tipu Sahib (sultan of Mysore) in the south encountered the dreaded disease, too. Their general, Hari Pant, mentioned in reports the terrible losses suffered by his troops on account of cholera.

Little is known about the course of the epidemic in between these major outbreaks. This may have been because few of the contemporary British physicians had identified this disease as cholera and also because hospital records were rarely preserved until a medical board was established in Bengal and Madras in 1786. During 1783, cholera was also reported from Burma. Over the next few decades until the Asiatic Cholera Pandemic of 1817–25 (q.v.), cholera outbreaks continued to occur in many parts of India.

Further reading: Macnamara, *A History of Asiatic Cholera*.

Indian Cholera Epidemic of 1817–18

Devastating epidemic that unleashed the fury of the first pandemic of cholera (see ASIATIC CHOLERA PANDEMIC OF 1817–23). It began in the town of Jessore (near Calcutta) in Bengal in August 1817 (the first case apparently occurred in Purneah in the Bihar state in 1816) when a civil surgeon reported the high incidence of a severe gastrointestinal disorder among many of his patients. Calling it *morbus oryzeus* (rice disease), he observed that it had been contracted from eating rice contaminated by water from heavy rains. Within weeks the seriousness of the disease became apparent when it spread 200,000 square miles across Bengal and the Ganges delta region and caused many to die on the same day they were stricken. In November 1817, British troops marching through Bengal collapsed in the hundreds, being seized by violent attacks of vomiting and diarrhea. Destruction on such a large scale had never been seen before, and it led some to conclude, albeit mistakenly, that this was indeed a new and largely unfamiliar disease.

It spread to Bihar and eastern Uttar Pradesh (formerly India's United Provinces), where the cold winter of 1817 held it in check. But, in March 1818, it flared into an epidemic at Allahabad. From here it spread along the commonly traveled routes to the northwest and central regions of the country, then down south and across peninsular India to Sri Lanka (formerly Ceylon) in December 1818. British forces fighting on India's northern borders transmitted the infection to their Afghan and Nepalese opponents. It continued to spread unchecked both to the east (see THAI CHOLERA EPIDEMIC OF 1820; INDONESIAN CHOLERA EPIDEMIC OF 1821; CHINESE CHOLERA EPIDEMIC OF 1820–22; JAPANESE CHOLERA EPIDEMIC OF 1822) and to the west (See ASTRAKHAN CHOLERA EPIDEMIC OF 1823), by sea and overland.

Cholera, caused by the bacterium *Vibrio comma* (*cholera vibrio*), is generally spread through contaminated food and water. It flourishes in unsanitary and overcrowded conditions and has thus been endemic in India for centuries. The vast congregation of people at many pilgrimage centers in the country has further facilitated its spread. Outside India, the annual pilgrimage made by devout Muslims to Mecca has often caused epidemics.

In India, unusually heavy rainfall in 1817 was followed by floods, crop failures and famine—ideal conditions for the spread of this disease. In fact, the epidemic continued to rage intermittently in various parts of the country (except for the hilly regions) until 1823. This, the first known spread of the disease outside the country, killed thousands of people in India alone and was followed by a wave of cholera pandemics through the rest of the century.

Further reading: Marks and Beatty, *Epidemics*; Stamp, *The Geography of Life and Death*; Akhtar and Learmonth, eds., *Geographical Aspects of Health and Disease in India*.

Indian Cholera Epidemic of 1826–27

Epidemic that ushered in the Asiatic Cholera Pandemic of 1826–37 (q.v.). Like its predecessor (see INDIAN CHOLERA EPIDEMIC OF 1817–18), it originated in the Lower Bengal region and spread rapidly across most of northern India.

Cholera incidence was reportedly on the rise in Bengal during the first four months of 1826; there were reports of outbreaks among the troops in the Presidency Circle (76 cases in April, 38 deaths), Dinapore or Dinapur (57 cases, 23 deaths), and Buxar (49 cases, 29 deaths). Meanwhile, cholera was apparently also raging across the surrounding districts. Banaras (Benares) was badly affected, losing 200 to 300 people to the disease every day; however, the troops and the jailed prisoners here remained mysteriously free of the infection. By June 1826, the epidemic had reached Kanpur (Cawnpore), where cholera was also reported among the troops (108 Indians and 64 Britishers taken ill); by August, the epidemic had temporarily subsided in the region.

In November, cholera was also prevalent among the troops in Delhi, Agra, and Mathura or Muttra. Earlier in the year, in April and May, the western India province of Gujarat was severely struck by the disease. While precise mortality figures are not available, there were a large number of deaths.

Early in 1827, cholera reappeared suddenly in the Ganges delta region, extending even farther east into Arrakan, Moulmein (now in Burma) and Chittagong (now in Bangladesh). The hospital in Calcutta was reportedly overflowing with cholera patients during this period.

In May and June 1827, British physicians reported extensive and often severe outbreaks of cholera in Delhi, Meerut, Bareilly, Moradabad, Hardwar, and Agra. The disease had a crippling impact on the local population in these towns and cities. Cholera even spread to towns in the foothills of the Himalayas and farther west into Punjab and Sind (now in Pakistan). In Rajasthan (Rajputana), Ajmer and Jaipur (two cities) suffered serious attacks, but Udaipur (Oodeypore) escaped. Kanpur, Allahabad, and the surrounding districts, which had endured cholera devastation in 1826, were only mildly affected during this second wave. India's Central Provinces (modern-day Madhya Pradesh) were spared during this epidemic.

From Punjab in the northwest, the epidemic is believed to have continued on its westward journey through Afghanistan, Iran (see PERSIAN CHOLERA EPIDEMIC OF 1829–30), the Arabian Peninsula, Russia, and eventually Europe and North America.

Further reading: Pollitzer, *Cholera*; Macnamara, *A History of Asiatic Cholera.*

Indian Cholera Epidemic of 1860–61

Scattered but intense cholera outbreaks during 1859–60, which coalesced into an extensive epidemic that spread across the northern half of India during 1860–61 (see ASIATIC CHOLERA PANDEMIC OF 1846–63).

Cholera was widespread over much of Bengal and peninsular India in 1859 and 1860. In July 1860, it invaded Agra and quickly swept through the city during August. The European contingent in nearby Mathura (Muttra) lost 24 members to the disease that month. According to eyewitness accounts, the disease generally assumed a more virulent form than on previous visitations, but it did not penetrate into the drought-stricken Punjab and the Northwest Provinces that year.

In 1861, cholera erupted once again all over the previously infected areas; natives and European troops were attacked in great numbers. Of Bengal's 52 jails, only 11 escaped the disease. Kanpur (Cawnpore) and Allahabad were attacked in May and Gwalior and Jabalpur in July. This time, cholera traveled through Bharatpur and southern Gurgaon district to arrive in Delhi on June 11, 1861. Very quickly, it spread through crowded regiments and jails (in Agra and Mathura as well), causing high mortality. Meerut was ravaged during late July and August, the prison there reporting 664 cases and 344 deaths during a one-month period. Ambala was infected in mid-July, Mian Mir (Meean Meer) at the end of July, and Lahore in August 1861.

One of the worst outbreaks of the epidemic occurred among the European troops in Mian Mir near Lahore. The first 15 European cases ended fatally, and cholera spread through almost all the regiments; 457 cases and 261 deaths occurred here over a 10-day period in late August. Total evacuation of troops was recommended but only a few units could actually be moved out to Shahdara (suburb of Lahore). Those left behind were panic-stricken as cholera continued its trail of destruction; nearly 50 percent of the hospital attendants contracted the disease as well. Overall, out of 2,452 Britishers in Mian Mir, 880 were struck by cholera and 535 died (Indian troops did not suffer to the same extent). The officers commanding the British regiments were praised for their courage and for trying to boost the sagging morale of their troops during this difficult fight with a dreaded disease.

Everywhere in India, villagers had developed their own rituals and ceremonies for warding off epidemics, which they had begun to associate with foreign conquest and rule. These rituals were often misinterpreted by the British authorities, just as their efforts to clamp down on these ceremonies were misinterpreted by the natives. Thus, the situation was not conducive to reform.

Although not India's most severe epidemic of cholera, it was nonetheless a major threat to British rule and forced a drastic reappraisal of colonial health policy in the region. For a start, the government appointed its first comprehensive inquiry (chaired by Sir J. Strachey) into the history of the disease in India. Also, a parliamentary commission was established to investigate the sanitary conditions of the army in India, resulting in the establishment of the Indian Sanitary Commission in 1861. The epidemic indirectly hastened the passage of England's Sanitary Act of 1866 and was one of the motivating factors behind the International Sanitary Conference held in Istanbul in 1866. Cholera's repeated onslaughts in various parts of the country led the government to appoint provincial sanitary commissioners in 1864.

Further reading: Macnamara, *A History of Asiatic Cholera*; Arnold, "Cholera and Colonialism in British India."

Indian Cholera Epidemic of 1864–65

Severe epidemic of cholera in central and western sections of India, an offshoot of the Asiatic Cholera Pandemic of 1865–75 (q.v.).

Cholera was rampant throughout Bengal and other parts of northern India during 1863–64. From Bengal, it invaded the provinces of central and western India. Another focus was the Hindu holy city of Pandharpur in Maharashtra state, where cholera broke out among thousands of people gathered for a pilgrimage in November 1863. As they returned home, they carried cholera to Pune, Bombay, and other cities in the area; many died en route. Between December 1863 and May 1864, about 3,000 people died of cholera in Bombay alone.

Reportedly, an extremely virulent form of cholera ravaged these central and western provinces that year; for instance, hundreds were killed every day in Berar, Khandesh, Surat, and the southern Konkan districts. Cholera's death toll in Bombay for 1864 was 4,588—exceeding the previous ten-year average by over 2,000. In 1865, cholera spread south along India's southwestern Malabar coast, killing some 40,000 people, according to one source. The Mysore and Bellary districts were severely affected as well. And 1865 was also one of the worst cholera years in the Bombay Presidency; about 84,000 civilian deaths were attributed to cholera that year, and even this is considered an underestimation. The epidemic also killed about 60 percent of the women who accompanied the soldiers in the European regiments.

From Bombay, the epidemic spread along the coast to Pakistan's seaport city of Karachi and to southern Persia (see PERSIAN CHOLERA EPIDEMICS OF 1866–70) and eventually into Yemen. See also MECCA CHOLERA EPIDEMIC OF 1865.

Further reading: Macnamara, *A History of Asiatic Cholera.*

Indian Cholera Epidemic of 1867–68   Severe epidemic of cholera illustrating the critical role played by pilgrimages in the spread of the acute intestinal disease in India.

One of the many recrudescences (reappearances) of the Asiatic Cholera Pandemic of 1865–75 (q.v.), this epidemic owed its beginning to the Hardwar Kumbh Mela (fair) held in April 1867. Pilgrims had begun streaming into Hardwar weeks before the auspicious time set for the ritual Hindu bath in the sacred waters of the Ganges River. When the day arrived, at least three million people were assembled there, with 19 confirmed cholera cases in their midst. Having completed the ceremonial mass bathing and other rituals (like scattering the ashes of dead relatives in the river), the pilgrims left on their slow journey home. Some were struck by cholera on the way and never made it. Those who survived carried the infection home to their villages across northern India along the normal routes of transportation. Likewise, cholera soon arrived in Peshawar in Pakistan and Kabul in Afghanistan, from where it traveled westward. Meanwhile, recently developed railroad arteries facilitated its dissemination through the central part of India and from Nagpur to Bombay.

Some areas suffered more than others. Cholera remained active in many drought-stricken areas (Rajputana, Punjab, the North West Provinces, the Central Provinces, and the Bombay Presidency) throughout 1968. In Amritsar, for instance, the com-

munity of Kashmiri shawl-makers suffered considerably during this outbreak. Bengal was also affected. Among the European troops stationed there, cholera alone accounted for nearly 44 percent of all deaths in 1867. According to one account, 117,181 cholera deaths were reported during this epidemic. The actual toll was undoubtedly much higher.

Further reading: Longmate, *King Cholera;* Arnold, "Cholera Mortality in British India, 1817–1947."

Indian Cholera Epidemic of 1875–77   Widespread and explosive cholera epidemic in India, one of the last outbursts of the Asiatic Cholera Pandemic of 1865–75 (q.v.).

The epidemic began, as the pandemic had, in Bengal's delta region toward the end of 1874. The onset of winter arrested its westward march in the state of Bihar and the eastern fringes of the state of Uttar Pradesh in northern India. But late in February 1875, cholera erupted to cause a violent outbreak in Allahabad, a city in Uttar Pradesh and a major Hindu pilgrimage center, which became an important cholera disseminating center through and from which the infection spread all over the country along the regular travel routes.

The northwest and central regions of the country were the next to be infected. Hindu pilgrims from Allahabad and Nasik (a holy town) introduced cholera into the heart of India. From Nasik, one wave of infection moved south toward the Malabar coast, while south India was also invaded by cholera in two other directions, from Ceylon (Sri Lanka). One penetrated the Tirunelveli district and spread north through Madurai and Tiruchirapalli, where it fused with another strain that had arrived from Ceylon via the port of Nagapattinam (Negapatam). The two strains of cholera were reinforced by streams of infection from Bombay and the Deccan region.

Cholera's diffusion through the country was gradual, in keeping with the modes of transportation. Its effect was devastating. According to R. Pollitzer (see below), a reported 364,755 people died during this epidemic in India.

Further reading: Akhtar and Learmonth, eds., *Geographical Aspects of Health and Disease in India;* Pollitzer, *Cholera.*

Indian Cholera Epidemic of 1891–92   Severe epidemic of cholera that erupted in British-ruled India and spread rapidly into some parts of Europe. A recrudescence (reappearance) of the Asiatic Cholera Pandemic of 1881–96 (q.v.), it originated in the province of Bengal during 1891 when 60,000 Hindu pilgrims arrived unannounced at a small village to celebrate a bathing festival. The authorities were not aware of this festival, which came once in 30 years, and were quite unprepared for the crowds. Not unexpectedly, cholera broke out among the pilgrims and was soon transported by them into distant places. More than 580,000 cholera deaths occurred that year; Assam, Bengal, and the United Provinces (Uttar Pradesh) were among the most severely affected areas. That year, the town of Hardwar was free of epidemic cholera, but in 1892 the disease edged closer and eventually erupted prior to the *Kumbh Mela* (fair) there.

In April 1892, therefore, the government of India's North-Western Provinces issued a ban on the Hardwar *Mela* and ordered over 200,000 Hindu pilgrims out of the area. The railway authorities were asked not to issue any more tickets for Hardwar. These measures were not actively resisted but were regarded by the anti-British movement as an infringement of the country's religious practices and beliefs. Nevertheless, the epidemic did erupt and spread across 14 districts within ten days. It continued westward—across Punjab (75,000 cholera deaths were recorded here), through Afghanistan and Persia (Iran), and within five months had penetrated Russia (see RUSSIAN CHOLERA EPIDEMIC OF 1892–93).

There were 724,384 deaths attributed to cholera that year (1892)—a death rate of 3.40 per thousand people. The mortality rate was particularly high in Assam (4.29 per thousand people), Bihar/Orissa (4.60 per thousand), and the United Provinces (4.15 per thousand people). Scholars have observed that in the latter half of the nineteenth century, famine and cholera were often inseparable companions. During 1892, famine loomed over many parts of British India because of insufficient monsoon rains the previous year, particularly in the Bombay, Bengal, and Madras presidencies (provinces).

Further reading: Arnold, "Cholera and Colonialism in British India"; Longmate, *King Cholera.*

Indian Cholera Epidemic of 1900

India's worst cholera epidemic ever, which served to foment the Asiatic Cholera Pandemic of 1899–1923 (q.v.). Like the Indian Cholera Epidemic of 1891–92 (q.v.), it was closely associated with widespread famine conditions caused by meager monsoon and winter rains over much of central, western, and southern India during 1899. It began, as had its predecessors, in the river delta regions of Lower Bengal and spread rapidly across much of the country and to the east (see PHILIPPINE CHOLERA EPIDEMIC OF 1902–04) and west of it. During 1900, cholera was epidemic in most of the provinces of India, and the death toll for the year was a staggering 805,698 people (3.72 per thousand)—the worst ever recorded for the disease in a single year.

The highest mortality rate—8.71 deaths per thousand people—was recorded in the province of Bombay, where cholera was particularly virulent in the labor camps at the relief works. Bihar/Orissa (6.46 per thousand people) and the Central Provinces (6.60 per thousand people) also suffered high mortality rates. The average mortality rate was 3.72 per thousand people.

Cholera mortality then declined somewhat until 1906, when 690,521 deaths were recorded and 1908, when mortality from the disease was nearly 600,000.

Further reading: Arnold, "Cholera and Colonialism in British India"; Klein, "Death in India, 1871–1921."

Indian Cholera Epidemic of 1964–66

Offshoot of the Asiatic Cholera Pandemic of 1961–75 (q.v.) that eventually (after the beginning of 1966) led to the displacement of classical cholera from India by the milder *el tor* biotype (see INDONESIAN CHOLERA EPIDEMIC OF 1961–62; PHILIPPINE CHOLERA EPIDEMIC OF 1961–62; TAIWANESE CHOLERA EPIDEMIC OF 1962).

The *vibrio el tor*, as the cholera's causative agent was called, apparently entered India during March 1964 through the port city of Madras in the southern state of Tamil Nadu. Another focus was established in Calcutta in April 1964. In both cases, repatriates arriving by sea from Mian Mar (Meean Meer), where *el tor* had been prevalent since 1963, were believed to have introduced the infection. In mid-1964, *el tor* appeared along the west coast, causing outbreaks in the cities of Surat and Baroda in Gujarat state and in Bombay and other cities in Maharashtra state. The Gujarat outbreaks in July 1964 were attributed to infection by sea from Pakistan. Parts of India's Bihar state also reported scattered outbreaks, and the infection even crossed over into Katmandu, Nepal. In June 1965, *el tor* reached Gurgaon district—perhaps by the overland route from Pakistan—and spread from here to Delhi, Karnal, Panipat, and Ballabhgarh in Uttar Pradesh. From Madras, *el tor* spread extensively to several cities in the states of Andhra Pradesh and Kerala and to the cities of Bangalore and Mysore in Karnataka.

Within one year of its arrival, *vibrio el tor* had spread rapidly overland throughout India, enveloping 17 states as opposed to the seven generally infected by classical cholera (caused by the *vibrio comma*). Where it encountered classical cholera, *el tor* progressively replaced it. *El tor* outbreaks were characterized by milder cases and many more carriers; the *vibrio* (bacteria) itself could survive much longer outside the human body, too. All these factors plus the geographical contiguity of Asian territory helped the *el tor* pandemic to spread rapidly westward. Cholera mortality in India at this point was a mere 0.1 percent of what it had been during the nineteenth century.

Further reading: Barua and Burrows, eds., *Cholera;* Mukherjee and Basu, "Cholera El Tor in India."

Indian Conjunctivitis Epidemic of 1971   Extensive epidemic of acute hemorrhagic conjunctivitis (AHC), part of the African and Asian Conjunctivitis Pandemic of 1969–71 (q.v.), which affected millions of people in India. The disease was nicknamed "Joy Bangla disease" or "Bangladesh conjunctivitis" because the epidemic coincided with the movement that led to the creation of the nation of Bangladesh (formerly East Pakistan) and was believed to have been introduced by refugees entering Bengal from there. The epidemic was first observed in the city of Bombay in March 1971. Muslims returning from their pilgrimage to Mecca, where they mingled with Indonesian pilgrims, are credited with importing the infection into Bombay, a port on India's west coast.

Given the crowded living conditions and unhygienic practices in Bombay, the epidemic spread rapidly throughout the city. From March to September 1971, some 500,000 cases were reportedly treated for AHC in this city alone. The actual figures were undoubtedly much higher; according to some sources, 95 percent of the city's population was actually infected. An unusual feature of this outbreak was that between May and August 1971, experts observed that AHC was occasionally accompanied or followed by neurological complications such as radiculomyelitis and infection of the cranial nerve. Similar observations were made during the AHC epidemics in Japan and Thailand. The disease's causative virus was later identified as the enterovirus type 70 (E70).

From Bombay, AHC spread rapidly all over India, causing large outbreaks in Calcutta, Lucknow, Amritsar, Pune, Madras, and New Delhi during April–June 1971. At least a million cases were reported from Calcutta alone, where, during the epidemic, almost everyone on the streets could be seen wearing dark glasses. Overall, the maximum number of cases occurred in people 20 to 30 years old. Generally, patients undergoing the prescribed treatment recovered within seven to ten days.

Further reading: Pramanik, "Joy Bangla—An Epidemic of Conjunctivitis in India"; Kono, "Apollo 11 Disease or Acute Haemorrhagic Conjunctivitis."

Indian Dengue Hemorrhagic Fever Epidemics   Series of outbreaks caused by dengue (breakbone fever) and dengue-related viruses in different parts of India during the 1960s. The country's first recorded epidemic of dengue hemorrhagic fever (DHF) occurred in the eastern city of Calcutta late in 1963. Similar in many ways to the DHF outbreaks that struck Thailand, Singapore, Burma, Malaysia, and the Philippines during the same period, the Calcutta epidemic affected people of all ages. However, children seemed to have suffered in greater numbers and from a more severe form of the disease. During the outbreak, 158 deaths were reported, but actual mortality may have been much higher. The causative agent was the dengue type 2 virus.

During 1964, Calcutta was again invaded by a dengue-like virus that was subsequently identified as the *chikungunya* virus (meaning "doubled up" in Tanzania, where the virus was first isolated in the 1950s). This virus is not generally implicated in the more severe or fatal forms of the disease, hence this outbreak was far milder than that of 1963.

Dengue had been endemic in the southern Indian state of Tamil Nadu (formerly Madras) during 1960–63. In 1964, the *chikungunya* virus caused a major outbreak in the city of Vellore in Tamil Nadu. Apparently, nearly 200,000 cases (representing more than 20 percent of the population) were reported during this outburst. The central Indian city of Nagpur also suffered an outbreak caused by the same virus in 1965. In some parts of the city, nearly 40 percent of the inhabitants came down with the illness.

During 1968, 200,000 people were infected by the dengue virus during an epidemic in Kanpur (Cawnpore) city in Uttar Pradesh state. People suffered from hemorrhagic symptoms and mortality was considerable.

Another Indian city, Ajmer (Ajmere) in the northwestern state of Rajasthan (Rajputana), reported a smaller outbreak caused by dengue viruses type 1 and type 3. Hemorrhagic symptoms were found in 55 cases. See also SINGAPORE DENGUE HEMORRHAGIC FEVER EPIDEMICS; THAI DENGUE HEMORRHAGIC FEVER EPIDEMICS.

Further reading: Howe, ed., *A World Geography of Human Diseases;* Horsfall and Tamm, eds., *Viral and Rickettsial Infections of Man.*

Indian Encephalitis Epidemic of 1977–78   Major outbreak of Japanese B Encephalitis (JBE) that was especially devastating in the state of Uttar Pradesh in northern India. The fatality rate is one of the highest for this disease.

Japanese B Encephalitis had been known to occur sporadically—initially in southern India (where it was first observed in 1955), but since 1973 also in the north and northeast. Epidemic JBE, however, was less common and generally minor in scope. In 1977, 31,995 cases of JBE were reported in the country, but since these were not concentrated in any one geographical area, the news of its presence did not cause much alarm. Cases were reported from Karnataka, Tamil Nadu, West Bengal, Bihar, and Assam. During the following year, 23,446 cases occurred—a large percentage of them in Uttar Pradesh, India's most highly populated state. Unofficially, it is estimated that between one million and two million people of all age groups were attacked by this virus in India in 1978. In October, the government-owned radio reported that 480 people had died of JBE in a one-month period, most of them in Uttar Pradesh.

JBE is transmitted by mosquitoes (*Culex tritaeniorhynchus* and *Culex gelidus)* from an intermediate host to man. It favors hot and dry weather, particularly after heavy rains. See also JAPANESE ENCEPHALITIS EPIDEMICS OF THE 1920S AND 1930S.

Further reading: Spink, *Infectious Diseases;* Swedlund and Armelagos, eds., *Disease in Populations in Transition.*

Indian Influenza Epidemic of 1918–19 Devastating epidemic that struck India during the second wave of the global pandemic of influenza (see SPANISH INFLUENZA EPIDEMIC OF 1917–19), causing an estimated 12,500,000 human deaths in India. Everywhere the influenza struck with unexpected severity (about 20,000,000 deaths were recorded worldwide), but no country suffered as much as did India.

The epidemic was first observed in Bombay, India, in June 1918 and subsequently in Madras and Karachi, but its virulence was not manifest until the second wave invaded in September. Bombay, with its teeming millions of people, crowded slums, and deplorably filthy living conditions, was the worst hit. Eight hundred influenza deaths were recorded in this city on one day—October 6, 1918.

By December 1918, the death toll was already in the millions: 800,000 victims in Berar and the Central Provinces, 800,000 in the Punjab, 900,000 in Bombay, 1,100,000 in the United Provinces, 23,000 in Delhi, and 60,000 in neighboring Burma. In the Punjab, trains were packed with dead and dying passengers, and the streets and cemeteries were strewn with corpses. Altogether, more people died in India during this epidemic than during 20 years of cholera or during the four years of World War I.

Far more severe than the previous influenza epidemic (see ASIATIC INFLUENZA PANDEMIC OF 1889–90), it was also distinguished by the variety and intensity of the complications that followed the onset of "flu." The disease's incubation period was often less than two days. In this case, following the usual symptoms of influenza (fever, headache, muscle ache, nausea, and dry cough), some patients coughed or brought up large quantities of sputum and turned bluish-purple. The excessively high mortality was generally attributed to complications, such as pneumonia, bronchitis, tuberculosis, hemorrhages of the nose and lung passages, malaria, and dysentery.

India's medical and administrative facilities—already strained by war duties and the failure of the 1918 monsoon—were unable to cope with a calamity of this magnitude. In fact, the epidemic quickly ran its course through the country before any significant preventive measures were introduced to combat it. Indonesia was the next Asian country to be affected: Influenza claimed about 1,500,000 victims here.

Further reading: Pyle, *The Diffusion of Influenza;* Stamp, *The Geography of Life and Death;* Marks and Beatty, *Epidemics.*

Indian Influenza Epidemic of 1957–58 Mild but widespread epidemic, an offshoot of the Asian Influenza Pandemic of 1957–58 (q.v.). It started when a luxury liner from Singapore arrived in India's southern port city of Madras on May 16, 1957; numerous influenza patients were on board. The ship was quarantined at sea, but four of the nurses who went on board to treat the passengers came down with the disease a mere 48 hours after being exposed to it.

It is uncertain whether the Indian cities of Bombay and Calcutta were simultaneously exposed or whether the Asian flu virus arrived from Madras, but outbreaks occurred in both cities during the week of May 21. More than 1,000 flu cases were reported in Calcutta in week 22, and the city's first two fatalities were on June 1. Passengers arriving on other luxury liners from Southeast Asia ports continually replenished the source of infection so that all four southern Indian states (Tamil Nadu, Kerala, Karnataka [Mysore], and Andhra Pradesh) were soon affected.

From May 18 until the end of June 1957, the virus (type A) had penetrated most areas of the country, starting with an explosive spread through the crowded main cities and then slowing somewhat in its journey to smaller towns and villages. Earlier in 1957, another influenza virus (type B) had caused localized outbreaks all over the country; in some areas, it still raged simultaneously with this new virus strain. During the 23rd week (June 2–8, 1957), the epidemic spread extraordinarily fast, infecting most of Kerala, Mysore City, and Kolar in Karnataka and many towns in Andhra Pradesh, Maharashtra, Orissa, Uttar Pradesh, and the Punjab. Pakistan's cities of Karachi and Lahore also reported influenza outbreaks during this period.

Starting from the 24th week, the epidemic generally intensified in previously affected areas. In New Delhi, 80,573 flu cases and 15 deaths occurred during June alone. When the 12-week-long main wave of the epidemic ended on August 10, 1957, most of the Indian states had recorded 75 percent of their cases. Doctors and nurses and children between six and 15 years of age recorded higher than average attack rates, 57 percent for the latter group. During a 38-week period (May 19, 1957–February 8, 1958), 4,451,785 cases and 1,098 deaths were reported. On the basis of the 1951 census, the attack rate was 12,366 per million and the mortality rate was three per million people. There were 242 deaths for every one million cases. The attack rate ranged from 0.4 percent (4,000 per million people) in some northern states to 2.8 percent (28,000 per million) in Bombay. The highest mortality was in West Bengal (40.5 percent).

Many people suffered a second attack of influenza either during the main wave or immediately after it. It is not known how many of these were due to the Asian virus and how many to the type B virus already prevalent in the country. Nausea and vomiting were noted in an unusually large number of cases during this epidemic. In some areas, the primary attack was either accompanied or followed by a dysenteric condition. Elsewhere in the country, there were reports that the virus had attacked the nervous system in varying degrees.

Further reading: Menon, "The 1957 Pandemic of Influenza in India."

Indian Kala-azar Epidemics, Early

Indian Kala-azar Epidemics, Early   Major epidemics of kala-azar (visceral leishmaniasis) that struck northeastern India during the nineteenth and early twentieth centuries. Some were so severe that entire villages were wiped out, and many areas were abandoned. They also led to a considerable decline in the hitherto steady population growth. In its epidemic form, kala-azar was confined to the Ganges and Brahmaputra River basins, extending from Lucknow in Uttar Pradesh, in the west, to Sylhet in Assam, in the east.

Little is known about the history of kala-azar in India prior to the nineteenth century, when it was often confused with malaria, and it is possible that some of the early outbreaks may have been a mixture of both diseases since parasitological diagnosis did not become widespread until 1910. It is now established that the *Phlebotomus argentipes*, a type of sand fly, is the principal vector of epidemic kala-azar in India. Locally, synonyms such as *kala-jwar, kala-dukh, Burdwan* fever, *Shirkari* disease, and *Sahib's* disease were used to describe kala-azar.

The first outbreak for which records are available occurred in 1824. Apparently a mixture of kala-azar and malaria, this epidemic killed 75,000 people in Jessore in the eastern province of Bengal. Over the next few decades, kala-azar became endemic in the region and spread slowly through Lower Bengal.

It invaded Burdwan in western Bengal in 1868 and, over the next five years, devastated its population. The year 1873 marked the peak of the kala-azar incidence in Bengal. The epidemic slowly subsided but kala-azar became endemic; it is a severe infectious disease marked by fever, progressive anemia, leukopenia, and enlargement of the spleen and liver.

It also spread eastward into Assam, where the Garo Hills region was severely affected between 1875 and 1883. Apparently, this was kala-azar's first incursion into Assam, and it traveled up the Brahmaputra River valley, invading the Nowgong district by 1891. During the next decade, until 1901, Nowgong and its environs suffered the ravages of an intense kala-azar epidemic. Within the first five years, more than a quarter of the arable land in the affected areas went out of cultivation, and whole villages vanished. In 1902, the epidemic infected the Sylhet district and remained there until 1907. Around the same time, kala-azar outbreaks were reported from Bihar, Uttar Pradesh, Orissa, and Tamil Nadu. Some scholars believe that kala-azar actually spread from Assam to Bengal in the 1870s.

In Assam, the second wave of kala-azar was accompanied by an epidemic of malaria. During this phase, between 1909 and 1912, kala-azar incidence rose dramatically in some districts.

The third wave of kala-azar established itself in Assam shortly before the Spanish Influenza Epidemic of 1917–19 (q.v.). It raged for ten years and, except for the mass treatment measures undertaken, would have been as deadly as the kala-azar epidemic of 1891–1901. Between 1924 and 1927, some 156,000 cases were treated in Assam. Without this treatment, the epidemic would have been devastating. By 1930, when this wave receded, kala-azar had penetrated as far east as the Sibasagar district.

Bengal, Bihar, and Assam experienced kala-azar outbreaks in the 1940s and again in the 1970s. During the 1950s and early 1960s, when malaria was eradicated through widespread spraying of DDT, kala-azar disappeared again, only to reemerge with redoubled fury in these areas in the 1970s.

Further reading: Davis, *The Population of India and Pakistan;* Peters and Killick-Kendrick, eds., *The Leishmaniases in Biology and Medicine.*

Indian Kala-azar Epidemics, Later

Indian Kala-azar Epidemics, Later   Epidemics of kala-azar (a mainly tropical and subtropical rural disease) across northeastern India during the 1940s, returning with renewed force during the 1970s. Kala-azar is a severe infectious disease caused by a flagellated, parasitic protozoan *(Leishmania donovani)*.

Kala-azar broke out in Assam, Bengal, and Bihar around 1943 and, for the first time, spread over into eastern Uttar Pradesh. In famine-ravaged Bengal, the epidemic lingered until 1949 (see INDIAN KALA-AZAR EPIDEMICS, EARLY).

During the 1950s, kala-azar disappeared thanks to extensive malaria eradication measures undertaken in the northeast regions of India. The spraying of DDT helped kill the *Phlebotomus argentipes,* a species of sand fly that is the accepted vector for the disease in these areas. However, as soon as the antimalaria campaign ended, kala-azar returned with even greater virulence, initially in Bihar and later spreading elsewhere. Bihar's earliest cases occurred in 1969, but the magnitude of the problem was not realized until 1973, when the epidemic was first brought to official attention. During 1974–77, over 70,000 cases of kala-azar were reported from four districts in the state of Bihar alone. The epidemic peaked in 1979 and, prior to its decline a few years later, had penetrated into areas where kala-azar had not been known before. In 1981, for instance, 700,000 cases reportedly occurred throughout India.

Kala-azar, or visceral leishmaniasis, is transmitted through the bite of the *Phlebotomus* sand fly carrying the infectious agent. The incubation period generally ranges between two and six months. In the early stages, diagnosis is difficult because the onset varies dramatically from the mild to the very severe and continues for days or months (six months on average). Kala-azar is characterized by recurrent malaria-like fever, severe anemia, enlargement of the spleen, and gradual emaciation and muscular wasting. Subsequently, all these symptoms become more pronounced, the liver swells, and jaundice and spontaneous hemorrhages may occur. Secondary infections may complicate matters in the latter stages of the disease. Post-kala-azar dermal leishmaniasis (PKDL) may occur years after the patient is cured and sometimes even in isolation. Nowadays, with early diagnosis and advanced treatment, patients rarely have to endure the more serious stages of the disease.

Some scholars have described kala-azar epidemics in India and elsewhere as being cyclical in occurrence. Others have observed that they tend to occur simultaneously with famine, other epidemics, earthquakes, or other such factors following an inter-epidemic period during which a susceptible population is established.

Further reading: Peters and Killick-Kendrick, eds., *The Leishmaniases in Biology and Medicine;* Henschen, *The History of Diseases.*

Indian Kyasanur Forest Disease Epidemics of 1957–58　Two epidemics of Kyasanur Forest Disease (KFD) that occurred in the Shimoga district of Karnataka state in southern India. KFD is a disease that affects humans and monkeys; in fact, the disease's virus was first isolated from a wild monkey *(Presbytis entellus)* in the Kyasanur Forest of the Shimoga district during March–April 1957. It is caused by a group B tick-borne virus belonging to the Russian spring–summer (RSS) viruses, and its clinical course is very similar to that of Omsk hemorrhagic fever. This was the first tick-borne virus disease to be recognized in India, and the first known incursion of an RSS-related virus into a tropical area.

Symptoms of KFD appear three to eight days after a person is bitten by an infective tick, often near where monkey mortality, following an epizootic, has been observed. Fever (lasting five to 14 days) and headache signal its onset, which is sudden. Vomiting and diarrhea start two to three days later. Severe pain in the neck, lower back, and the extremities leads to extreme prostration, lassitude, drowsiness, and in rare cases to coma. Inflammation of the conjunctivae is pronounced. Sometimes, diagnosis is aided by an eruption on the soft palate. Leucopenia and thrombocytopenia and hemorrhagic symptoms (sometimes lasting weeks) usually set in during this stage, the latter leading to possibly fatal complications around the second week. The central nervous system is not implicated and complete recover from KFD is usually a very slow process.

Both the KFD epidemics occurred within a 100-square-mile zone of the Kyasanur Forest, where the disease had not been heard of before December 1955. The first cases occurred during January–April 1956 in four villages. Early in January 1957, more cases occurred but were reported as enteric fever. In February, the incidence of such cases began to increase and laboratory investigations were launched at the end of March 1957. Meanwhile, the steady rise in the reported KFD cases continued from over 20 villages until the arrival of the monsoon rains in early June, when the human cases abruptly ceased. Coincidentally, this was also the period (spring–summer) when the ticks (*Haemaphysalis spinigera,* the dominant species locally) were most active. Monkeys and birds were found to be the most common carriers of the infected ticks. A few more cases occurred once the rains ended in September. Overall, from September 1956 to August 1957, 466 cases of KFD were reported; it is estimated that just as many cases escaped notification. The mortality rate from KFD was around ten percent.

The second epidemic, slightly smaller than the first, occurred between late 1957 and August 1958. From January to July 1958, 181 cases were observed, three percent of them ending fatally. That year, premature rains in early April helped limit the case incidence greatly. The cases began declining in April and the outbreak was over by May. Except for the earliest cases, most of them covered the same area as the previous epidemic. Incidence was higher among teenagers, children, and the elderly, perhaps because much of the local adult male population was already immune.

The KFD virus attacked mainly young adult males working in the Kyasanur Forest. With so many of them sick and unable to work during one of the busiest times of the year, the manpower situation in the locality became critical. Since then, residents have been taught to prevent tick bites and also how to control the tick population. Also, a recently developed vaccine is proving fairly effective in preventing the infection.

Further reading: Work et al., "Virological Epidemiology of the 1958 Epidemic of Kyasanur Forest Disease"; Work, "Kyasanur Forest Disease."

Indian Malaria Epidemic of 1974–75

Extensive epidemic of malaria that ravaged various parts of India during 1974 and reportedly escalated in 1975, thereby erasing some of the gains made by the country's 20-year malaria eradication campaign.

During 1974, India was the most highly infected country in the world; its 2,400,000 reported malaria cases (considered a fraction of the actual cases) accounted for a third of the globally reported malaria cases that year. The 1973 hike in world crude oil prices had made the purchase and domestic production of petroleum-based insecticides prohibitively expensive. In addition, the malaria parasite had developed a capacity to withstand the normal dosage of chloroquine, a drug used to treat malaria, just as the mosquitoes were becoming resistant to DDT. Moreover, India could not afford the $75,000,000 needed annually to effectively control the disease (as it was, some $26,000,000 of its $46,000,000 health budget was reserved for malaria control alone).

The infection was apparently brought into the country by refugees streaming in from Sri Lanka and Pakistan, but it did not spread evenly in all parts of the country. For instance, in 1974, the Indian state of Andhra Pradesh reported about 125,000 cases, Karnataka had 150,000 cases, and Tamil Nadu reported only 19,687 cases. Nearly 10,000 cases were reported from Madras alone during the first six months of 1975, and 12,000 cases occurred in New Delhi until September 1975. Overall, some five million people were apparently infected during 1975. In the Assam region, some people had developed chloroquine-resistant malaria so quinine had to be used in their treatment instead. There were fears

that this strain might spread elsewhere in the country.

India's annual production of 100,000,000 chloroquine pills could not meet the needs of its 600,000,000 people, so the antimalaria treatment was recommended only for those performing essential services. Arrangements were also made to divert funds from other health projects so that domestic production of chloroquine could be increased. Despite these efforts, malaria continued to spread through the next two years; six million cases apparently occurred in 1976 and nearly 30,000,000 in 1977.

Further reading: Altman, "Malaria Surges in India Despite Vast Drive"; Ramesh, *Cholera and Malaria Incidence in Tamil Nadu, India.*

Indian Plague of 1896–97

Epidemic that started in Bombay's dock area in the summer of 1896—the city's first recorded incidence of bubonic plague in 184 years. Part of the Third Plague Pandemic (q.v.), the disease was transmitted via the shipping channels from Hong Kong (see HONG KONG PLAGUE OF 1894) and claimed about 300,000 lives in India over the next two years.

From the docks in Bombay the disease spread rapidly across the city, killing 2,000 people in 1896; 11,000 in 1897; and 17,000 in 1898. Officials initially denied the existence of plague in the city and later tried to suppress any information about it, but it was already common knowledge. Terrified, some 200,000 citizens hurriedly fled into the interior, carrying the disease with them. In September–October 1896, the disease became more virulent, killing 20,000 people in six months. By 1898, the epidemic had covered the Bombay and Mysore presidencies (now the states of Maharashtra and Karnataka, respectively) and the adjacent areas of the Hyderabad state (now Andhra Pradesh), where it did not take a serious turn until 1911, and even the city of Calcutta in the east. After 1898, Calcutta's annual death toll from the plague remained in the range of seven thousand to eight thousand for a few years.

Though the city of Bombay was hit the hardest, fear of the epidemic spread all over the country. Attributing its fury to the power of evil spirits, Muslims hung sacred inscriptions on the streets to ward them off, while Hindus believed it to be a just punishment for their sins. During this epidemic, 80 percent of those who contracted bubonic plague died from it, but the number of actual plague cases was grossly underreported. In the 50 years between 1898 and 1948, over 12,000,000 people died of the plague in India, half of them in the first ten years alone.

Further reading: Pollitzer, *Plague;* Gregg, *Plague: An Ancient Disease in the Twentieth Century;* Winslow, *The Conquest of Epidemic Disease.*

Indian Plague of 1904–07   Recrudescence of the Indian Plague of 1896–97 (q.v.), part of an ongoing pandemic of plague sweeping across much of the globe during the late nineteenth and early twentieth centuries (see PLAGUE PANDEMIC, THIRD).

The epidemic began in Bombay and soon spread into India's interior, aided by fleeing masses of people. The mortality was staggering, particularly in the provinces of Bombay and Punjab (the rural death rate far exceeded the urban death rate here). According to one estimate, 9,210 plague deaths occurred in Bombay (population one million) over a 12-month period in 1905–06. Punjab bore the brunt of this epidemic, with 650,000 plague deaths (27 per 1,000) during 1906–07 and two million deaths during 1901–11. The recorded nationwide death toll between July 1, 1904, and June 30, 1905, was 1,328,249. It is believed that at least three million to four million Indians died of plague during 1896–1906, and nearly two million in 1907 alone. During the course of this epidemic, the newly established Plague Research Commission confirmed the decade-old findings of the French scientist P. L. Simond, who had been ridiculed for his explanation of the role of the rat, the flea, and *Yersinia pestis* (the plague bacillus) in the transmission of the disease.

News of the epidemic caused panic in many countries, which dispatched commissions to investigate and report on the situation in India. Locally, the public health authorities launched a massive preventive campaign aimed at the eradication of the rat population. For instance, the Bombay Council had 31,000 employees engaged in cleaning and disinfecting the streets. The city's sewers were treated with three million gallons of disinfectant. Homes were sprayed with carbolic acid. While these efforts helped control the rat population in the city, they also helped the spread of the disease inland.

Clearly, this was one of the most devastating outbreaks of plague in this century. The incidence of plague in India declined noticeably after this period.

Further reading: Lien-teh et al., *Plague: A Manual for Medical and Public Health Workers*; Hobson, *World Health and History.*

Indian Plague of 1994.   Unexpected outburst of bubonic and pneumonic plague in India in September 1994. Transmitted by fleas that infest rats, the bubonic form of the bacterial disease first erupted in Maharashtra state in west central India, where many rats were drawn by relief grain and other stockpiled food sent there after severe earthquakes in 1993 that killed some 10,000 people.

Public health officials at first seemed to downplay the danger of the disease, undoubtedly to avoid panic in Bombay, the capital of Maharashtra and India's largest city with more than 12.5 million inhabitants. However, on September 20, 1994, Indians began dying from pneumonic plague (a more deadly strain of the bubonic plague) which is spread via coughs and droplets of contaminated saliva exhaled by infected individuals, in the port city of Surat, about 150 miles north of Bombay. In less than a week, about 200,000 panicky residents of Surat (with a population of more than 1.5 million) fled the city in jammed trains and buses, usually heading south to Bombay. Even doctors fled Surat by the hundreds.

Alarmed that the Surat refugees would carry the plague into Bombay's rat-infested shantytowns and slums, health officials undertook swift rat-control and disease-control measures, such as stockpiling tetracycline and other antibiotics. Officials urged calm, but cases of plague began to be reported in Bombay, New Delhi (north central India), and Calcutta (northeast India). There were increased efforts to find and treat the sick, along with increased availability of antibiotics in pharmacies.

By October 1, health officials and the World Health Organization reported that plague had eased and was under control in India, and yet many citizens and authorities remained fearful that the estimated 400,000 people who had fled Surat by then would continue to spread the disease throughout the country. At least 54 people had died of plague in Surat, and unofficial estimates put the death toll as high as 300. Some families reportedly cremated or buried suspected plague victims without reporting the deaths.

This epidemic of plague once again raised much concern about the old Hindu practice of rat worship in India. Like cows, rats are deified in Hindu temples; no Hindu worship is complete without an offering to the elephant-headed god Ganesha (or Ganeśa), who is accompanied by a rat whenever he travels about. In the early morning in many towns and cities in India, men and women can be seen carrying rats in traps and releasing them at a distance from their homes. Indians rarely kill rats, which many health officials consider a deadly menace that must be eradicated to escape plagues in the future.

Further reading: John F. Burns's articles on India, *The New York Times*, September 24–October 3, 1994.

Indian Poliomyelitis Epidemics of World War II   Outbreaks of poliomyelitis (infantile paralysis) that occurred among soldiers and natives in India during World War II, from 1942 to 1944. Prevalent in parts of India, poliomyelitis or polio was an important concern for British troops stationed there. From one reported case in 1941, the incidence rose dramatically in 1942 to 1.7 per 1,000 among British officers, 0.3 among the general ranks of British soldiers, and 0.01 among the Indian troops. The case fatality rate was 17 percent among the Britishers. The incidence fell off slightly in 1943—0.5 per 1,000 for British officers, 0.1 for other ranks, and 0.01 for the Indians in combat. However, the case mortality among the British was a staggering 33 percent. In 1944, 1.4 cases per 1,000 were reported among British officers, 0.3 among the British ranks, and 0.01 among the Indian soldiers. The case mortality rate was 30 percent.

Polio's initial symptoms—influenzal, catarrhal, or gastrointestinal—persisted from two to ten days. Some patients were struck by a second wave of these symptoms within days of recovering from the initial attack. In most of the cases, the lower dorsal and lumbo-sacral sections of the spinal cord were affected. Also, the muscles governing hip and knee movement were more prone to attack than the distal muscles. Localized paralysis was observed in some cases. In approximately five percent of the cases, the cerebrospinal fluid remained uninfected during the meningitic or paralytic phases of the disease. Many abortive cases were reported.

As in the Middle East theater, British officers suffered a higher incidence of the disease than the rest of the troops, British or Indian. The disease appeared to attack those who had been in the region less than two years and, therefore, had not developed sufficient immunity. It is believed that the unsanitary and irregularly inspected conditions in the officers' mess and the officers' greater contact with India's civilian populations may have increased their chances of contracting the disease. See also MIDDLE EAST HEPATITIS EPIDEMICS OF WORLD WAR II.

Further reading: Cope, ed., *History of the Second World War: Medicine and Pathology;* World Health Organization, *Poliomyelitis.*

Indian Smallpox Epidemic of 1769–70

Devastating epidemic of smallpox that ripped through Bengal and perhaps much of India. The British had taken Bengal from Muslim control in 1764.

In Bengal (northeast British India), the epidemic capped a season of drought, floods, and eventually famine and added its own toll to an already ravaged countryside. The cumulative impact of the famine, which began in 1769, was so disastrous that it lasted through two generations. Smallpox struck Bengal early in the year; Murshidabad, the Bengali capital, was invaded in March, and mortality in the city was staggering. Eyewitnesses have recorded that the bodies of the dead and the dying were piling up so rapidly in the streets of Murshidabad that the authorities were unable to deal adequately with their

disposal. Groups of people were engaged just to remove the dead bodies from the streets. The epidemic apparently wiped out entire families.

Even Bengal's Muslim nawab (viceroy) Syefuddowla could not escape smallpox's fury and died after four years in office in 1770. It is estimated that about 63,000 people died of smallpox in Murshidabad alone. Bengal lost one third of its population—nearly three million people according to some—to smallpox. Another view is that three million human deaths were recorded from all over India during the epidemic. However, historians are divided on whether it spread elsewhere in India and its impact there if it did. With inoculation (which is known to spread natural smallpox among the uninoculated) more popular in Bengal than in the rest of India, it is possible that Bengal endured the worst of the epidemic.

Further reading: Hopkins, *Princes and Peasants: Smallpox in History;* Hunter, *Annals of Rural Bengal.*

Indian Smallpox Epidemic of 1973–74

Last great smallpox epidemic in the world, whose origin was traced to the industrial city of Jamshedpur in the southern part of the Indian state of Bihar. The constant movement of migrant laborers to and from the township led to localized outbreaks in four eastern states (Bihar, Uttar Pradesh, Madhya Pradesh, and West Bengal) in late 1973. These outbreaks soon flared into an epidemic even as international efforts were under way to detect, report, and prevent any incidence of the disease in India, its principal endemic home. When it peaked in mid-1974, 188,000 people in 8,664 villages had been infected, the highest number recorded in over two decades.

In February 1974, 1,170 new outbreaks were reported from villages in Bihar, 18 from its urban areas, most of them confined to its eastern districts. Within a couple of weeks, it had spread to neighboring West Bengal and Nepal, and the number of active cases increased dramatically. While each search period revealed a higher incidence than the previous one, eradication efforts suffered severe setbacks because of a series of natural and man-made calamities (particularly political unrest) that struck Bihar. Floods in the northern part of the state and drought in the south caused thousands of migrant workers to flee, many carrying the disease with them. Twenty-five percent of the villages in Bihar's three northeastern districts were infected.

Uttar Pradesh recorded the second highest incidence of smallpox cases. From West Bengal, the disease spread slowly to Orissa, Madhya Pradesh, and Maharashtra. In May 1974 alone, a record number of 48,833 cases were reported in the country, over 11,000 every week. Of these, 35,000 were reported in

Bihar with 10,000 deaths in that month alone. During the first half of 1974, an estimated 30,000 people lost their lives to smallpox in the country. Reportedly, three quarters of the world's smallpox cases were concentrated in Bihar and Uttar Pradesh at that time, while India contained 82 percent of the world's incidence that year.

India has had a long history of smallpox epidemics, but this severe epidemic was brought to international attention only when reporters covering India's first atomic blast in Rajasthan in May 1974 gave it extensive coverage. From then on, international, government, and private agencies redoubled their efforts and resources to eradicate smallpox from India. An intensive campaign, Operation Zero Smallpox, was launched later that year. Its great success (the last smallpox case recorded in India occurred in May 1975) can be considered one of the triumphant chapters in the global history of public health.

Further reading: Brilliant, *The Management of Smallpox Eradication in India*; Fenner et al., *Smallpox and Its Eradication*; Hopkins, *Princes and Peasants: Smallpox in History*.

Indonesian Cholera Epidemic of 1821

Offshoot epidemic of the Asiatic Cholera Pandemic of 1817–23 (q.v.), tearing quickly through the island of Java, killing some 125,000 people within a short period. The islands of Sumatra and Borneo were also affected in Indonesia.

The cholera was believed to have been imported into Semarang, a coastal town in north Java, in April 1821 from India (see INDIAN CHOLERA EPIDEMIC OF 1817–18). In Semarang, it wreaked considerable havoc in a short time. In 11 days, 1,255 deaths were reported. The epidemic entered Batavia (now Djakarta) on April 27, but there the fatalities were much lower—778 deaths in 11 days. Shortly thereafter, epidemic cholera had invaded 14 residencies (official administrative divisions of representatives of the governor general) and provinces in north Java. All except one were coastal regions. Within these provinces, the lowlying areas were more severely affected. The average duration of the epidemic in most provinces was three to four months. By December 1821, cholera had virtually disappeared from the island. However, it reappeared in three residencies in 1822, in one residency in 1823, and in three residencies in 1824.

From Java, the epidemic moved to China (see CHINESE CHOLERA EPIDEMIC OF 1820–22) and Japan (see JAPANESE CHOLERA EPIDEMIC OF 1822). Indonesia was subsequently struck by other severe cholera outbreaks.

Further reading: Owen, ed., *Death and Disease in Southeast Asia*; Marks and Beatty, *Epidemics*.

Indonesian Cholera Epidemic of 1961–62

Epidemic that spread across many Indonesian islands and marked the beginning of the Asiatic Cholera Pandemic of 1961–75 (q.v.). The so-called *el tor* cholera began on the Indonesian island of Sulawesi (formerly Celebes), endemic home of the bacterium *Vibrio el tor*, which had caused outbreaks there in 1937–38, 1939–40, 1944, and 1957–58. In January 1961, the disease erupted again in the port city of Makassar on Sulawesi and subsequently spread to the central and northern parts of the island, where 109 cases and 29 deaths occurred during the epidemic.

In May, visitors from Makassar carried the disease to a coastal area near the town of Kendal in central Java, where the island's first cases were reported. The epidemic then spread to Java's cities of Semarang and Djakarta in June. Apparently, it was also introduced into the city of Bandung but did not spread there. The island of Kalimantan (Borneo) was infected in August. Over the next few months, cholera coursed through East Java, East Sumatra, and one of the small islands in the vicinity of Timor. The volatile political situation in Indonesia and the resulting movement of troops and civilians no doubt hastened its spread. Until February 1, 1962, the local authorities had been notified of 4,107 clinically confirmed cases and 897 deaths (mortality rate of 21.9 percent). The actual number of cases may have been much more than this; also included in this figure are the 92 cases that broke out across ten wards of the Central Hospital in Djakarta. The epidemic persisted in parts of Indonesia until March 1962.

As in the Philippine Cholera Epidemic of 1961–62 (q.v.), the disease predominantly infected coastal, riverside, and lakeside communities and poor people living in urban squalor. Hilly and forested areas were spared. Indonesia's Chinese community was not infected to the same extent as the other communities, perhaps because of prevalent customs like drinking tea and eating fresh-cooked vegetables.

Subsequently, the *el tor* vaccine was introduced into Sulawesi, along with four different types of cholera vaccine elsewhere in Indonesia.

Further reading: Barua and Burrows, eds., *Cholera*; Felsenfeld, "Some Observations on the Cholera (El Tor) Epidemic in 1961–62."

Indonesian Influenza Epidemic of 1918

Major epidemic, part of the global Spanish Influenza Epidemic of 1917–19 (q.v.), which claimed an estimated 1.5 million human lives in Indonesia.

The first wave of the epidemic entered Indonesia, apparently from Bombay (see INDIAN INFLUENZA EPIDEMIC OF 1918–19), at Pankattan on Sumatra's east coast, late in June 1918. Several areas of western Java and Kalimantan (Borneo) reported outbreaks by late July, but the islands to the east remained untouched. This first wave recorded a high attack rate (for instance, at the Central Jail in Batavia [Djakarta]), but mortality was generally low.

The second wave struck in October 1918 following a long, dry spell when respiratory ailments had rendered the populace vulnerable; it was more widespread and lethal. The eastern part of the Indonesian archipelago, spared by the first wave, was particularly hard hit. Provinces that had been attacked earlier, however, generally escaped the worst of this onslaught. In Java, where 1.8 percent of the Indonesians died, the eastern provinces were seriously affected. The islands of Sulawesi (Celebes), the Moluccas, and Timor registered high mortality. An observer in southeast Sulawesi reported widespread destruction; for instance, in a village of 900 residents, 177 died within a three-week period. The death toll on the island of Lombok was 36,000 people, representing almost six percent of the population.

As elsewhere in the world, the influenza epidemic was virulent and struck without warning. High fever, dry cough, severe headaches, backaches, and muscle pains were common symptoms. Frequently, complications such as pneumonia, malaria, hemorrhages of the nose and lungs, dysentery, and tuberculosis set in with great intensity.

In most places where a large number of people congregated, absenteeism was high and shops, offices, and schools had to be closed. A high proportion of children under 15 years of age were among those killed. Normal life, especially in the eastern islands, was seriously disrupted since there was a shortage of manpower to carry out many routine but necessary tasks. On the small island of Buton (Butung or Boetoeng), corpses were reportedly lying beside the roads, there being no one to bury them.

By late January 1919, the epidemic had almost faded—almost as quickly as it had struck. Its impact was, however, so substantial that it was soon incorporated into the local folklore. It also forced the enactment of an Influenza Ordinance in 1921, which required doctors to report any outbreak of influenza with a high death rate; then civil authorities could immediately introduce precautionary legislation regarding restrictions on public gatherings, school closures, and the establishment of temporary shelters that could provide free food and medicine and, if required, funerals. Violation of the ordinance meant a six-day prison term or a fine of up to 50 guilders. Since passengers on ships had transmitted the disease to the eastern Indonesian islands, strict controls were imposed on shipping through the affected areas. Violation resulted in a one-year prison term or a fine up to 10,000 guilders.

Further reading: Owen, ed., *Death and Disease in Southeast Asia.*

Indonesian Plague of 1910–14

See JAVANESE (INDONESIAN) PLAGUE OF 1910–14.

Indonesian Smallpox Epidemics of 1965–67

Series of major but scattered smallpox epidemics whose actual impact was grossly underreported in Indonesia.

In 1965, two different and widely separated areas of Indonesia reported a dramatic rise in smallpox incidence. During that year, the country reported 56,359 cases of smallpox. Of these, East Java alone contained 36,120 cases. In the same year, a smallpox epidemic was also reported from Central and South Kalimantan (Borneo). It may have begun well before 1965, but exact details are not available since reporting was inadequate. Mass vaccination campaigns had been conducted all over the country during the early 1960s. Perhaps in response to these, the epidemic in Kalimantan subsided gradually over the next two years. Another epidemic was reported from West Nusa Tenggara in 1966.

Then, in August 1967, Djakarta (Jakarta), the capital of Indonesia, reported an outbreak of the disease that quickly flared into an epidemic; by November, over 50 cases of smallpox were being reported each week. In 1967, Java alone reported more than 100,000 cases of smallpox. This figure, it is believed, represented only ten percent of the actual number of cases. Elsewhere in the country, the reporting was even more inadequate.

In 1968, Indonesia launched an ambitious smallpox eradication program and was the first of five Asian countries—where smallpox had been endemic—to declare itself free of the dreaded disease.

Further reading: Fenner et al., *Smallpox and Its Eradication.*

Indonesian Typhoid Epidemic of 1846–50

See JAVANESE (INDONESIAN) TYPHOID EPIDEMIC OF 1846–50.

Iranian (Persian) Typhus Epidemic of 1942–44

Extensive outbreaks of louse-borne typhus fever occurring in Iran (known as Persia until 1935) during military operations in World War II.

Typhus had been prevalent in Iran for many years; cases were reported mainly from the cities, but the data from the rest of the country was incomplete. Given Iran's strategic location and importance during the war, the authorities became alarmed when typhus erupted there on a large scale in 1942. It was apparently brought into the country by some 28,000 Polish refugees and soldiers who crossed over from typhus-ridden concentration camps in Russia. Malnourished and lacking adequate medical care, many of them developed typhus during a serious outbreak in their camp. This outbreak (1,102 cases) was reportedly brought under prompt control and did not lead to further outbreaks. This may have been because Iran had been designated as a testing ground for new delousing techniques and for further studies of the disease.

The epidemic in 1943–44 was more severe and widespread, registering 19,321 cases with an estimated mortality rate of 18 percent. Its virulence led some experts to suspect (wrongly, as it later turned out) that a new strain of *Rickettsia* was responsible. British Colonel Sachs of the Royal Army Medical Corps recorded over 25,000 cases of typhus with mortality ranging from 12 percent to 37 percent. He also reported 160 typhus cases (36 deaths) among the British and Indian troops fighting in Iran between January and July 1943. This forced the British Command there to vaccinate its troops against typhus.

The Iranian town of Andimeshk (population 8,000), near one of the American camps, reported about 1,000 cases of typhus during 1943. While these cases apparently spread rapidly among the growing civilian population in the area, the Americans recorded only ten typhus cases with no fatalities. They were well protected through the use of vaccination and delousing procedures, which were extended in 1944 to cover thousands of civilians. Between 1943 and 1946, the United States Typhus Commission (see JAPANESE-KOREAN TYPHUS EPIDEMIC OF 1945–46) worked tirelessly to educate the people of the Middle East regarding typhus prevention and supplied them with vaccines and insecticides. As a result, typhus outbreaks had declined in most of these countries by the end of this period.

Further reading: Moulton, ed., *The Rickettsial Diseases of Man.*

Iraqi Schistosomiasis Epidemics of c. 1910–30

Three outbreaks of schistosomiasis (bilharziasis) that occurred among foreign troops stationed in Iraq during and just after World War I (1914–18). The debilitating infection schistosomiasis (or "snail fever"), caused by certain separate species of blood flukes or parasitic worms called *Schistosoma*, seriously attacks the human gastrointestinal or urinary tract. The fluke eggs can live within certain freshwater snails (hosts). The organisms emerge from the snails as free-swimming larvae to enter another host (a human being who may be working or swimming in water); the larvae can penetrate the human skin and move to the internal organs via the bloodstream.

The first outbreak occurred among Indian troops based in Basra in southern Iraq during the war. The second and third outbreaks affected British troops at the towns of Minaidi and Al Kufa in 1921 and 1924. These two outbreaks were apparently caused by the *Bulinus truncatus*, a molluscan intermediate host inhabiting the water in which the troops bathed. All three outbreaks were responsible for creating an awareness of the disease and a desire to control its spread. Immediate steps were taken in this regard. For instance, canals were regularly dried out, the water supply was treated with cresol and copper sulphate, and its flow rate increased. Also, troops were urged to avoid any contact with untreated water.

In Iraq, the incidence of schistosomiasis had been particularly high in the central and southern parts of the country. During the first four months of 1928, 887 cases of schistosomiasis were reported; 62 percent from Basra province alone. The causative agent, *Schistosoma haemotobium,* had apparently been present in the basin of the Tigris and Euphrates rivers since ancient times. Children above ten years of age and workers exposed to water where infected snails abound were most susceptible to the disease. Its transmission in Iraq was seasonal, June to October being the period of highest incidence.

Recognizing the disease as a major health hazard, the government subsequently established a bilharziasis unit within the Department of Endemic Diseases to control its incidence. Special dispensaries and mobile units were also set up to diagnose and treat cases in areas of highest prevalence.

Further reading: Ansari, ed., *Epidemiology and Control of Schistosomiasis (Bilharziasis);* Simmons et al., *Global Epidemiology.*

Irish Pestilences of 1519–25

Series of epidemics that scourged many areas of Ireland almost continuously for a period of six years, probably beginning with an eruption of bubonic plague in Dublin in the autumn of 1519. After subsiding in the winter, the disease recrudesced in the spring, a seasonal pattern that suggests bubonic plague. During July it was found in many places throughout the English Pale (the large area of English occupation on the east coast of Ireland).

The following summer the English Earl of Surrey wrote from Ireland to Cardinal Thomas Wolsey in London that "there is a marvellous death in all this country, which is so sore that all the people be fled out of their houses into the fields and woods, where they likewise die wonderfully; so that their bodies be dead like swine unburied." This indicates a probable epidemic of typhus fever, which is transmitted by the human body louse. The plague-infected, house-dwelling rat would remain behind in a town as its inhabitants fled, so bubonic plague is almost certainly not the pestilence the Earl of Surrey witnessed in the summer of 1521.

It is probable that smallpox and influenza, in addition to bubonic plague and typhus fever, comprised the mix of diseases that continued to invade Dublin, Limerick, Munster, and other places in Ireland through 1525.

Further reading: Creighton, *A History of Epidemics in Britain*; Shrewsbury, *A History of Bubonic Plague in the British Isles.*

Irish Pestilences of 1535–36

English chronicles report "a raging pestilence" in Ireland for the year 1535, in the Pale, the area around Dublin occupied by the English, and in other parts of the country as well, particularly in Cork. As the term "plague" was used at that time to designate a number of distinct diseases, the epidemic of 1535 remains unidentified, although bubonic plague may certainly have been the disease in question. Smallpox is specifically mentioned as one of the epidemics scourging Ireland that year. The following year was evidently equally disastrous for Ireland, when "a general plague, galar breac, the flux, and fever" continued to afflict the population. The general plague may have been bubonic plague accompanied by the effect of famine; galar breac is an Irish name for smallpox, and the flux is dysentery. The fever referred to may have been typhus or relapsing fever. Because bubonic plague and dysentery are mainly warm-weather diseases and typhus is most prevalent in winter, Ireland during these years was apparently subjected to one wave of sickness after another with no seasonal intermission.

King Henry VIII of England was advised during this time that few men would be forthcoming from Ireland to staff his army because so many men had died "in consequence of plague."

Further reading: Creighton, *A History of Epidemics in Britain*; Shrewsbury, *A History of Bubonic Plague in the British Isles.*

Irish Plague of 1348–50

See PLAGUE OF IRELAND, GREAT.

Irish Plague of 1574–76

Epidemic of bubonic plague that erupted in Dublin in the summer of 1574 and spread to many parts of eastern and southern Ireland during the next two years. Subsiding with the onset of cold weather, the plague reappeared in the spring of 1575 and continued through the summer, probably along with an outbreak of dysentery caused by extreme heat and drought that lasted till the end of August. By June so many wealthy citizens and city officials had fled Dublin to escape infection that the townspeople ordered that they either return themselves or send a deputy to discharge their civic obligations—or else face permanent loss of citizenship.

Concealing family plague victims was common, and city authorities regularly issued strictly enforced orders with stiff penalties to prohibit such concealment because it was believed that isolation of the plague-sick was necessary to prevent contagion. This belief was erroneous because bubonic plague is spread only through the bite of a plague-carrying or "blocked" rat-flea. Temporary housing for infected persons, to segregate them from healthy citizens, was provided by the city.

A physician was appointed and recompensed to tend "the Maire and every other that shalbe in danger or neede of phisicke or surgrye." This was the first such appointment made in Ireland and represented a step forward in the public provision of health care for the underprivileged.

The last quarter of the sixteenth century was apparently free from any major occurrence of bubonic plague or any other epidemic disease in Ireland.

As in England and Scotland, the busy ports along the eastern coast of Ireland, as well as inland river ports, were most susceptible to plague, as it was introduced from abroad by ships carrying plague-infected rats, which would quickly infest the houses of the town wherever the ships landed. Plague might be imported from England or from the many ports of continental Europe.

Further reading: Creighton, *A History of Epidemics in Britain*; Shrewsbury, *A History of Bubonic Plague in the British Isles.*

Irish Plague of 1604–05

Visitation of bubonic plague in Ireland—part of a long and widespread epidemic that afflicted the British Isles from about 1600 to 1610 (its most violent period spanning the years 1603 to 1608). Dublin was suffering by the early spring of 1604, and was quickly abandoned by its well-to-do citizens, who could afford the expense of fleeing to uninfected locations. As in prior epidemics, the remaining townsfolk threatened disenfranchisement to those who had fled. Records indicating mortality do not exist, but the many ordinances issued by Dublin's officials to deal with the epidemic suggest its extent. The sick were segregated in a pesthouse built outside the city, and men were appointed to supervise its inmates and bury the dead. Proof was demanded of travelers that they were coming to Dublin from a plague-free location, to ensure that further infection was kept out of the city.

The pain suffered by plague-victims, especially during suppuration of the buboes located in the groin, armpits, and neck, sometimes caused them to run from their houses in a state of delirium; this prompted the directive to the plague officials to "stop the infected from running abrode" through the streets of Dublin. The mayor ordered citizens to light fires before their doors three nights a week "for better purgeing of the aire" (see LONDON PLAGUE OF 1578).

After subsiding in the winter months, plague reappeared in Dublin in the spring of 1605 and apparently continued throughout the summer and fall of that year. Ireland did not experience another visitation of plague until 1650.

Further reading: Creighton, *A History of Epidemics in Britain*; Shrewsbury, *A History of Bubonic Plague in the British Isles*.

Irish Plague of 1650–51   Bubonic plague appeared in Ireland in the spring of 1650 for the first time since the outbreak of 1604, possibly introduced to the island by a Spanish ship landing at the western port of Galway, from which the disease spread eastward to Dublin. This epidemic, which evidently lasted for two plague seasons (the spring, summer, and fall of 1650 and 1651), was the final visitation of plague in Ireland.

The sick were isolated in a pesthouse outside the city of Dublin, and the plague victims were cared for at the city's expense. A surgeon (whose family succumbed to plague) was appointed by the town assembly, which also complained of "the absence of the able inhabitants of this cittie," who had apparently fled Dublin to escape infection, as they customarily did whenever the plague struck.

The death toll for this outbreak cannot be calculated because of lack of historic records, but its severity is revealed in a document of June 1651 that mentions "the heavie plague whereby this cittie is exceedingly depopulated."

No sooner did the plague subside than Ireland experienced a disastrous famine that caused high mortality during the next few years. Ireland's population, especially the poor, continued to suffer, not only from starvation but also from diseases, such as dysentery, that normally accompanied periods of dearth.

Further reading: Byrne et al., eds., *A New History of Ireland*; Creighton, *A History of Epidemics in Britain*; Shrewsbury, *A History of Bubonic Plague in the British Isles*.

Irish Typhus and Dysentery Epidemic of 1740–41
Epidemic of typhus fever and dysentery that accompanied the most terrible famine Ireland experienced in the eighteenth century. The misery of the poor was recorded by many contemporary observers, whose writings document the prevalence of both diseases during this time. One witness writes that "Multitudes have perished, and are daily perishing, under hedges and ditches, some by fevers, some by fluxes [dysentery], and some through downright cruel want in the utmost agonies of despair."

The early and exceptionally cold winter of 1739–40 caused the destruction of the potato harvest of the fall of 1739 and ruined the following spring planting. Typhus fever flared quickly among the large numbers of poor who wandered about in search of food, unknowingly spreading the disease through its vector, the human body louse, the constant companion of these unwashed, destitute people.

Many fever victims were left unattended as physicians refused to visit patients for fear of infection. The Irish philosopher Bishop George Berkeley wrote about the calamity, and graciously distributed money, food, and medicine to the poor who appeared at his house, near Cork, each week.

Dysentery became widespread in Ireland during the hot and dry summer of 1740 and continued throughout the year, intensifying again during the drought conditions of the following spring.

Little or no public resources were available to meet crises such as this in eighteenth-century Ireland, and private charity could help only a relative few. Large-scale emigration, which provided an escape route for hundreds of thousands of people during the great famine of 1846–49, was not a possibility in the 1740s.

The most reliable estimate of human deaths resulting from famine and disease during this period, based on the observations of a physician working in the county of Munster, is 80,000 for all of Ireland, out of a population of less than two million.

Famine conditions and epidemic illness declined in the later months of 1741. Typhus fever and dysentery continued to appear sporadically throughout the remainder of the eighteenth century, although they did not reach epidemic proportions again for another 80 years (see IRISH TYPHUS AND DYSENTERY EPIDEMIC OF 1817–18).

This epidemic in Ireland coincided with a similar outbreak of typhus fever in England and Scotland (see LONDON TYPHUS EPIDEMIC OF 1741–42).

Further reading: Creighton, *A History of Epidemics in Britain*; Foster, *Modern Ireland, 1600–1972*.

Irish Typhus and Dysentery Epidemic of 1817–18
Outbreak of epidemic typhus fever that affected an

estimated 700,000 to 1,500,000 people throughout Ireland in a population of about six million. Dysentery also struck many of them at the same time.

This epidemic, following the typical pattern of typhus fever, occurred as a result of a ruined harvest in 1816, which caused families all over Ireland to abandon their homes and wander through the countryside and into towns and cities in search of food. Large numbers of vagrants, carrying about the human body-louse, which transmits the disease, thus spread the infection through their contact with others in crowded and dirty workhouses, lodging places, soup lines, and hospitals. This large-scale vagrancy was made worse by the usual yearly migration of harvest workers. Special "fever huts" were constructed along the roads to accommodate field laborers sick with typhus. It was observed by many contemporaries that the warm hospitality the Irish normally showed to paupers was denied them during the epidemic, due to fear of infection, and that ordinary feelings of concern for the suffering were often lacking, even within families, so acute was the distress, particularly among the poor.

Contemporary reports tell of incredibly dirty and lice-ridden people huddling together in their cabins, or admitted as fever-patients to hospitals. Near the end of 1818, as food-supply problems eased and people could sustain their families at home and by doing so avoid spreading their lice far and wide, the incidence of typhus fever declined.

Curiously, although the number of cases during this epidemic was extremely high, mortality was uncommonly low, perhaps at approximately 65,000 human deaths. It was reported, however, that the case-mortality rate among the more privileged classes was quite high, around 25 percent to 35 percent.

Dysentery, an enteric disease usually prevalent in times of food scarcity, caused an estimated 45,000 deaths.

Like most other significant outbreaks of epidemic typhus fever in the British Isles, Ireland's experience during these years was shared by England and Scotland, although in this instance on a less dramatic scale (see ENGLISH TYPHUS EPIDEMIC OF 1816–19).

Further reading: Creighton, *A History of Epidemics in Britain*; Zinsser, *Rats, Lice and History*.

Irish Typhus and Dysentery Epidemic of 1846–50

Devastating epidemic of louse-borne typhus fever and dysentery that accompanied the worst period of destitution in Ireland's history, the Great Famine of 1846–49. A partial harvest in 1845 followed by a completely ruined crop in 1846, another partial harvest in 1847 and yet another totally blighted crop in 1848 left hundreds of thousands of Irish laborers, small tenant-farmers *(cottiers)*, and others with literally no means of subsistence. Their weakened constitutions and disrupted lives made them particularly susceptible to illness.

Typhus fever flared all over Ireland, reaching epidemic proportions by the spring of 1847. As countless families abandoned their homes to wander the roads in search of food, the human body-louse, which the poor of Ireland commonly hosted and which transmits typhus fever, was spread far and wide. More than 200 special fever hospitals accommodated 450,000 patients in the four years 1846–50; at least 47,300 died.

According to 1851 census figures, more than 2,680,500 destitute people flowed into Ireland's dirty and overcrowded workhouses, where at least 223,500 died. Typhus fever and dysentery accounted for many if not most of these deaths. Relapsing fever, a common "famine fever" that weakens the body but is rarely fatal, afflicted many thousands as well. Even the public works projects the government set in motion to provide employment were places where infection could easily spread, as large numbers of unwashed, lice-ridden people worked and slept together.

Private charities and public assistance provided food and medical services for some, but the social mechanisms necessary to meet such a large-scale calamity were not in place or even thought to be the responsibility of government. Thousands of people were simply left to starve or die of disease. Many contemporaries wrote heartbreaking accounts of the suffering they witnessed. A magistrate visiting western Cork recorded his encounter there with "famished and ghastly skeletons . . . such frightful spectres as no words can describe, either from famine or from fever." This harrowing picture was unfortunately a common sight throughout Ireland. Traditional burial rites were often ignored because people feared contagion from corpses, and it was not unusual for bodies to lie for days in deserted cabins. Burial pits, into which 30 or more bodies were placed, were not uncommon in Ireland during these years.

Census figures for 1847–50 record nearly 166,000 human deaths from fever and over 100,000 from dysentery and diarrhea. These numbers are low because many deaths were not officially recorded. Estimates of mortality for the entire famine period range from 800,000 to 1,100,000 (including deaths that would normally have occurred in the course of each year). Emigration, mostly to the United States but also to England and Scotland, provided an escape from Ireland for about one million people. Irish emigrants fleeing to England brought typhus, or "Irish fever" with them, contributing to the epidemic afflicting that country in the same years (see ENGLISH TYPHUS EPIDEMIC OF 1847–48).

The epidemic of 1846–50 was the last major outbreak of typhus fever in Ireland.

Further reading: Creighton, *A History of Epidemics in Britain;* Boyce, *Modern Ireland: The Search for Stability;* Hoppen, *Ireland since 1800: Conflict and Conformity.*

Irish Typhus Epidemics of 1708–10, 1718–20, and 1728–30

Three severe outbreaks of epidemic typhus fever in Ireland, each lasting about three years and appearing at rough intervals of eight years. Each period of abnormally high deaths from fever followed poor harvests and corresponded to similar outbreaks of typhus fever in England (see LONDON TYPHUS EPIDEMICS OF 1709–20; LONDON TYPHUS EPIDEMIC OF 1726–29). A physician who attended well-to-do families in the city of Cork, Ireland, during these two decades documented the clinical aspects of the disease that afflicted most of his patients. These valuable medical writings provide evidence that the prevailing illness was typhus fever.

Epidemic typhus fever is a louse-borne disease, and thus is especially likely to occur during times of social dislocation such as war, high unemployment, and famine. Large numbers of people leave their homes in search of safety or food and spread lice through their continual movement and contact with portions of the population they would not ordinarily meet. The bad harvests Ireland experienced during this period, especially in 1726, 1727, and 1728, and the resultant spreading of infection caused by families wandering from place to place, ensured that typhus fever would become rampant throughout Ireland. Moreover, dysentery, a perennial famine-disease, was also quite widespread during these years, especially in the typhus epidemic of 1728–30.

The great Dublin-born English satirist Jonathan Swift wrote his infamous *Modest Proposal for preventing the Children of Poor People in Ireland from being a Burden to their Parents or Country* during these famine years; he memorably describes the appalling conditions of poverty and disease in which the destitute of Dublin lived.

Further reading: Creighton, *A History of Epidemics in Britain;* Zinsser, *Rats, Lice and History.*

Irish Typhus Epidemic of 1836–40

Four-year visitation of typhus fever that reached epidemic numbers in many areas of Ireland, especially in counties in the north and west. The worst years were 1837 and 1840. As is usual for typhus fever, fatalities were proportionately highest among people over the age of 40.

Unlike many other serious outbreaks of typhus fever in Ireland, the epidemic of 1836–40 was not precipitated by crop failures or economic stagnation. These conditions usually caused extensive social dislocation and thus accelerated the spread of infection, as vagrants transferred their body-lice, which carry the disease, to people with whom they came into contact in their wanderings in Ireland. Outbreaks of typhus fever, however, were not dependent upon, but merely worsened by, acute economic and farming calamities. Fundamentally a disease of the poor, whose unclean and crowded living conditions encouraged the spread of lice, typhus fever was almost continuously present in Ireland, if not always in epidemic proportions, until the latter nineteenth century.

Other parts of the British Isles experienced major epidemics of typhus fever during these years as well (see SCOTTISH TYPHUS EPIDEMIC OF 1836–40).

Further reading: Creighton, *A History of Epidemics in Britain;* Foster, *Modern Ireland, 1600–1972.*

Iroquois Indian Smallpox Epidemic of 1662

Outbreak of smallpox that killed more than a thousand Indian members of the Iroquois confederacy known as the Five Nations (made up of the Cayuga, Mohawk, Oneida, Onondaga, and Seneca Indians inhabiting New York state). The well-organized Iroquois Confederacy or League was markedly struck by infectious diseases after 1609, the year Henry Hudson sailed up the river later named for him, as far as present-day Albany. With the procurement of European trade goods, the Indians suffered more bouts of epidemic illness, and the Iroquois Confederacy's population fell from about 20,000 (prior to 1630) to no more than 10,000 by 1662.

The source of the 1662 smallpox epidemic among the Iroquois is not certain. However, the year before, a small band of Susquehannocks, neighbors of the Onondagas in central New York, was apparently decimated by the disease, which they may have spread to the Onondaga nation through trade. Nonetheless, any Indian in the Five Nations could have been infected from smallpox-carrying Canadian Indians in the north or Lenni-Lenape (Delaware) Indians in the south.

The Iroquois lived in crowded dwellings housing three or four generations and had no concept of sanitation or quarantine. They traditionally visited sick relatives and friends—a custom detrimental to the healthy Indians, because the infection is normally transmitted by close contact with patients through respiratory discharges or by contaminated articles. The sick Indians complained of high fever, aching limbs, and a burning rash of pustules that covered most of their bodies. Many of those who survived were left blind, while nearly all who became infected were disfigured (notably pockmarked). Smallpox was especially fatal to the children and the elderly, many of whom died from dehydration. The large number of deaths among the elderly men deprived the confederacy of its most experienced leadership in politics and ritual information.

Further reading: Dobyns, *Their Number Becomes Thinned: Native American Dynamics in Eastern America;* Trigger, *Handbook of North American Indians, Northeast.*

Israeli Diphtheria Epidemics of 1950–51

Two outbreaks of diphtheria in Israel, following a massive influx of immigrants in 1948 (when the state of Israel was proclaimed).

Diphtheria, long endemic in the former state of Palestine, received little official attention because it was not regarded as an important disease. In 1950, the recorded incidence was more than 1,660 cases—a 25 percent increase over the previous year. Nearly 50 percent of these occurred in non-urban localities, particularly in the camps and settlements where the new immigrants were housed. Eight percent of the cases were reported from Haifa, nine percent from Jerusalem, and 34 percent from the Tel Aviv-Jaffa area. The incidence rate was estimated at 148 per 100,000 people, the case fatality rate at 0.6 percent.

Diphtheria, an acute bacterial disease, primarily infects the tonsils, pharynx, larynx, nose and occasionally other mucous membranes, the skin, and the conjunctiva or the genitalia. It spreads from person to person mainly by direct contact but sometimes also through infected articles and raw milk. There are various types of diphtheria, but the characteristic feature is patches of inflamed grayish lesions caused by the release of a certain cytotoxin. Its incubation period is two to five days; it is highly contagious for about two weeks and generally affects children or adults who have not been immunized.

Immunization against diphtheria, while not mandatory then, was a routine procedure in most Israeli camps and child welfare centers. During 1950, however, diphtheria immunization was withdrawn because the authorities feared that it might aggravate an ongoing poliomyelitis epidemic, which is believed to have helped trigger the diphtheria outbreaks of 1951.

During September–December 1951, diphtheria again became epidemic in Israel. There was a sharp and sudden rise in the reported diphtheria cases in the last four months of the year. A total of 2,445 cases of diphtheria, a case rate of 190 per 100,000 people, reportedly occurred in 1951. Israel's Ministry of Health responded by launching a mass immunization campaign in 1952, intended to immunize every child under 12 years of age. See also ISRAELI POLIOMYELITIS EPIDEMICS OF 1950–52.

Further reading: Simmons et al., eds., *Global Epidemiology;* Benenson, ed., *Control of Communicable Diseases in Man.*

Israeli Leptospirosis Epidemic of 1949–50

Apparently the first recorded human outbreak of leptospirosis.

The term leptospirosis refers to a group of zoonoses (diseases communicable from animals to man) caused by spirochete bacteria of the genus *Leptospira.* The bacteria are transmitted to man through the urine or tissues of infected animals, such as dogs, livestock, rodents, and wild animals, which are the reservoirs or carriers of the disease. It is thus an occupational hazard for those persons (mainly males) whose work brings them into contact with the infected matter of such animals, as well as for those who enjoy outdoor activities. The symptoms of this group of diseases are varied and vast, often complicating the diagnosis.

The outbreak in Israel began when cases of leptospirosis were observed among the human population in some of the agricultural districts of the Sharon plain. Although only 448 cases were reported between June 1949 and April 1950, the actual incidence is believed to have exceeded 1,000 cases. Mortality (usually due to complications) was estimated at one percent to two percent. The highest incidence occurred in the Beth Itzhak area (34 per 1,000 people). Incidence in the adjoining agricultural areas was eight per 1,000 persons, while in Nathanya and the surrounding immigrant camps it was only one per 1,000 people. The vegetable farmers suffered the highest attack rates. The outbreak, it was found, was caused by the *Leptospira geffeni* through its chief rodent reservoir, a vole, *Microtus guentheri.*

The Israeli authorities took immediate steps to destroy rodent populations. Only sporadic cases occurred in 1951. Subsequently, men in potentially hazardous occupations were immunized against certain prevalent strains of the bacteria. Leptospirosis is also known as Weil's disease, canicola fever, infectious jaundice, hemorrhagic jaundice, mud fever, pea picker's disease, swineherd's disease, and the Stuttgart disease.

Further reading: Simmons et al., eds., *Global Epidemiology;* Benenson, ed., *Control of Communicable Diseases in Man.*

Israeli Poliomyelitis Epidemics of 1950–52

Epidemics of poliomyelitis (infantile paralysis) that struck Israel for three consecutive years.

Until 1950, poliomyelitis (or polio) had been known to occur only sporadically in Israel. However, late in 1949, the monthly incidence of poliomyelitis began to show an increase and in 1950 developed into an intense epidemic. Forty percent of the 1,604 cases reported in 1950 occurred in May and June. During July and August, nearly 250 cases were reported every month. Initially, most of the cases were observed in the larger towns, but the epidemic subsequently spread all over the country. Overall, four percent of the cases were reported from Jerusalem, 24 percent from the Tel Aviv-Jaffa area, and 11 percent from Haifa. Only one percent of the polio cases involved the Arab community in Israel. Thirty percent of the cases occurred in children below one year old, 55 percent in children below two years of age, and 93 percent in children under five years of age.

The 1950 epidemic was quite intense as evidenced by the large number of paralytic cases (see BANGKOK POLIOMYELITIS EPIDEMIC OF 1952). It claimed 154 human lives, a case fatality rate of 9.6 percent.

Polio struck again in 1951. This time there were 919 reported cases and 127 deaths. The case fatality rate was considerably higher at 13.8 percent. The following year, polio incidence declined slightly—851 reported cases—but the mortality rate was still high, with 116 registered deaths.

In January 1956, Israel's Ministry of Health established a special laboratory for the manufacture of the polio vaccine. Mass vaccination got underway early in 1957.

Further reading: World Health Organization, *Poliomyelitis*; Simmons et al., eds., *Global Epidemiology*.

Israeli West Nile Fever Epidemics of the 1950s

Series of outbreaks of West Nile fever.

The clinical course of the disease was marked by fever, rash (pronounced in young children), severe headache, pain behind the eyeballs, back pain, anorexia, vomiting, and abdominal pain. Occasionally, enlargement of the lymph nodes, angina, and diarrhea were present. In the early days when the disease was not adequately understood, it was apt to be diagnosed as a mild, dengue-like illness.

Israel's first recorded outbreak of West Nile fever occurred in 1941, but the etiology of the disease was not understood until the 1950s, when the virus was isolated and identified as a group B mosquito-borne togavirus of the arbovirus family. All the outbreaks discussed here occurred in two main areas—one 40 miles north of Tel Aviv and the other about 15 miles southeast of the city. They were brief (no more than eight weeks long), explosive, and seasonal (occurring between July and October).

In 1950, a large outbreak occurred at a military camp near Pardes Hannah, north of Tel Aviv. The first two cases were discovered in mid-July. Over the next month, the incidence escalated into an epidemic. During its most intense period (three weeks), about 500 people were hospitalized. In the following two weeks, 120 more cases were observed. Then the outbreak tapered off and no new cases were reported after the third week of September. Of the approximately 1,000 people at the camp, 636 were treated for the disease.

West Nile fever became epidemic again during the summer of 1951, the target this time being the kibbutz of Maayan Zvi, south of Haifa. Milder than the previous epidemic, it had two peaks, the first at the end of July, the second in mid-September. Of the 303 people at the kibbutz, 123 of them (41 percent) were affected; all the infants below two years of age were infected. Morbidity among the other age-groups was as follows: 81 percent in the 3–5-year-olds, 34 percent in the 6–11-year-olds (a group away from the kibbutz at that time), 56 percent in the 12–16-year-olds, and 21 percent among adults (mainly 20–35-year-olds). It was during this epidemic that the causative virus was isolated from the blood of an infected child.

Late in the summer of 1952, another more dispersed outbreak of West Nile fever was reported from various communities along the Israeli coast. Several hundred people were estimated to have been infected during outbreaks at the Pardes Hannah camp (50 cases in two weeks), Givat Brenner kibbutz (30 cases late in August), and in many coastal communities during September.

A severe epidemic centered around the Hadera and the Ramlah-Lydda areas broke out during August–September 1953. Over its brief, five-week spell, it infected over 200 people in both these areas and 42 others elsewhere in the country. A detailed study of 70 patients undertaken at the Tel Hashomer Government Hospital during this epidemic yielded important information about the disease.

A smaller outbreak, also involving communities in the north and south of the country, was recorded in 1954. Approximately 100 cases are estimated to have occurred. The next two years (1955 and 1956) were non-epidemic. However, another severe outbreak occurred in 1957 when more than 200 cases were reported from the northern part of Israel.

In neighboring Egypt, West Nile infection was primarily a childhood disease and adults seemed basically immune to it. In Israel, both children and adults were prone to attack, perhaps because the virus, barring the outbreak of 1941, was relatively new to the country.

Further reading: Klingberg et al., "Certain Aspects of the Epidemiology and Distribution of Immunity of West Nile Virus in Israel"; Bernkopf et al., "Isolation of West Nile Virus in Israel."

Italian Cholera Epidemic of 1866–67

Devastating outburst of Asiatic cholera, an acute bacterial, intestinal disease characterized by its sudden onset, that killed about 130,000 inhabitants of Italy in 1867. It was part of the Asiatic Cholera Pandemic of 1865–75 (q.v.) then sweeping through Europe and other continents.

Spread by human carriers, by infected feces, food, or water, and by flies, cholera was conveyed to Italy mainly by ships. Also, the movement of troops during the Seven Weeks' War (Austro-Prussian War) in the summer of 1866, as well as pilgrimages and fairs, helped spread the disease. The historic town of Acqui in Piedmont, northwest Italy, first reported cholera's outbreak in mid-September 1865. The communicable disease was soon recorded in Trento and other northern towns, particularly in seaports like Trieste on the Adriatic. In southern Italy, the disease was noticed during this time in San Giovanni Rotondo and nearby Naples on the Mediterranean. The epidemic gradually spread throughout the Italian peninsula in 1866–67, causing much morbidity and death.

Numerous Italian physicians had been aware of potential methods of cholera control (like cleaning up their communities) since 1849, when British scientist John Snow discovered that the disease was spread by infected water and that epidemic control could be achieved by stopping the distribution of infected water. During the cholera pandemic in Europe (1866–67), international medical conferences were held in various leading cities, including Venice, and concluded that cholera in Europe since 1830 had been transmitted by unusual activity of the disease in the Indian subcontinent. In addition, during this period, many European scientists abandoned the anti-contagionist theory concerning cholera. Dr. Snow and others held that specific contagia (like living organisms) were the causes of infectious epidemic diseases; some others held the miasmatic theory stating that epidemics were the result of atmospheric conditions (including poor sanitary conditions); and still others held to a compromise (a limited contagionism), saying that contagia operated in conjunction with atmospheric and social conditions. See also BRITISH CHOLERA EPIDEMICS OF 1848–49 AND 1853–54; BRITISH CHOLERA EPIDEMIC OF 1865–66; U.S. CHOLERA EPIDEMIC OF 1866.

Further reading: De, *Cholera: Its Pathology and Pathogenesis*; Siegfried, *Routes of Contagion*.

Italian Cholera Epidemic of 1884–85   Devastating outbreak of cholera, killing approximately half of the estimated 100,000 persons who contracted this acute, infectious intestinal disease, principally characterized by diarrhea, cramps, and dehydration and spread by polluted water and food. In the early 1880s, Italian physicians and sanitarians had little definite knowledge of cholera, and their views were sometimes shaded by commercial and political interests. During the Italian Cholera Epidemic of 1866–67 (q.v.), scientists had examined the possibility that water supplies for drinking and cooking could become cholera contaminated; however, they had not considered food as another transmitter of the disease. Prevention measures and sanitation control in Italy were inadequate then.

In the summer of 1884, during the early part of the Asiatic Cholera Pandemic of 1881–96 (q.v.), the disease evidently entered a number of small Italian ports aboard contaminated trading ships from Alexandria, Egypt. The contamination infected raw mussels, which were unwittingly sold in large amounts by Italian street vendors. Thousands of people in coastal and inland towns and cities, including Genoa, Naples, Rome, and Venice, became infected; the city of Turin in the Po River valley, La Spezia in Liguria, and towns along the Adriatic coast were notably attacked during the epidemic, during which the overall mortality rate was at least 50 percent. Without modern rehydration therapies, coma and death often resulted on the day of infection.

After German bacteriologist Robert Koch's discovery of the comma bacillus as the cause of Asiatic cholera (1883), an international conference on cholera (held in Venice in 1885) concluded that the outbreaks in Europe (see SPANISH CHOLERA EPIDEMIC OF 1884–85) had originated in India, arriving on the continent via Egypt or North Africa. Italian scientists then studied cholera in depth, which resulted in extensive improvements in water purification systems, sewage disposal, and public health. Consequently, Italy experienced only small outbreaks of imported cases and aboard ships in various ports afterward.

Further reading: Chambers, *The Conquest of Cholera*; Siegfried, *Routes of Contagion*.

Italian Diphtheria Epidemic of 1618   Major outbreak of diphtheria that killed at least 8,000 persons in Naples and many more in other parts of southern Italy.

In June 1618 "male in canna" (what Italians then called diphtheria, caused by a bacterium that primarily infects the throat) was introduced into southern Italy via Spain (people may be carriers without suffering from the illness themselves). The first diphtheria cases occurred among the children in the village of Chiaia near Naples. At the time Italian physicians observed that the pharynx of those infected became reddish and inflamed and, in some cases, glands and tonsils became swollen; also, patients experienced difficulty in swallowing and breathing, and sometimes a shiny mucus (pituita) erupted from a patient's head. Suffocation resulted at times. Death usually occurred on the fourth day of infection, but sometimes sooner, according to some accounts. Because the deadly disease affected more than one member of a household, Italian doctors rightly considered it contagious (diphtheria is transmitted mainly via human discharges from the nose and throat).

From Chiaia, the infection spread to Naples, where it claimed some 8,000 human lives, most of them children. The disease then moved from Naples to the city of Messina in Sicily, where doctors observed some kind of white matter (which turned blue and then black) on the surface of the throats of infected patients; many of these patients perished as a result of attempts made to remove these "false" membranes by means of an instrument or a finger. The epidemic also spread in 1618 to Palermo, Sicily, whose inhabitants named the disease "morbus gulie" (or gullet disease).

During the 1618 epidemic, Italian physicians maintained records about the disease and fairly accurate observations about its effect on victims. Their "findings" were published between 1620 and 1632. During the 20 years following the 1618 epidemic, serious diphtheria outbreaks struck the Italian peninsula at least five times; Naples was once again severely infected in 1642.

Further reading: Andrews et al., *Diphtheria;* Styler, *Plague Fighters.*

Italian Influenza Epidemic of 1580

Outbreak of influenza that evidently left a high human death toll on the Italian peninsula. This acute infectious viral disease of the respiratory tract spread from Asia Minor (Turkey) to the islands of Malta and Sicily and to North Africa during the summer of 1580.

The Italian city of Naples was severely attacked by influenza by August, at which time it moved northward to Rome, Florence, Genoa, Milan, and Venice. King Philip II of Spain, who also ruled over southern Italy and several North African ports, had generated extensive commerce and political ties among numerous Mediterranean and Italian regions. Thus trade had facilitated the diffusion of influenza, which is transmitted by direct human contact and newly soiled articles (carrying the infection) or through airborne droplets (particularly among crowded populations). Because of Spain's great and widespread power in Europe at this time, some authorities have said that the 1580 influenza deserved to be called the "Spanish flu," maybe even more so than the worldwide Spanish Influenza Epidemic of 1917–19 (q.v.). Muslim pirates from Asia Minor and other parts of the eastern Mediterranean also helped spread the disease through their raids on southern and central Italian coastal towns. By September 1580 the inhabitants of the Lombard towns in northern

Italy were infected, as were many in the Piedmont region to the west, bordering southern France (which was also affected by the flu).

The northward spread of influenza was more lethal to Italy in 1580, in the pre-antibiotic period, especially among the very young and the elderly (as is the usual case with flu epidemics). Later, influenza generally spread from east to west across Europe, and Italy was attacked later in the outbreak, from northern regions. In addition, the Pyrenees and Alps acted as partial barriers to the spread of severe epidemics into Italy. See also VENICE PLAGUE OF 1575–77.

Further reading: Patterson, *Pandemic Influenza, 1700–1900;* Pyle, *The Diffusion of Influenza.*

Italian Meningitis Epidemics of 1839–45

Outbreaks of cerebrospinal meningitis (CSM) that killed untold thousands of persons. This acute bacterial disease, which came to be called "Tito Apoplettico" by Italians, tends to afflict children and adolescents more often than adults, but a remarkably large proportion of the cases in Italy in 1839–45 were among adults in early to mid-life.

Italy first recorded CSM in the period 1805–15, when the disease was prevalent worldwide, occurring in military garrisons as well as in rural and crowded urban areas. During another worldwide CSM outbreak (1837–50), Italy first recorded cases in the Adriatic seaport of Ancona in 1839. French infantry and artillery troops had been stationed in Ancona since 1832 and had been constantly replaced or reinforced by new recruits from France, where CSM had been active since 1837. CSM infection is by the respiratory route; pathogenic bacteria inhabit the mucous membranes of the nose and throat and are commonly transmitted in droplets by sneezing or coughing. The introduction of CSM carriers from France enabled the "wasting" disease to establish itself in Ancona, from where it moved both north and south along the Adriatic coast, infecting the ports of Senigállia, Fano, Pésaro, San Benedetto, and Pescara.

During the winter of 1840, the inhabitants of Naples and the region of Calabria in southern Italy were seriously infected and suffered the brunt of the CSM epidemic until 1845. Inhabitants of Sicily also contracted CSM in the winter of 1840 and endured epidemics again during the warmer months of 1843 and 1844. (In 1840 Italians infected at Senigállia carried CSM to the Greek island of Corfu [Kerkira], and afflicted French troops carried it to Algiers in North Africa.) During the epidemics in Italy—an era before the use of sulfa drugs and antibiotics—medical measures taken against CSM did little or nothing to reduce the toll in suffering and death; in some places, 80 percent of those infected perished. Southern Italy again suffered CSM epidemics between 1874 and 1876.

Further reading: Foster and Gaskell, *Cerebro-Spinal Fever;* MacNalty, *Epidemic Diseases of the Central Nervous System;* Hirsch, *Handbook on Geographical and Historical Pathology.*

Italian Plagues of 1477–79   Devastating outbreaks of mainly bubonic plague that claimed the lives of more than 40,000 persons (perhaps more) in parts of northern Italy from 1477 to 1479. There was a severe famine in Italy during this period, so that many of the plague cases may have been misdiagnosed and may actually have been typhus fever, according to recent conclusions of some historians. Nevertheless, many plague infections displayed buboes (inflammatory swellings of glands in the groin or armpit) and other common plague symptoms. The estimated 80,000 human fatalities attributed to the epidemic appears too high, but more than half that number, at least, seem to have expired from plague.

The Italian city of Milan (capital of Lombardy) was attacked by the contagious, bacterial disease in the spring of 1477, and more than 22,000 inhabitants had perished from it by year's end. The commensal black rat, which lived in proximity with the inhabitants, was the rodent host of the disease, which was generally passed to humans by the bite of an infective rat flea. At the time, an Italian diarist from Parma described some Milanese citizens so feverishly delirious with plague as being suicidal (they threw themselves out of windows); entire families were wiped out.

The Lombard city of Brescia was also struck by plague in 1477 and lost more than 200 people each day during the epidemic's first four months. An Italian chronicler in Brescia reported that many priests and friars, fearful of the lethal disease, refused to aid the sick and instead encouraged processions that only helped to spread the plague bacillus *(Yersinia pestis).* Physicians in the lazaretto (hospital for the treatment of plague) were unable to cope with the overwhelming number of patients; the mortality rate was as high as 90 percent in the untreated bubonic cases, and almost all with the pneumonic form of plague died, some within hours of contracting it from a highly contagious bubonic patient. Most of the physicians succumbed to the disease themselves. Piles of dead bodies awaiting burial were set upon by roaming dogs, and gravediggers were accused of robbing and even sexually molesting corpses. In Brescia, where plague was called "mal del zucho," total disease fatalities rose to about 34,000 by the end of 1477 (however, many of these were likely attributable to typhus). In Milan, the plague (and typhus) lingered epidemically but much less fatally until 1479.

Plague also reached the large seaport of Venice in northeast Italy, where it affected mainly the poor and killed about 30,000 people in 1477–78. From Venice, the pestilence was transmitted to the Croatian region of Dalmatia in 1478. That same year Mantua, a city in eastern Lombardy, suffered moderately from a plague outbreak. Once again the poor suffered the most; they were segregated in unsanitary quarters and left to starve by the rich, who fled Mantua at the start of the epidemic. In the nearby commune of Sondrio, the poor and hungry threatened to rob the homes of the wealthy for food. To the south, the Italian communes of Modena, Parma, and San Marino were also affected by plague, but not as devastatingly as Venice, Milan, Brescia, and other places. See also PLAGUE OF FLORENCE (BLACK VOMIT); PLAGUE OF FLORENCE IN 1417; PLAGUE OF FLORENCE IN 1630–33.

Further reading: Carmichael, *Plague and the Poor in Renaissance Florence;* Cloudsley-Thompson, *Insects and History;* Winslow, *The Conquest of Epidemic Disease.*

Italian Plagues of 1629–31   Catastrophic outbreaks of mainly bubonic plague that claimed the lives of about 280,000 persons in Lombardy and other territories in northern Italy.

In 1629, during the Thirty Years' War (1618–48) in Europe (see THIRTY YEARS' WAR EPIDEMICS), German and French troops carried the plague disease to the city of Mantua in eastern Lombardy, where France was waging war against Austria and Spain. Some Venetian soldiers, who contracted plague and fled Mantua, carried it throughout northern and central Italy. Brescia in central Lombardy became the first Italian city seriously attacked by plague that year. The plague bacillus also spread in 1629 to other northern Italian cities, including Bologna, Padua, Parma, Turin, and Genoa on the coast.

When plague reached Milan (Lombardy's major commercial center) in October 1629, strict preventive measures were mandated there, including the burning of all items suspected of harboring the dreaded infection and the quarantining of all persons who had come in contact with plague-infected people. These unpopular measures are thought to have helped keep the outbreak isolated among those who had acquired supposedly contaminated articles from German soldiers. Plague-infested fleas (responsible for spreading the disease to rodents and humans) can survive wherever there are an abundance of rodents; they can live from six weeks to a year lodged in clothes, carpets, grains, and other goods.

In March 1630, as a result of relaxed precautionary measures during a carnival in Milan, plague erupted severely in various quarters of the city and then spread to such an extent that about 3,500 inhabitants were reportedly dying every day. Milanese officials erected two additional lazarettos (lazarets, hospitals for contagious diseases) and some 800 straw huts outside the city to shelter relatives of the sick. In Milan and 14 other cities in northern Italy, plague broke out in two major waves: in the autumn and winter of 1630 and the spring and summer of 1631. Ignorant of the cause of the disease, Italian physicians administered various ineffective treatments to their patients, including bloodletting, emetics, and ointments. Death sometimes occurred on the first or second day of infection for those who contracted the more infectious pneumonic or septicemic forms of plague; bubonic plague patients generally died within two to seven days.

Overall, Milan (Lombardy's largest city, with a population of about 130,000 people prior to 1630) suffered approximately 60,000 fatalities. Mantua recorded some 25,000 human deaths; Cremona some 17,000 deaths; and Brescia about 11,000 deaths. The mortality rate in each of these three Lombard cities has been estimated at around 46 percent. In Bergamo (northwest of Brescia) there were about 10,000 plague fatalities (40 percent mortality); in Como (north of Milan) there were 5,000 deaths (42 percent mortality). Monza (near Milan) had the highest mortality rate of Lombardy's cities: about 57 percent (some 4,000 out of a population of 7,000 perished).

East of Lombardy, the republic of Venice, which had barely recovered from the Venice Plague of 1575–77 (q.v.), was again severely struck in 1630–31, when reportedly about 46,000 inhabitants out of a population of 140,000 died from plague. Some historians contend that the 1630–31 epidemic of plague in Venice helped cause the subsequent downfall of this city-state as a world power. After the epidemic, the Venetians erected the Santa Maria della Salute, a magnificent church on the Grand Canal, in gratitude for their deliverance from the terrible sickness. The city of Verona (under the rule of Venice) suffered a mortality rate of 61 percent, with about 38,000 inhabitants dying from plague. East of Verona, Padua (also under Venetian rule) reported similarly terrible human losses: about 19,000 deaths out of 32,000 inhabitants (59 percent mortality) during 1630–31. The nearby city of Vicenza (under Venetian rule too) suffered about 12,000 fatalities at the time from the disease.

In north-central Italy, the papal-ruled city of Bologna lost an estimated 15,000 citizens to plague (24 percent mortality), while nearby Modena lost some 4,000 out of its 18,000 citizens and Parma, another neighbor, saw half its population succumb (15,000 victims) during this plague period. The disease was not as devastating to populations in northwest Italy; for instance, the city of Carmagnola (south of Turin) reported about 1,900 deaths (25 percent mortality in a population of 7,600). Plague also spread farther north into Tyrol (Tirol), an Alpine region of western Austria and northern Italy, to afflict even more inhabitants. See also PLAGUE OF FLORENCE IN 1630–33.

Further reading: Cipolla, *Fighting the Plague in Seventeenth Century Italy*; Prinzing, *Epidemics Resulting from Wars*.

Italian Plagues of 1656–57 Catastrophic outbreaks of mainly bubonic plague, killing about 218,000 persons in Naples, Rome, and Genoa out of a total population of 498,000 in these three cities. Much of the rest of Italy remained plague-free, partially due to events dating from before 1652.

For more than 100 years prior to 1652, the health magistracies (offices of the magistrates) in the capital cities of the republics and principalities in northern Italy had firmly established a policy of regularly informing each other about plague outbreaks in Italy and the rest of Europe, as well as in North Africa and the Middle East. In 1652 these northern Italian cities set up an official "circle of communications," called the *concerto*, and invited Rome and Naples to the south to participate in such joint actions as not doing business with any plague-infected cities and states. Naples (then under Spanish rule) kept corresponding with the northern cities but refused to suspend or restrict its trade with Spain and Spanish territories, where plague occurred in 1652; thus Naples was forced to remain outside the "circle," as was Rome.

Exactly where plague came from in 1656 and how it spread in Italy are not known. Some say the disease spread from Naples to Rome to Genoa, and others say it moved in the opposite direction, from north to south. After plague erupted in Genoa in 1656, the *concerto* fell apart, with the city of Florence in central Italy barring all business with Genoa (plague did not enter Florence in 1656 and 1657). Venice in northern Italy also took strict precautionary measures, remembering the disastrous Venice Plague of 1575–77 (q.v.)

Naples was rather lax in its restrictions and precautions, and its health board consisted of only two persons, a commoner known to take bribes to break the law and an aloof nobleman. Various ineffective methods of treatment (notably bloodletting and emetics) were administered to plague-suffering Neapolitans, who were victims primarily of the bubonic form, although the pneumonic and septicemic forms ("plague with blood spitting") did occur. Naples apparently suffered approximately 150,000 human deaths (half its population) during the epidemic; also killed by plague were some 45,000 people in Genoa (about 60 percent of the city's inhabitants) and about 23,000 people in Rome (about 19 percent of its population).

Further reading: Cipolla, *Fighting the Plague in Seventeenth Century Italy*; Hirst, *The Conquest of Plague*.

Italian Smallpox Epidemics of 1814

Variola outbreaks that affected thousands of people mainly in Italy's northern region of Lombardy, as well as in Rome. As French Emperor Napoleon I's hold on Italy weakened in 1813, invading Austrian forces carried the smallpox virus with them to the duchy of Milan, the commerial center of Lombardy, which suffered an outbreak the following year. Thousands of Milanese were vaccinated in a process employed by a Milanese scientist, Luigi Sacco, who had been using it since discovering natural cowpox infections in area cattle in 1800. Smallpox spread eastward to Cremona, another duchy in Lombardy.

However, Sacco's arm-to-arm cowpox vaccine had a dangerous side effect: Other diseases could be transmitted in the process, such as syphilis and erysipelas (acute skin infection). That fear was realized in Cremona in 1814, where 63 children in the rural village of Rivalta received vaccinations with material taken from the vaccinal pustule of an infant thought to be healthy but carrying syphilis, caused by a spirochete (single-celled, spiral germ). Forty-four of the vaccinated children contracted overt syphilis, and several immediately died of it; it also spread to some of the victims' mothers and nurses.

The movement of infected Austrian troops spread smallpox to other northern Italian cities, such as Brescia, Mantua, Parma, and Modena. Precautions to fight the disease varied from almost nothing to serious measures, such as in Rome, where the Pope endorsed vaccination in 1814 after a serious outbreak that year. Despite the dangers of arm-to-arm vaccination, the cowpox vaccine reduced considerably the number of infections and helped control smallpox in Italy. See also ITALIAN SMALLPOX EPIDEMIC OF 1900–02.

Further reading: Dixon, *Smallpox*; Hopkins, *Princes and Peasants: Smallpox in History*.

Italian Smallpox Epidemic of 1870–72

Serious smallpox outbreak killing untold thousands of persons in the newly united kingdom of Italy.

The deadly smallpox virus had evidently been smoldering in many parts of Italy since 1861. Many Italian patriots led by Giuseppe Garibaldi had contracted the disease while fighting the French for control of Sicily and Naples in 1861; these volunteer patriots had become infected in the district of Côte-d'Or in eastern France, where the disease was then very prevalent. After achieving the unification of Sicily and Naples, they carried the virus home with them to the Italian peninsula.

Before 1870, the northern Italian city of Milan in Lombardy reported about 200 to 300 cases of smallpox annually. The spread of smallpox significantly increased in July 1870 when the Franco-Prussian War (1870–71) broke out. (War is traditionally a breeder of disease, which is easily spread when soldiers are herded together in camps and barracks, exposed to hardship, fatigue, vermin, and inclement weather, and involved in mass movements.) After France's Emperor Napoleon III withdrew his troops from Rome and elsewhere in Italy (whose unification was thus completed), the highly communicable smallpox virus spread among the inhabitants of numerous Italian cities. Milan was particularly hard hit, reporting an estimated 6,000 cases of smallpox and more than 1,000 deaths before the epidemic in the city ended in 1871. The new Italian capital of Rome suffered a severe outbreak between October 1871 and about mid-1872, during which more than 1,000 persons perished from smallpox.

Variolation (inoculation with the smallpox virus) had long been practiced in Italy but was replaced in 1798 with Edward Jenner's more effective method of inoculation with cowpox; however, neither the germ for smallpox nor the immunity process of vaccination (Jenner's method) was clearly understood in much of Italy in 1870. Vaccination with Jenner's vaccine, which can not be transmitted to a second subject, was entirely voluntary in Italy during this time. Smallpox continued to be a serious problem in the country into the early years of the twentieth century.

Further reading: Shurkin, *The Invisible Fire*; Prinzing, *Epidemics Resulting from Wars*.

Italian Smallpox Epidemic of 1900–02

Outbreak of smallpox (known medically as variola) that claimed the lives of almost a quarter of the 60,532 persons reported infected. It struck especially severely in the major Italian cities of Genoa, Milan, Naples, and Rome.

This ancient European scourge, a disease known to have afflicted Italy since the sixth century A.D., had become endemic in regions of the country by the sixteenth century, when outbreaks began to occur sporadically, and in the following centuries. The highly contagious viral disease, which is transmitted directly from person to person through respiratory discharges and by contaminated material, claimed nearly 50,000 Italian lives during a serious, three-year-long outbreak throughout the country (1887–89). However, smallpox vaccination remained entirely voluntary in Italy well into the twentieth century, despite the Italians' general endorsement since the early 1800s of English physician Edward Jenner's cowpox vaccine as a deterrent. Confusion about the efficacy of the smallpox vaccine helped the anti-vaccinationists' movement, which raised questions about the duration of immunity, among other things.

Italian officials reported 14,951 human fatalities from smallpox during the 1900–02 epidemic. France, Germany, and Great Britain—countries then with larger populations than Italy (which had an estimated 35,000,000 people)—reported morbidity and mortality from the disease in far fewer numbers. For instance, in Germany (which had about 65,000,000 people at that time), only 386 human deaths from smallpox were reported between 1900 and 1910, undoubtedly due to the development of an effective vaccination program. During this same decade in Great Britain, where anti-vaccinationists were still strong, there were an approximate 5,000 deaths from the disease (see BRITISH SMALLPOX EPIDEMIC OF 1901–02). In Italy, the variola virus claimed another 4,049 victims from 1904 to 1910. It would take the devastating Italian Smallpox Epidemic of 1920–21 (q.v.) before Italian authorities would undertake mass smallpox vaccination and thus free the country from the disease's ravages.

Further reading: Hopkins, *Princes and Peasants: Smallpox in History*; Shurkin, *The Invisible Fire*.

Italian Smallpox Epidemic of 1920–21

Severe smallpox (variola) outbreak that killed 12,433 persons out of 31,097 who were reported infected. This highly contagious viral disease, which is transmitted normally by close contact with patients through respiratory discharges, had been prevalent in Russia, Poland, and parts of Austria-Hungary during World War I (1914–18). Sick soldiers returning home after the war brought the disease back to Italy.

During World War I, smallpox had not been epidemic among the Italian military forces, who had been vaccinated. However, being in contact with various populations in which the disease was prevalent caused a number of infections and some deaths among the soldiers in combat. Enough of the smallpox virus was present in bodies and clothing of the returning Italian soldiers to constitute a serious threat to the Italian civilian population by 1920. This was not the first time returning Italian troops were responsible for infecting the home populace; in 1870 volunteer patriots of General Giuseppe Garibaldi, working to unite Italy, brought smallpox into Italy from France.

During the first two decades of the twentieth century, there were approximately 18,000 human deaths

from smallpox in Italy, whose population was not well vaccinated despite the introduction of compulsory vaccination in parts of the country since 1806. In 1920 Italy was especially hard hit by smallpox, recording 26,453 cases and 11,073 deaths. Mass vaccinations in 1921 reduced smallpox morbidity (incidence of disease) to 4,644 reported cases and total fatalities to 1,360. Women accounted for a large proportion of the cases during the 1920–21 Italian epidemic, which permeated into regions of Austria, Switzerland, and France that border Italy. Many of the 1,740 smallpox infections that were reported in well vaccinated Germany in 1920–21 were among Italian visitors to that country.

Italy had only 534 cases of smallpox with 37 fatalities in 1922, and for the next 20 years, the morbidity continued to decline dramatically (no cases were reported for many of those years); in 1943 and 1944 (during World War II) an upsurge occurred when a total of 5,704 smallpox infections were reported in the country.

Further reading: Dixon, *Smallpox*; Shurkin, *The Invisible Fire*.

Italian Typhoid Epidemics of 1950–52

Outbreaks of typhoid fever and paratyphoid fever (intestinal disease resembling typhoid but caused by a related but slightly different *Salmonella* bacterium) that infected a reported 87,276 persons (3,572 of them died). Both typhoid and paratyphoid (much less fatal than the former) are spread in a number of ways having to do with poor sanitation. Populations in rural Italian areas, where water supplies, sewage, garbage, and polluted streams could carry the infection, were most susceptible, though city dwellers in Naples and elsewhere sometimes became infected by contaminated shellfish, salads, milk, and dairy products, as well as drinking water.

In the mid-eighteenth century, typhoid fever was cited as a "new disease" in Italy, and afterward the infectious disease (characterized by severe abdominal pain, diarrhea, high fever, intense headache, and a splotchy rash) occurred in the country during periods of social breakdown. In 1943, during World War II, typhoid was prevalent in Italy's central and southern regions, in places ravaged by air raids and bombings. After the war, famine and hardship continued, with flooded fields and polluted water and food supplies in numerous areas; more than 50,000 cases of typhoid and paratyphoid fever were reported between 1943 and 1949.

Typhoid escalated in Italy in 1950 and 1951, mainly in rural areas where the standards of hygiene remained low due to poverty and neglect (parts of Italy were still garrisoned by foreign troops). The island of Sicily was also attacked by typhoid then. More men than women were infected, and most of the infections occurred in those between age five and 30. In 1950 Italian fatalities for typhoid and paratyphoid numbered 1,347, a 2.9 percent death rate per 100,000 persons. The following year 1,267 persons died from the two typhoids, a 2.7 percent mortality rate per 100,000. Both of the diseases decreased in 1952, with the mortality rate dropping to two percent per 100,000. However, Italy continued to suffer the most of all European countries from typhoid and paratyphoid infections from 1953 to 1957, during which time 108,798 cases (a total of both diseases) were reported. Later, improved sanitary engineering in rural regions and widespread immunization against the diseases reduced the total number of infections to 11,898 between 1962 and 1967; since then typhoid has almost disappeared from Italy.

Further reading: Huckstep, *Typhoid Fever*; May, *The Ecology of Human Disease*.

Italian Typhus Epidemic of 1505

Subject of the first complete description of typhus, written by Girolamo Fracastoro, who also mentioned an epidemic that swept Italy two decades later (see FRENCH ARMY TYPHUS EPIDEMIC OF 1528). Erupting in Europe in epidemic form during the late 1400s, typhus caused numerous outbreaks throughout the next century, as armies spread the disease while fighting the near-constant wars of the time. An Italian physician with an interest in theories of contagion, Fracastoro observed the 1505 and 1528 epidemics firsthand and described typhus accurately, certain that he had seen nothing like it before.

As he noted, its distinguishing feature was a rash of spots like flea bites—called "lenticulae" (small lentils), "punctículae" (small pricks), or "petechiae"—which appeared on the arms and torso on the fourth or seventh day of the illness. Before then patients had such a mild fever that most doctors did nothing to treat them. After the rash broke out, however, the victims became extremely fatigued, unable to do anything except lie on their backs while their minds wandered. Once the crisis passed in a week or two, many recovered, but death was sure for those who manifested certain symptoms, such as sudden weakness, hemorrhaging from the nose, inability to urinate, or the disappearance of the spots. The disease was also selective in that it rarely struck women or old people. Young men and boys were the likely victims, especially those of the noble classes, who, as Fracastoro points out, were usually spared by other epidemics.

Fracastoro, who lived long before the role of viruses as disease carriers was known, believed that typhus was spread not through the air or by objects like clothing or furniture but only by direct handling of the sick. Although it would be centuries before the true route of typhus transmission was understood, Fracastoro was correct in suggesting that war and famine contributed to outbreaks of the disease.

By 1505 Italy had suffered from ten years of warfare, starting with the invasion by the French king Charles VIII in 1495. In renewing the Italian campaigns, his successor captured Milan, while Ferdinand II of Spain conquered Naples. Foreign rulers were not the only ones responsible for war in Italy. Caesar Borgia tried to subdue the central part of the country, Florence battled unsuccessfully to take Pisa, and other city-states and local rulers fought among themselves. As various armies, sometimes including foreign mercenaries, crisscrossed the peninsula, they could easily have brought typhus in their wake. Fracastoro was aware that the disease could travel long distances. He not only claimed that it came from Cyprus and the surrounding islands, but also noted that people going from Italy to other countries where spotted fevers were not present sometimes died anyway, "as if they carried the infection with them."

Further reading: Major, *Classic Descriptions of Disease*; Castiglioni, *A History of Medicine*; Salvatorelli, *A Concise History of Italy*; Zinsser, *Rats, Lice and History*.

Italian Typhus Epidemic of 1528

See FRENCH ARMY TYPHUS EPIDEMIC OF 1528.

Italian Typhus Epidemics of 1796–1800

Devastating outbreaks of typhus fever (epidemic typhus) that swept through much of Italy, killing more than 20,000 persons during the French Revolutionary Wars (1792–1802). Typhus, a rickettsia-caused disease transmitted by lice from person to person, occurs frequently during famines and wars. Italians had suffered severe outbreaks of the disease, which they named "petechiae," since the early sixteenth century.

In 1796, Napoleon Bonaparte's French armies in Italy defeated the Austrians and took control of the Piedmont region of northwest Italy; the cities of Nice and Genoa surrendered and French garrisons occupied Piedmontese fortresses. After defeating the Austrians at the Battle of Lodi (May 10, 1796), Napoleon controlled most of Lombardy in northern Italy. Later, during fighting at Mantua in Lombardy, there was a severe eruption of typhus among both the Austrian and French forces (who may have carried the rickettsial organism with them from France, where a major outbreak had occurred at Nantes). Typhus then spread to civilians in Mantua and other cities and towns in northern Italy in 1796 and 1797; Sicily also was infected by the disease during this stage of the war.

Two years later in 1799, during the War of the Second Coalition (1798–1801), Austro-Russian armies defeated the French in Piedmont and in Naples in the south. In the fall, epidemic typhus overwhelmed the retreating French Army in Nice, where it had taken refuge; in addition, a third of Nice's population fell victim to the infection (characterized by chills, high fever, severe headache, muscular pains, and often a spotted rash over the entire body). From Nice typhus spread along the Ligurian coast to San Remo, Impéria, and Savona, as well as to other towns in Liguria. Genoa, in Liguria, was already fighting off the disease (since June and July 1799), which was attacking military troops, commercial travelers, and fugitives from northern Italy. Genoa's civilian population was not seriously affected until February 1800, when its poor and unsanitary citizens were the main victims of typhus. After winter, fatalities began to soar in Genoa and, during an epidemic six-month period ending in August 1800, totaled an estimated 14,000.

Further reading: Prinzing, *Epidemics Resulting from Wars*; Ackerknecht, *History and Geography of the Most Important Diseases*.

Italian Typhus Epidemic of 1816–18   Devastating epidemic of louse-borne typhus fever that spread over the whole Italian peninsula, killing untold thousands of people. An estimated ten percent of those infected perished; among those hospitalized, the death rate was 16 percent to 20 percent overall (40 percent for those 40 to 50 years old and nearly 100 percent for those over 50).

After the Napoleonic Wars (1803–15) and the end of Napoleonic rule in Italy, a wave of typhus infection swept into Italian areas on both sides of the Adriatic Sea in the north. The rickettsial disease, carried by human body lice and thriving under dirty, crowded conditions, traveled from Rovigno (Rovinj, Croatia) north to Trieste at the head of the Adriatic and from Venice south along the coast to Ancona. Later that same year (1816), the infection spread to Italy's Alpine area, particularly Lombardy, which had been devastated by harvest failures as a result of cold and wet weather and severe flooding. Impoverished Italians, crowded together and exhausted by hunger, had little concern about personal and communal cleanliness. There was also a lack of fuel to build fires and heat water for the bathing and washing of clothes and bedding, on which body lice lived and bred. And roving bands of destitute beggars and migrants helped diffuse the epidemic in the larger Lombard cities of Bergamo, Brescia, and Milan.

By 1817 the epidemic had spread to Florence, Rome, and Naples to the south. It then traveled farther south into the island of Sicily, notably to Ragusa, where many were afflicted. Vessels entering Sicily's main ports of Messina and Palermo were placed in quarantine. The epidemic least affected the Piedmont region in northwest Italy, but the inhabitants of Savoy (bordering Piedmont) were ravaged by typhus; ships entering ports such as Genoa in the kingdom of Sardinia (composing Savoy, Piedmont, and the island of Sardinia) were quarantined, as were ships in many other Italian seaports. (At the time typhus was also known as "ship fever," the scourge of seamen and navies, spreading from ships to hospitals on land to the surrounding communities.)

Further reading: Ackerknecht, *History and Geography of the Most Important Diseases*; Post, *The Last Great Subsistence Crisis in the Western World*.

Italian Whooping Cough Epidemics of 1901–05
Series of serious annual outbreaks of whooping cough (pertussis), where a total of about 60,000 persons (mostly very young children) died from this highly contagious, bacterial respiratory infection. During these years, whooping cough killed more children in Italy than did diphtheria and scarlet fever combined—two other extremely infectious diseases commonly attacking children.

In the winter of 1901 an epidemic occurred throughout the Italian peninsula that was most severe in the large cities of Venice, Florence, Genoa, Milan, and Rome. There were a total of about 250,000 cases of whooping cough in the country that winter. No age group was immune, but most of the cases involved children aged two to five; more females of all ages were attacked by the pertussis bacillus (*Bordetella pertussis*) than were males (doctors provided no reason for this occurrence, which is the opposite of the trend in most infectious diseases). Many of the young, fatal patients lost their breath and turned blue after repeated coughing, which ended in forced intakes of breath, or "whoops," and lasted sometimes as long as three weeks.

In 1901 more than 50 percent of the approximate 15,000 deaths from whooping cough were among Italian children under three years old. This high death toll was caused by bronchopneumonia and diarrheal diseases accompanying complications of whooping cough. The overall fatality rate was higher among females; this was thought to be due to the difference in the structure of the female larynx, making females more susceptible to bronchopneumonia.

Whooping cough continued to break out yearly from 1902 to 1905, killing a total of approximately 45,000 Italians, mainly children. Though the disease remained prevalent and extremely troublesome in Italy, health authorities gradually understood the dangers of whooping cough and the preventive measures to be taken. The fatalities from the disease steadily declined. Since the 1930s there has been an effective inoculation that will almost completely prevent whooping cough, but the use of the pertussis vaccine has never been made mandatory in Italy, where whooping cough (while no longer a devastating childhood disease) has continued to appear.

Further reading: Lapin, *Whooping Cough;* Parton and Warlaw, eds., *Pathogenesis and Immunity in Pertussis.*

J

Jamaican Yellow Fever Epidemic of 1655 First reported outbreak of yellow fever on the island of Jamaica in the West Indies, killing at least a thousand native Indians and hundreds of Spaniards and English (rivals for control of the island).

Yellow fever (an infectious viral disease of warm climates) was apparently introduced to Jamaica by European ships transporting either black slaves from West Africa or commercial cargo from Cuba, which became infected after 1648. When the epidemic erupted in Jamaica in 1655, the African slaves appeared relatively immune to the virus (recovery from the disease confers immunity) and suffered small losses. But the natives were vulnerable, along with the English forces that were attacking the Spanish troops on the island. The English under Admiral Sir William Penn captured Jamaica in May 1655 but lost an average of 140 men per week from yellow fever before the epidemic died out later that year.

After yellow fever and other diseases were supposedly brought by Europeans to the New World, native Indian populations in the West Indies vanished in large numbers, and more and more West African slaves were imported to work on the European plantations. This increased the black population in Jamaica and much of the rest of the Caribbean, where yellow fever epidemics decimated the natives of Guadeloupe in 1635 and 1648, St. Kitts in 1635, and Barbados in 1647 and 1691 (see BARBADIAN YELLOW FEVER EPIDEMIC OF 1647; BARBADIAN YELLOW FEVER EPIDEMIC OF 1691). Jamaica again suffered from an epidemic in 1671, when a victorious British fleet returned to the island with the disease from Panama.

Further reading: Cloudsley-Thompson, *Insects and History*; Scott, *A History of Tropical Medicine*.

Japanese Army Beriberi Epidemic of 1904–05

Thousands of cases of beriberi that occurred in the Japanese Army during the Russo-Japanese War of 1904–05 (won decisively by Japan).

Beriberi is a nutritional deficiency disease now known to be caused by the lack of vitamin B_1 (thiamine) in one's diet. In 1904–05, that precise nutrient had not been discovered and isolated, although it was known that the disease was connected with the lack of something in one's diet. In the Japanese Navy, Surgeon-General Takaki had succeeded in controlling the incidence of beriberi among sailors by altering their rations. Some of his recommendations were adopted by the Japanese Army but apparently were not strictly or regularly enforced, perhaps on account of wartime emergencies. Hence, the high incidence of beriberi among Japanese soldiers during this war with Russia.

Surgeon-General Takaki reported 97,572 cases of beriberi in the Japanese Army from the start of the war (February 1904) up to August 31, 1905. There were 3,956 recorded deaths caused by the disease. Another report put the number of beriberi cases at 200,000 and observed that it was the army's number-one health problem. Takaki pointed out that while beriberi was raging through the Japanese Army camps during the siege of Port Arthur (Lü-shun), the navy did not report even one case. This has been attributed to the difference in their respective daily rations: 5 oz. of meat and 30 oz. of rice for each soldier and 1 lb. of meat, 10 oz. of barley and 20 oz. of rice for each sailor.

Beriberi, known as *kakke* or *ashike* in Japanese, had plagued the Japanese Army for years. For instance, in 1875, 26 percent out of 17,500 soldiers were affected and, in 1876, 11 percent out of 35,300 soldiers. There are three forms of the disease: wet beriberi, dry beriberi, and infantile beriberi. Generally, the disease manifests itself in a combination of the first two forms.

Further reading: Williams, *Toward the Conquest of Beriberi*; Ackroyd, *Conquest of Deficiency Diseases*.

Japanese Cholera Epidemic of 1822

Outburst of the Asiatic Cholera Pandemic of 1817–23 (q.v.) in the east, causing massive destruction in western Japan. It was first observed in the Japanese port of Nagasaki in 1822 and is believed to have been imported there either from Java or from China (see CHINESE CHOLERA EPIDEMIC OF 1820–22) and Korea via the island of Tsushima and the seaport of Shimonoseki (at the southwest extremity of Honshu Island, Japan).

From the Nagasaki, the epidemic disease spread to the island of Kyushu and the province of Choshu (in southern Honshu) and simultaneously along the Inland Sea to Osaka. A sharp increase in mortality was noted in the cities of Hagi (in Choshu), Hiroshima, Nagasaki, and Osaka during September–October 1822. The city of Kyoto also suffered but not as much. Apparently, the epidemic did not spread beyond Hakone (a resort region) in the east—thanks to the mountainous terrain and the onset of winter. Precise mortality figures are not available for this epidemic, but it is clear that Nagasaki and Osaka were the hardest hit.

Known in Japan as the *Korera* epidemic of Bunsei 2, its arrival in late autumn was an important factor in halting the eastward movement of the infection and in leading to its early disappearance from the country. Had it reached Japan early in the summer it would have wreaked havoc across more of the country. As it was, this epidemic provided a mere hint of the more severe pandemics to come.

Further reading: Jannetta, *Epidemics and Mortality in Early Modern Japan;* Gallagher, *Diseases that Plague Modern Man.*

Japanese Cholera Epidemics of 1858–59 and 1862
Two major cholera epidemics, both connected with the Asiatic Cholera Pandemic of 1846–63 (q.v.), which swept through Japan causing widespread mortality.

The scholar August Hirsch in his *Handbook on Geographical and Historical Pathology* believed that the first outbreak of cholera during this pandemic in Japan occurred in 1854. Japanese sources, however, do not mention such an epidemic.

Most sources agree that the first epidemic struck the Japanese port city of Nagasaki in June of 1858, a few weeks after the signing of a treaty with Western powers that opened Japanese ports to foreign trade. The infection was apparently brought into town by a cholera patient on board the United States warship *Mississippi*, which had arrived from China. Not surprisingly, many Japanese associated the disease with the Western invasion. Far more severe than the Japanese Cholera Epidemic of 1822 (q.v.), it spread rapidly toward the northeast and reached the capital of Edo (Tokyo), then Japan's largest city, by the end of July. During September–October 1858, cholera raged in the city, causing unusually high mortality. With the onset of cooler winter weather, it declined in Edo.

The epidemic spread (with varying intensity) across all of Japan by land and sea. In the Sendai region, for instance, Edo, Osaka, and Ishinomaki were infected by sea. The latter port was the first to be invaded. From here the epidemic traveled along the coast and later inland along the Kitakami River. Cholera was fairly widespread in the Sendai region in 1858 and 1859 and apparently more virulent in the second year. Known in Japan as the cholera epidemic of Ansei 5 and 6, it was neither mentioned in Ogenji's death records nor indirectly reflected in a noticeably higher death rate in 1858–59 in the Hida region.

According to some scholars, the epidemic of 1859 struck more districts and caused higher mortality. An estimated three million people (adults and children) died of cholera in 1858–59. Between July and September 1860, nearly 250,000 cholera victims were cremated in Edo alone. Clearly, it was a major disaster, and the government responded by introducing relief measures to help those who were left without support.

In 1861, cholera virtually disappeared from the country. However, in 1862, it erupted again. Some scholars consider the 1862 outbreak as a continuation of the 1858–59 epidemic. Like its predecessor, the epidemic of Bunkyu 2 also began in Nagasaki. It was apparently more severe and widespread than that of 1858–59. Mortality statistics for 1862 are somewhat misleading because Japan was also ravaged in that year by a severe outbreak of measles (see JAPANESE MEASLES EPIDEMIC OF 1862), during which many died of diarrhea and related complications. See also PERSIAN CHOLERA EPIDEMICS OF 1846–63.

Further reading: Jannetta, *Epidemics and Mortality in Early Modern Japan;* Taeuber, *The Population of Japan.*

Japanese Dengue Epidemics of 1942–45
Severe and widespread outbreaks of dengue fever that occurred mainly in and around Japan's port cities during World War II. Also called breakbone fever, dengue was apparently nonexistent in Japan prior to 1942. However, during the second phase of the war, Japanese ports served as entry points for passengers arriving from Shanghai, Singapore, and the Malayan states, where dengue was endemic. Also, the wartime scarcity of water forced people to store water in every container they could find. The *Aedes albopictus* mosquito, later identified as the sole vector of the disease in Japan, bred abundantly in these water-filled containers. The dengue type 1 virus was isolated as the predominant virus of the acute febrile disease.

Some two million cases of dengue reportedly occurred in Japan (mainly in the ports of Nagasaki, Kure, Sasebo, Kobe, and Osaka) during 1942–45. For instance, Osaka (about two million people) reported about 5,000 cases in 1942, some 3,000 to 4,000 cases in

1943, and close to half a million cases in 1944. Statistics are not available for 1945 because the air raids in the cities led residents to seek refuge in neighboring villages. Many other ports suffered similarly.

The Japanese dengue epidemics were part of a massive regional outbreak of dengue that affected most of the countries of the Pacific zone.

Further reading: Sabin, "Research on Dengue during World War II"; Howe, *A World Geography of Human Diseases.*

Japanese Encephalitis Epidemics of the 1920s and 1930s
Series of epidemics of Japanese B Encephalitis (JBE). The disease, whose causative arbovirus was not isolated until 1935, had been prevalent in Japan since the summer of 1871. It had also been reported in the Philippines, Korea, Singapore, Taiwan, India, Burma (Myanmar), and Thailand (the Chiang Mai or Chiengmai valley region).

The first major outbreak was reported during the summer of 1924, with 6,125 cases of JBE and 3,797 deaths, a mortality rate of 62 percent. Tokyo and its surroundings were particularly hard hit, as was the coast of Japan's Inland Sea, just south of the 35th parallel. Small outbreaks were reported from certain eastern districts but Hokkaido was spared. JBE apparently preferred the hot, dry climate of Honshu Island; its incidence was highest in August in the south and in September in the northeast.

Another epidemic occurred in 1927, when 1,006 cases and 716 deaths were recorded, a 71 percent fatality rate. The epidemic of 1929 attacked 2,058 people and killed 1,340 (65 percent mortality). Scattered outbreaks were reported from the city of Fukuoka in 1932 and from the island of Okinawa in 1933. In the Okinawa epidemic, mainly children were affected.

The next major JBE epidemic struck in 1935; 5,370 people were affected and 2,264 died—a case fatality rate of 42 percent. Unlike the other outbreaks, this one raged in Tokyo even after the weather had turned cooler. The arbovirus that causes the disease was discovered and isolated during this epidemic and found to be different from the related St. Louis virus.

Two more JBE epidemics were recorded in Japan during the decade. The first, in 1936, attacked 1,305 people and caused 696 deaths (53 percent fatality rate), and the second, in 1937, attacked 2,030 and killed 1,115 people (55 percent mortality).

JBE generally attacks people above 50 years of age, among whom the fatality rate is higher, and favors men slightly more than women. During the period between 1924 and 1937, there were reported a total of 21,355 cases of JBE and 12,159 deaths (57 percent mortality rate). This may not be a very accurate figure since many mild cases, especially in children, often escaped notification. During World War II, JBE broke out among civilians in Okinawa and in Korea and posed a real threat to the American troops who would be stationed there.

Further reading: Spink, *Infectious Diseases;* Simmons et al., *Global Epidemiology.*

Japanese Epidemic of A.D. 585–87
Severe epidemic, believed to be smallpox, which invaded Japan from the Korean mainland in A.D. 585, the fourteenth year of Japanese Emperor Bidatsu's reign. If the epidemic was indeed smallpox, it may rank as the country's first recorded smallpox epidemic. Historians consider an earlier epidemic in A.D. 552 one of plague or measles.

The opening of contacts with the mainland had resulted in the advent of Buddhism in Japan. The Koreans sent Buddhist literature, texts, priests, a temple architect, and several images of Buddha to Japan. Consequently, Emperor Bidatsu urged his subjects to worship Buddha. Many blamed the severe disease outbreak that followed on the introduction of this new religion. The people, believing that the pestilence was a punishment from the Shinto deities for embracing the new faith, reacted violently as they had in A.D. 552. They flung the images of Buddha into the canals, burned temples, and stripped and beat the Buddhist nuns.

Obviously, these violent measures had no effect on the epidemic, which, according to chronicles, was widespread. Thousands of people were afflicted with the disease, their bodies covered with sores, and many died. Even the emperor and the chief of the clan leaders were infected. The pro-Buddhist elements let it be known that they believed the outbreak was in retribution for desecrating images of Buddha. Many of the public privately agreed.

In the autumn of 585, the emperor ordered that the Buddhist temples be rebuilt but banned conversions. He died shortly thereafter, becoming perhaps Japanese royalty's first smallpox victim. He was succeeded by his brother Yomei, who became a Buddhist himself. He too was stricken by smallpox in 585 and died in the continuing epidemic two years later. Yomei's son, Shotoku, subsequently erected a temple to the "Buddha of Medicine," which became the center of Japanese culture. See also JAPANESE SMALLPOX EPIDEMIC OF A.D. 735–37; JAPANESE SMALLPOX EPIDEMICS OF THE EIGHTH AND NINTH CENTURIES A.D.; JAPANESE SMALLPOX EPIDEMICS OF THE TENTH CENTURY A.D.

Further reading: Hopkins, *Princes and Peasants: Smallpox in History;* Farris, *Population, Disease, and Land in Early Japan, 645–900.*

Japanese Epidemic of A.D. 994-95

Major epidemic of an unidentified disease that struck Japan with tremendous virulence in A.D. 994-995. Historical sources are agreed on the severity of this epidemic, which apparently killed many in the elite ruling class over a brief two to three month period. Among the victims were seven or eight ministers and noblemen at the court and countless numbers belonging to the lower ranks. Overall, it is estimated that more than half Japan's population died during this epidemic—perhaps the result of an unknown disease striking a highly susceptible population for the first time. According to some scholars, the disease involved was smallpox, but there is no consensus on this owing to lack of corroborative evidence.

Further reading: Jannetta, *Epidemics and Mortality in Early Modern Japan;* McNeill, *Plagues and Peoples.*

Japanese Influenza Epidemic of 1957-58

Offshoot of the Asian Influenza Pandemic of 1957-58 (q.v.), which affected Japan in two distinct waves during 1957-58 (see INDIAN INFLUENZA EPIDEMIC OF 1957-58).

The disease, apparently introduced into one or more Japanese cities from either Singapore, Taiwan, or Hong Kong, was first observed in a school in Tokyo on May 10, 1957. It quickly assumed epidemic proportions, spreading first throughout the large cities, then to the smaller towns and rural areas. The precise route of transmission was not determined, but it is clear that the virus spread simultaneously from several large cities, aided, in many instances, by schoolchildren on educational trips. At the end of May, the virus was isolated in Tokyo and identified as the so-called A/Asia/57 virus.

The first wave of the epidemic peaked around the end of June 1957 and, by late July, had subsided in most of Japan's prefectures (provinces). The average attack rate was 26 percent overall and rose to 50 percent to 60 percent in schools and camps. Seventy to eighty thousand cases were reported at the height of this first wave, and more than 20,000 schools were believed to be affected. At its peak, more than 1,000 deaths occurred.

The epidemic's second phase occurred during November–December 1957 and affected an estimated 80,000 people and 20,000 schools at its most intense period. Nearly 6,000 people died; the increase over the first wave has been attributed more to the time of year than to the virulence of the virus.

During the first two weeks of 1958, barely a week or so after the second wave had begun to subside, another minor outbreak of influenza (sometimes considered an extension of the second wave) was reported. At its worst, more than 8,000 people and 300 schools were infected and about a hundred fatalities were recorded.

Nationally, the average attack rate was about 20 percent in the first wave and 50 percent after the second wave. During the first wave, the highest attack rates were observed in those between five and 20 years of age. The death rate was exceptionally high in infants and the elderly. Most of the deaths were due to secondary complications. For instance, of the 580 deaths recorded in Tokyo, 316 were from acute pneumonia and 133 from cardiac insufficiency. Other complications noted during this epidemic included various types of asthma, pulmonary edema, meningitis, encephalitis, enteritis, nephritis, hepatitis, and dyspepsia.

Since the flu virus was not isolated until the end of May when the epidemic was already quite widespread, commercial production could not begin until July. The first batch of the vaccine was ready for use in November 1957, when the second wave of the epidemic had already peaked. Vaccinations were given in certain prefectures during November–December but only on a limited scale since the initial supplies were quickly exhausted.

Further reading: Fukumi, "Summary Report on the Asian Influenza Epidemic in Japan, 1957."

Japanese-Korean Typhus Epidemic of 1945-46

Massive and widespread epidemic of louse-borne typhus in Japan and Korea during 1945-46.

Typhus had been reported from both countries prior to this large epidemic, but Japan's last major outbreak occurred in 1914, while Korea had suffered a series of small outbreaks every year for the previous two decades. In 1945, however, while typhus cases were reported from Korea, no major outbreaks occurred in any Korean city. On the other hand, the disease raged in Hokkaido, Japan's northernmost island, where over 1,000 cases were reported from January to August 1945. Typhus fever had established itself in Hokkaido at the start of World War II with the advent of Korean laborers to work in the mines there. When the hostilities ended, mass repatriations of prisoners and citizens resulted in the rapid dispersal of typhus across Japan and Korea.

The seriousness of the situation became apparent when nearly 150 typhus cases were reported from Hokkaido, mainly from the Yubari coal mines, during the first week of November 1945. Dusting with DDT and using the typhus vaccine helped bring this outbreak under control. Since many of the miners were being repatriated, the area was quarantined and every person leaving Hokkaido was deloused with

DDT. This ensured that the disease did not spread elsewhere in Japan from this endemic focus.

But, a month later, typhus broke out in three different areas in Japan—Yamagata, Tokyo, and Osaka—with all three outbreaks originating in Korea. In the Yamagata prefecture in north-central Honshu, typhus began in some of its mountain villages among the Japanese repatriated from Korea. Once again, strict measures, including quarantine, were imposed and the spread of the disease was arrested.

The Osaka outbreak began in a city jail when a Japanese civilian, imprisoned for selling Japanese Army blankets obtained in Manchuria and Korea, caught typhus. His case escaped notification for over two weeks, and when he and his fellow prisoners were released, cholera-infected lice entered the city with them. The number of typhus cases rose rapidly, and a mass delousing exercise was promptly launched in Osaka city. The outbreak was eventually contained but not before the disease had already spread to neighboring cities such as Kobe, Kyoto, Nagoya, and Tokyo, and even farther away Nagasaki in southern Kyushu and Aomori in northern Honshu. The enforcement of rigid quarantine and remedial measures succeeded in suppressing these outbreaks.

By far the biggest outbreak occurred in the Tokyo area. Until early March 1946, stray typhus cases had been reported in the city, beginning with a Japanese family recently back from Korea. Suddenly, however, the number of cases escalated to epidemic proportion coinciding with the peaking of the Osaka outbreak. Many cases went unreported and the introduction of half-hearted and ineffective control measures did little to halt the spread of this epidemic to Yokohama and Nikko. Eventually, more stringent action was taken by the Tokyo health authorities and the outbreak subsided.

In Korea, where typhus was also reported during this period, the situation was somewhat different. No major outbreaks were reported from any Korean city in the latter half of 1945 and the early months of 1946, thanks to a coordinated typhus control strategy launched jointly by the military government and the United States Typhus Commission late in 1945. In all the major cities, typhus control procedures were taught to Korean and American personnel. Specific areas within the cities where typhus had raged during previous epidemics were identified, and its residents vaccinated and dusted with DDT on a monthly basis. Most of the cases occurred in the American zone and were imported from Manchuria and northern Korea, as well as a few from Japan.

Overall, 30,000 cases were reported from both countries, and the mortality rate ranged between six percent and ten percent. But for the rigorous and stringent control measures launched by the various authorities, it is believed that the epidemic would have affected over two million people. Its spread was aided by the overcrowded and unsanitary living conditions during World War II and the massive repatriations following it. Also, the public health departments in both countries were not organized or equipped to deal with such widespread outbreaks.

Thanks to the effectiveness of the control measures, typhus did not take root among the American military even as the disease was intensifying among Korean and Japanese civilians. Only 28 cases were reported among the American soldiers, since most had been vaccinated earlier; these were quite mild and no deaths occurred.

Further reading: Moulton, ed., *The Rickettsial Diseases of Man.*

Japanese Malaria Epidemic of 1945–46

Major outbreak of malaria following the end of World War II (1939–45) and the start of the massive repatriation of Japanese soldiers.

The problem began when the war ended and Japanese soldiers, including units from the Pacific Theater, where malaria had ravaged troops on both sides, started returning home (see SOUTHWEST PACIFIC MALARIA EPIDEMICS OF 1942–45). Overall, about 600,000 Japanese soldiers came home, many bringing malaria with them. More than 14,000 new cases of malaria were reported during 1945–46, mainly *Plasmodium vivax* (malaria parasite) infections mixed with a few *Plasmodium falciparum* infections. The Yaeyama Islands in the Okinawa prefecture were also severely hit, and about 50 percent of the population was taken ill with malaria and many died.

During 1947, Japan and the United States Army jointly launched a malaria control program involving residual spraying of DDT. The effectiveness of this measure was soon reflected in a noticeably reduced infection rate.

Further reading: Cross and Cross, eds., *Human Ecology and Infectious Diseases*; Spink, *Infectious Diseases.*

Japanese Measles Epidemics of A.D. 998 and 1025

Japan's first recorded epidemic of measles, which affected much of the population. The *Eiga (Eigwa) monogatari* (Tales of Splendor), a chronicle of events by an anonymous woman attached to the Heian court, carries a brief description of this epidemic. According to it, the epidemic infected everyone regardless of age or social class and also claimed some victims. The chronicle distinguished between the familiar smallpox (*mogasa*) and the lesser-known measles, which was then referred to as *aka-mogasa* (red rash pox) because of the bright red color of the spots. Subsequently, measles became popularly known as *hashika*. Some sources mention the concurrent presence of smallpox in the country during the same year.

Measles, a contagious viral disease, has a high attack rate as it moves rapidly through a community. The onset of the disease is marked by headache, fever, and general listlessness. Soon thereafter, the eyes start burning and respiratory problems (sneezing, cough, cold) appear. A few days later, the fever rises and a reddish-purple rash appears on the face and spreads all over the body. All the symptoms usually begin receding around the tenth day. Most of the fatalities are caused by complications arising from the disease and, very rarely, by the disease itself.

The measles epidemic of 1025, also mentioned in the *Eiga (Eigwa) monogatari*, apparently infected all those spared by an earlier epidemic—mainly people born since the epidemic of A.D. 998. The author expressed concern about the well-being of Japan's emperor and younger members of the royal family, all of whom were in their teens and twenties and, therefore, most susceptible to the disease. This statement led some scholars to conclude that measles may have been responsible for some of the earlier unidentified epidemics in Japanese history. Measles struck in epidemic form again in 1077 and 1093–94.

Further reading: Jannetta, *Epidemics and Mortality in Early Modern Japan*; Fujikawa, *Japanese Medicine*.

Japanese Measles Epidemic of 1690–91

Measles epidemic that swept through much of Japan, apparently infecting a large cross section of its population.

The epidemic broke out early in the third month of 1690 and was prevalent until the fifth month of 1691. It affected both young and old, men and women, and few escaped its fury. Edo (Tokyo) reportedly suffered the epidemic during the fourth month of 1691. Local records from Sendai refer to a widespread measles outbreak in the region in 1691. Since there was no corresponding increase in the region's mortality records for that period, scholars have concluded that it probably did not lead to a large number of deaths. In Hida, measles raged in 1691. There are no references to the seasons during which the epidemic attacked the Hida and Sendai regions, so its course cannot be traced with certainty.

Epidemic measles again invaded Japan in 1708–09, 1730–31, 1753, and 1776.

Further reading: Jannetta, *Epidemics and Mortality in Early Modern Japan*.

Japanese Measles Epidemic of 1708–09

Apparently a severe and widespread epidemic of measles, recording high mortality.

According to a contemporary account, the epidemic began in the fall of 1708 and, by the spring of 1709 (when it ended) had affected all of Japan's 60 provinces. It affected everyone regardless of age, sex, or social status. We are told that it struck Edo (Tokyo) on Honshu Island in the winter. Nowhere in the Sendai temple records is the epidemic mentioned, nor is there any noticeable rise in registered deaths during this period. Whether this is because the records were lost or because the epidemic was much milder than the previous one (see JAPANESE MEASLES EPIDEMIC OF 1690–91) and affected mainly those under 18 years of age, is open to conjecture. The epidemic was not recorded in the remote Hida region on Honshu Island either, where, judging by another account, it did not penetrate.

Further reading: Jannetta, *Epidemics and Mortality in Early Modern Japan*.

Japanese Measles Epidemic of 1730–31

Relatively mild epidemic of measles, spreading across Japan from the southwest to the northeast.

First reported from the island of Kyushu in 1730, the measles epidemic attacked the highly populated region of Kinki (on Honshu Island) in the tenth month. In the winter of 1730, it arrived in Edo (Tokyo), where it lingered until the following spring. Measles also invaded Kyushu's Sendai region sometime in 1731, but it is not known when it began or how long it lasted. It is also clear that this epidemic, unlike its predecessor (see JAPANESE MEASLES EPIDEMIC OF 1708–09), reached Honshu's Hida region in 1730. In both regions, however, the epidemic apparently did not lead to any perceivable increase in mortality. Japan was visited by another and more severe epidemic of measles in 1753 (see JAPANESE MEASLES EPIDEMIC OF 1753).

Further reading: Jannetta, *Epidemics and Mortality in Early Modern Japan*.

Japanese Measles Epidemic of 1753

Epidemic of measles that invaded all of Japan, from southwest to northeast, over an eight-month period in 1753.

It began on the island of Kyushu in April and by the summer had moved east to the cities of Kyoto and Osaka. Edo (Tokyo) was severely affected during the summer and fall months and recorded high mortality. An examination of some local temple records in the Sendai region reveals that both adults and children succumbed to the measles epidemic in large numbers between August and October. The epidemic was so widespread it even reached the northernmost island of Hokkaido by fall. Hokkaido, usually less threatened by measles epidemics than its bigger neighboring island of Honshu, also recorded many fatalities during this epidemic.

Further reading: Jannetta, *Epidemics and Mortality in Early Modern Japan*.

Japanese Measles Epidemic of 1776 Epidemic of measles that spread throughout the country, following the traditional southwest to northeast route of most measles epidemics (see JAPANESE MEASLES EPIDEMIC OF 1753).

The city of Osaka reported the epidemic in the third month of 1776. Later that month, Edo (Tokyo) was affected, and measles continued to rage there until the start of autumn. The death records from the Sendai and Hida regions indicate that the disease was in epidemic form here between the sixth and eighth months. Temple records from six Sendai temples also point to heavy mortality in that area. Seven Ogenji villages recorded nine deaths due to measles during 1776. We know that even Hokkaido (northernmost of the four main islands of Japan) was invaded in 1776, but no further details are available.

Further reading: Jannetta, *Epidemics and Mortality in Early Modern Japan.*

Japanese Measles Epidemic of 1803 Nationwide epidemic, raging during the Tokugawa era in Japan between the spring and fall of 1803. The measles infection was introduced into the country by a Korean ship, either through the port of Nagasaki or Tsushima island. Following the traditional dissemination pattern of most measles epidemics (see JAPANESE MEASLES EPIDEMIC OF 1730–31; JAPANESE MEASLES EPIDEMIC OF 1776) in the country, this one also moved from southwest Japan to the densely populated centers of Honshu island and its interior and then to the northeast.

The epidemic peaked in Nagasaki in the spring and then raged in Osaka over the next two months. In Edo (Tokyo), the epidemic started slowly but suddenly gained in intensity in May and affected almost everybody. The province of Hida was invaded around April, and Ogenji and Sendai provinces a month later. The epidemic continued for three to four months in Ogenji. In Sendai province, there was a marked rise in fatalities during the following two months.

One of the more severe epidemics of measles (see JAPANESE MEASLES EPIDEMIC OF 1862) in Japanese history, it was widely described in contemporary Tokugawa literature. These accounts outlined the symptoms of the disease and highlighted some of its observed complications. They also noted that many of the fatalities resulted from these complications rather than from the disease itself.

Further reading: Jannetta, *Epidemics and Mortality in Early Modern Japan.*

Japanese Measles Epidemic of 1823–24 Epidemic disease generally believed to be measles, prevalent in parts of Japan in 1823–24 (see JAPANESE MEASLES EPIDEMIC OF 1803).

There are conflicting accounts of when the epidemic actually began. Some say it began during the eleventh month of 1823 in western Japan. It is not clear when Edo (Tokyo) was first invaded, but measles apparently raged there between the fourth and sixth month of 1824. Some believe it began even earlier. According to the *Buko nenpyo* (Japanese chronicle of events in Edo during the Tokugawa period, 1603–1867), it lingered in Edo until the autumn.

In the Sendai region, there was a dramatic rise in mortality in some areas during the seventh and eighth months. Records indicate the prevalence of a measles epidemic of great magnitude in the northern extremes of the region. There is no mention of the epidemic in local records of the Hida and Ogenji areas. The outbreak there may have been a mild one. Some scholars believe that the disease involved may not have been measles but another similar disease. Whatever the illness, it was clearly an imported epidemic with an uneven impact across the country.

Further reading: Jannetta, *Epidemics and Mortality in Early Modern Japan.*

Japanese Measles Epidemic of 1862 Most devastating epidemic of measles in Japanese history, affecting an estimated 63 percent of the population. Like the Japanese Measles Epidemic of 1803 (q.v.), this one also apparently entered Japan on a foreign ship docked at the port of Nagasaki. It began during February of 1862.

Within the next two months, the epidemic traveled to Kyoto and Osaka. Edo (Tokyo) was the next city to be affected; the epidemic lingered there for several months and even Shogun Iemochi (Japan's military ruler) was not spared the infection. The city of Sendai reported its first cases in the sixth month, but the disease spread rapidly into the surrounding areas and peaked two months later. Measles also invaded Hida around this time, causing heavy mortalities in the region. While Ogenji sources do not actually mention the presence of a measles epidemic, they do record a noticeable rise in fatalities among the younger population during this period.

As the epidemic traveled north through the country, it affected both the young and the old and dislocated normal community life. The previous measles epidemic, a relatively mild one, had struck 26 years earlier; the long interval no doubt explains why the 1862 epidemic came down heavily on those below 26 years of age. It was the last measles epidemic recorded during Japan's Tokugawa period (1603–1867).

Further reading: Jannetta, *Epidemics and Mortality in Early Modern Japan.*

Japanese Rubella Epidemic of 1684

Perhaps the first identified rubella (German measles) epidemic of the Tokugawa period (1603–1867). The epidemic struck Nagasaki during the fourth and fifth months of 1684, and more than 7,000 people reportedly died in the city as a result. Apparently, rubella also caused many deaths in Kyushu and Chugoku. It spread to Naniwa and Kyoto in the sixth and seventh months. In Kyoto, residents took to the streets in the evening waving hand-made dolls and beating drums in an effort to drive away the disease. The epidemic claimed the lives of over 1,000 traders in Sakai. Thereafter, the disease reached Kanto and Nagoya (mid-July), where many fell sick but generally recovered over a three- to five-day period. Rubella then spread to Omi, Settsu, Mino, Mikawa, and Edo (Tokyo).

Rubella, a mild eruptive viral disease usually of childhood or early adulthood, was not considered serious until it was discovered that rubella early in pregnancy could cause congenital birth defects in the baby (see AUSTRALIAN RUBELLA EPIDEMIC OF 1938–41). One attack confers lifelong immunity.

There were two more rubella epidemics during Japan's Tokugawa period—in 1779 and 1835.

Further reading: Jannetta, *Epidemics and Mortality in Early Modern Japan*; McGrew, *Encyclopedia of Medical History.*

Japanese Smallpox Epidemic of A.D. 735–37

Devastating epidemic of great historical importance, killing four brothers of the powerful Fujiwara family, which virtually ruled Japan; it paved the way for the spread of Buddhism in the country. A Japanese fisherman shipwrecked on the Korean coast developed smallpox on his return to the island of Kyushu (in southwest Japan) late in A.D. 735. This started a series of severe outbreaks that soon reached the main island, Honshu, and peaked around the capital in A.D. 737. Nara (home of the Fujiwaras) was particularly hard hit, losing many of its 500,000 citizens.

The third known smallpox epidemic to have hit Japan, it spread rapidly throughout the country, causing widespread destruction among all classes of society and disrupting day-to-day activities at the individual and governmental level. As the epidemic continued to rage, the surviving farmers became too sick to plant new crops, and this led to severe famine. The farmers were granted tax relief while prisoners were given amnesty. For a while, people in the worst ravaged areas were supplied with food and medicine. Eventually, many government officials were also afflicted.

The epidemic awakened religious fervor in the public. As a peace offering, Emperor Shomu, a Buddhist, ordered the erection of a monastery and a seven-storied pagoda in each of Japan's 71 provinces. Meanwhile, the Shinto priests sought to blame the epidemic on the new religion (Buddhism) taking root in the country. As a last resort, Shomu announced that he was building a massive statue of Gautama Buddha. The bronze and gold statue, one of the largest in the world, was finally completed in A.D. 748. The epidemic was followed by two more epidemics in the same century (in 763 and in 790).

Further reading: Sansom, *A History of Japan to 1334*; Brinkley, *A History of the Japanese People*; Jannetta, *Epidemics and Mortality in Early Modern Japan*; Hopkins, *Princes and Peasants: Smallpox in History.*

Japanese Smallpox Epidemics of the Eighth and Ninth Centuries A.D.

Smallpox epidemics about which few details are available (see JAPANESE SMALLPOX EPIDEMIC OF A.D. 735–37).

The disease in A.D. 790 apparently infected everyone under 30 years of age in Nara, Japan's ancient capital in west-central Honshu. The disease was thought to have been imported from China, perhaps via Japanese merchants trading at China's seaports, many of which had suffered frequent epidemics during this period. As in the Japanese Smallpox Epidemic of A.D. 735–37, this outbreak also affected the rest of the country, leading to high mortality. In A.D. 814, Japan was invaded by another smallpox epidemic, which followed a dissemination pattern similar to that of the massive epidemic of A.D. 735–37. Smallpox was first reported from the Japanese port of Dazaifu, where it apparently arrived either from China or from Korea. From Dazaifu, it traveled along the coast of the Inland Sea (between Honshu and Shikoku islands) up to the Eastern Mountain Route (Tosando). Fatalities there reportedly included nearly half the population. The southernmost island of Kyushu, already ravaged by famine, was the worst hit by the epidemic; its peasants suffered terribly.

Smallpox again struck Japan during the second month of A.D. 853. According to a chronicler, it affected residents of the capital (Nara) and the provinces surrounding the Kinki region on Honshu Island. He referred to many fatalities during this epidemic.

Further reading: Farris, *Population, Disease, and Land in Early Japan.*

Japanese Smallpox Epidemics of the Tenth Century A.D.

Series of smallpox epidemics of varying intensity that ravaged Japan during the tenth century.

The first epidemic of the century struck in A.D. 915 and must have been a major outbreak, because a grand purification ceremony was held and Buddhist prayers chanted to try and ward off the disaster. Japan's Emperor Daigo was infected too; this perhaps prompted the introduction of strict containment measures. He ordered that the people be absolved of all unpaid tributes due in kind and from paying their taxes. He even forgave them half of their yearly quota of forced labor.

Little is known about the second epidemic, except that it invaded Japan in A.D. 925. Perhaps it was a relatively mild outbreak.

Smallpox appeared again in epidemic form in A.D. 947. Among those who suffered during this onslaught were the former emperor, Suzaku, and the current emperor, Murakami. Provincial authorities were urged to pay obeisance at nearby Shinto temples and pray for the health of the emperors.

The next three epidemics occurred in A.D. 974, 993, and 998. The *I Shinho*, a Japanese medical book published in A.D. 982, reveals that the practice of isolating smallpox patients in special hospitals was introduced during this period. Apparently, Japanese physicians also recommended that red cloths be hung in the sick-room and also wrapped around the patient as an important step in the cure of the disease.

Improved travel conditions between China and Japan may have been responsible for the sudden increase in the frequency of epidemics during this century. See also JAPANESE SMALLPOX EPIDEMIC OF A.D. 735–37.

Further reading: Hopkins, *Princes and Peasants: Smallpox in History.*

Japanese Syphilis Epidemic of 1512 Japan's first recorded epidemic of syphilis. Syphilis, unknown in Japan until this time (1512), was apparently introduced into the country by Chinese traders/pirates arriving at Nagasaki.

According to the *Gekkai-roku*, a Japanese medical treatise, syphilis was present in epidemic form in 1512. In this and in other contemporary works, the disease was referred to as the "T'ang Sore" (the Chinese were called "men of Tang" since contact between the two countries was established during the T'ang dynasty), the "Liu Chiu Sore" (named for the islands between Japan and Taiwan where the disease was believed to have originated), or the "Chinese ulcer." A few decades later, it became known as *karakasa* (Chinese pleasure disease). During the epidemic (ninth year of the Eisho era), people were described as suffering from oozing ulcers and pustules all over the body. Writing in 1585, a Jesuit priest

pointed out that in Japan, unlike in Europe, syphilis was not regarded as an affliction to be ashamed of but as a disease like any other.

Syphilis, a chronic venereal disease affecting both men and women, is caused by the spirochete *Treponema pallidum*, which is transmitted by sexual contact, including kissing (uncommonly). Within two to three weeks, a slow-growing chancre appears at the site of contact. It usually disappears with or without treatment within two months but not before the organism has penetrated the lymphatic system. The second stage is marked by the eruption of mild to oozing skin lesions, which may disappear within weeks or persist for a year or more. The person continues to be infectious during the subsequent latent phase even though no external lesions are visible. In severe or untreated cases, syphilis can cause major damage to the nervous, cardiovascular, and other key systems.

It is not clear whether the sixteenth century outbreaks of syphilis were the result of the organism's first contact with a susceptible population or whether syphilis was an ancient disease that erupted briefly into widespread epidemics during the sixteenth century before settling back into a chronic state.

Further reading: Quétel, *History of Syphilis;* Bollet, *Plagues and Poxes: The Rise and Fall of Epidemic Disease.*

Javanese (Indonesian) Plague of 1910–14 Demographically relatively minor as an epidemic of plague, but noted for galvanizing Indonesia's public health services into action.

Plague, apparently unknown in Indonesia until 1910, was imported into the Javanese port of Surabaya by a cargo ship transporting rice from Burma. The first cases were noticed in November 1910 in Turen village, Malang district; by year's end, 17 human casualties were reported. The town of Karanglo was next in line of infection, and very soon (March 1911) all of the areas in Malang were reporting cases of plague. Spreading also to Kediri and Surabaya, the disease claimed 2,000 lives in 1911. Moving slowly from east to west along the island's volcanic zone in 1912, it quickly infected Java's eastern interior section. Fearing mass devastation if the epidemic spilled out over the rest of the island, Java's European (Dutch) government swung into action.

Travelers in the affected areas were suddenly confronted by road blocks at all the major intersections, where they and their belongings were forced to submit to disinfection. The findings, which were sent to a laboratory for analysis, revealed the presence mainly of common parasites and, very rarely, of rat fleas. The government also ordered the quarantining of victims, evacuation of villages, and rat-proofing of all houses in the affected areas.

Despite these efforts, the plague infection gradually moved toward central and western Java in 1913 and fatalities climbed. The cities of Surakarta and Madura reported cases, brought in by cargo or travelers. As the death toll rose, the need for a coordinated prevention and containment strategy became apparent. Until late in 1914, three different agencies—the Civil Medical Service, the local government, and the Technical Service—had been involved in the anti-plague campaign. In January 1915, the governor general combined the three agencies to form the Special Plague Service, authorizing it to take full control of the anti-plague campaign. Headquartered in the city of Malang, the service was declared to be autonomous in plague-ridden areas.

Already the disease had claimed 15,000 victims in Java and the new service promptly announced several new measures. It ordered that suspected cases be reported immediately and that a victim's funeral be delayed to allow a postmortem to confirm the diagnosis. Thereafter, burial was to be undertaken quickly, and the family members moved to a temporary shelter so that they and their clothing could be disinfected. Thatched roofs were replaced with tiles, and rafters were redesigned to discourage rats from building nests in them. Trained health workers were sent to live in the villages so they could serve as trusted contacts for the local population.

These measures, it seemed, were effective. By the end of 1915, East Java's reported mortality figures were one third of what they had been in 1914. Total mortality from plague continued to decline even though small outbreaks were reported from Surakarta (1,406 victims), Rembang, Semarang, and Yogyakarta over the next few years. Plague incidence once again rose to epidemic levels during 1930–34 (see JAVANESE (INDONESIAN) PLAGUE OF 1932–34).

Further reading: Owen, ed., *Death and Disease in Southeast Asia.*

Javanese (Indonesian) Plague of 1932–34

Severe epidemic of plague, generally considered the third and final phase of a massive outbreak that began with the Javanese Plague of 1910–14 (q.v.).

When plague first broke out in 1910, it did so in the eastern part of the island of Java. During the second and relatively milder phase of the epidemic, between 1920 and 1927, central Java was the main focus and 8,000 to 10,000 deaths were reported annually. With the third phase (1932–34), it hit West Java; the province of Priangan (where plague incidence had been slowly rising) bore the worst of the onslaught. The reported death toll for 1932 was 4,366

persons, and in 1933 it soared to over 15,000. In 1934, 23,267 cases of plague were reported; the death toll for that year was a staggering 23,239 persons. Case mortality figures during this epidemic were very high; of every 10,000 victims, less than two survived the disease.

Most of the outbreaks were of the bubonic variety; only six percent to eight percent were pneumonic. The dense population and salubrious mountain climate of Priangan apparently aided the rapid spread of the disease in the province.

The Plague Service, established in 1915, was unprepared and unable to cope with a disaster of this magnitude. Thus, more people died of the plague in Priangan during 1933–35 than were affected by the disease in all of East Java during 1910–39. Troubled by serious economic problems, the service also faced tremendous opposition in many areas, particularly because of the spleen-puncture method used to determine plague deaths. Some refused the procedure, while others secretly buried plague victims. The intelligence unit of the service was bolstered by additional manpower to enable it to find and report new cases. A newly developed live-plague vaccine, found to be more effective than that used earlier in central Java, was finally sanctioned for use in a mass-inoculation campaign beginning January 1935. More than two million people were inoculated in that year alone. Over the next few years, several million people were revaccinated. This new strategy helped slow down and eventually arrest the spread of the disease in Java.

Further reading: Owen, ed., *Death and Disease in Southeast Asia*; Gregg, *Plague: An Ancient Disease in the Twentieth Century*; Pollitzer, *Plague.*

Javanese (Indonesian) Typhoid Epidemic of 1846–50

Massive epidemic that swept through the Indonesian island of Java, leaving scarcely anyone unscathed by typhoid fever.

The years 1844 and 1845 were particularly disastrous for most of the residencies (administrative divisions) in Java. Harvest failures and the ensuing food shortages were widespread. The misery was further compounded during the second half of 1845 by heavy rains and flooding, which destroyed the crops in seven residencies. The situation was repeated in the early months of 1846. Conditions were thus ripe for the outbreak of an epidemic of typhoid fever (an acute, infectious disease).

The illness was first noticed in the mountainous inland zone. An official report for the month of February 1846 referred to the disease as prevalent in Kedu. By June it had flared into an epidemic; by the end of 1846, it had already invaded three neighboring residencies and Surakarta, all of them already reeling from the natural disasters of famine and/or flooding. The epidemic spread to eight residencies in 1847. In 1848, six residencies were still suffering from the disease.

Of those who were infected, 30 percent died in 1846, 47 percent in 1847, and 41 percent in 1848. Despite a satisfactory rice harvest in 1848, the epidemic continued on its course that year and the year after. In eastern Semarang, hard hit by typhoid fever in 1846, 1847, and 1848, harvest failures and famine struck again in 1849. People tried escaping into adjacent provinces, taking the cycle of shortages and epidemics with them. By 1850, the typhoid epidemic suddenly subsided.

Further reading: Owen, ed., *Death and Disease in Southeast Asia.*

Joachim's Army Typhus Epidemic of 1542

Outbreak of typhus fever that killed many of the 55,000 soldiers in the army led by Joachim, Margrave of Brandenburg, before they could even engage the enemy—Turkish forces that had occupied the city of Buda (later Budapest) since the preceding summer.

Control of Hungary had been a goal for Ottoman Sultan Suleiman I (the Magnificent) since his accession in 1520. After the Turks defeated the Hungarians at Mohacs in 1526—a battle at which the Hungarian king lost his life—the country was plunged into civil war. Two rivals now claimed the throne: John Zápolya, elected by the majority of the Hungarian nobles, and Ferdinand I of Austria, a Habsburg and the brother of Charles V, the Holy Roman emperor. The two factions were locked in a power struggle for a

dozen years; in 1538 they reached a compromise that nevertheless did not hold after Zápolya's death two years later.

The Ottoman sultan encouraged the disunity, even to the point of concluding separate alliances with both sides, since a strife-torn Hungary limited Habsburg power in eastern Europe and allowed the Turks to push northward. Finally, in 1541, Suleiman I decided that the time was right to strike at Buda. Claiming he came to protect the rights of Zápolya's infant son and chosen successor, the sultan marched to the capital and occupied it, capturing much of central Hungary as well.

Hungarians and Habsburgs now put aside their rivalry in an attempt to drive the invaders out of Buda. Both sides contributed soldiers, equipment, and financial support for an army to be led by Joachim. The preparations were in vain, since typhus fever struck down the imperial forces before the Turks could. Also known as "Hungarian disease," typhus had probably become endemic in the country after being brought there from Asia Minor by successive Turkish campaigns. In the 1542 epidemic the Germans suffered more heavily than did the Hungarians, many of whom had likely been exposed to the disease before and had the temporary immunity it confers. In any case, the imperial troops withdrew from Buda, carrying typhus to the rest of Europe. The Hungarian capital was left in Turkish hands, where it remained for over a hundred years.

Further reading: Prinzing, *Epidemics Resulting from Wars;* Zinsser, *Rats, Lice and History;* Shaw, *History of the Ottoman Empire and Modern Turkey;* Sinor, *History of Hungary.*

Justinian, Plague of   See PLAGUE OF JUSTINIAN.

K

Kenyan Cholera Epidemic of 1974–75 Outbreak of cholera in southwestern Kenya from December 1974 to April 1975, killing 770 persons out of 2,773 reported infected. The more than 25 percent mortality rate was high for modern times, and exactly what type of precautions were taken in Kenya during the four-month epidemic are not known (antibiotics and an effective vaccine for the serious intestinal disease were then available).

Kisumu, a port town on the northeastern shore of Lake Victoria, reported the epidemic's first cases of cholera, which is caused by a spiral-shaped bacterium *(Vibrio comma)* and is spread by improper or unsanitary disposal of human waste that contaminates drinking water and food (unwashed hands and shared food also play a large part in spreading the disease). Victims complain of severe diarrhea and cramps. The epidemic that began after mid-December 1974, affecting urban and rural people in the Kisumu area, was unrelated to a previous outbreak of cholera in 1970–72 in East Africa (see ASIATIC CHOLERA PANDEMIC OF 1961–75). During those years the disease had diffused into Kenya from several directions, supposedly carried mainly by nomadic herders and trading caravans; by April 1972 this cholera outbreak had ended in Kenya. The 1974–75 epidemic was confined within a 50-mile radius of Kisumu, except for an outbreak occurring to the east in the Kiambu district near Nairobi, Kenya's capital.

The source of the Kisumu cholera infection was not identified, but it is possible it arrived in Kisumu via a traveler from Mecca, where some African Muslim pilgrims contracted it several days before the outbreak in Kisumu. There is also the possibility the epidemic originated from an undiscovered, endemic cholera site in East Africa. During the dryer months in southwestern Kenya (December–March), the organism for cholera may have survived in more or less stagnant water bodies, such as unprotected alkaline water holes located in the rural areas around Kisumu and Kiamba. Also, the concentration of people and the increase in travelers helped spread the disease, which remained endemic in certain African regions after Kenya's epidemic ended in April 1975.

Further reading: Barua and Burrows, eds., *Cholera;* Stock, *African Environment Special Report 3: Cholera in Africa.*

Kenyan Plague of 1941–42 Outburst of bubonic and pneumonic plague that killed 529 persons in the British East African colony of Kenya in 1941 and 1942. Since the disease was first recorded in Kenya in 1902, it had erupted in varied proportions annually (see KILIMANJARO PLAGUE OF 1912).

In January 1941 several cases of plague were reported in the western section of Nairobi, Kenya's capital city, where the disease had long been endemic. There were 340 reported cases of plague (240 of which were fatal) in Nairobi from January 1941 to April 1942. Heavy rainfall and the increase in grain storage—where wild rats, the natural reservoirs of plague, seek food and shelter—helped bring on the epidemic. The disease was easily transferred to human beings through the bite of infective rat fleas, and most of the infections in Nairobi occurred in the unsanitary Indian section of the city; very few Europeans were infected.

The western Kenya town of Kisumu, a port on Lake Victoria and a major center for the grain and cotton seed trade, was also attacked by plague, which especially struck the rundown and overcrowded Indian bazaar area there. The disease also spread to some native villages on western reservations (or reserves) and eastward to the port city of Mombasa on the Indian Ocean. In Mombasa, all of the plague infections were of the pneumonic form, in contrast to those in Nairobi and western Kenya, most of which were of the bubonic form (causing acutely inflamed and painful swellings [buboes] of the lymph nodes). Bubonic plague frequently leads to death from pneumonia (inflammation of the lungs from the inhalation of exhaled droplets from plague patients).

Although morbidity (incidence of disease) and mortality (loss of life) for plague in Mombasa alone are not really known, there were a total of 1,195 plague cases and 289 plague deaths reported outside Nairobi, including cases and deaths in Mombasa. Many persons in infected urban areas and villages were given inoculations of an anti-plague vaccine, and rat control measures were also carried out in these areas. Nairobi and Mombasa remained free of plague from 1943 to 1952, but the rest of Kenya reported 275 infections and 93 fatalities from plague during that time. In 1950 in the village of Rongai in western Kenya, the plague bacillus (*Yersinia pestis* or *Pasteurella pestis*) was found entrenched in wild rodents, which were subject to periodic epizootics and thus a source of infection to human beings.

Further reading: Pollitzer, *Plague;* Simmons et al., *Global Epidemiology.*

Kenyan Relapsing Fever Epidemic of 1945–46

First known epidemic of the louse-borne type of relapsing fever to occur in East Africa, killing about 800 of some 2,000 persons infected in Mombasa and other Kenyan coastal areas, as well as in the hinterland.

Relapsing fever, caused by the microorganism spirochaete, was introduced into Kenya from Seihut, South Arabia, in February 1945; several Arabian dhows (sailing vessels) arrived at Mombasa Island with sick persons on board. British medical authorities in Kenya (then a British colony) diagnosed the illnesses as louse-borne relapsing fever after finding passengers and crew infested with lice; no ticks were found on board the vessels so the tick-borne form of the disease (endemic to East Africa) was not discernible. Despite the dhows being quarantined and the sick isolated on shore, the infection spread into Mombasa and elsewhere.

Two women who had visited an infected man in Mombasa brought the disease home with them to Marjakani in the native reserve; four days later, they became sick with symptoms of high fever, severe headache, aching joints and muscles. By late July 1945 the same symptoms of the disease were noticed by 18 family members and friends of the two women; 14 of them died. At first, because the sick patients in the reserve were jaundiced, they were thought to have yellow fever; by August 1945 medical authorities diagnosed the cases as louse-borne relapsing fever.

In September 1945 the disease reached epidemic proportions in Kenya's hinterland, traveling north as far as Vitengeni. It also spread south to Ndavaya and west to Taru, mainly affecting the Giriama and Duruma tribes. In these areas, there were about 1,500 cases and 380 deaths from the disease. Women were infected more frequently than were men and children, apparently because the women customarily slept in the same house as the diseased corpses during the native funerals, which lasted several days (the men and children slept outdoors). Nonetheless, there was a higher mortality rate for men than women, due to the higher incidence of the disease among older men, who were more louse-infested and less resistant to the disease. It appeared that the disease moved along trade routes and was particularly carried by trucks and the railways.

Kenya's louse-borne relapsing fever epidemic was linked to an epidemic of the disease that originated and was centered in Libya in late 1942. From Libya, the disease had moved northwest to Tunisia by October 1943 and west to Algeria by November 1944 and Morocco by February 1945, and east to Asyut (Assiout) on the Nile in Upper Egypt by October 1944. Spreading to the Middle East, the disease reached Seihut on Arabia's southern coast, from where it was carried to Kenya in 1945. (Reportedly, by 1946, more than 125,000 persons had been infected with the louse-borne relapsing fever.) Some of the control measures initiated in Kenya and other places were the quick removal of the sick to hospitals, boiling clothes to kill lice, suspension of native funeral ceremonies, discouragement of travel, and disinfestation of louse infested houses.

Further reading: Davies et al., "An Epidemic of Louse-Borne Relapsing Fever in Kenya"; Hartwig and Patterson, *Disease in African History.*

Kenyan Smallpox Epidemic of 1897–99

Catastrophic outbreak of smallpox that infected untold thousands of natives in the British East Africa protectorate. In some Kenyan regions, particularly in the interior, the fatality rate was higher than 40 percent, due to the lack of immunity to the disease as well as the limited amount of Edward Jenner's smallpox vaccine available.

Smallpox first appeared in Kenya in the southern coastal city of Mombasa about 1300, apparently arriving aboard trading vessels from India, China, or Arabia. Other parts of Kenya remained free of smallpox until the 1800's, when the Arab-dominated slave trade brought infected slaves into the newly established colonies in East Africa. The construction of the first railroad in East Africa (1896–1901) played an important role in the transmission of this highly contagious viral disease into Kenya's interior. As tracks were laid from Mombasa inland to Lake Victoria and Uganda, the smallpox scourge was brought to these remote regions.

A powerful and militant East African tribe in the interior, the Masai, had managed to escape the smallpox infection until this time. The Masai, who lived off the milk, blood, and meat of their cattle, had earlier (about 1893) been severely weakened by a terrible outbreak of rinderpest (also called cattle plague), an acute viral intestinal disease of cattle and sometimes sheep and goats and wild game animals. Smallpox struck the weakened Masai and wiped out about three-quarters of them by 1899.

About the same time, another tribe of pastoralists, the Kikuyu, who lived in the remote highlands north of Nairobi (Kenya's capital), were seriously attacked by the disease; in the Kiambu district, the mortality rate among the Kikuyus was 70 percent. From the Kikuyus, the virus spread south into the German protectorate of Tanganyika (Tanzania), and those Kikuyus who survived the epidemic fled to Fort Hall and elsewhere to escape the horrible ravages of smallpox (disfigurement and blindness). By 1902, many of the Kikuyu had still not returned to the Kiambu highlands; abandonment of their land may have made it easier for the British to settle this region.

In 1898 the epidemic struck Mombasa, whose native African population was more seriously infected than the European and Indian populations during the following year. By 1899, half a dozen native villages in northern Kenya were gravely depopulated, including the Rendile tribe, which was nearly exterminated by smallpox. Since then Kenya has alternated sharply between outbreaks and periods free of smallpox; in 1943–45 the populace suffered many infections and a 31 percent mortality rate.

Further reading: Hallett, *Africa Since 1875;* Hopkins, *Princes and Peasants: Smallpox in History.*

Kenyan Typhoid Epidemic of 1954

Severe outbreak of typhoid fever that killed 103 persons out of 870 who were infected in the scrub desert region of southern Kenya in East Africa.

Typhoid fever was endemic in Kenya before 1954; the incidence of the disease ranged between 300 and 500 cases each year, with an annual fatality rate of 10 percent to 20 percent. In January 1954 cases of typhoid were reported in an isolated community inhabited by wandering, native African tribes in an outlying district of Nairobi, Kenya's capital. The water supply in the area, which the natives regularly used, was apparently contaminated and impure. Poor sanitary habits allowed for the spread of the disease in the region. The typhoid bacillus, *Salmonella typhi,* is found in water and food contaminated by urine or feces of a patient; it lives in the human digestive system and is carried from place to place by human beings. Infected persons develop fever, lassitude, loss of appetite, muscular pains, constipation more commonly than diarrhea, and delirium.

Overcrowded Kenyans helped spread the disease during the ongoing Mau Mau Uprising (1952–56) in the country. (The Mau Mau, a secret organization led by Kikuyu and other black tribesmen, carried on a terrorist fight against white settlers to restore the area to the native Africans.) Typhoid grew more serious during the hot, dry months of February and March 1954, and many of those infected, as well as an approximate five percent who were typhoid carriers, brought the disease into Nairobi in April and May. More than a thousand people throughout Kenya contracted typhoid by November 1954. Most of those infected were African natives; the disease's incidence was minimal among Europeans and Asians, who practiced higher standards of hygiene (sanitary processing of food and water; good disposal of human excreta). In addition, many whites and blacks (particularly in the community of about 17,000 where the outbreak originated) had acquired some immunization with a vaccine, given to them at least once, in the months before and during the epidemic, which subsided as medical and sanitary measures were set up.

Further reading: Huckstep, *Typhoid Fever;* Simmons et al., *Global Epidemiology.*

Kilimanjaro Plague of 1912

Epidemic of plague lasting about one month in the small village of Gassenia on the Kenya-Tanzania border, near Mount Kilimanjaro, killing three persons of bubonic plague and 55 of pneumonic plague. Although plague may have originated in Central Africa centuries earlier, it had been absent there for more than 50 years before this outbreak (see PLAGUE PANDEMIC, THIRD).

In 1912, after the plague disease broke out in Nairobi, the capital of Kenya, it spread to the eastern slope of Mount Kilimanjaro (Africa's highest peak) and the village of Gassenia during the spring rainy season. As a result of flea bites, three natives in Gassenia became infected with bubonic plague. Unless persons with bubonic plague are treated medically immediately, they will usually die within three to six days, as did the three natives in Gassenia.

Without an accompanying "bubo" (hard lump), it is difficult to distinguish the feverish symptoms of plague from some other tropical and subtropical diseases. Persons with this form of plague are not infectious to others, unless they come in contact with an open and infected "bubo" (bubo is a Greek word for groin, where many persons are bitten by disease-carrying fleas). Septicaemic plague may also affect victims severely even before bubos have had time to develop, when victims' lungs are invaded by the disease organism.

Basically a disease of wild animals, plague begins with a bacillus that infects fleas. Rats, the best-known animal hosts of plague, are usually responsible for transmitting it into densely packed human populations. While wild rats in Africa and other warm areas of the world live far from human habitation in forests and deserts, when they die with plague, fleas from them seek out the "closest" animal to live on—man's house rats or man himself.

During the first week of the Kilimanjaro epidemic, a woman trained as a nurse came to Gassenia from a neighboring village to help treat those afflicted. She too contracted pneumonic plague, dying shortly thereafter, but not before she had spread the disease to 16 others in her village, all of whom perished along with the 55 in Gassenia; all of them contracted plague from the breath of a sick person, not from a flea bite. Instead of isolating the sick natives in Gassenia, consoling relatives and friends were in direct physical contact with the sick, who coughed out the deadly microorganism, thus infecting others with pneumonic plague, which is highly contagious.

Dr. Richard Lurz, a medical officer of the Imperial German Army who was assigned to Gassenia during the epidemic, published a paper in 1913, claiming that the plague disease was carried by house (black) rats as well as tree (wild) rats native to the region. However, it was not until 1952, when plague was discovered in the Rift Valley in both the house rat and the tree rat, that the theory that there had never been a plague transmitted by wild rodents in Central Africa was discarded. Dr. Lurz's 1913 report had apparently remained obscure because of the outbreak of World War I.

Further reading: Gregg, *Plague: An Ancient Disease in the Twentieth Century; Oxford Textbook of Medicine.*

Kiribati Measles Epidemics of 1890 and 1936
See GILBERT AND ELLICE ISLANDS MEASLES EPIDEMICS OF 1890 AND 1936.

Korean Cholera Epidemics of 1821–22 and 1895
Two of the many epidemics of cholera that attacked the Korean Peninsula during the nineteenth century; 1821 was the beginning of the kingdom of Korea's first major recorded epidemic, an offshoot of the Asiatic Cholera Pandemic of 1817–23 (q.v.). The acute intestinal disease then raging in China (see CHINESE CHOLERA EPIDEMIC OF 1820–22) traveled overland to arrive in Pyongyang at the end of July 1821 and quickly tore through this city, killing more than 1,000 people in a ten-day period. It reached the city of Seoul in August, and by the end of September, cholera had invaded the southern part of the Korean Peninsula, including all the cities in Kyongsang province.

By all accounts, it was a devastating epidemic that apparently killed nine out of every ten people it

struck and left even the medical community helpless; doctors were unable to either treat or prevent the disease even as untold numbers succumbed to it. Across the kingdom, various feasts and ceremonies were conducted by the superstitious king and commoners alike in an effort to appease the gods. The epidemic subsided briefly with the onset of winter. However, it resurfaced in April across Seoul and once again spread through the country. In mid-August, it reached Japan (see JAPANESE CHOLERA EPIDEMIC OF 1822).

Until the 1870s, epidemic cholera often visited Korea, usually in conjunction with visits to China and Japan. Cholera outbreaks were also recorded in 1881, 1885, 1886, 1890, and 1891 in Korea, where a significant epidemic took place as a consequence of the Sino-Japanese War raging in neighboring Manchuria during 1895. Cholera spread slowly from Manchuria across the Korean Peninsula to Seoul, where it caused an extremely severe outbreak. At the height of the six-week-long epidemic in Seoul (population 220,000), about 300 people died of cholera every day. Overall, Seoul's death toll exceeded 5,000. The city's first cholera hospital was shut down after 75 percent of the first 135 patients died of the disease. Another hospital reported a 35 percent mortality rate among its 173 cholera patients. It is not known how many people were struck by the disease in Korea, but it is estimated that at least 300,000 people lost their lives during this epidemic.

Further reading: Magner, "Diseases of the Premodern Period in Korea."

Korean Hemorrhagic Fever Epidemic of 1951–54
Strange, new disease—hemorrhagic fever with renal syndrome (HFRS)—that struck numerous United Nations (UN) troops fighting in Korea.

The infection was first observed in the spring of 1951 when many UN soldiers lay prostrate with a flushed face, chills, high fever, anorexia, severe headaches, muscle and joint pains, vomiting, and varied hemorrhagic symptoms. During the disease's second stage, the soldiers' condition suddenly worsened accompanied by shock, cardiovascular instability, and renal failure. Physicians, confounded by these symptoms, realized that this was indeed a new and unfamiliar disease.

Also known as Epidemic Hemorrhagic Fever (EHF) or Far Eastern Hemorrhagic Nephroso Nephritis or "Hemorrhagic Fever," prefaced by the geographical locality of its occurrence, the infection was later found to be one of a group of hemorrhagic fevers occurring in many areas of the Eurasian land mass. The Hantaan virus, which caused the 1951–54 Korean epidemic, is transmitted to man through the excretions and aerosols of healthy rodent carriers—in this case, the wild mouse *Apodemus agrarius*.

Nearly 1,000 UN soldiers were attacked by this virus by the end of 1951; 80 of them died as a result. All through 1952 another 1,000 cases were treated; soldiers of every nationality were affected. Cases were reported even after the hostilities had ended (the Korean War, 1950–53). For instance, in 1953 and 1954 there were another 1,000 cases, bringing the total number of cases among the United Nations forces to 3,000.

To facilitate treatment and research, the United States Army Medical Service set up a Hemorrhagic Fever Center near Uijongbu, South Korea. Suspected cases were airlifted to this center for diagnosis and treatment. Meanwhile, the disease was also spreading southward through civilian populations, affecting, in some cases, even children under ten years of age. When the South Korean Army assumed charge of the Demilitarized Zone after the war, HFRS was the major infectious disease it had to contend with. An HFRS epidemic was reported from China in 1980–81.

Further reading: Mackenzie, ed., *Viral Diseases in South-East Asia and the Western Pacific.*

Korean Hepatitis Epidemic of 1950–51
Outbreak of infectious hepatitis among United States troops at the beginning of the Korean War (1950–53).

Hepatitis was present among the Americans, albeit in a scattered form, during the first few months after their landing in June 1950. The troops moved north, and in November the disease began to spread rapidly. The virus was already widespread in the Korea civilian population through which the highly susceptible Americans moved. In December came a retreat, and subsequently the troops gathered just below the 38th parallel. Within the crowded and insanitary military camps and under combat conditions, hepatitis quickly assumed epidemic proportions. During the first three months of 1951, 573 sick soldiers were evacuated from their infantry units and transported to a hepatitis center in Kyoto, Japan. The epidemic peaked in February 1951 when 229 cases were reported; hospital admissions were the highest this month—35 per 1,000 troops.

Even at the height of this epidemic, the hepatitis cases were evenly distributed among all infantry companies; 65 percent to 70 percent of the companies that were infected had only one case each month. In an effort to control the spread of the disease, the authorities began treating the water supply with chlorine in April 1951. By then, however, disease incidence was already declining and continued to decline further during the rest of the year, as did the intensity of military activities. Hepatitis was not a major problem again until 1954, when cases began to increase.

Further reading: Hartman et al., eds., *Hepatitis Frontiers;* Havens Jr., "Viral Hepatitis."

Kumasi Plague of 1924–25
See ASHANTI PLAGUE OF 1924–25.

L

Libyan Plague of the First Century A.D. Earliest certain instance of bubonic plague in the Mediterranean world. The fourth-century A.D. Greek physician Oribasius quotes an account by Rufus of Ephesus that describes the epidemic. Rufus (a Greek anatomist) refers to a treatise by Dioscorides and Posidonius, probably Alexandrian doctors who recorded an epidemic they witnessed early in the first century A.D. Despite the fragmentary textual tradition, the diagnosis of the outbreak is clear. According to Rufus, the two Alexandrians observed not only acute fever, intense pain, agitation, and delirium, but also large, hard, non-suppurating buboes (swellings) that developed behind the knees and around the elbows as well as "in the usual places." Most of those afflicted with the "pestilential" buboes died.

Rufus also tells us that similar buboes were mentioned by Dionysius Curtus, who is hard to identify but who may have practiced medicine in Alexandria in the third century B.C. If that date is correct, bubonic plague would be older than the Christian era. In any case, the appearance of the plague in Libya—and in Egypt and Syria, where Rufus says that buboes were also common—makes sense. All three areas were crossed by travel and trade routes that extended throughout Africa, Asia, and Europe. Such commercial centers could easily bring together black rats, bacteria, and humans—the combination needed for bubonic plague.

Further reading: Simpson, *A Treatise on Plague*; Patrick, "Disease in Antiquity: Ancient Greece and Rome"; Crawfurd, *Plague and Pestilence in Literature and Art.*

Livorno-Lucca Yellow Fever Epidemic of 1804 Serious outbreak of yellow fever that infected hundreds of persons in two Italian Tuscan cities. A disease of warm climates, yellow fever was carried by infected *Aëdes aegypti* mosquitoes aboard trading vessels from Havana, Cuba, in the summer of 1804. Ships' water supplies, good breeding grounds for the mosquitoes, made long distance transmission of the disease from the Caribbean possible. Occasional cases of yellow fever in Italian ports had occurred during the 1700s, when trade with the Caribbean islands and Africa was rapidly expanding, but no grave outbreak was reported until 1804 in Livorno (Leghorn), a seaport in western Italy on the Ligurian Sea.

Authorities believe the disease came either on a Spanish ship with mosquitoes directly from Havana or aboard an Italian ship that traded earlier at Barcelona, Spain, where infective mosquitoes had arrived and slipped aboard various vessels. Livorno recorded about 700 to 800 cases of yellow fever, of which at least 70 percent were fatal. Italian physicians were shocked and could do little for the sick. They were, however, accustomed to dealing with malaria, another mosquito-borne infection, and so treated their patients with traditional purges and bleedings; quarantine and other measures were also taken to avoid contact with victims of the fever.

Before Livorno's epidemic came to an end with the cooler weather in the late fall, the disease had made its way inland to Lucca, an important commercial city about 12 miles north of Livorno. It infected and claimed about the same number of people in Lucca in 1804 as it had in Livorno. There is no substantiation that other Italian cities in the region became infected at the time.

Further reading: McGrew, *Encyclopedia of Medical History*; Scott, *A History of Tropical Medicine.*

Londonderry and Dundalk Typhus and Dysentery Epidemics of 1689 Major outbreaks of epidemic typhus fever and dysentery in Ireland at Londonderry and at a military encampment near Dundalk; caused high mortality among both townsfolk and soldiers during the campaigning of the English and Irish armies in 1689.

Epidemic typhus fever is transmitted from person to person by the human body louse and therefore thrives when personal and public hygiene are absent, such as in poverty-stricken urban areas, in cramped and filthy quarters in ships and prisons, and in times of war. Londonderry, a town in the north of Ireland, was besieged by Catholic Jacobite troops for 105 days in the spring and early summer of 1689. Of approximately 30,000 inhabitants and a garrison of 7,020 Protestant soldiers, an estimated 10,000 people died during the siege, some from the effects of battle but many more of disease, mostly the "flux," or dysentery, and typhus, also called the "Irish ague." It is recorded that the besiegers of Londonderry remarked upon the extraordinary odor emitted from the 500 or so ill people who were forced to leave the city on July 2, an indication of typhus fever, which produces in its victims a quite sickening smell. The besieging army, exposed to cold and wet weather, also suffered many thousands of losses from dysentery, "French pox" (syphilis), and typhus fever.

In the second major instance of "camp fever" during the hostilities of 1689, Protestant troops encamped near the town of Dundalk on the east coast of Ireland were ravaged by typhus in August, September, and October. The marshy camping ground and the cold, rainy weather added to the miseries of the men and to the spread of the disease. When the camping site was moved in the hopes of escaping infection, the sick were left behind. When the commanding officers finally decided to abandon the campaign, the sick were loaded onto wagons, from which those who died along the way were tossed off onto the roads. Marching soldiers who were ill simply fell out of rank and died by the roadside. Several of the ships that received the sick to remove them to Belfast became true ghost ships, floating in the bay at the town of Carrickfergus with every man on board dead. It was noticed that many of the corpses were covered with lice, an observation that at the time indicated lack of personal cleanliness but was not linked by observers in any way with the disease that killed them.

The disaster at Dundalk, which destroyed approximately 6,000 men of an army of 12,000, was probably the most virulent and mortal attack of typhus fever ever recorded in British military history.

Further reading: Creighton, *A History of Epidemics in Britain*; Shepherd, *Ireland's Fate*.

London Plague of 1499–1500   First major epidemic in England in the sixteenth century, and in fact the only mortality crisis caused by plague until 1563; began in London in June 1499. The contemporary English chronicler Raphael Holinshed writes that "men died in manie places verie sore; but specialle and most of all in the citie of London," so evidently, although concentrated mostly in London, this visitation of plague reached other parts of England. The epidemic lasted through the winter of 1500, indicating either a mild winter—this would permit plague-carrying rat-fleas, which hibernate in cold weather, to remain active—or the presence of pneumonic plague, which attacks the lungs and is transmitted from person to person, mostly in low temperatures, through plague bacilli emitted through sneezing or coughing.

Although contemporary observers placed the death toll from this epidemic at as much as 30,000 persons, or half the estimated population of London at that time, official city and state records do not reflect that enormous figure. Mortality rates were consistently exaggerated throughout this period of history.

Because English records show that no more than one third of the population die in a plague epidemic, and usually much less, it can be assumed that this outbreak was not quite as drastic as chronicles indicate. Nonetheless, this sickness—assumed to be plague because of the season in which it appeared, but not substantiated through descriptions of symptoms—caused thousands of deaths. Unfortunately, the absence of statistical data, which after 1538 becomes available with the institution of parochial burial records, and the absence of eyewitness accounts by contemporary writers, give us very little information about this important and apparently widespread epidemic.

Further reading: Creighton, *A History of Epidemics in Britain*; Mullet, *The Bubonic Plague and England*; Shrewsbury, *A History of Bubonic Plague in the British Isles*; Slack, *The Impact of Plague in Tudor and Stuart England*.

London Plague of 1563   First major mortality crisis caused by bubonic plague in sixteenth-century London. Perhaps the worst incidence of plague experienced by metropolitan London in its history, the city and its outlying parishes lost an estimated one quarter to one third of their estimated population of 80,000 persons.

The disease erupted in epidemic form in June 1563, and, following the usual pattern of bubonic plague, the death toll rose steadily from July through October and declined in November with the onset of cold weather, when the plague-carrying fleas, which transmit the disease, began to hibernate for the winter. Plague deaths reported in December were in all probability caused by complications and sequelae (aftereffects) due to plague infection acquired earlier rather than fresh cases, and by the end of January deaths from plague ceased altogether. Approximately 1,000 people died of plague weekly in mid-August, 1,600 per week in the second half of September, and 1,800 per week at the peak of its virulence in the first week of October. Altogether the death figure is estimated at about 20,000 for London and its outlying parishes, representing about 85 percent of deaths from all causes in 1563.

Fleeing from a town or city in time of plague was common, especially by wealthier families who had country homes or could otherwise afford the expense of staying elsewhere. When this exodus is taken into account, the proportion of people dying from plague rises to a possible one third of London's population, which is the maximum percentage of a given population bubonic plague killed in the British Isles, according to records.

Parish burial records, upon which knowledge of the plague's effect are primarily based, show clearly the unpredictable and haphazard way bubonic plague attacks a community. Some London parishes were decimated during the epidemic of 1563, while others were barely touched. This demonstrates the relationship between rat-infestation and incidence of plague: the higher the number of plague-infected rats in a given locality, the higher the number of plague-carrying fleas that will desert their dead rodent hosts to get their blood-meal from human beings, and thereby transmit the disease. Epidemiologists do not know, however, what determines the activity of the plague bacillus, *Pasteurella pestis,* within a community of rodents. It is the unpredictable nature of plague—singling out some parishes, or even just a few families within a parish, and leaving others free—that contributed to the terror people felt at the first hint of this disease.

Queen Elizabeth I took strong precautions to protect herself and her court from plague, which posed a constant threat in England throughout her entire reign (1558–1603). When plague broke out in London in 1563 she removed to Windsor Castle, and erected a gallows in the town marketplace where anyone coming from London was to be hanged. She also prohibited goods from London to be brought to Windsor, and although no one had any idea that plague was carried by fleas, this was a wise precaution as it prevented stray fleas imbedded in merchandise from being let loose. Parliament prorogued its meeting from October 1562 to October 1563, an action it took whenever plague was present or its arrival feared.

Measures to stem the epidemic, most of which had become standard by this time, included confinement of the stricken to their homes, airing or burning of garments worn by the sick, cleaning of the streets, and destruction of stray dogs, which were believed to transmit the plague. Plague-infected houses had to be marked by a blue cross, and bonfires, to "consume ye corrupte ayers," were to be set in the streets three times each week at sundown. Plays, fairs, and other public gatherings were prohibited to help pre-vent contagion, a measure that was, unfortunately, of little use for bubonic plague, except in so far as plague-infected fleas—which constituted about 12 percent of any given flea population—might jump from one person to another and bite another victim. Closely packed groups of people were also believed to generate pestilence through the confluence and concentration of foul bodily vapors corrupting the air. In this regard, parts of church windows were removed to create better circulation, and parishioners were encouraged to worship privately at home.

The second half of the sixteenth century, plague-ridden as it was, saw the publication of many translations and original English works explaining causes, suggesting precautionary actions, and recommending cures. A tract entitled *Dialogue against the Fever Pestilence,* which appeared in 1564 in response to the London crisis, is one of the most interesting, containing social commentary that reveals the distrust and contempt many people felt toward surgeons and apothecaries. It also sets forth the basic medical theories of the day, ideas that had been current for centuries. Both corrupt air and immoderate personal habits caused pestilence, and could be anticipated by close attention to cosmological events such as comets and planetary conjunctions. Like many medical writers, the author of this *Dialogue* admonishes every man to be of good cheer so that they might more effectively ward off sickness. A typical plague remedy runs as follows: "Take the best Yellow Aloes, twoo unces, Myrrhe and Saffron, of eche one unce, beate them together in a Morter a good while, putte in a little sweete wine, then roll it up, and of this make five Pilles." Other ingredients in plague recipes included many kinds of herbs, rose water, white vinegar, garlic, walnuts, and eggs.

The plague of 1563 reached far beyond the boundaries of metropolitan London to many areas in the north and south of England. It continued to appear in many towns and villages during the following two years, including Stratford-upon-Avon, where William Shakespeare was born in April of 1564.

Further reading: Mullet, *The Bubonic Plague and England;* Shrewsbury, *A History of Bubonic Plague in the British Isles;* Slack, *The Impact of Plague in Tudor and Stuart England.*

London Plague of 1578 Outbreak of bubonic plague experienced by London in the summer and early fall of 1578. Although virulent enough to cause an estimated 8,000 human deaths, this was only one of several outbreaks that occurred in various parts of England throughout the 1570s. Burial records of London parishes show that in the years 1578 through 1582 deaths from smallpox, measles, and dysentery also reached epidemic proportions.

England's Queen Elizabeth I, having witnessed the enormous destruction that plague caused in London in 1563 (see LONDON PLAGUE OF 1563), issued many orders designed to prevent the disease from spreading and, for those who were already infected, to help ease their suffering. She instructed the College of Physicians to devise ways for providing inexpensive and readily available preventive and curative medicines for use particularly by the poor. Each parish was assigned two female "nurse-keepers" to tend the sick people confined in plague-infected houses, and monetary "plague-relief" was given to the poor.

By 1578 it had become usual for civic authorities to prohibit public assemblies in time of plague to help minimize contagion. In August 1577, in response to a minor outbreak, all plays, which drew large crowds in London, were suspended, and in November "all suche innes, taverns, and ale-houses as are known to have been infected since Michaelmas (29 September) laste" were ordered to be closed. Other measures included the confinement of the sick to their homes and the marking of their houses with blue crosses as a warning to others. Because bubonic plague is transmitted from plague-infected rats to human beings through the bite of fleas carrying the plague bacillus, segregation of the sick was of no use in preventing the spread of the disease, having no effect whatsoever on the movements of the rats. Plague-carrying or "blocked" fleas will sometimes crawl into clothing and bedding, and the queen's orders to dispose of such items used by the stricken could have resulted in the destruction of some of these deadly fleas.

Further steps, taken in other towns as well as in London, included removing refuse, destroying stray animals, and setting bonfires to purify the air, which was thought to carry infection and to enter the body through the pores of the skin.

People gradually became aware that bubonic plague was imported into the British Isles from foreign places, and it is interesting to observe that large outbreaks in the Low Countries and Germany preceded those in Britain. London, as England's busiest port, was especially vulnerable. Always alert to news of plague from abroad, the London authorities placed all ships with their passengers and cargoes under quarantine if they came from a city known to be afflicted with plague. Unfortunately such quarantines were totally ineffective, because any plague-infected rats on board would scurry off the ships and enter the city as soon as the ship docked.

Several new medicinal and homiletic works were published between 1577 and 1580, all containing theories and remedies that had been current for generations. Plague, and pestilence in general, was caused by God's displeasure, by corrupted air, and by the movement of the planets. Moderate personal habits and a cheerful disposition could help ensure good health, and praying was deemed essential. The question of flight in time of plague from both family and civic duty was discussed by several writers, as fleeing from one's town at the first hint of plague had become common, and some considered it a cowardly avoidance of personal and social obligations.

Plague either spread from London or was introduced independently from abroad into Norwich in 1578, where mortality was very high. Plague was active in East Anglia, Cambridgeshire, Hertfordshire, and Essex that year; Newcastle in the north, Salisbury in the south, and Plymouth in the west also suffered badly in 1579. Many other towns, and some London parishes, saw cases of plague during the next several years. Earlier outbreaks during the decade include Cambridge in 1574, Stamford and Hull in 1575, Shrewsbury and the Cornwall moors in 1576, and many parts of the north of England in 1577. In 1592 the disease once more began to seriously threaten the entire country (see LONDON PLAGUE OF 1593).

Further reading: Mullet, *The Bubonic Plague and England*; Shrewsbury, *A History of Bubonic Plague in the British Isles*; Slack, *The Impact of Plague in Tudor and Stuart England*.

London Plague of 1593

Outbreak of bubonic plague that destroyed an estimated 17,000 people out of an approximate population of 150,000 for London and its suburbs. The disease first appeared in London, which had last experienced a major visitation of plague in 1578 (see LONDON PLAGUE OF 1578), in September 1592, causing alarming mortality until cold weather began to diminish the activity of the plague-carrying rat-fleas that cause the disease. After their usual pattern of hibernating for the winter, the fleas broke loose in April 1593, an indication that the weather was unusually mild, as typically the plague season does not begin until midsummer. Deaths reached a peak about the third week of August, continued at the same rate through September, and declined as usual with the onset of frosty weather. Parish burial records demonstrate an especially high mortality in the slum areas around the London docks, the most vulnerable area of any city, where rats were most likely to settle upon landing from the ships that had transported them from plague-infected foreign cities. Packed closely together in dreadful rat-infested hovels, and far less able to flee the city than wealthier citizens, the poor always experienced the highest mortality from plague.

Parish records also reveal the unpredictable nature of bubonic plague, which is due entirely to the density of the rat population in any given area of a city, and how many rats in that population might be infected with plague. Some parishes suffered tremendous losses, while others lost only a few individuals. This apparently haphazard selection (the connection between rats, fleas, and man was not discovered until the early twentieth century) was noted in some parishes. The seemingly capricious character of plague caused serious controversy about the part men should play in attempting to control or avoid disease: Since nothing seemed to protect a person from infection, except good luck, perhaps men should acquiesce to God's will and await their time of death. In contrast, Queen Elizabeth I's privy council ordered that no clergyman or lay person must preach against taking action to prevent the plague. Far from denying divine involvement, however, the queen acknowledged that the nation was being punished with the epidemic in retribution for its sins. The author of *The Haven of Health*, speaking of pestilence in general, wrote "When nature will no longer work, then farewell physic . . . The physician may do his endeavor, but the success is in God," a view that expresses the helplessness people felt despite the measures taken and the medicines prescribed to combat disease. It was also thought uncharitable to refuse to tend the sick for fear of being infected oneself; the loneliness suffered by plague-stricken people is attested to in many surviving documents.

Plague remedies from earlier times circulated widely and new ones were concocted. *A Defensative against the Plague* recommended applying plucked chicken rumps to plague blotches. Queen Elizabeth I had a recipe of sage, rue, elder leaves, red bramble leaves, white wine, and vinegar, while English author Francis Bacon used a confection of cardamom seeds, treacle, and wine.

Dozens of ordinances appeared, some merely reissued from earlier years, some newly devised, such as the order addressed to the head of the Admiralty to prevent the plague from spreading in his fleet, and the order to halt the manufacture of starch because hogs, thought to be infectious, were used in the process. The usual prohibitions against public gatherings were enforced court terms were adjourned, and goods suspected of carrying infection were confiscated. Streets had to be cleared of refuse, bonfires lit to cleanse the infected atmosphere, and segregation of the sick strictly observed. Monetary help was given to the plague-stricken poor. The queen was protected in the usual way by the barring of access to the royal court without special permission and the forbidding of her attendants to visit London and other infected places without a license.

The epidemic abated in London in October 1593, but it had spread during the summer and fall to the counties surrounding the city, through Middlesex to Essex, Hertfordshire, and Buckinghamshire. At Cambridge, which was attacked severely at the end of the year, the plague-sick poor were confined to a pesthouse, while wealthier victims were permitted to remain in their homes. Most of the larger towns in England erected temporary buildings on grounds outside the town to isolate their plague-infected citizens. Unfortunately these measures were useless in preventing the spread of bubonic plague. Tewkesbury, Derby, Leicester, Lichfield, York, and Durham suffered severe outbreaks in 1593 as well. Both 1596 and 1597 saw a resurgence of plague in many places, particularly the Lake District and the north of England, where Durham lost one quarter to one third of its population. Cranbrook and Hastings in the south were fiercely attacked in 1598.

The London plague of 1593 was preceded by many outbreaks in various parts of England from 1590 to 1592, particularly in the southwestern counties. Epidemiologists have concluded that any major outbreak requires the introduction of a fresh strain of the plague bacillus (*Pasteurella pestis*) virulent enough to spread widely through a given population of rats. It is possible that plague entered England through a port in Devon on the southern coast, imported from Portugal, where the disease was epidemic in 1589, engendering the national outbreak that then ensued. Until the twentieth century, this bacillus was indigenous only to India and Asia, and perhaps Africa, which meant that epidemics in Europe and Britain came ultimately from those areas. The precise biological laws governing the activity of *Pasteurella pestis* remain unknown.

Further reading: Mullet, *The Bubonic Plague and England*; Shrewsbury, *A History of Bubonic Plague in the British Isles*; Slack, *The Impact of Plague in Tudor and Stuart England*.

London Plague of 1603 First of four major outbreaks of bubonic plague to afflict London in the seventeenth-century. The epidemic of 1603, according to one estimation, killed more than 22 percent of the city's estimated population of 141,000, the highest percentage of deaths from plague among all four epidemics. Other estimates put the population of London at this time, including its suburbs, at 250,000, with deaths from plague at about 35,000 or slightly more.

Probably introduced into the port of London from Amsterdam, the plague first appeared in the suburb of Southwark in early March, although the death of England's Queen Elizabeth I delayed official reaction until the end of April. The epidemic reached its peak at the end of August, but continued with little loss of virulence through September, subsiding only in

December when cold temperatures inhibited the activity of the plague-carrying rat-fleas (see PLAGUE OF ENGLAND, GREAT). Throughout the spring and summer of the following two years, the plague appeared sporadically in various parts of the city but mortality did not reach epidemic numbers.

Anti-plague measures ordered by the city authorities included the destruction of stray dogs, which were believed to carry the disease, the marking of infected houses with red crosses and the words "Lord have mercy upon us," and the removal of non-Londoners from the city who were not there for business or other special purposes.

An especially interesting aspect of the London epidemic of 1603 is how visibly the plague's concentration among the poor was revealed. More reliable parish record-keeping and the publication of official Bills of Mortality demonstrated this fact statistically, while written works, both religious and secular, showed that people were well aware of the far greater incidence of plague among the underprivileged social classes. Death figures clearly show that the plague was deadliest in the overcrowded neighborhoods of the poor, which were located mostly outside the walls of the wealthier inner city. The resentment exhibited by the poor was a natural consequence of the regulations forced upon them by the elite members of society, who could escape infection by fleeing the city, a precaution that the poor for the most part could not afford. Enforced confinement of the plague-sick as well as exposed household members, was particularly cruel, especially when these virtual prisoners watched as city officials, wealthy citizens, and even clergymen abandoned them to their fate.

Resistance to enforced segregation, closing of alehouses, restrictions on the number of people permitted to attend a funeral, and other anti-plague measures increased, and the government responded to this threat to social order by imposing harsh punishments on those who disobeyed them. In addition to being shut up forcibly in their houses, a person found walking about with plague-sores could be fined, whipped, and put in the stocks. Death by hanging was officially threatened for such offenses, but unlike the Scots, the English did not in practice impose this final penalty.

Thomas Dekker and other English pamphleteers found a large audience for their writings about the plague, which combined stark realism with comforting doses of pathos and humor. Preachers also became highly visible, many espousing the view that, as only God determines the time of a man's death, all medical efforts and social policies to cure or avoid the plague were in vain. Such critics found many supporters and were vigorously silenced by govern-mental authorities, who were determined to continue enforcing their policy of segregation of infected persons.

Disruption of commerce and widespread unemployment followed in the wake of this terrible disaster. The epidemic of 1603 was very widely dispersed, affecting many areas of England outside London. Sporadic outbreaks in various places occurred until about 1610.

Further reading: Shrewsbury, *A History of Bubonic Plague in the British Isles*; Slack, *The Impact of Plague in Tudor and Stuart England*; Wilson, *The Plague in Shakespeare's London*.

London Plague of 1625   Epidemic of bubonic plague that was preceded by floods and famine in 1622 and 1623, and by high mortality due to outbreaks of dysentery, typhus fever, and smallpox in 1623 and 1624.

It was fortunate that the early spring of 1625 was unusually cold, as low temperatures inhibit the activity of plague-carrying or "blocked" fleas, which transmit the plague bacillus (*Pasteurella pestis*) from rats to human beings (see PLAGUE OF ENGLAND, GREAT). Plague cases, therefore, began appearing in noticeable numbers only toward the end of May, while heavy rains in June also curtailed the fleas' activity. By July, however, the plague was at full force, reached its peak in August, and declined steadily through the fall months, until cold weather at the end of November marked the virtual end of the epidemic. Because of this somewhat short plague season, effectively only July through September, the epidemic was less destructive than it might have been under warmer weather conditions, although with its death-count of at least 20 percent of London's population (perhaps as much as 300,000), it was among the worst outbreaks of bubonic plague in England's history. This infection, like all major outbreaks of plague, was undoubtedly imported to England by ships from a port in continental Europe, probably from Holland.

People had begun to differentiate bubonic plague from other diseases, most notably from typhus fever, with which it was often confused, and death figures from plague alone thus became more reliable. Combined with deaths from other diseases (including starvation and other causes as well), mortality quite possibly reached 100,000 persons in metropolitan London in 1625.

City authorities issued the usual anti-plague measures, which were in fact a reprinting with only slight changes of a set of orders published during the epidemic of 1578 and used in each succeeding outbreak. Their action, however, was delayed by the death of England's King James I on March 27, the arrival of the new queen on May 1, and the king's funeral on May 7. The usual exodus to the uninfected countryside by the wealthier citizenry was delayed by the royal ceremonies connected with these events, although everyone who could afford to do so left as soon as they could thereafter. In June the Lord Mayor fled, in July the royal court removed to Hampton Court, and Parliament adjourned to Oxford. The poor were used to the desertion of the nobility, civic officers, well-to-do merchants, and others of the more privileged classes during outbreaks of plague, but their abandonment by many parish priests, whose duty it was to help their suffering parishioners, was especially bitter.

The badly constructed wood and thatch dwellings of the poor made excellent habitats for the black house-rat, whose plague-infection spread easily and quickly to families crowded together in tiny rooms. Man and rat lived in close quarters in the slums of the city, where plague deaths were always most numerous. Plague was in fact recognized as a disease of the poor, and in the outbreaks of the seventeenth century it was increasingly present in the suburbs of London and other cities, where the poor population generally lived.

A letter written from London on September 1, 1625, reveals the desolation of the city:

> The want and misery is the greatest here that ever living man knew; no trading at all; the rich all gone; housekeepers and apprentices of manual trades begging in the streets, and that in such a lamentable manner as will make the strongest heart to yearn.

Citizens began returning to the city in October, and on December 30 the anti-plague regulations were officially withdrawn. The effects from disruption of trade, loss of population, and acute social distress continued long afterward. The sufferings of the poor were heightened even further by a bad harvest in 1626.

Further reading: Shrewsbury, *A History of Bubonic Plague in the British Isles*; Slack, *The Impact of Plague in Tudor and Stuart England*; Wilson, *The Plague in Shakespeare's London*.

London Plague of 1636   Outbreak of bubonic plague that was not as devastating as the two London epidemics that preceded it (1603 and 1625) or the final disastrous visitation of 1665 (see PLAGUE OF LONDON, GREAT). Nonetheless, more than 10,000 people of an estimated population of 350,000 died in London and its suburbs from the disease.

Plague was introduced into England's eastern coastal ports of Hull and Yarmouth in the spring of 1636, probably from Holland, and made its way southwestward toward London (into which plague was probably imported in foreign ships as well). The eastern out-parishes began reporting deaths in mid-April. It spread slowly through the spring and early summer, perhaps due to chilly weather that suppressed the activity of the plague-carrying rat-fleas (see PLAGUE OF ENGLAND, GREAT); death figures rose steadily in August and September. Thereafter mortality declined, but remained constant through October, November, and well into December, an unusual occurrence probably due to an unseasonably mild fall. Cases continued to be reported throughout the winter, many of them possibly confused with typhus fever, a cold-weather disease that displays some plague-like symptoms. Plague again appeared in London in the spring of 1637, causing perhaps at least 3,000 deaths.

Concentration of plague in the poor population crowded together in tenements on the outskirts of the city had become by 1636 the usual pattern of plague epidemics in London and other English cities. The usual exodus from London of government officials, wealthy citizens, and even clergymen depopulated the inner city, where superior living conditions would have protected them to a large degree had they chosen to remain and attend to their civil and ecclesiastical duties.

The cruelty and ineffectiveness of enforced confinement, largely restricted to the poor, merely promoted social resentment and caused more deaths, as plague-carrying fleas infesting a dwelling jumped from person to person in a segregated, closed-up house. Some English preachers even asserted that quarantine was part of the overall punishment that God devised for those sinners who had contracted plague. Many clergymen found themselves in the embarrassing position of having to reconcile their panic flight from their parishes with their obligation to stay and succor their parishioners, and with their theological claims that God, and not haphazard nature, ordained the death of each individual.

Minor outbreaks of plague continued to occur in London during the next five years, and other areas of England experienced visitations of varying severity during these years as well.

Further reading: Shrewsbury, *A History of Bubonic Plague in the British Isles*; Slack, *The Impact of Plague in Tudor and Stuart England*.

London Plague of 1655   See PLAGUE OF LONDON, GREAT.

London Smallpox Epidemics of 1667–68, 1674, and 1681   Three of the worst outbreaks in the second half of the seventeenth century; claimed approximately 3,200, 2,500, and 3,000 human lives respectively. Although these epidemics stand out because of the high numbers of deaths involved, they were by no means isolated instances. With few exceptions, smallpox mortality was very high in every year beginning around 1660, as well as having reached epidemic proportions many times before that date, notably in 1628, 1634, and 1641.

The English diarist Samuel Pepys noted in February 1668 that "It also hardly ever was remembered for such a season for the smallpox as these last two months have been." Thomas Sydenham, a great English clinician, said he observed more cases of smallpox during the epidemic of 1667–68 than he had ever seen, remarking also that, because the infection itself was of a mild nature, it "cut off comparatively few among the immense number of those who took it." Thus, the death figures for these years, looked at in isolation, understate how extensive the epidemic was. The case-mortality rate was, on average, one in every five or six cases, a statistic that remained constant until inoculation with smallpox virus began to be employed extensively in the 1750s (see ENGLISH SMALLPOX EPIDEMIC OF 1751–53).

Sydenham introduced the so-called cooling treatment to combat the fevers of smallpox patients. This radically challenged the traditional "sweat therapy" whereby the patient was wrapped in blankets in a stultifying room in the hopes of expelling supposedly fermented, disease-causing bodily "humors." Both these treatments remained controversial, especially because there is no known cure for smallpox in any case. Sydenham's real importance lies in his distinction between discrete and confluent smallpox. Noticing that patients whose pustules had not conflated usually recovered, he recommended no treatment at all in such cases. Because medical procedures often worsened a patient's condition, Sydenham's deceptively simple advice undoubtedly saved many lives. Bloodletting as well as vomits and purges were topics of great controversy among physicians in the treatment of smallpox.

Many royal personages died of smallpox in the seventeenth century, including Queen Mary (died 1694), one of whose physicians wrote a detailed account of her illness that reveals the terrible effects the disease has upon the body and the suffering the patient endures in a severe case. The usual pustules and spots appeared all over her face and most of her body. Spitting blood, breathing with difficulty, and delirium were among the other common symptoms the queen experienced. Queen Mary had "black" smallpox, a hemorrhagic type that is nearly always fatal.

The London Bills of Mortality, which were published from 1629 on, are the only documents containing figures on death from smallpox in seventeenth-century England. It may be assumed that other parts of England experienced serious outbreaks of smallpox, which is a highly contagious disease, at about the same time as London.

Further reading: Creighton, *A History of Epidemics in Britain;* Hopkins, *Princes and Peasants: Smallpox in History;* Shurkin, *The Invisible Fire.*

London Smallpox Epidemic of 1721   Highly fatal epidemic that is historically important as the stimulus for the first public experimentation in England with the then recently discovered procedure of variolation. London's epidemic spread to other parts of England during the next two years.

Variolation, or inoculation with the virus of smallpox, confers immunity to the disease for life. An incision is made in the skin, and viral matter taken from a pustule or dried scab of an infected person is inserted into the recipient's cut. In successful inoculations, the inoculee contracts a mild case of smallpox, from which he or she recovers easily. Widely practiced in China and Africa, probably for many centuries, the procedure was first noted by English visitors to China in the early 1700s, and by British residents of Constantinople (Istanbul) during an outbreak of smallpox there in 1706.

In 1717 Lady Mary Wortley Montagu, wife of the British ambassador to Constantinople and herself a recovered smallpox patient, enthusiastically drew the attention of her countrymen and -women to this life-saving procedure by sending detailed reports to England and enlisting the help of respected physicians. Lady Montagu had her young son variolated in Constantinople, and in London, shortly after the outbreak of smallpox in the spring of 1721, she had her young daughter variolated as well. This was the first variolation to be officially performed in England. Because this epidemic in 1721 was perceived as especially fatal to children, the Prince of Wales allowed his two young daughters to be variolated in 1722. With these highly publicized and successful cases the practice began to gain wide attention.

But variolation was not completely trusted. Some people died, either from exposure to natural smallpox itself as a result of the inoculation, or by catching the infection from a person who recently had undergone the procedure. With the risk of death between one percent and three percent, and that of secondary complications even greater, many people were reluctant to have themselves or their children inoculated. Preachers warned against it as being dangerous and sinful, and many physicians were opposed as well. The practice gradually gained popularity, but was not publicly endorsed by Britain's prestigious College of Physicians until 1755 (see ENGLISH SMALLPOX EPIDEMIC OF 1751–53). Interestingly, smallpox inoculation had long been practiced among the peasantry in Europe and England; but "buying the pox" was considered merely a folk practice and was ignored by the medical establishment.

Other notable smallpox epidemics afflicted London in 1710 (3,138 recorded deaths), 1714 (2,810 recorded), and 1719 (3,229 recorded deaths).

Further reading: Hopkins, *Princes and Peasants: Smallpox in History*; Shurkin, *The Invisible Fire*; Smith, *The Speckled Monster*.

London Typhus Epidemic of 1661–65

Epidemic of typhus fever, mixed with other largely unidentified fevers and illnesses. The cause of death in many cases was attributed to "spotted fever," indicating the characteristic red spots of typhus. Other symptoms as described by the famous English physician Thomas Sydenham (1624–89) strongly point to typhus as the type of fever most prevalent during these five years. The virulence of the fever intensified at the end of 1663, and the death toll continued to climb through the next year and into the spring of 1665. Unusually cold weather helps explain the dramatic rise in mortality that occurred in the winter of 1664–65, as lice-borne typhus fever tends to spread quickly when lice-ridden people huddle together for warmth and clothes remain unchanged for long periods of time. Such conditions were common to the lower classes, and typhus was thus the scourge of the underprivileged population. Although people of the more privileged classes were equally inattentive to personal cleanliness and were often victims of typhus fever, they did not live in squalid, crowded dwellings, and thus their risk of infection was less.

Approximately 15,700 human deaths were attributed to "spotted fever" and "fever" from 1661 through 1665. Among the more illustrious fatalities was the governor of New England, Sir William Phipps, who died in February 1664 during a visit to London.

Bubonic plague began to appear in London in the spring of 1665, and soon burst into full fury, displacing and far surpassing deaths from typhus fever (see PLAGUE OF LONDON, GREAT).

Further reading: Creighton, *A History of Epidemics in Britain*; Zinsser, *Rats, Lice and History*.

London Typhus Epidemic of 1685–86

Severe outbreak of typhus fever which, together with unusually high mortality from smallpox, constituted two devastating epidemic years for the people of London, England. The fever was so widespread and fatal that it provoked the fear that bubonic plague, which had

decimated London in 1665, was returning (see PLAGUE OF LONDON, GREAT). On March 12, 1685, a worried Londoner wrote: "A fever rages that proves very mortal and gives great apprehension of a plague." Thomas Sydenham (1624–89), the pioneering physician who had described an epidemic of typhus fever that preceded the Great London Plague of 1665 (see LONDON TYPHUS EPIDEMIC OF 1661–65) described this illness as a "new fever," a puzzling fact in view of his clinical observations that point almost certainly to typhus. The characteristic red spots or blotches of typhus fever were noted by Sydenham and other contemporary observers. Sydenham at this time was attempting to disprove the effectiveness of Peruvian bark as a treatment for fever. Because many influential medical figures were convinced of its efficacy, Sydenham's identification of the fever of 1685–86 as a "new" disease could have been a deliberate tactic to allow him to credibly demonstrate that the application of bark to suffering patients was useless.

Parish burial registers record 3,512 human deaths from "fever" and 317 deaths from "spotted fever" in 1685. The figures for 1686 are 4,107 and 299 respectively.

Further reading: Creighton, *A History of Epidemics in Britain*; Zinsser, *Rats, Lice and History*.

London Typhus Epidemics of 1709–20

Period of exceptionally high mortality caused by various types of fever, among which typhus fever was probably the most prevalent. Although deaths from fever as recorded in the London Bills of Mortality were consistently high throughout the period, the worst years were 1710, 1714, and 1719.

An unusually hard and long winter followed by a poor harvest in 1709 was undoubtedly a factor in the epidemic, evidently of typhus, that began in the fall of 1709 and lasted throughout 1710, in which year 4,740 human deaths were attributed to "fever" (4,397) and "spotted fever" (343). Spotted fever refers to the red or purple spots, sometimes as small as a fleabite but often much larger, that appear in many cases of typhus. A contemporary witness, Sir David Hamilton, described the fatal illness of the son of a well-to-do London gentleman who "about the 5th of October, 1709 . . . was seized with a fever; at which time, and for some weeks before, a malignant fever raged in London." The symptoms he listed, including red and purple spots on the patient's chest and legs, a terribly foul-smelling breath and perspiration, and "convulsive motions," are all characteristic of typhus fever. Treatments included liquid medicines and "doses of bark" (see LONDON TYPHUS EPIDEMIC OF 1685–86).

Deaths from fever, most of which were probably due to typhus, reached nearly 4,781 in 1714, exceeding the previous three years by about 1,000 to 1,600 deaths per year. Deaths climbed to about 3,750 in 1715, and in 1716 and 1717 declined to around 3,100 per year. The years 1718, 1719, and 1720 saw an upsurge in fatal cases to 3,607, 3,927, and 3,976 respectively. The next few years, with deaths from various types of fever ranging from about 3,000 to nearly 3,500 a year, were somewhat less drastic, especially in comparison to London's next notable epidemic of fever, which started in 1726 (see LONDON TYPHUS EPIDEMIC OF 1726–29). In addition to typhus, relapsing fever and an illness that attacked mainly young children comprised a portion of the fever deaths during these years.

Further reading: Creighton, *A History of Epidemics in Britain*; Zinsser, *Rats, Lice and History.*

London Typhus Epidemic of 1726–29

Four-year period of epidemic fevers, among which louse-borne typhus fever was probably the most widespread and fatal. According to the London Bills of Mortality, human deaths from fever were about 4,700 for each year from 1726 through 1728, and 5,335 for 1729. The title of an essay written by a prominent physician in 1728 on the pestilential condition of London— "Practical Observations on the Epidemical Fever which hath regined so violently these two years past . . ."—reveals the severity of the epidemic.

Although typhus fever erupted in epidemics frequently during the first half of the eighteenth century (see LONDON TYPHUS EPIDEMICS OF 1709–20; LONDON TYPHUS EPIDEMIC OF 1741–42), it was evidently present in London in endemic form throughout this time. In any given year, parish burial registers record many cases of "spotted fever," referring to the characteristic red or purple spots of typhus. Contemporary accounts also reveal the continual presence of deadly fever. The celebrated Dr. John Arbuthnot wrote in 1733: "I believe one may safely affirm that there is hardly any year in which there are not in London fevers with buboes and carbuncles; and that there are many petechial or spotted fevers is certain."

Other febrile illnesses present during these years were relapsing fever, a fever that attacked mostly infants, and an unidentified fever characterized by lethargy and hysteria.

Further reading: Creighton, *A History of Epidemics in Britain*; Zinsser, *Rats, Lice and History.*

London Typhus Epidemic of 1741–42

Extensive and highly fatal epidemic of louse-borne typhus fever that caused over 7,500 deaths in London, England, in 1741 and nearly 1,200 deaths in January and February of 1742. These figures, of course, are not totally reliable, as record-keeping in the eighteenth century was not uniform, and precise cause of death was not always accurately assessed. They do, however, provide an approximate measure and reflect the unusually high incidence of fever during these years.

The epidemic followed an exceptionally cold winter in 1740, subsequent crop failure, and critical unemployment, conditions that contributed to the misery of London's poor population. This general situation of want and illness extended to all parts of the British Isles.

Symptoms as recorded by two contemporary physicians, particularly the frequent presence of red or purple spots and the onset of delirium in the second week of the illness, point definitely to typhus fever as the major component of this epidemic. Typhus cases tend to proliferate in cold weather, when unwashed people huddle together for warmth in lice-ridden clothing and bedding, a fact reflected in the steady rise in deaths through the fall and winter of 1741.

This visitation of epidemic typhus was the last of a series of major epidemics of fever in London and other parts of Britain in the first half of the eighteenth century (see LONDON TYPHUS EPIDEMICS OF 1709–20; LONDON TYPHUS EPIDEMIC OF 1726–29).

Further reading: Creighton, *A History of Epidemics in Britain*; Zinsser, *Rats, Lice and History.*

London Typhus Epidemic of 1750 (Black Assize)

Most famous incidence of an outbreak of louse-borne typhus fever at a court session in eighteenth century England. The 1750 Black Assize of the Old Bailey courthouse in London recalled the circumstances of three similar cases during the sixteenth-century (see CAMBRIDGE TYPHUS EPIDEMIC OF 1522; OXFORD TYPHUS EPIDEMIC OF 1577; EXETER TYPHUS EPIDEMIC OF 1586). In 1750 Sir Michael Foster, a justice of the King's Bench who had presided at the Old Bailey just a few months before, recorded that the court and the passages leading to it were unusually crowded, that these passages, which led directly from Newgate Prison, were particularly filthy, and that a foul smell was present in the courtroom. He stated that "within a week or ten days at most, after the session, many people who were present . . . were seized with a fever of the malignant kind; and few who were seized recovered." As was the case at the Exeter Black Assize of 1586, few women were affected. The Lord Mayor of London and the presiding judge, as well as many other gentlemen of position, died of the fever. In addition to several jury members, at least 40 other people who attended the trial were fatally infected. The incident set off a reaction of panic, and there are reports, some greatly exaggerated, that many Londoners fled the city to escape infection. Evidence indicates, however, that the fever affected only those who had attended the assize.

Because foul air was thought to cause disease, the strong smells present at the Old Bailey on this occasion promoted an interest in the problem of indoor ventilation. The simple solution of fitting buildings with more windows was discouraged by a window-tax, which was especially burdensome to the poor, who blocked up windows to avoid assessment. This severely limited their access to fresh air and increased their susceptibility to contagious, airborne diseases, as well as diseases, such as louse-borne typhus fever, that are transmitted from man to man by insects. Prisons, with few windows and grossly insanitary conditions, were commonly rife with typhus, or "gaol fever," as it was also called.

Further reading: Creighton, *A History of Epidemics in Britain*; Zinsser, *Rats, Lice and History*.

London Typhus Epidemic of 1862–65

Outbreak of epidemic typhus fever that probably caused at least 10,000 human deaths in London. Although deaths from typhus climbed suddenly in 1856 upon the return of English soldiers from the Crimean War (1853–56), the disease had remained at a lower, endemic rate of mortality since the last great outbreak 15 years before (see ENGLISH TYPHUS EPIDEMIC OF 1847–48). Unusually high numbers of deaths occurred in other areas of Britain as well, mostly in the north of England until about 1867, and in Scotland.

Always a disease of the poor, whose overcrowded living quarters and lack of personal cleanliness encouraged the breeding and spread of the human body louse that transmits the disease, this 1862–65 epidemic was most fatal in London's working-class areas, particularly the poverty-stricken East End. An economic depression causing social displacement and unemployment probably contributed to the spread of the infection.

The extended epidemic of the 1860s was the last decade in which cases of typhus fever were uncommonly numerous in Britain. Starting in the 1870s the disease began to decline, until its virtual disappearance at the turn of the century. No one knows precisely why typhus fever vanished from the British Isles. Whereas new or improved sewage and water supply systems installed in destitute urban areas may have facilitated its decline, typhus fever in fact began to wane before these improvements in public sanitation were uniformly introduced throughout Britain. The discovery that lice are the vectors of epidemic typhus fever did not take place until 1909, and the gradual awareness of the importance of personal cleanliness was a coincidental social improvement, apparently having little to do with the disappearance of the disease. The plausible suggestion that a change in the nature of the causative microorganism itself (*Rickettsia prowazeki*) accounted for the decline of typhus has never been satisfactorily demonstrated. The waning of epidemic typhus fever in the British Isles remains as puzzling as that of bubonic plague and the English sweating sickness, which vanished in the eighteenth and sixteenth centuries respectively.

Further reading: Creighton, *A History of Epidemics in Britain*; Wohl, *Endangered Lives: Public Health in Victorian Britain*; Woods and Woodward, eds., *Urban Disease and Mortality in Nineteenth-Century England*.

Los Angeles Plague of 1924–25

Worst U.S. outbreak of pneumonic plague (also the last such occurrence in an American urban environment) and the last time an American plague epidemic would involve rats. During the outbreak, 31 of the 33 pneumonic plague cases were fatal, while five out of the eight people infected with bubonic plague died. The epidemic took place in the Mexican section of Los Angeles, where the first victim, a Mexican, fell ill on October 1, 1924, and developed a femoral bubo originally diagnosed as venereal disease. Although he recovered, his daughter and others in his neighborhood fell ill and died. By October 28, 15 people were infected, and all of them died within three days. There were seven more plague victims on October 29. The epidemic in Los Angeles was underway. The victims complained of plague symptoms like stupor, high fever and chills, headaches, and, most important, very large, lymphatic swellings under their arms, in the neck, or in the groin.

A doctor examined a patient in Los Angeles's Mexican section in 1924 without diagnosing the plague; the patient and 13 others were then sent to the Los Angeles County General Hospital, which contacted the state and federal government for vaccine and plague serum. Later, a local health official informed the U.S. government of the ongoing epidemic. Only very distorted accounts appeared in newspapers, which frequently classified the disease as "malignant pneumonia."

Most of the deaths from plague had already occurred by the time sanitation and public health measures were instituted. The plague-ridden area of the city was isolated and food portions given to the frightened residents, who were informed of their predicament. Although the serum arrived, it was used on only one patient. By November 1924, a campaign against rats was undertaken in the city close to the harbor, rather than in the Mexican section, to forestall a port quarantine that could disrupt business. Eventually, a harbor quarantine took place, anyway. By early 1925, the plague epidemic had ended. See also SAN FRANCISCO PLAGUE OF 1900–04; SAN FRANCISCO PLAGUE OF 1907–09; NEW MEXICO PLAGUE OF 1965.

Further reading: Gregg, *Plague: An Ancient Disease in the Twentieth Century;* McGrew, *Encyclopedia of Medical History;* Veseltear, "The Pneumonic Plague Epidemic of 1924 in Los Angeles."

Los Angeles Poliomyelitis Epidemic of 1934

Outbreak of poliomyelitis (or infantile paralysis) caused by the rare type 2 poliovirus; but certain authorities believe that some other disease and/or hysteria played an important role in the epidemic, which caused much fright, despite the mildness of most polio cases.

Physicians and others at Los Angeles County General Hospital treated 1,301 cases of confirmed polio from May through November 1934; originally, 2,499 persons received treatment at the hospital as polio victims, but more than a thousand of them could have been suffering from related or other illnesses. This epidemic attacked children and adults of all ages (the poliovirus type 2 usually affects the youngest age group) and compelled Los Angeles's chief health officer, Dr. George Parish, to contact Dr. Simon Flexner, who was then director of the Yale Poliomyelitis Study Unit and who sent a research team to Los Angeles.

Although hospital personnel exposed to polio's paralytic cases especially dreaded the disease, abortive or unrecognizable cases (not paralytic ones) were the principal means of transmission of polio. The public also was not well informed by the medical community, and as a result, the contagious unit at Los Angeles County General Hospital was grimly looked upon as a pesthouse (shelter for those infected by a pestilential disease). Many of the staff members were gripped by terror of the disease.

Among the supposed polio victims (the 2,499 cases), there were 198 doctors and nurses who worked at Los Angeles County General Hospital; most were soon considered hysterical cases resulting from the presence of the disease in the hospital; no staff members died or were paralyzed, and only two had abnormal test results for polio. Most of them displayed either influenzal or rheumatoidal symptoms with significant emotional characteristics. Contributing to the tense atmosphere surrounding the hospital staff cases was a then typical treatment for the slightest muscle weakness: encasement of limbs in plaster casts suspended above hospital beds. Wards sometimes seemed like wartime disaster areas. See U.S. POLIOMYELITIS EPIDEMIC OF 1931; U.S. POLIOMYELITIS EPIDEMIC OF 1942–53.

Further reading: McGrew, *Encyclopedia of Medical History;* Paul, *A History of Poliomyelitis;* Marks and Beatty, *Epidemics.*

Lyon Plague of 1564   See PLAGUE OF LYON IN 1564.

Lyon Plague of 1628–29   See PLAGUE OF LYON IN 1628–29.

M

Madagascan Plague of 1924–25 Outbreak of plague (bubonic, pneumonic, and septicemic) that killed an estimated 2,000 natives and others infected on the French-controlled island of Madagascar, off the east coast of Africa.

The province of Antananarivo (Tananarive), on Madagascar's central plateau, reported numerous cases of plague pneumonia (transmitted person-to-person by droplet infection) in the early 1920s (the province has a comparatively inclement climate and the inhabitants are susceptible to pneumonia). Plague entered Antananarivo via the seaport of Tamatave (Toamasina) on the island's east coast, and between January and May 1924 it flared up particularly in the city of Antananarivo, Madagascar's capital and largest city, which recorded five bubonic, 22 pneumonic, and 22 septicemic cases during that period (the rest of the province reported 231 bubonic, 67 pneumonic, and 365 septicemic cases); about 650 persons died of plague in the entire province. Bubonic patients who developed secondary plague pneumonia transmitted the disease to others through coughing (the bubonic form is carried from rats to persons by the bite of a flea). In many of the septicemic cases (also caused by a flea bite), death occurred within hours after contracting the disease, before the development of buboes (swellings of the lymph glands in the groin or armpit). There were 454 plague cases (415 of them resulted in death) in Antananarivo province between September 1 and December 31, 1924. The province of Moramanga (east of Antananarivo) suffered severely in November 1924, when 37 out of a reported 43 plague cases proved fatal. The total plague infections and fatalities on Madagascar in 1924 were 1,270 and 1,163 respectively.

Between January 1 and August 31, 1925, Antananarivo province again suffered from plague of all forms and recorded 852 infections and 725 deaths. Afterward and during the following seven years, the disease declined in prevalence and was not epidemically serious until 1933, when Antananarivo and other regions were once again attacked (see MADAGASCAN PLAGUE OF 1933–37).

Further reading: Hirst, *The Conquest of Plague;* Lien-teh, *A Treatise on Pneumonic Plague.*

Madagascan Plague of 1933–37 Devastating period of epidemic plague (mainly the bubonic form) that killed at least 12,000 persons out of 13,953 reported infected on the island of Madagascar, some 200 miles off the east coast of Africa.

Outbreaks of the deadly disease had occurred continuously on the island after plague entered the seaport of Tamatave (Toamasina) in 1921. Afterward an endemo-epidemic focus was centered around Antananarivo (Tananarive), the capital city, and Ambositra, Fianarantsoa, Emyrne, and Vakinankaratra. Unlike the South African Plagues of 1935 and 1936 (q.v.), there was no evidence that wild rodents were responsible for harboring and transmitting the disease in Madagascar, where it broke out mainly in the rural bushlands.

In 1933 the deadly plague bacillus (the infectious agent) increased unexpectedly in incidences on the island. All three forms of plague (bubonic, pneumonic, and septicemic) broke out sporadically in isolated cases in both the dry, cooler season (May to October) and the hot, wet season (November to April), when a large number of domestic rats sought shelter in native dwellings. Many of the plague cases occurred among small families or in villages and appeared to be unconnected. About 60 percent of the 3,933 infections were bubonic in 1933. In the cooler months of August and September, many of the bubonic patients also developed pneumonic plague, which is usually fatal if untreated. Thirty percent of the cases in 1933 were pneumonic, and about ten percent of them were septicemic, which is also usually fatal if not treated (death sometimes occurring within hours after contracting the disease).

Madagascan officials reported 3,605 plague infections in 1934 and 3,493 in 1935, and overall mortality from 1933 to 1935 ranged between 85 percent and 91 percent. Native concealment of plague infection (in order to ensure observance of traditional funeral rites) was one of the reasons for the high mortality rate. The incidence of plague decreased to 2,006 cases in 1936, when it was most serious in the central Madagascan zone, where there were 1,363 cases (663 were bubonic, 442 pneumonic, and 258 septicemic).

Plague was then controlled through the enactment of active medical programs on the island: isolation of the sick, internment of the dead in special cemetaries, disinfection of contaminated dwellings and clothing, immunization of persons in infected areas, and destruction of rodents. The incidence of the disease declined to 916 cases in 1937. A live plague-bacillus vaccine, which had been developed in Madagascar's medical laboratories, was used by the government in a mass immunization program since November 1935. The number of plague cases dropped (though not consistently every year) to 143 by 1949, rising slightly to 153 in 1950.

Further reading: Simmons et al., *Global Epidemiology;* Pollitzer, *Plague.*

Madagascan Smallpox Epidemic of 1817–18

Serious epidemic of smallpox, not improved by the practice of variolation (vaccination with the smallpox virus), that killed hundreds of people.

Before the first Portuguese Catholic missionaries arrived in Madagascar, off the southeast coast of Africa, in the early part of the seventeenth-century, the native inhabitants were frequently in contact with the Arab slave-trading communities on the east coast of Africa, where smallpox was fairly common. Madagascar soon became a popular stopover for ships plying between Europe and the Far East. When smallpox became endemic on the island, ships coming and going helped spread the disease to other lands, such as the islands of Réunion and Mauritius, to the east in the Indian Ocean.

At the onset of the Madagascan smallpox epidemic in December 1817, two standard methods were practiced to deter the spread of the variola virus (the smallpox infectious agent). One method—inoculation against the disease by inserting scabrous matter from a smallpox patient into a portion of a person's cut skin—was used on the native ruler of Madagascar's central region, King Radama, who contracted a milder form of the disease from which he recovered; however, his sister's inoculation resulted in her death on December 23, 1817. Since transmission of the disease normally occurs by close contact with patients, there is today little surprise that five other members of King Radama's royal family and 13 oth-

ers in his court died of smallpox by January 5, 1818.

The second method to eliminate smallpox on Madagascar was a policy established earlier by Radama's father, King Adrianampoinimerina, who ordered all persons with smallpox to be buried alive. Hundreds of infected people were left to die in this merciless manner before King Radama abolished this burial law.

Smallpox also spread because of native funeral customs: Contaminated corpses were left in the open for several days while mourners sat or feasted nearby, and expensive contaminated shrouds or wraps covering the corpses were stolen and sold by grave robbers. Eventually the more effective cowpox vaccine (discovered by English physician Edward Jenner), which protected persons against smallpox without inoculating them with a contagious infection, was administered to the island's population, and the epidemic subsided after February 12, 1818.

Further reading: Cartwright, *Disease and History;* Hopkins, *Princes and Peasants: Smallpox in History.*

Mainz Typhus Epidemic of 1813–14

Epidemic of lice-borne typhus fever that broke out among the garrison of 30,000 French soldiers defending the Rhine River city of Mainz (Mayence) during a siege by the Allies from November 1, 1813, to May 3, 1814.

Quartering of the lice-infested soldiers in the homes of the poorer citizens of Mainz helped spread the disease among the civilian population, which numbered about 25,400 plus an unknown number of refugees from the surrounding area who fled to the city before the siege (near the end of the Napoleonic Wars). Far from giving comfort or true medical assistance, hospitals were simply places where sick soldiers were hoarded together under conditions that only increased and prolonged their sufferings. Because large stores of wine were in the city, employees of the hospitals were nearly always drunk, while soldiers under arrest who had been forced to clean the sick rooms had all died. Patients thus lay unattended. A physician serving in Mainz described the conditions he witnessed:

> I found the living and the dead, the wounded and the sick, scattered in confusion all over the place. The sick were stretched out on the floor, without even straw under them, covered with ordure. . . . The sick men told me that they had been in that same position for two, three, and even four days, without having had a drop of water.

The situation in Mainz deteriorated steadily as typhus fever continued to spread: "The infection carried away all the grave-diggers one by one, and it was impossible to find anybody who was willing to do that dangerous work. Thousands of dead bodies of citizens and soldiers lay for weeks in front of the Münstertor [town gate], where they were piled up like logs pending burial." By the time the siege ended and the epidemic began to abate, typhus fever had killed 17,000 to 18,000 French soldiers, and one tenth of the civilian population. Places along the military roads leading from Mainz were also rife with typhus fever. See also FRENCH TYPHUS EPIDEMICS OF 1813–14; GERMAN TYPHUS EPIDEMICS OF 1813–14, NORTHERN AND CENTRAL.

Further reading: Lautzas, *Die Festung Mainz im Zeitalter des Ancien Regime, der Französischen Revolutions und des Empire*; Prinzing, *Epidemics Resulting from Wars*.

Malaysian Poliomyelitis Epidemic of 1971–72

Large outbreak of poliomyelitis that marked the transition of polio (or infantile paralysis) from endemicity to epidemic proportions in Malaysia. It began in the western part of the country in September 1971. In the previous decade, the poliovirus type 1 was found to be responsible for the scattered polio cases, but in the first half of 1971, there was a noticeable rise in paralytic polio cases caused by the type 3 virus. Since the majority of children in the country lacked immunity to this type of poliovirus, Malaysia's Ministry of Health promptly announced the launching of a mass immunization campaign. However, before the campaign could get underway, epidemic poliomyelitis spread throughout the country. Unexpectedly for the country's health authorities, the culprit (infectious agent) was identified as the type 1 poliovirus.

The epidemic resulted in more than 1,600 paralytic cases and peaked in January 1972. During the outbreak, a higher incidence was recorded among males, among Malaysia's Indian community, and among urban dwellers. Children under four years of age were the chief targets, and a mass vaccination campaign began in January and lasted until May 1972. All infants were routinely immunized. As a consequence of this rigorous campaign, the incidence of the disease declined considerably. However, in 1977, a smaller outbreak occurred and was attributed primarily to difficulties in preserving and transporting the polio vaccine in viable condition for use in the outlying rural areas. This problem was subsequently addressed; after 1980, no paralytic poliomyelitis cases were reported in the country.

Further reading: Warren and Mahmoud, eds., *Tropical and Geographical Medicine*; Mackenzie, ed., *Viral Diseases in South-East Asia and the Western Pacific*.

Maldivian Cholera Epidemic of 1978

Severe outbreak of cholera, offshot of the Asiatic Cholera Pandemic of 1961–75 (q.v.). The Republic of Maldives, a group of 1,300 islands (only 202 permanently inhabited) in the Indian Ocean, had been cholera-free for almost five decades. The disease, reportedly imported via ship from an Asian country, therefore spread with great intensity amid a highly susceptible population. The outbreak, believed to have been caused by contaminated well water, lasted from the end of March 1978 to early May 1978. The causative bacterial agent was the biotype *el-tor*, serotype *Ogawa*, of the *Vibrio comma* or *cholera vibrio*.

Apparently, sporadic cases of gastroenteritis had been reported in the country since January 1978. However, the epidemic began its explosive journey when Maldivians returning to their islands after celebrating their national day (March 29) in the capital, Malé, carried the infection home with them. Records indicate that 11,303 people on 123 islands were infected, an attack rate of 7.7 percent. Some of the islands suffered more than others, with up to 30 percent of the population coming down with the disease over a two- to three-week period. There were 252 deaths on 62 islands, a case fatality rate of 2.2 percent. Overall mortality was 1.9 percent. Many of the deaths were recorded barely a few hours after onset, before hospitalization could be arranged. Some families lost several members to cholera.

The health authorities, aided by the World Health Organization (WHO) and a team from India's National Institute of Communicable Diseases, successfully responded to the crisis on several fronts. Surveillance units were set up to identify cholera patients, admit them to hospital, and gather epidemiological data. Patients were treated with tetracycline and oral rehydration therapy. In addition, the country's 35,000 water wells were chlorinated—a process that killed the larvae-eating fish that had helped control the mosquito population. Thus, the Maldive Islands were unwittingly left open to threats from dengue hemorrhagic fever.

Further reading: Evans and Feldman, eds., *Bacterial Infections of Humans*; World Health Organization, *WHO Chronicle*.

Malian Cholera Epidemic of 1970–71

Acute epidemic of cholera diffused along the Niger River area in Mali (formerly French Sudan), West Africa, killing thousands of people from November 1970 to March 1971. Mali's epidemic derived from the West African Cholera Epidemics of 1970–71 (q.v.), which began in Guinea in August 1970 and penetrated many parts of West Africa.

On November 5, 1970, a cholera-infected trader from Abidjan (the Ivory Coast) bought fish in a popular market in Mopti (a town on the Niger River in Mali); he apparently spread the disease through his contaminated urine in public latrines. When shoppers in Mopti returned home to villages along the river, they carried cholera with them; within three weeks outbreaks of the disease were reported in several places downstream from Mopti, including the town of Ségou. Two weeks later inhabitants of Timbuktu (Tombouctou), one of the major river ports in Mali, contracted cholera, as did many living downstream in Gao (the easternmost terminus of the Niger River navigation system in Mali).

During the fourth week of the epidemic (in early December 1970), the region containing Mali's capital, Bamako, became infected; the town of Koulikoro, downstream from Bamako (westernmost terminus of the Niger River), reported infections, and from there the disease gradually penetrated into the valley areas of the Bani River. It was impossible to estimate mortality among the nomads and fishermen in the region. Nara, in arid northwestern Mali, recorded 1,129 cholera cases (with 332 deaths) in 13 weeks; from Nara the disease moved into southeastern Mauritania. Because Bamako's authorities instituted a thorough anti-cholera vaccination program and protected the water supply, the capital city's population of about 300,000 people was spared painful devastation; only 158 cases of cholera were reported in Bamako.

However, because the disease spread so rapidly and many of the infected areas were inaccessible, the majority of cases went unrecorded; inadequate preparation by health officials contributed to the high incidence of cholera. In some villages with up to 1,000 inhabitants, as many as 500 became diseased, and fatality sometimes reached 50 percent. Some 2,000 of 5,000 infected Malian farmers died.

By late December 1970 cholera had spread down the valley of the Niger River in Mali and entered Upper Volta (Burkina Faso), western Niger, and Nigeria. The epidemic also extended into Guinea from Mali's southern border (about 100 miles from Bamako) and into Senegal from Mali's western border by mid-1971.

Further reading: Cartwright, *Disease and History;* Stock, *African Environment Special Report 3: Cholera in Africa.*

Malian Relapsing Fever Epidemic of 1921–22   Major outbreak of louse-borne relapsing fever that killed about 15,000 persons out of an estimated 108,000 who became infected in what was then called French

Sudan, in West Africa. It was the first epidemic of the disease known to have occurred in any part of tropical Africa.

Louse-borne relapsing fever spread into Mali from the town of Kouroussa in French Guinea (now Guinea), which borders Mali. It may have been introduced into French Guinea by soldiers returning home from the Mediterranean, Morocco, and Algiers (where the disease was prevalent) after World War I. Some authorities believe the disease may already have existed in Guinea and that the large number of troops who traveled to and assembled at Kati (near Bamako, Mali's capital) before their discharge from the army may have provided suitable conditions for the development of epidemic relapsing fever. The disease is common in wartime, famine, or other situations where malnutrition, overcrowding, and bad hygiene help to multiply and spread lice. The disease can also be spread by ticks.

Caused by a spirochetic infection of the blood, relapsing fever is not directly transmitted from one person to another. It is contracted by crushing an infective louse (*Pediculus humanus*) over a bite wound or through an abrasion of the skin or by way of the conjunctiva. Infected persons at first have symptoms common to other febrile disease: headaches, general weakness, chills, high fevers; later many of them become jaundiced and suffer from external and internal hemorrhages. Protection from louse-borne relapsing fever involves personal cleanliness, avoidance of lice-infested patients, and destruction of the lice; the infection can be cut short by antibiotics, notably penicillin and tetracyclines.

There are hardly any records available regarding morbidity and mortality in French Guinea for 1921, when relapsing fever moved northeastward into Mali, into the area of the headwaters (tributaries) of the Niger River. The disease seriously infected the region around San, from which it moved to the more densely populated town of Mopti on the Niger River in central Mali. This became the center of the epidemic during 1921–22. Medical authorities, for the most part, were inexperienced in dealing with the infection, and in one year, the mortality rate in Mali rose to 14 percent. In 1922 relapsing fever advanced from Mali southward into Upper Volta (now Burkina Faso), where it reportedly claimed more than 21,000 human lives by 1924. From Upper Volta, the disease diffused south to the Gold Coast (now Ghana) and east into what is now Niger, Nigeria, Chad, and Sudan (see SUDANESE RELAPSING FEVER EPIDEMIC OF 1926–28).

Further reading: Scott, *Epidemic Disease in Ghana, 1901–1960;* Shattuck, *Diseases of the Tropics.*

Maltese Plague of 1675–76 Devastating epidemic of mainly bubonic plague on the Mediterranean island of Malta, killing an estimated 11,300 persons out of a population of about 70,000.

Located 58 miles south of Sicily, Malta had strong trading ties with North Africa, Syria, Palestine, and Italy; in all these places, the plague bacillus (*Yersinia pestis*) had been habitually present in varying intensities since the Middle Ages. The disease evidently arrived in Malta about 1575, and a serious outbreak occurred there in 1592. It is not certain where plague came from in 1675, when the first cases occurred in December. Some diseased rats or rodents (primary hosts of plague) may have traveled with merchandise to the island and transmitted the disease to man (infected fleas seek out another host [maybe man] after rodents die from the disease). The plague epidemic (mainly bubonic, but also pneumonic and septicemic in form) grew in early 1676, with infected fleas carrying plague from one victim to another. Patients have severe headaches, fevers, and painful buboes (swellings) in the groin, armpit, or neck, along with other complications. Many of the sick were treated in lazarets or lazarettes (hospitals for contagious diseases and for quarantining the infected) and in new Catholic churches, dedicated to Saint Roch (a Franciscan monk who devoted himself to tending the sick and plague-stricken in the fourteenth century), erected at Valletta, Birkirkara, Balzan, and other places on Malta.

After eight months, the epidemic receded in August 1676. Among the many thousands who perished were ten physicians, 16 surgeons, more than 1,000 hospital attendants, and many priests. Later in 1677, the first Maltese medical work on plague (written in Latin) was published by Laurentius Haseiah (or Haseiac), who referred to the treatment of victims' buboes in 1675–76 (the infection issued from the pus from a broken bubo) and "the worst epidemic on record." The practice of quarantine and disinfection of letters (paper was thought to carry plague) was then instituted in Malta, where no serious outbreaks of the disease occurred until 1813 (see MALTESE PLAGUE OF 1813).

Further reading: Hirst, *The Conquest of Plague*; Scott, *A History of Tropical Medicine*; Marks and Beatty, *Epidemics*.

Maltese Plague of 1813 Severe epidemic of bubonic plague that killed 4,486 persons in seven months (1813) on the Mediterranean island of Malta, located between Sicily and North Africa.

Since the ravaging Maltese Plague of 1675–76 (q.v.), plague had receded on the island, but by mid-April 1813 the dreaded disease had once again engulfed Malta in epidemic proportions. Evidently,

several Egyptian ships, carrying passengers and cargoes from the Levant (regions bordering the eastern Mediterranean), where serious plague outbreaks had occurred since 1812, brought the disease into Malta's seaport and capital of Valletta in April. Cargoes of grain, fodder, clothing, and other goods harbored plague-infested rats and fleas; numerous passengers and crew members were stricken with the disease upon arrival in Malta (occupied by the British).

By July 1813 the plague was killing 50 and sometimes more persons each day. The Maltese village of Manderaggio suffered so severely that its residents had to be evacuated. Until November 1813 the epidemic was confined to the island of Malta, which had seen 4,486 people out of a population of 96,400 perish from the disease during the previous seven months. By early 1814 plague had spread to the less-populated Maltese island of Gozo—with Comino, Cominotto, and Filfla (as well as the largest island—Malta) comprising the Maltese Islands. In 1815, the epidemic moved to infect the Ionian Islands off Greece's west coast.

Many plague-stricken Maltese people were treated in lazarets or lazarettes (hospitals for contagious diseases and for the detention of persons in quarantine) during the 1813 epidemic, which was related in a treatise written in Latin by Agostino Naude, a Maltese physician. Several army surgeons also published their observations and comments about the 1813 "scourge."

An interesting outcome of this Maltese epidemic was an acrimonious debate that continued until the mid-nineteenth century as to whether plague was really a contagious disease. The anti-contagionists maintained that quarantines, lazarets, and all attempts at "police" control of the disease were useless and that epidemics declined naturally as fast as preventive measures were adopted. (Some serious European plagues did indeed die down with little or futile attempts to control them.) Anti-contagionists also denied there was valid evidence that plague was communicated by goods. The contagionists, however, maintained that there was strong evidence that the traffic in goods from plague-infected places played an important role in the spread of the disease in Malta.

After 1813 Malta was relatively free of the disease until 1936, when a minor outbreak occurred that killed 11 out of 28 infected persons.

Further reading: Hirst, *The Conquest of Plague*; Scott, *A History of Tropical Medicine*.

Maltese Poliomyelitis Epidemic of 1942–43 Outbreak of 483 cases, the majority on Malta, the rest on its neighboring island, Gozo. Although polio epidemics usually take place in the summer, the Maltese outbreak began in November 1942, reached a peak with 108 cases during the week of December 20, and then rapidly abated and disappeared by the beginning of March 1943. As was common with the polio virus, most victims were young: 82 percent were Maltese children under the age of five. Nearly two thirds of the remaining cases, however, occurred among British servicemen (over age 20) who had been sent to defend the islands during World War II. In contrast, only four Maltese adults—and no Maltese soldiers—were affected, even though native and British troops worked together.

The unusual seasonal appearance and the distinctive pattern of infection were only two of the reasons the limited epidemic attracted attention. Not only was it the first of any size on Malta (an earlier outbreak in 1902 had been relatively small), but it was also located in the tropics. Since most previous polio outbreaks had occurred in temperate zones, researchers believed that the disease was a feature of cooler climates. Once British and U.S. troops arrived in the Mediterranean basin during World War II, however, some of them came down with polio. At first military physicians assumed that the soldiers had carried the disease with them from their home countries, but the Maltese outbreak proved that native Mediterranean populations could be reservoirs of the polio virus.

The epidemic started among civilians, with the first cases reported on November 15 on Malta and November 21 on Gozo; the first serviceman did not fall ill until November 27. The servicemen who eventually were afflicted had been stationed on Malta for an average of 12 months. Only four had been on the island for four months or less, and all of these came in December 1942 or later—after the first cases appeared among civilians. It seems likely, then, that the disease was carried from the natives to the foreign troops. Contacts between the military and civilian populations could not be traced precisely, but they were not rare: Maltese cooks and laborers worked in the military camps, and several servicemen fathered children during their tour of duty on Malta.

Further details of the epidemic strengthen the likelihood that the virus was indigenous to the islands. Despite the fact that the epidemic hit every major town, Maltese adults were almost entirely spared; they must have acquired immunity from earlier, practically undetectable bouts with the virus. These exposures were so mild that they never flared up into an epidemic. During the fall of 1942, however, something happened to create a polio virus somewhat more virulent than the one that usually circulated on

Malta, and young children, who had no immunity whatsoever to polio, were infected in great numbers. There were 397 patients under the age of five (all of them suffering from paralysis—it was not possible to count minor cases), of whom 3.7 percent died.

The relatively low mortality rate among children contrasted sharply with that among the foreign servicemen. Of the 57 cases, 19.3 percent were lethal—a much higher percentage than among corresponding age groups in Britain. Nor did the survivors have it easy. They experienced a much greater degree of disability than their cohorts at home. Because of the high morbidity and mortality among the British troops, researchers concluded that the strain of polio virus on Malta was different enough from the one known in Britain that many servicemen had no immunity from it.

Life on Malta before the epidemic was harsh because of the war. Ever since Italy had declared war on Britain in June 1942, the island (at the time a British colony) had come under constant aerial attack. The Maltese people were forced to crowd into makeshift, often unsanitary quarters as their homes were bombed. Food supplies were so low that in the summer of 1942 the Maltese government authorized the use of untreated sewage to fertilize the crops. Yet medical investigators working for the British armed forces could find no proof that the virus was spread through overcrowding, contaminated food or water, or flies. In only seven households did more than one child fall ill, while the near-simultaneous outbreaks on Malta and Gozo (which had its own water supply and had not used sewage as fertilizer) suggests that food and water played no role in disease transmission.

Further reading: Seddon et al., "The Poliomyelitis Epidemic in Malta, 1942–3"; Paul, *A History of Poliomyelitis*; Taylor, *Poliomyelitis and Polioencephalitis*.

Manchurian Cholera Epidemic of 1919

Epidemic that entered Manchuria from southern China in July 1919 and claimed 10,000 victims, 4,500 in Harbin (Pinkiang) alone. It is believed to have originated in India in the spring of 1909 and traveled to southern China via the shipping routes across the South Seas. Scattered cases had been reported frequently from Hsientou, Fuchou, and Shanghai districts during June, so ships coming in from Shanghai were subjected to strict quarantine and inspection. Dairen (Talien) recorded its first case of cholera on July 9, while several cases broke out in Newchwang on July 8. The virus then traveled rapidly along railway routes to Mukden (Shen-yang), then north to Changchun, Kirin, Harbin, and Tsitsihar and eastward to Antung. From Dairen, the infection crossed into the

Japanese Leased Territory and the southern part of the Railway Zone.

The Manchurian Plague Prevention Service immediately swung into action (see MANCHURIAN PLAGUE OF 1910–11; MANCHURIAN PLAGUE OF 1920–21). Isolation and detention centers were established at all major railway junctions, including Port Arthur (Lüshun), Dairen, Mukden, and Newchwang. Disinfection was ordered for all public transport and strict supervision introduced at burial grounds. When the epidemic worsened, an Extraordinary Epidemic Headquarters was set up at Mukden to coordinate and direct preventive measures.

Treatment was provided for the sick at various hospitals in the region. Mortality rates varied: 14 percent in Harbin, 56 percent in Dairen, 34 percent, 58 percent and 67 percent in the three Russian hospitals in Harbin and Vladivostok. According to one source (entitled *Report on Progress in Manchuria, 1907–1928*), the epidemic affected 45,251 people, killing 27,288. It was suppressed in October 1919.

Further reading: Nathan, *Plague, Prevention and Politics in Manchuria, 1910–1931*.

Manchurian and Mongolian Plagues of 1928–30

Series of bubonic plague epidemics that struck southern Manchuria and the Tungliao region of Fengtien (formerly part of eastern Inner Mongolia).

Bubonic plague had been known to be endemic to the region since the early 1920s. The outbreaks occurred every year from 1928 to 1930 and followed the laying of new railway lines in the region. However, the disease avoided the bustling railway towns (see MANCHURIAN PLAGUE OF 1910–11) and concentrated its fury on scattered villages, where flea-infested rodents ensured the transmission of the disease to man. Each outbreak reportedly extended over a few months and killed several hundred people. According to Dr. Wu Lien-teh (see below), 268 people died of bubonic plague in various districts of southern Manchuria in 1930. He and his staff apparently found corpses of plague victims abandoned in open fields far away from laboratory facilities.

The Plague Prevention Service (see MANCHURIAN PLAGUE OF 1920–21) was summoned to deal with the outbreaks. It quickly brought in trained personnel and set up a laboratory and field headquarters at Chengchiatun (Liaoyuan), the junction of both railway routes (Ssup'ingkai-Taonan and Ssup'ingkai-Tungliao). With the cooperation of the Chinese-owned railway management and of the local Fengtien government, the service was able to contain the outbreaks and prevent them from penetrating the more heavily populated regions of southern Manchuria. The service also built a new chain of hospitals.

The villagers, whom the Plague Prevention Service was trying to help, were openly hostile. In the 1929 outbreak, a gang of riflemen attacked the field headquarters and had to be driven away by railway guards. Rather than heed medical advice, many offered animals in sacrifice in the hope that it would cure them of the dreaded disease.

Further reading: Nathan, *Plague, Prevention and Politics in Manchuria, 1910–1931*; Lien-teh, *Plague Fighter*.

Manchurian Plague of 1910–11

Unprecedented outbreak of pneumonic plague that originated in the Trans-Baikal region in August 1910 and spread over a thousand miles across Manchuria to Shantung, killing 60,000 people.

Stray cases of bubonic plague (see HONG KONG PLAGUE OF 1894) had been reported among the Mongol and Buriat hunters on the Siberian steppe. These had been contracted from infected marmots—wild rodents trapped for their fur, which was highly valued on the international market. In 1907, an influx of Chinese migrant laborers arrived in Manchuria to cash in on the booming fur trade. Inexperienced in hunting, they began trapping marmots indiscriminately and then transporting them to Siberian railway towns for sale. It was in Manchouli (headquarters of the trappers) that one of the hunters caught the infection (fever, bloody sputum) and died within three days. The infection spread rapidly through the crowded migrant camps and along the Chinese Eastern Railway in September 1910.

On October 27, it reached Harbin (Pinkiang) in northern Manchuria, where it became more virulent. Of the 25,000 residents in Fuchiaten (Harbin's Chinese quarter), 140 to 180 people died every day. Corpses lay scattered everywhere, and special imperial sanction had to be obtained for mass cremations (for 2,000 lying dead in the streets) in January 1911. Despite precautionary measures (e.g., detaining and isolating travelers from plague-ridden areas) instituted by the Japanese-controlled South Manchuria Railway in cooperation with the Kwangtung provincial government, the disease spread to Changchun (December 31, 1910), Mukden (Shen-yang), and Wafangtien. Dairen (Talien) reported its first case on January 5, 1911.

Within their respective zones, Chinese, Japanese, and Russian authorities immediately implemented their own prevention and containment strategies, but the mapping of a well-coordinated scheme of action took a little longer to negotiate. Passengers and cargo were subjected to strict inspection at outgoing ports to ensure that the plague did not spread via shipping. Korean and Japanese authorities took special precautions to prevent the infection from entering their countries. By March 1911, when plague was exterminated from Manchuria, it had reportedly (according to Chinese authorities) claimed 60,000 victims (including 7,000 in Harbin; 6,000 in Changchun; and 5,000 in Mukden).

An International Plague Conference was held in Mukden from April 3 to April 28, 1911, to discuss future strategies. To implement its recommendations, the North Manchurian Plague Prevention Service was established. That agency was responsible for laying the groundwork of China's public health system. In 1920–21, Manchuria was again visited by an epidemic of pneumonic plague, but thanks to strict preventive measures, the fatalities were much lower.

Further reading: Nathan, *Plague, Prevention and Politics in Manchuria, 1910–1931; Report on Progress in Manchuria, 1907–1928;* Lien-teh, *Plague;* Pollitzer, *Plague;* McNeill, *Plagues and Peoples.*

Manchurian Plague of 1920–21   Less severe than the Manchurian Plague of 1910–11 (q.v.), starting as an outbreak of bubonic plague (see HONG KONG PLAGUE OF 1894) at Abakait (near Manchouli) in August 1920. Some say the outbreak began in Hailar (Hulun) and Dalainor (Hulunnor) in September, from where it spread rapidly thanks to the deliberate thwarting of anti-plague measures by hostile Chinese troops stationed in northern Manchuria. By December, the disease had turned pneumonic. In January 1921, it spread from Harbin (Pinkiang) along the Chinese Eastern Railway to Vladivostok, where it continued to rage until October. The plague's casualties numbered 9,300—including 6,957 persons in the Chinese Eastern Railway zone, 640 in Vladivostok, 29 in Changchun, 35 from outside the railway zone between Changchun and Mukden (Shen-yang) and 30 from the railway zone itself.

Taking prompt action, the Manchurian Plague Prevention Service convened a meeting of Chinese, Japanese, and Russian authorities on January 6, 1921. A central office was established at Harbin to coordinate various plans of action. Railway sidings were laid and freight cars readied to accommodate plague victims at certain railway junctions. Detention stations with a housing capacity of 2,000 patients were set up at Changchun. Those traveling third class and intending to change trains (mainly Chinese coolies) had to stay in detention for five days and were allowed to proceed only when certified as being in good health.

Over a million dollars were spent on suppressing this epidemic, which would have intensified but for the cooperative action undertaken by the concerned authorities.

Further reading: Nathan, *Plague, Prevention and Politics in Manchuria, 1910–31; Report on Progress in Manchuria, 1907–1928;* Lien-teh, *Plague.*

Mandan Indian Smallpox Epidemic of 1837   Grave epidemic of smallpox that nearly wiped out the Mandan Indian tribe during three months in 1837. White Europeans carried the variola virus into what is now south and central North Dakota, where the Mandan lived along the Heart and Knife rivers (tributaries of the upper Missouri) in close association with the Hidatsa (or Gros Ventre) and Arikara Indians, two tribes also dwelling in and near the region.

In 1780–81 the Mandan Indians were first infected by smallpox (which evidently came to them by way of Mexico) and were reduced to about 1,500 to 2,000 in number after a devastating epidemic that killed thousands of them. Called the "People of the Pheasants," the Mandan were later visited and described by the American explorers Meriwether Lewis and William Clark in 1804.

In June 1837 the highly contagious smallpox disease was transmitted to the Mandan from infected passengers and traders aboard an American Fur Company steamboat traveling westward up the Missouri River from St. Louis. Members of the Hidatsa and Arikara tribes were also infected at the same time. Nearly all the Indians who were infected and survived the smallpox epidemic were disfigured; many victims were blinded. According to the American artist and traveler George Catlin (1796–1872), who painted these North American Indians of the Plains, his friend the Mandan chief Ma-to-toh-pa (also called "The Four Bears") starved himself to death after watching his wives and children die of smallpox. However, another source claims that the Mandan chief died of the disease himself on July 30, 1837, after making a speech to his people concerning his disdain over having to die with his face so "rotten" (a deeply pockmarked face, characteristic of smallpox).

At the close of the 1837 epidemic in September, the Mandan and Hidatsa groups were so reduced in number that they were forced to amalgamate at Like-A-Fishhook village. Some claim that only 27 Mandan were left; others say there were 100 to 150 survivors. The Mandan remnant later moved with the Hidatsa north to the Fort Berthold area, and later (1870) these two groups, along with the Arikara, were placed on a nearby, large Indian reservation. But in the late 1830s, smallpox spread from the Mandan to the Dakota (Sioux) Indians in the region and to the Crow and Assiniboin tribes in what is now Montana. From these groups, the disease spread by 1839 to the Kiowa and other tribes in the southwest, moving into present-day New Mexico. Traders from Santa Fe apparently brought the smallpox virus to the eastern United States.

Further reading: Hopkins, *Princes and Peasants: Smallpox in History*; Ramenofsky, *Vectors of Death*.

Marburg Virus Epidemic of 1967 Outbreak of a previously unknown type of hemorrhagic fever that appeared in Germany and Yugoslavia during the late summer of 1967. The infections were confined to three cities (notably Marburg, Germany) and primarily to people whose work involved contact with African green (vervet) monkeys. Although the total number of cases was small, the epidemic created alarm because the mortality rate was high (over 25 percent) and treatments such as antibiotics were powerless against the disease.

In demand at laboratories, which found their kidney cells ideal for growing viruses, nearly a quarter of a million vervet monkeys had been imported into Europe and the United States by the late 1960s. On August 8, 1967, however, researchers got their first indication that something dangerous might be lurking in those shipments. Employees of a German pharmaceutical company in Marburg began suffering from fever, vomiting, diarrhea, severe headache, and body aches. Doctors suspected dysentery, but none of the patients responded to antibiotic treatment. The intestinal complications were accompanied by other symptoms: a widespread rash of bright red spots, reddening of the genitals, enlargement of the liver, and hemorrhaging. Blood seeped out of the gastrointestinal tract, the lungs, the nose, the gums, and spots where patients had been pricked by needles.

While Marburg had the greatest number of victims, several nearly identical cases were observed in laboratory workers in Frankfurt at about the same time, and in Belgrade in September. Of the 31 total patients, 25 had directly handled monkey blood, either while dissecting the animals, working with their organs or cells, or cleaning culture containers; seven of these patients died. There were also six secondary infections among spouses and health care providers in contact with the workers, but all of these people recovered. Many of the survivors complained of exhaustion, weight and hair loss, sweats, and even psychiatric disturbances for weeks to come.

Epidemiologists traced all three outbreaks to several shipments of green monkeys from the same area of Uganda in east-central Africa. Yet in that country there was no evidence of an epizootic or of illness among monkey trappers. The monkeys must therefore have become infected en route, most likely in London, where they were held in custody for a number of hours along with several dozen other species of animals and birds.

Within days of the first case several important steps were taken to stop the epidemic. Public health authorities in Marburg ordered that all lab workers wear gloves and masks even when performing routine cleaning procedures. They alerted all doctors to the symptoms and carefully observed people who had been in contact with the lab workers. Soon afterward the infectious agent was isolated. A new virus larger than known viruses and of a different shape, it would prove remarkably similar to the Ebola virus, which was responsible for the Zairian Ebola Epidemic of 1976 (q.v.). By the end of August, the monkeys in Marburg had been put to death and their bodies burned.

Because of the epidemic, laboratories turned to other species of animals for experiments, and Marburg virus infection seemed to disappear entirely. In early 1975, however, an Australian tourist died of the disease in a hospital in Johannesburg, South Africa. A friend who had been traveling with him and a nurse who took care of both patients also came down with the infection, but both recovered. Since then, no further cases of Marburg virus infection (sometimes called green monkey disease) have been observed anywhere.

Further reading: Martini and Siegert, eds., *Marburg Virus Disease*; Simpson, *Marburg and Ebola Virus Infections*.

Marseilles, Plague of See PLAGUE OF MARSEILLES.

Massachusetts Smallpox Epidemic of c. 1617–19 Introduction of smallpox by Europeans on the American continent north of Mexico; this great outbreak destroyed 90 percent of the Massachusetts Bay Indians. English and Dutch fishing boats regularly visited the Massachusetts coast and could have brought the infection. Also, English explorer Bartholomew Gosnold visited Martha's Vineyard in the early 1600s. Destruction of the Indians eliminated one of the problems that would beset the Puritans when they erected their colonial settlement in Massachusetts in 1620. By then, there were only a few Narragansetts remaining of a tribe that, six years earlier, had commanded 3,000 braves. In their writings, the Puritans portrayed themselves as God's chosen sent to the New World following His will. At the same time, God destroyed the infidel savages who could obstruct the Christian pathway. Concepts of the heroic colonizer and evil savage pervaded colonial writings about the establishment and development of New England settlements. Later, some colonists even instigated and thrilled in the spread of smallpox among the Indians.

The Indians could not have resisted invasion. This disease was a mighty weapon, terrifying in its power. After Plymouth Plantation was established, an exploratory party went to Patuxit, where they found multitudes of Indians long dead, probably from the epidemic of 1617–19, which they concluded was plague, despite the decay. Although historians disagreed about whether the epidemic was smallpox or bubonic plague (both rampant in Europe), the preponderance of the evidence suggested smallpox, as recorded by the French at the time. Captain Thomas Dermeer, who witnessed the 1617–19 epidemic, reportedly saw pockmarks on some of the Indians.

Smallpox caused the greatest destruction among populations never before exposed, wiping out up to 90 percent of the infected. The disease had so lethal an effect on the Indians that they often died before the rash appeared, according to one nineteenth-century commentator. Also known as variola, smallpox was a highly contagious virus that a victim either inhaled or picked up via particles contaminated by a diseased person's nasal or oral mucous membrane. Victims could get the infection indirectly by touching contaminated objects. Because of their total vulnerability, Indians would have contracted the most virulent form of smallpox, although even the lesser variety (variola minor) would have proven fatal. After infection and an incubation period of about two weeks, victims would exhibit the symptoms of high fever, aches and pains, headaches, and, sometimes, vomiting. Later, spots appeared that became eruptions filled first with clear lymph and then pus, which would break, after which scabs would form and then fall off, causing scars, pockmarks, and spotty pigmentation. Accompanying or resulting infirmities could include blindness, heart problems, and arthritis, among many others.

In 1620, the Puritans settled in Plymouth, struggling to surmount deprivation, exposure, and sickness. They might not have been able to withstand any real resistance from the Indians. Instead, the recent epidemic left them plenty of space and opportunity to start their new civilization. To the Puritans, the decimation of the Indians to their own benefit came to be interpreted as part of God's plan. In the seventeenth century, diseases like smallpox, influenza, typhus, and measles were as significant a factor in conquering the new land as any other. See also MASSACHUSETTS SMALLPOX EPIDEMIC OF C. 1633; CONNECTICUT SMALLPOX EPIDEMIC OF 1634.

Further reading: Bollet, *Plagues and Poxes*; Bradford, *Of Plymouth Plantation*; Hopkins, *Princes and Peasants: Smallpox in History*.

Massachusetts Smallpox Epidemic of c. 1633

Pestilence that struck both the Massachusetts Bay Indians, decimating any possible resistance to the onslaught of new settlers, and the Plymouth Colony inhabitants; initiated a westward-moving wave of smallpox. Ships brought smallpox along with the settlers to the New World in the 1630s. A child died on one ship; 14 died on another. Religious leader Increase Mather later interpreted the routing of the Indians as God's judgment on the Indians' dispute over the amount colonists paid for the land. Whole towns of Indians were destroyed. By comparison, only 20 Plymouth Colony inhabitants died, and those had been original settlers brought by the *Mayflower*.

Also known as variola, smallpox was a highly infectious virus that victims either inhaled or picked up via contaminated particles. Symptoms included high fever, aches and pains, headaches, and sometimes vomiting. Later, skin eruptions formed that finally left scars, pockmarks, and spotty pigment.

Immunity explained the marked contrast between the effects of smallpox on European settlers as opposed to that on the Indians. Europeans, hailing from an area where infestation was endemic, had a high degree of immunity. In general, the disease was often fatal to the previously unexposed, and the Indians' innocence of the disease was complete. Nine out of ten Indians usually died in an epidemic, according to many accounts. A nomadic way of life, as well as panicked flights to escape contact with the diseased, both contributed to the widespread destruction of Indian nations. See also MASSACHUSETTS SMALLPOX EPIDEMIC OF C. 1617–1619; CONNECTICUT SMALLPOX EPIDEMIC OF 1634.

Further reading: Bradford, *Of Plymouth Plantation*; Hopkins, *Princes and Peasants: Smallpox in History*; Winslow, *A Destroying Angel: The Conquest of Smallpox in Colonial Boston*.

Massachusetts Smallpox Epidemic of 1648–49

One of the major outbreaks of smallpox in the English colonies in America. Most of the early outbreaks of the disease were confined to one settlement or area, but the 1648 epidemic spread to numerous towns and varied widely in severity from town to town in the Massachusetts Bay Colony. Boston was affected, but nearby Roxbury saw many more of its inhabitants perish from the disease, which was perhaps black smallpox (*purpura variola*), a highly fatal form, according to some reports.

The English colonists—men, women, and children—who had not been exposed to smallpox previously and thus developed an immunity to it, were greatly alarmed when many of them suddenly complained of splitting headaches, backaches, chills, fevers, nausea, and sometimes convulsions and delirium. Over the next few days, these symptoms faded as the characteristic, deep-seated smallpox rash appeared (a rash usually leaving a survivor with a permanent reminder of his or her bout with the disease); some were left with pockmarked faces, blindness, or infertility.

The town of Scituate, south of Boston, was especially hard hit, as was Cape Cod, where an outbreak of whooping cough was concurrently afflicting many settlers. The combined diseases (smallpox and whooping cough) may have led observers to perceive the smallpox epidemic as more severe than it actually was. Nevertheless, the epidemic seriously affected so many children in Scituate and Barnstable (on Cape Cod) that the church fathers in these towns declared a "Day of Humiliation" on November 15, 1649.

Further reading: Duffy, *Epidemics in Colonial America;* Shurkin, *The Invisible Fire;* Winslow, *A Destroying Angel: The Conquest of Smallpox in Colonial Boston.*

Mauritian Influenza Epidemic of 1919 Outbreak of influenza on Mauritius, a British crown colony until its independence in 1968, where about 100,000 inhabitants were infected and over 10,000 of them died between May and October 1919. The origin of the "Spanish influenza" on Mauritius is not known; the island, the main one of the colony, was then a strategic British stronghold in the Indian Ocean. The flu may have been imported from India, China, or a European country with strong trading ties to the island, or the infection could have been transported with troops from Britain.

The respiratory illness, which had been raging throughout much of the world since late 1917 (see SPANISH INFLUENZA EPIDEMIC OF 1917–19), entered Port Louis, Mauritius's capital, in early May 1919 and infected the native, Chinese, Indian, and European populations with equal intensity. Onset of the infection was frequently sudden (sometimes within a few minutes), with victims complaining of the ordinary influenza symptoms: headache, malaise, congested nose, cough, fever, chills, and body aches; most patients remained sick for three days. In about six weeks in May–June 1919, at least 80,000 people were infected on Mauritius, where British and other physicians were unable to adequately treat the sick and thousands perished. Most of the deaths were because of complications such as staphylococcal pneumonia and empyema (collection of pus in a bodily cavity), both secondary infections and lethal prior to the use of penicillin.

The "Spanish influenza" continued to strike Mauritians severely until early July, when cases began to decline more and more until the epidemic ended in October. Fatalities were especially high among the elderly, many of whom died from heart problems.

Further reading: Burnet and Clarke, *Influenza;* Crosby, *America's Forgotten Pandemic: The Influenza of 1918.*

Mauritian Malaria Epidemic of 1866–68 One of the earliest malaria epidemics reported in detail, before the mosquito was identified as the disease-infecting vector. A severe epidemic, it swept the island of Mauritius in the Indian Ocean for three years, killing almost one fourth of the resident population of about 300,000.

The epidemic disease first broke out in early 1866 at the Albion sugar estate just south of Port Louis, the capital of Mauritius. The sugar trade had made Mauritius one of Great Britain's most lucrative colonial possessions. Laborers from India, as well as British troops, had brought malaria parasites to the island two decades earlier; yet the fever had never spread nor had the disease ever been deadly prior to 1866. It changed from endemic to epidemic seriousness that year, sometime after the infectious vector (the *Anopheles gambiae* and *Anopheles funestus* varieties of mosquito) arrived in Port Louis from Madagascar or from India, most likely on board one of the ships that docked there.

The vector, which preferred a sunny and human environment, found an ideal one in Mauritius, where more Europeans at that time lived than in the whole of Africa. The recently cleared jungles and forests (for the planting of sugar cane) provided a perfect breeding ground for these anopheline mosquitoes, while the rapidly increasing workforce on the sugar plantations became an ideal repository for the malaria parasite. When the heavy rainfall of December 1865 caused widespread flooding in the newly cleared lands, many weedy streams and stagnant pools of water were created, thus making perfect breeding habitats for the malaria-carrying mosquitoes.

In the epidemic's first year, 1866, it extended over a 40- to 50-square-mile area, slowly spreading, with one wave of the disease moving south of the Albion estate while another traveled to Port Louis, where some 6,000 people (out of a population of about 47,000) died of malaria during that first year. Thousands fell ill, and there were not enough healthy men left to bury the corpses. During the following two years, the disease invaded all the coastal and low-lying areas on this 720-square-mile island, a British crown colony. There were 31,920 deaths in 1867, the peak epidemic year. More than 10,000 victims were claimed the next and final year of the epidemic; after that, it started subsiding.

Not until 1880 did a French Army surgeon, Alphonse Laveran, discover malaria's causative, parasitic organism, now called *Plasmodium,* which mosquitoes pick up from the blood of infected people and transfer to healthy people. The mode of infection, however, was not substantiated until 1897, when Ronald Ross, a British military surgeon, proved that malaria is transmitted by mosquitoes. Subsequently, in 1898, the Italian zoologist G. B. Grassi identified the vector to be the *Anopheles* genus of mosquitoes.

Though it was proved even later that only one tenth of all known *Anopheles* species will transmit malaria, the communicable disease, with its recurring symptoms of severe fever and shivering, still claims the lives of about one million infants and children in Africa every year. Those who survive gradually build up an immunity. This was the case in Mauritius, where the disease remained endemic, but where, after 1868, there was no repetition of what has been called "The Great Mauritius Epidemic."

Further reading: Ackerknecht, *History and Geography of the Most Important Diseases*; Harrison, *Mosquitoes, Malaria and Man*; Russell, *Man's Mastery of Malaria*.

Maximilian II's Army Typhus Epidemic   Outbreak of typhus fever that struck the army of the Habsburg Holy Roman Emperor, Maximilian II, in the summer of 1566; weakened by disease, the troops could not aid their Hungarian allies, who were fighting the Ottoman Turks. Like their predecessors in a 1542 war against the Ottomans (see JOACHIM'S ARMY EPIDEMIC OF 1542), the imperial soldiers were quite susceptible to typhus, which they called "the Hungarian disease" and which probably came to Hungary during the numerous Ottoman campaigns of the sixteenth century. Once the disease became endemic in Hungary, the country would serve as the origin for many subsequent epidemics that spread throughout Europe, as the one of 1566 did (which lasted until 1568).

For much of the 1500s, Hungary was the battleground on which imperial troops of the Holy Roman Empire contended with Ottoman armies. The frontier between East and West kept shifting because of near-constant skirmishes, raids, local conflicts, and all-out campaigns. By attacking in 1566, the aged sultan Suleiman I (Sulayman I) hoped to extend the borders of Ottoman-controlled Hungary (the center portion of the country) and strike at Vienna itself, in Austria. With an army 100,000 strong, Maximilian marched out to defend his eastern territories, but the epidemic rendered his troops useless. Sick and dying, they encamped along the Danube on the island of Komorn while a vastly outnumbered Hungarian garrison at Szigetvar held out for more than a month before being killed by the Turks. However, during the siege, Suleiman died, and the Turks soon went home without capitalizing on their victory.

Thomas Jordanus, a German surgeon who accompanied the imperial troops, described the epidemic, which was clearly typhus. Like so many soldiers before and since, those under Maximilian suffered from food shortages, poor water and sanitation, and unbearably hot weather—all of which led to dysentery, scurvy, and malaria. Typhus soon followed; after an onset of chills, victims came down with abdominal pain, delirium, and extreme thirst, and nearly all whom Jordanus observed had the characteristic skin eruption.

The disease did not remain confined to the soldiers in Hungary. The country had been devastated by the endless fighting and by Habsburg demands for money to pay soldiers, obtain weapons, and build and maintain a series of border forts against the Ottomans. Their country ruined, and their agricultural system in shambles, many Hungarian civilians caught typhus from the troops, who then carried it even farther afield. Vienna was hit with the most severe typhus epidemic it ever knew; the residents of entire streets, not just of individual houses, were afflicted. For the next two years local typhus outbreaks flared up in many parts of Europe, including Austria, Italy, Bohemia, Germany, France, Belgium, and the Netherlands, as the imperial troops returned home. The Austro-Turkish wars of the 1500s created circumstances that gave typhus a chance to pass from one person to another, instead of the infection being carried by fleas from infected rats (this phase of transmittal was thus bypassed).

Further reading: Prinzing, *Epidemics Resulting from Wars*; Sugar, ed., *A History of Hungary*; Zinsser, *Rats, Lice and History*.

Mecca Cholera Epidemic of 1831   Epidemic marking cholera's first devastating invasion of Mecca, site of Islam's holiest shrine.

An offshoot of the Asiatic Cholera Pandemic of 1826–37 (q.v.), it began in the spring of 1831 when Muslims from modern-day Iraq and the Arabian Peninsula brought cholera into Mecca in western Arabia during their annual *hadj* (pilgrimage). Prior to that, a few cases of cholera had been reported in Mecca and were believed to have been imported from India. Amid the vast gathering of humanity assembled at the shrine in Mecca, the disease broke out with tremendous virulence and spread very rapidly. Apparently, nearly half of those gathered there were struck by cholera and thousands of Muslims, including dignitaries such as the governors of Mecca and Jeddah and the pasha of Syria, succumbed to it. There were so many human corpses and so few persons to bury them that the idea of separate burials was abandoned. Over the next three weeks, about 3,000 pilgrims on their way home from Mecca reportedly died of cholera.

From Mecca, one branch of the epidemic traveled to Syria and Palestine while another offshoot crossed the Suez Canal and devastated Cairo (July 1831) and Alexandria (August 1831) in Egypt, before moving westward to Tunis later in the year. During the next few years, Ethiopia, Somaliland, Zanzibar, Algeria, and Sudan were hit. Mecca continued to suffer the onslaught of cholera almost every year during pilgrimage time until 1912.

Further reading: Macnamara, *A History of Asiatic Cholera.*

Mecca Cholera Epidemic of 1865

Offshoot of the fourth cholera pandemic (see ASIATIC CHOLERA PANDEMIC OF 1865–75), the holy city of Mecca's most severe cholera epidemic broke out in the jubilee year of the annual *Hadj* (pilgrimage). The epidemic sped the transmission of cholera throughout the African and European continents along new routes of transportation (see MECCA CHOLERA EPIDEMIC OF 1831).

By all accounts, the epidemic was devastating in its intensity; it began during the third week of March 1865 among the hordes of Muslim pilgrims assembled at the Kaaba, Islam's holiest shrine. According to some, cholera may have been present in Mecca already and flared up with the advent of the Muslim crowds. The disease was then very virulent over many parts of India and apparently also along Saudi Arabia's nearby Red Sea coast. Undoubtedly, pilgrims arriving in Mecca from these infected regions could have brought the disease with them. Some historians are even more specific and state that cholera arrived in Mecca from Singapore via Bombay on the ships *Persia* and *North Wind.* The commanders of these vessels later testified in front of the British consul in Jedda (Jidda) that cholera did not break out on board until the ships had left the port of Malacca.

Regardless of the route, the epidemic was very severe in Mecca, where 90,000 or so pilgrims had gathered. About 30,000 reportedly died of cholera in Mecca, Meenha, Arafat, and later Jedda. In mid-May the pilgrimage ended and thousands of Muslims left for home, via such ports as Suez and Alexandria. Many perished en route; some of those who did not, brought cholera with them.

Further reading: Pollitzer, *Cholera*; Macnamara, *A History of Asiatic Cholera.*

Memphis Yellow Fever Epidemics of 1878–79

See U.S. YELLOW FEVER EPIDEMICS OF 1878–79.

Metz Typhus Epidemic of 1552

See CHARLES V'S ARMY EPIDEMIC AT METZ.

Mexican and Central American Dysentery Epidemic of 1970

See GUATEMALAN DYSENTERY EPIDEMIC OF 1969–70.

Mexican Cholera Epidemic of 1833

Serious early outbreak of cholera. Cholera entered Mexico on May 24, 1833, through the seaport of Tampico, from Cuba or New Orleans. It quickly spread to the upland areas of central Mexico, where San Luis Potosí was the first city to suffer from the disease. Reports from the seaport of Campeche on the Yucatán Peninsula indicate that a ship from Tampico had spread the disease there.

The disease, caused by the bacterium *cholera vibrio* and found in contaminated drinking water, first strikes people with an acute attack of diarrhea and vomiting, which results in extreme dehydration. In severe cases, death is immediate—sometimes within a matter of hours. At San Luis Potosí, 4,366 people died between June and October 1833. Death carts would make their rounds to pick up the human dead; after the last round, corpses would be dumped and left heaped on the ground to be tumbled into a massive burial ditch the next morning.

From San Luis Potosí, the cholera epidemic moved northwest to the town of Zacatecas and south to Guadalajara, where 3,275 people died in two months. In Mexico City, with its crowded and unsanitary conditions, an approximate 10,322 people died from the disease.

Further reading: Marks and Beatty, *Epidemics*; Cartwright, *Disease and History*; Mathews and Mosley, "Cholera."

Mexican-Guatemalan Smallpox Epidemic of 1797

Outbreak of smallpox that began on the Atlantic Coast of Mexico and spread throughout Mexico and Guatemala. Of historical note is the fact that doctors made the first real attempt to variolate the native population.

The epidemic is generally dated 1797 (when it reached its peak); yet it evidently originated about 1792–93, when existing smallpox outbreaks were reported in the states of Chiapas and Tabasco in southeastern Mexico. There were 602 smallpox cases (105 persons died) in the coastal town of Campeche in 1793–94. The disease then traveled south into Guatemala, following trade routes, and north-westward into the interior, striking the Mexican cities of Orizaba, Puebla, and Mexico City.

Mexico had no public health agents to ordinate a relief program in 1797, and small towns and villages relied on aid from large cities during epidemics. At that time there was a serious effort by the medical profession to introduce variolation to all segments of society in both Mexico and Guatemala. It is estimated that there were between 100,000 and 150,000 smallpox cases and between 14,000 and 25,000 deaths during this epidemic; the majority of the cases were children under 18 years of age.

Variolation is an obsolete practice of transferring the smallpox virus from one human being to another by inoculation. It was hoped that a mild smallpox case would occur that would then give immunity to the patient. The inoculation process was not always sterile, and frequently the virus infected a healthy person with a severe case of smallpox. Although crude, variolation was somewhat successful. Of those patients that were inoculated, there was an estimated 3.5 percent death rate and of those not inoculated, an 18.5 percent death rate.

The first obvious signs of smallpox are fever and backache. A rash develops after three to five days and then develops into pustules that erupt. It is at this stage that the patient is contagious. There has never been a cure for smallpox, and before variolation came into wide use, quarantine and isolation were the most effective way to stop the spread of infection.

Quarantine proved hard to enforce in Mexico and Guatemala because it interrupted business, and isolation of patients in poor hospitals meant almost no care and almost certain death. The practice of hiding smallpox cases became widespread, and riots erupted when the government resorted to using military force to bring the sick to hospitals. People overcame the military at times to break into hospitals to remove patients.

Eventually, the smallpox disease traveled outward to more rural areas and slowed down its rate of infection. The epidemic ceased altogether in 1798.

Further reading: Cook, "The Smallpox Epidemic of 1797 in Mexico"; Baxby, *Jenner's Smallpox Vaccine*; Shurkin, *The Invisible Fire.*

Mexican Smallpox Epidemic of 1520–21   Pernicious epidemic decimating millions of Aztecs, including their emperor, Cuitlahuac, during the conquest of Mexico by Hernando Cortes. Smallpox (*viruela* [Spanish], *hueyzanuatl* [Aztec]) was introduced to the American mainland by Francisco de Baguia, a black slave to Pánfilo de Narváez. Narváez had been dispatched to Mexico in March 1520 by the Spanish governor of Cuba, where smallpox was rampant. The Narváez expedition was meant to supersede that of Cortes, who had left for Mexico the previous November. Narváez and his men arrived near the present-day seaport of Veracruz on April 23, 1520. The smallpox spread like fire to the Indian population. In most provinces it was reported that more than half the Aztec population died. Many victims actually died from starvation; so many had taken sick or had died that there was no one well enough to

tend to the stricken or to prepare bread for food. To quell the stench from the many corpses, houses were collapsed over whole families of dead.

The pestilence spread to the edge of Mexico's inland plateau during the summer and pervaded the inland plateau by September. Smallpox was introduced to Tenochtitlan, the Aztec capital (now Mexico City), in June 1520, during the battle between Aztecs and Spaniards that followed the brutal massacre of the native population at the great feast of Huitzilopochtili. The massacre and ensuing battle provoked by it led to a retreat by Cortes; the smallpox virus, possibly on the corpse of a Spaniard or one of Cortes's Tlaxcalleca Indian allies, was left behind in Tenochtitlan. Within two weeks, a plague of the most virulent, infectious variety ensued, with a very high death rate. In August half the city was dead of smallpox. By September, the disease had swept through Anahuac (the central plateau) as far as Chalco. The epidemic lasted approximately 70 days, taking Cuitlahuac, the new emperor who had succeeded the slain Montezuma and had ruled for only 14 days, along with much of the other effective leadership. A young, inexperienced nephew of Montezuma, Cuauhtemoc, became the new emperor. Most of the city was infected; victims were immobilized by pain. Corpses lay in the roads and were described as "sticky, compacted and hard grain." It was a much weakened Tenochtitlan that Cortes returned to and eventually conquered during June through August 1521. Cortes himself is quoted as saying "a man could not set his foot down except on the corpse of an Indian."

More than 250 years before Edward Jenner's cowpox vaccination was discovered (1798), childhood exposure to the virus was the sole means of protection from the disease. It was said that virtually every Spaniard had experienced smallpox as a child. The Indians had never before been exposed to the disease. That smallpox devastated the Aztec population and helped Cortes bring about the destruction of the Aztec empire is clear. What is not certain is how many of the natives were felled by the disease. Some historians have claimed that half the Mexican population, estimated then to have been about 30 million, succumbed to the disease. Other sources have estimated that 2 million to 3.5 million of the Aztecs died. Smallpox was still present over a full year after the arrival in Mexico of Narváez's infected slave. The account of Bernal Diaz de Castillo, describing the scene at Tlaltilco in August 1521, states:

> The streets, the squares, the houses . . . were covered with dead bodies; we could not stop without

treading on them, and the stench was intolerable . . . all the causeways were full, from one end to the other, of men, women and children, so weak and sickly, squalid and dirty, and pestilential that it was as misery to behold them.

Smallpox moved along with the Spaniards to devastate the Mayan population farther south, the Cakchiquels in Yucatan, and the Incas in Peru.

Further reading: Hopkins, *Princes and Peasants: Smallpox History*; Ashburn, *The Ranks of Death: A Medical History of the Conquest of America.*

Mexican Typhus Epidemic of 1576 First specifically recognized epidemic of typhus fever in Mexico, where Aztec Indians and many others fell victim to it. At the time typhus was very prevalent in Spain, where it was known as *tabardillo* or *tabardete* or *pintas*; in Mexico it was known by the vernacular term of *hueyzanuatl* or *matlalzahuatl* by the natives.

This frequently fatal disease, carried by rat fleas and body lice, reportedly first occurred in Mexico in 1570. It is believed that typhus-infected rats most likely carried the disease aboard Spanish ships sailing to Mexico and elsewhere in Latin America. There was constant ocean traffic and communication between Spain and the New World in the sixteenth century. And ships frequently made trips between Havana, Cuba (an important Spanish port), and the coast of Yucatán and part of Veracruz, Mexico. Typhus-carrying rats probably were transported aboard ships from Cuba to Mexico, where undoubtedly rat fleas transmitted the disease to lice-infested native peoples. The disease was clearly recognized by friars, who carried Roman Catholicism to the natives in the Mexican interior and central high plateaus and who recorded a fearful epidemic in 1576. At about the same time, Spaniards in Peru made note of many incidents of typhus among the natives. Authorities conclude that the disease was a dreadful "gift" from white Europeans to the Indians in the Americas. See also MEXICO CITY TYPHUS EPIDEMIC OF 1813.

Further reading: Zinsser, *Rats, Lice and History*; Ramenofsky, *Vectors of Death: The Archaeology of European Contact.*

Mexico City Smallpox Epidemic of 1779 Epidemic of smallpox (*variola major*) that killed an estimated 20 percent of the population (about 18,000 people out of 90,000).

Smallpox had been occurring periodically in South America since the 1500s. By the 1700s, it had become endemic to Mexico City and also existed within the interior, breaking out about every seven years.

The 1779 epidemic started with sporadic outbreaks in August of 1779 and gathered momentum each month. By December, there were 44,286 cases and 8,821 deaths reported. The hospitals were overflowing and corpses filled the streets. It was one of the most devastating epidemics to strike Mexico City, where about 80 percent of the people lived on the edge of destitution. The unsanitary conditions, the close quarters, and the lack of quarantine measures allowed the disease to thrive.

Smallpox is a highly infectious disease; the first obvious signs are fever and backache. After three to five days, a rash develops covering the human body and sometimes attacking the eyes (at its peak, smallpox was the leading cause of blindness in the world). The lesions progress to pustules that are infectious. The sores form crusts and fall off, often leaving the person scarred.

The Mexican epidemic in 1779 killed or infected so many people that successive epidemics were considered mild—the result of the adult population having already acquired immunity. The form of smallpox that constituted the 1779 epidemic is known as *variola major*, the deadliest strain of the disease; *variola minor* is a milder form, usually with a fatality rate of about one percent. (As a disease and a population exist together, a mutual tolerance develops, and the disease loses its severity.) *Variola major* was replaced by *variola minor* in the 1900s.

There were very few outbreaks of smallpox reported in Mexico City in the 1780s. The next epidemic to strike the city was in 1797; it would mainly affect young people under the age of 20. During the outbreak, physicians made the first real attempt at variolation (vaccinating with the smallpox virus) of the natives. See MEXICAN-GUATEMALAN SMALLPOX EPIDEMIC OF 1797.

Further reading: Cook, "The Smallpox Epidemic of 1797 in Mexico"; Fehrenbach, *Fire and Blood*; Cowley, "The Great Disease Migration"; Hopkins, *Princes and Peasants: Smallpox in History.*

Mexico City Typhus Epidemic of 1813 Devastating epidemic that killed an estimated 20,385 persons. At the time Mexican natives called typhus by the vernacular name of *matlalzahuatl*, from which they had suffered in epidemic form in 1576, 1736, and 1762 in rural and mountainous regions.

In January 1813 epidemic typhus broke out in the highland town of Puebla and soon spread to Mexico City (80 miles northwest of Puebla). Located on the site of a former lake bed, Mexico City's waterways or canals were used for garbage disposal; even its outer-lying lakes were often filled with city garbage, creating a very unhealthy environment. A Junta (Council) of Health was organized to manage the city's defenses against the spread of the disease.

Officials quickly ordered a quarantine of persons infected with typhus, which had already struck poor Mexicans in low-lying areas. By mid-April 1813 typhus was a threat to all city inhabitants and was spreading rapidly. The cost of the ongoing Mexican struggle for independence (against Spanish rule) drained funds needed to pay physicians and buy food for victims of the epidemic. By soliciting the wealthy, the junta raised 27,000 pesos to fight the disease, but the money ran out in a month and a half. Public granaries ran out of money to buy maize, and the city government had to rely on private charity to supply public food kitchens. Relief efforts had become minuscule by June 1813, when it was reported that 65,512 people had contracted typhus.

A critical labor shortage occurred as Mexican workers fell ill, died, or fled the city. The dead were buried in the streets and in vacant lots, and the government was forced to use convicts to dig graves and to carry on sanitation work. Officials could do little, and the epidemic was left to run its course. It slowed with the coming of cooler weather. The final death toll reportedly amounted to one out of every eight citizens of Mexico City, which experienced a record loss of life from an epidemic.

Further reading: Anna, *The Fall of the Royal Government of Mexico City*; Marks and Beatty, *Epidemics*.

Middle East Hepatitis Epidemics of World War II

Outbreaks of infectious hepatitis among the Allied troops fighting in the Middle East theater from 1940 to 1943.

Hepatitis had been steadily spreading among the British troops in Palestine since the latter half of 1940 and was beginning to acquire a reputation as a fast-moving, sometimes fatal, disease. It intensified into a major epidemic during the fall of 1942, shortly before the Allies' one-million-strong Middle East army advanced to El Alamein, Egypt. When the epidemic struck in September 1942, the British Eighth Army occupied the western desert up to El Alamein, the Ninth Army was stationed in Lebanon and Syria, and there were Allied bases in Cyprus, Malta, Palestine, Egypt, Sudan, Aden, and Ethiopia. Following the front line, the epidemic spread rapidly throughout the Middle East Command, even to besieged Malta, but the incidence varied from place to place and group to group. It was highest where the conditions were extremely filthy, such as among the fly-ridden, half-buried corpses of the German or Italian enemy.

The front line of the Eighth Army was one of the worst affected. In fact, the epidemic began there in September 1942 within the New Zealand division stationed in the southern area near the El Alamein line. The outbreak, which was concentrated in a five-square-mile area, peaked in October and affected 14 percent of the men in this division. Early in October, hepatitis broke out among the Australian division in the north, which was separated from the New Zealand unit by the British division. This outbreak subsided by the end of October. Troops in the British division were affected later in the campaign, the epidemic peaking there in December. The outbreaks faded in the region by March 1943.

Overall, it is estimated that many regiments lost eight percent or nine percent of their members and up to one third of their officers to hepatitis. More than half a million man-days were lost because of the disease in the entire British Command. Generally, British troops were more likely to be attacked than troops from other countries, and British officers four times as likely to contract it than the men under their command. In December 1942, the reported incidence per 1,000 men was 8.2 overall, 9.83 in Egypt (including the Eighth Army based there), 15 in the Eighth Army as a whole, and 9.86 in the Ninth Army. Highest attack rates were in the 21- to 25-year-old category. Despite their relatively small strength, American troops in the Middle East (including Egypt) reported an annual hospital admission rate of 16.7 per 1,000 during the period June–December 1942. Meanwhile, morbidity among the civilian populations in Egypt, Syria, or Lebanon did not increase proportionally.

The Middle East forces of the Allies were again invaded by hepatitis late in 1943. The resulting epidemic, which spread concurrently with a similar epidemic in Italy, was widespread but did not have the same impact as the epidemic of 1942 since the Allied Command was not militarily active.

Hepatitis, along with malaria, was one of the major causes of morbidity in the Middle East theater during World War II. Studies conducted during the war by the medical authorities in the military have greatly contributed to our understanding of the disease and how it is transmitted.

Further reading: Cope, ed., *History of the Second World War: Medicine and Pathology*; Hoff, ed., *Preventive Medicine in World War II*.

Milan Plague of 1629–31   See ITALIAN PLAGUES OF 1629–31.

Mongallan Meningitis Epidemics of 1918–24 and 1926–31

Serious outbreaks of cerebrospinal meningitis (CSM) that killed about eight out of ten victims stricken in Mongalla, a province in southern Sudan. At first, the epidemics were peculiarly confined to the central region of Mongalla, an area previously free from CSM, which is characterized by inflammation of the membranes of the spinal cord and brain. Symptoms of CSM include fever, dizziness, delirium, rash, numbness, headache, and stiff neck.

In early 1918 the disease erupted in central Mongalla, to which apparently it was carried by Ugandan natives from the south. (Some Ugandan porters, who served in German East Africa during World War I, had contracted the infection and introduced it to their people in 1916.) CSM spread from one Mongallan community to another in the central region before moving northward, causing high mortality over six years.

A less damaging CSM epidemic hit Mongalla's central region in 1926. Improved medical services enabled the number of deaths from CSM to be counted: 335 in 1928, 446 in 1929, and 356 from January through March 1930; only six victims perished from it in the remaining months of the year. Once again, the disease traveled a northward route of contagion after leaving central Mongalla.

Dr. Alexander Cruickshank, a member of the Sudan Medical Services, recognized that the epidemics in Mongalla were partly the result of poor housing conditions. He claimed that the Azande native people, who lived in the western area, had escaped the airborne, bacterial disease because they were nutritionally healthier and lived in less crowded housing than the Dinka and Nuer natives in the central area.

The Dinka and Nuer tribes, affected by a famine in 1927, had occupied the black cotton plains of Mongalla's cattle country, which was badly infested with mosquitoes and fleas and, during the hot dry season, was whipped continually by gusty winds that raised a fine gritty dust. To protect themselves from the insects, cold, and wind, the natives crowded into their poorly ventilated dwellings and covered themselves with ash, a deterrent against insect bites. Evidently, droplets and discharges through coughs and sneezes of infected persons were mainly responsible for spreading the meningococcal bacteria.

Although modern chemotherapy and available antibiotics have helped to improve the treatment of CSM, this epidemic disease remains one of the most dangerous in Africa and one that is still puzzling to medical authorities.

Further reading: Hartwig and Patterson, *Cerebrospinal Meningitis in West Africa and Sudan in the Twentieth Century;* Burnet and White, *Natural History of Infectious Disease.*

Montreal Smallpox Epidemic of 1885 Catastrophic outbreak of smallpox (variola) that killed 3,164 persons, mainly French-Canadians. Children under ten years old comprised 2,717 of the fatalities.

From 1872 to 1880 there had been a total of 4,910 human deaths from smallpox in the Quebec city of Montreal, whose mostly French-Canadian population had violently opposed vaccination at the time. Fostered by a prominent Montreal physician, opposition to inoculation rested on the possibility of serious ulcerations as a result, possibly because of a syphilitic origin for the disease. In late February and early March 1885 the hospital Hôtel Dieu reported the first smallpox cases and fatalities of the impending epidemic in Montreal, whose unprotected populace was soon being threatened by the disease. Twenty-two persons died form smallpox in Montreal in June; by the time the epidemic peaked in August, there were 1,243 deaths reported. Yet opposition to vaccination continued, culminating in a major riot in the streets on September 28, 1885, at the end of a week when 226 out of 245 smallpox fatalities had been among French-Canadians. On that day, a mob of anti-vaccinationists wrecked the east end of the medical health officer's department and threatened to burn down the mayor's house and those of others supporting vaccination. Military intervention was needed to quell the riots.

The seriousness of the Montreal epidemic caused U.S. officials to refuse the entry of unvaccinated emigrants from Canada into the country. When several smallpox cases occurred in Toronto, Ontario's authorities imposed even stricter measures to prevent the disease from entering the province; they feared that smallpox-contaminated goods produced or manufactured in Montreal (where families of many factory workers were particularly hard hit by the disease) could easily enter Ontario by railway freight. Therefore goods entering the province were carefully inspected and those suspected of contamination were fumigated. Also, public health officials in Montreal arranged with some 80 merchants who shipped goods to Ontario to have their workers' homes inspected, vaccinations administered, and smallpox patients isolated. All passengers on railways traveling west from Montreal were ordered checked for evidence of vaccination; if not vaccinated, they were arrested and pulled off the trains to Ontario.

This last serious smallpox epidemic in Montreal ended in late 1885. From then on, vaccination in Quebec was carried out without opposition, and the province has since remained more free from smallpox than any other in Canada.

Further reading: Heagerty, *Four Centuries of Medical History in Canada;* Roland, ed., *Health, Disease and Medicine.*

Moroccan Meningitis Epidemics of 1967–70 Two serious outbreaks of cerebrospinal meningitis (CSM), killing a total of at least 1,230 persons out of

an estimated 10,000 infected. Previously, between 1930 and 1965, this country in northwestern Africa had reported only about 4,170 CSM infections. During those earlier years, the disease had occurred sporadically, with as few as seven cases in 1933 and as many as 489 in 1961; there is no available data concerning CSM in 1966.

It is not known why CSM, an acute bacterial inflammation of the meninges (membranes) surrounding the brain and spinal cord, suddenly broke out in epidemic proportions in Morocco in the winter of 1967 (although CSM began escalating that year in many West African countries south of the Sahara Desert). Caused by specific bacteria closely related to the infectious agent of gonorrhea, CSM was confined to the more populated Moroccan cities of Casablanca, Marrakesh, and Rabat, the capital. These urban centers, where the majority of the country's population lived in overcrowded and unsanitary conditions, were well suited for transmission of the pathogen by aerial droplets during the cold, dry weather; asymptomatic carriers played a major role in the spread of the infection. Sulfonamide therapy, as well as diagnostic and therapeutic measures, kept the number of fatalities to about 950 before the epidemic ended in the spring of 1968. Unofficially, more than 7,000 people had contracted CSM.

The following winter a second CSM epidemic erupted in the dirty slums of Morocco's main cities and continued into the spring of 1969. About ten percent of the 2,821 reported cases were fatal. In 1971 the incidence of CSM in Morocco declined to 475 cases. See also NIGERIAN MENINGITIS EPIDEMICS OF 1949 AND 1950.

Further reading: Ackerknecht, *History and Geography of the Most Important Diseases;* Hartwig and Patterson, *Cerebrospinal Meningitis in West Africa and Sudan in the Twentieth Century.*

Moroccan Plague of 1911

Outbreak of mainly bubonic plague striking the historic Doukkala district and adjacent areas in French Morocco, claiming the lives of 8,000 to 10,000 persons. For nearly a century, this infectious, bacterial disease had been absent in Morocco, but it unexpectedly reappeared in 1909–10 in the Casablanca area, where the outbreak was minor, with a total of 25 cases observed in military stations there (see PLAGUE PANDEMIC, THIRD).

The 1911 epidemic was most likely of maritime origin: Commensal black rats initially became plague-infected in the Atlantic ports of Casablanca (Morocco's largest city) and Rabat (the capital) and then spread the disease inland. Between May and June and again in October 1911, plague raged in Doukkala and adjacent hinterlands. The black rat carried the infection, and when it died, its diseased fleas sought another host, which frequently became a human being, particularly in areas where people lived close to rat populations. With the bite of an infective flea, persons contracted plague. Human-flea infestations, prevalent in North Africa, had long been a parasitic annoyance in many Moroccan houses, and the human flea as well as the body louse were implicated in the transmission of plague to humans. Although most of the plague cases in 1911 were bubonic (the glandular type), there were numerous pneumonic cases (the lung type, contracted directly from the highly infectious bubonic victims). Among the Moroccan Muslims infected, the fatality rate averaged 70 percent in the epidemic areas, whereas among the stricken Europeans, the fatality rate was less severe, averaging 50 percent.

After 1911 plague was endemic in some Moroccan regions; outbreaks of varying intensity occurred from 1912 to 1919 in the interior, spreading also to Casablanca and Rabat.

Further reading: Hirst, *The Conquest of Plague;* Pollitzer, *Plague.*

Moroccan Relapsing Fever Epidemic of 1945–46

Serious epidemic of relapsing fever (a systemic spirochetal disease) that killed at least 2,000 persons of the 43,900 cases reported. Other parts of North Africa were struck, too (see ALGERIAN RELAPSING FEVER EPIDEMIC OF 1943–46).

The disease entered Morocco (divided then into French and Spanish protectorates) at the city of Oujda, near the Algerian border, in January 1945. There was overcrowding, poverty, and much vermin infestation in Oujda, whose 20,000 inhabitants were also feeling the ravages of World War II. Thus, the disease, spread by human head and body lice (as well as rodents' ticks), became epidemic, thriving in the filth and poverty (as does typhus, which had infected Morocco since 1942 and would kill thousands of Moroccans by the end of 1946).

In 1945 Morocco's population was weak and susceptible to disease because of poor nutrition and successive years of mediocre harvests. Thus relapsing fever rapidly spread southward and westward from Oujda and reached the more populous, interior cities of Fez (Fès), Marrakesh (Marrakech), and Meknès and the large coastal city of Casablanca (about 500,000 people) by the fall of 1945. The disease also was entrenched in the coastal city of Rabat (north of Casablanca), headquarters of the sultan and the French. Thousands of people suffered from recurring bouts of high fever lasting two to nine days.

In the ancient rival cities of Fez and Marrakesh, relapsing fever was particularly severe in January

1946, when the colder climate and lower temperatures (about 50° F in winter) forced people to wear heavier clothing that became lice-infested. The mortality rate in both these cities was the highest, at ten percent; other urban areas, which were hard hit by the disease epidemic, recorded fatality rates ranging from two to ten percent. About 435 Europeans in Morocco contracted relapsing fever; this was a minuscule percentage of the approximately 325,000 Europeans (predominantly French) living mainly in coastal Moroccan cities. Among Morocco's population of Berbers, Arabs, and Jews, the disease infected 43,465 (most likely more, but records are scarce). Antibiotic medical treatment and isolation of patients and disinfestation measures helped prevent the infiltration of the disease into populated rural communities, and systematic use of DDT powder also proved effective in suppressing its spread. The epidemic died out by August 1946.

Further reading: Shattuck, *Diseases of the Tropics;* Simmons et al., *Global Epidemiology.*

Moroccan Typhus Epidemic of 1942–45 Severe epidemic of louse-borne typhus fever during World War II, killing a reported 8,040 persons out of some 40,200 infected. Other North African countries, such as Algeria, Tunisia, and Egypt, fought typhus outbreaks at the same time (see ALGERIAN TYPHUS EPIDEMIC OF 1942–44). Morocco had also suffered from epidemic louse-borne typhus fever in 1927–28 and 1937–39.

From January to October 1942, the Moroccan urban centers of Casablanca, Fez (Fès), Marrakesh, Meknès, and Rabat (the capital)—whose populations totaled about 1,182,000 out of Morocco's estimated 8,616,000 people (mainly rural)—began enduring epidemic typhus, which is carried by human body lice and thrives in crowded, dirty conditions. (The body louse becomes infected by feeding on a typhus patient's blood and excretes rickettsiae in its feces, which infect a human being through a bite or wound.) In Marrakesh, where temperatures in the winter can drop below 50° F, people frequently leave their clothes on for long periods, seldom wash, and live in overcrowded and unsanitary housing; this only prolongs the survival of the rickettsiae of the dried louse feces, which may remain infectious for many months. Moroccans in areas not as cold as Marrakesh tend to live the same way—and specifically so during wartime, notably World War II, when there was a lack of soap, clothing, and insecticides, as well as the presence of drought and social stress.

Moroccan authorities in 1943 instituted typhus control measures that included the enforced isolation of cases and contacts, the determination of infected individuals and contaminated dwellings, and the immunization of urban populations. Consequently, typhus infections dropped from about 25,000 in 1942 to 4,000 in 1943 to 3,000 in 1944, but they unexpectedly rose to about 8,200 in 1945, when another louse-borne disease, relapsing fever, broke out simultaneously in numerous districts. During the typhus epidemic, the fatality rate among Morocco's Muslim population (the country's largest ethnic group) was ten percent to 20 percent; the death rate was about the same for the Jewish population (about 203,000 people). Among the approximately 325,000 Europeans in Morocco, the fatality rate averaged from 20 percent to 30 percent in various regions. The subsequent, systematic use of DDT powders helped reduce typhus cases to 126 in 1947, the smallest annual number ever recorded in Morocco.

Further reading: Spink, *Infectious Diseases;* Cloudsley-Thompson, *Insects and History.*

N

Naples Syphilis Epidemic of 1494–95 See FRENCH ARMY SYPHILIS EPIDEMIC OF 1494–95.

Naples Typhus Epidemic of 1528 See FRENCH ARMY TYPHUS EPIDEMIC OF 1528.

Naples Typhus Epidemic of 1943–44 Serious outbreak of louse-borne typhus fever (classical or epidemic typhus) that killed 199 civilians out of 1,423 who were infected from December 1943 through February 1944, during World War II.

The rickettsial infection, transmitted mainly by body lice, was carried by Italian troops returning to Naples from fighting in North Africa and Sicily in mid-1943. By the time the Allies were liberating and occupying the city (October 1943), epidemic typhus was spreading seriously among Tunisian and Yugoslavian captives in Italian-operated prison camps, where the disease thrived under dirty, crowded conditions and developed into epidemic proportions.

Not directly transmitted from person to person and not conveyed by the bite of a louse, epidemic typhus spreads by the contaminative method. Infection arises from crushed lice or their rickettsiae-infected feces being rubbed into a wound or superficial skin abrasion of a person. Clothing, bedding, or dust containing dry, infected lice feces can remain infectious for many months. The symptoms, appearing generally after an incubation period of one to two weeks, include high fever, headache, numbness, vomiting, and blood in the stool and urine; eventually red spots (resembling flea bites) break out on a patient's skin, and there may be delirium.

In early December 1943 typhus fever spread from the prison camps to the civilian population in Naples, where men, women, and children of all ages were infected in this badly overcrowded and heavily bombed city. The morbidity (incidence of disease) and mortality (loss of life) in the prison camps are not clearly known. However, in Naples' civilian female population, there were a reported 718 infections and 105 fatalities; morbidity was highest among women aged 12 to 20 (166 cases with ten deaths). Among women aged 39 to 47, infections numbered 116, with 28 deaths. There were 705 cases with 94 deaths among Naples' civilian males; the highest incidence of infection (221 cases) occurred in males aged 12 to 20. Men between 39 and 47 years old suffered the highest mortality rate (29 died out of 59 cases). Children under age three had the lowest morbidity (one death out of 38 reported cases).

After mid-December 1943 the Allies took preventive measures against the disease—mainly dusting with the insecticide powder DDT to destroy lice. The typhus epidemic peaked in January 1944 and ended at the end of the next month; overall mortality was about 14 percent. DDT powder was dusted on more than 3,260,000 persons in Naples between December 15, 1943, and May 31, 1944—the first time in history that a typhus epidemic had been arrested by direct action.

Further reading: Horsfall and Rivers, eds., *Viral and Rickettsial Infections of Man;* McGrew, *Encyclopedia of Medical History.*

Napoleon's Army Epidemics in the Near East Devastating and repeated outbreaks of bubonic plague that beset Napoleon Bonaparte's forces in Egypt and Syria between 1798 and 1801. Endemic to the Near East, plague infected Napoleon's Turkish opponents and killed some of the British troops who were also trying to oust him from the area. The French, however, suffered the most; by the time they completely left Egypt in 1801, their number had been cut in half by disease and losses in combat.

After his spectacular conquests in Italy, Napoleon wanted to seize control of Egypt and the Levant (the eastern Mediterranean) and eventually push the British out of India. Within weeks of landing in Egypt in early July 1798, Napoleon had defeated the Mamelukes (who administered Egypt under the Ottoman Empire) and had begun to institute French rule in the country. Success was quickly followed by defeat, however: the British destroyed the French fleet at the mouth of the Nile River and set up a highly effective blockade. Now short on supplies and reinforcements, the French land forces were also contending with continual revolts among the Egyptians and with bubonic plague.

The epidemic, which broke out in full force in December, was comparatively mild at Damietta, but the French units at the coastal towns of Alexandria, Rosetta, and Aboukir (Abukir) were severely afflicted. At Alexandria, the epidemic began slowly, but at its height in January 1799, about 17 men died each day.

To deal with the outbreak, Napoleon—who never fell ill himself from the plague—tried a number of measures. He would not allow the term "bubonic plague" to be used because he was convinced that the fear it generated made people more susceptible to the disease; the contagion was simply called a fever with buboes. Personal hygiene and laundering of clothes were strictly observed. Doctors and orderlies were required to attend the sick on penalty of being shot; buboes that did not open by themselves were lanced because Napoleon believed that lancing lowered the death rate.

To forestall a Turkish attack on his weakened forces in Egypt, Napoleon decided to invade Syria, but the plague was rampant there. After their easy conquest of the port city of Jaffa in March 1799, dozens of the French soon fell victim to the disease. Hoping to maintain his army's morale, Napoleon visited the plague-stricken at the hospital, and even cared for them and moved the corpse of one victim.

If Napoleon could not escape the plague in Syria, neither could he turn his military luck around. Expecting that the coastal city of Acre would be as easy a target as Jaffa, he found instead that the city's defenses had been strengthened by the British. When repeated French assaults on the fortress were repulsed, Napoleon tried to use the plague to disguise his failures. In letters to Paris, he claimed that fear of catching the infection, which he said was killing more than 60 people a day in Acre, kept him outside the city walls. The truth is that, while plague was raging among the Turkish defenders of Acre, it was also attacking the French. When Turkish reinforcements arrived, the French had to retreat to Jaffa, many of the sick being sent on quarantine ships to Damietta.

Back at Jaffa, plague was still taking the lives of French soldiers in the garrison or at the hospital; 50 patients remained when Napoleon was ready to return to Egypt. Unwilling to take them along or to leave them to be killed by the Turks, Napoleon ordered his doctors to give them fatal doses of opium. Since several men were known to have vomited up the opium and recovered, it seems likely that sublethal doses were actually administered.

On his return to Egypt Napoleon learned that Russia and the Ottoman Empire had declared war on France and that Russia had invaded Italy. Although he sailed home to deal with the latest crisis, the French Army stayed on in Egypt for two years longer, enduring repeated attacks not only by the British and the Turks but also by plague. The disease occasionally struck the British—whose fleet at Aboukir, for example, lost 13 or 14 men to plague in 1801—but it continued to hit the French harder. The French commander at Cairo decided to surrender in 1801 when he realized that his soldiers (30 or 40 of whom were dying of plague each day) could hold out no longer. When the British defeated the French garrisons at Aboukir and Alexandria that same year, Napoleon's Near Eastern campaign drew to a close.

Further reading: Herold, *Bonaparte in Egypt*; Marks and Beatty, *Epidemics*; Savant, *Napoleon in His Time*; Wright, *Napoleon and Europe*.

Napoleon's Army Epidemics in Russia

Serious attacks of typhus, dysentery, and other diseases that killed untold thousands of soldiers in Napoleon's Grand Army during 1812 and early 1813. Along with fierce battles, starvation, and extreme winter cold, these diseases helped render French Emperor Napoleon's attempted invasion of Russia a dismal failure. Of more than half a million soldiers who began the campaign, only about 30,000 survived. Wandering homeward, often alone or in small groups, they carried typhus with them and touched off local outbreaks in Prussia and Germany.

Napoleon's invasion of Russia was the most ambitious attempt in his decade-long struggle to control Europe. In late 1811 and early 1812 in Germany, he assembled his Grand Army, a total of nearly 600,000 soldiers from all parts of his empire. The large and multilingual group was beset by supply shortages and poor discipline from the start; it also suffered from disease, mostly dysentery and diarrhea. On the army's march through Prussia and Poland, about 60,000 soldiers died or became seriously ill—well before they engaged a single Russian opponent in battle.

The campaign began in earnest in late June, when the Grand Army crossed the Niemen River and easily captured Lithuania. The Russians chose not to fight but to keep moving, thereby forcing Napoleon's troops to advance. On their way the Russians devastated the countryside, leaving no crops or supplies for their pursuers. The progress of the French was slow. Baggage trains could not keep up; stragglers continually fell behind; more and more soldiers became ill, especially with typhus, which began to appear during the summer. The Grand Army left behind hundreds of the sick in overcrowded, makeshift hospitals along their route, but there were few doctors and almost no medicine to help them.

Although typhus outbreaks and combat had cost the Russians dearly, Napoleon's army was in worse condition. When the soldiers arrived in Moscow in mid-September 1812, they found that their opponents had already fled and had taken most of the civilians, and the food, with them. A day or two later some of the remaining Russians set fire to the city, burning two thirds of it. Realizing that in the ruined city he could not get enough food and clothing to keep his soldiers through the winter, Napoleon left Moscow in mid-October.

The horrors of the Grand Army's retreat are known through memoirs written by several French officers. They were among the very few lucky ones. Losses on the journey out of Moscow were astoundingly high because of cold, famine, and fatigue. Horses died by the hundreds, injured from traveling on ice and snow or starving from lack of grain. The fewer horses the army had, the fewer provisions it could carry, yet food was to be found scarcely anywhere. Harassed by pursuing Russians and Cossacks, the Grand Army was forced to return on the same route it had taken into Moscow, rather than on another one where supplies might have been greater. The soldiers subsisted mainly on horsemeat and melted snow, sometimes with a bit of flour or honey. With their boots worn through from marching and their uniforms in tatters from combat, many of them simply froze to death when they collapsed from hunger and fatigue. It is no wonder that disease was a constant companion.

Many of the hospitals the French had set up en route to Moscow were now filthy and overcrowded; dead bodies lay strewn in corridors. Yet these ill-provisioned buildings were forced to accept soldiers who had fallen ill on the retreat. Typhus and other infectious diseases spread rapidly through the hospitals, overwhelming any efforts to control them. The Grand Army moved on, leaving the sick behind again, either to die or to be taken prisoner by the Russians.

As extreme privation forced each soldier to think only of himself, the army's ranks became more and more disorganized. Many soldiers left the line of march to pillage the countryside on their own; others got lost in the blinding snow or were abandoned by their comrades when they became ill. Napoleon decided in early December to return at once to Paris, but the remnants of his army still staggered behind. Traveling westward through Prussia and Germany,

they—and the Russians who followed them—spread typhus as they went. Many of these local outbreaks continued into 1813; Napoleon's invasion of Germany later that year and his subsequent battles with Russia, Austria, and Prussia helped reignite typhus outbreaks in central Europe.

Further reading: Fezensac, *The Russian Campaign, 1812;* Nicolson, *Napoleon 1812;* Prinzing, *Epidemics Resulting from Wars;* Wright, *Napoleon and Europe.*

New England Diphtheria and Scarlet Fever Epidemics of 1735–40

Severe outbreaks of "throat distemper" (later identified as either diphtheria or scarlet fever) in various parts of New England, when a "disease corridor" ran through the entire area.

In May 1735 the first cases of "throat distemper," which was actually diphtheria, occurred in the town of Kingston, New Hampshire, where a recorded 26 children died from the disease in the month of August alone. The epidemic moved northeastward, affecting many small towns in New Hampshire and Maine. From July 1735 to July 1736 the death records of 15 New Hampshire towns show that 954 persons perished from the disease, and most of the victims were children. The epidemic also moved south to Haverhill, Massachusetts, in November 1735; records indicate that 116 people in Haverhill died of "throat distemper" in 1736, and 130 perished the following year (out of all these fatalities, 98 were children and youngsters under 20 years old). Bostonians to the south feared that the deadly disease would soon strike their city; the first case of "throat distemper," which was actually scarlet fever, was reported on August 20, 1736. While human deaths had occurred almost immediately after the outbreak of "throat distemper" in the New Hampshire towns, Boston experienced a considerable time lag between the first case of the disease and the first fatalities, which occurred in October 1736.

The so-called "throat distemper" epidemic in New England was said to have peaked in March 1736. Fatalities in Boston were comparatively low during the epidemic, which killed 114 city residents out of more than 4,000 who reportedly contracted the disease (scarlet fever). Boston's surrounding towns were hit much harder, with about one in three to six cases proving fatal at the time. Newport, Rhode Island, also reported that about one person out of 50 died from "throat distemper." Evidently scarlet fever affected Boston and Newport much less than diphtheria affected the smaller towns.

Connecticut also suffered from attacks of diphtheria between 1735 and 1740, but its mortality rate from the disease was not nearly as high as that of the northeastern New England regions. Two possible explanations have been proposed for this difference: one, that the epidemic in Connecticut spread from the southwest to the northeast, thus making it unlikely that Massachusetts' epidemic had moved into Connecticut and more likely that Connecticut had a different strain of diphtheria (which originated there or was part of a New Jersey outbreak at the time). The second explanation for Connecticut's lower mortality rate is based on the theory that human beings can build up immunity to diphtheria. Because the disease had attacked Connecticut previously, much of the population may have acquired some immunity to it.

At the time physicians did not understand fully how the "throat distemper" was transmitted; many thought that human beings did not spread the disease, evidently because many who were exposed to it never contracted either diphtheria or scarlet fever. Moreover, many people who had never been exposed to infected persons came down with the disease. Hence, the New England physicians failed to realize that healthy persons were also carriers of scarlet fever and diphtheria, both of which share many of the same symptoms, making physicians easily confused in the 1700s. A very sore throat and fever are characteristic of both scarlet fever and diphtheria. However, scarlet fever produces a rash, while diphtheria produces ulcers in the glands or throat. Thus, the difference in the severity of the "throat distemper" outbreak in Boston compared to the outbreaks in surrounding areas greatly puzzled many early physicians and scientists. They did not know that scarlet fever had attacked Boston while diphtheria had struck the other towns. Boston doctors at first attributed the city's lower fatality rate to their superior medical treatment, and clergymen believed that Massachusetts laws requiring adequate pay for ministers saved the people there from a more terrible wrath of God. Because these laws did not exist in New Hampshire, the clergy thought that God was punishing the heathen in New Hampshire.

Surprisingly, the epidemics did not produce much confusion or hysteria, largely because most New Englanders' faith in God led them to accept their diseased fate quietly. And it may not have been entirely coincidental that a period of intense religious renewal known as "The Great Awakening" occurred at the same time and afterward in New England and other British American colonies.

Further reading: Duffy, *Epidemics in Colonial America;* Top, ed., *The History of American Epidemiology; Disease and Society in Provincial Massachusetts: Collected Accounts, 1736–1939.*

New England Influenza Epidemic of 1789 Widespread outbreak of influenza that affected thousands of people in the fall of 1789. The contagious disease, which attacks the respiratory system and can result in pneumonia and pleurisy, also struck many inhabitants in neighboring New York State and Nova Scotia and various other places in North America, including Philadelphia and Georgia (see EUROPEAN INFLUENZA PANDEMIC OF 1788–89).

The flu virus first entered New England through Connecticut seaports with infected traders and travelers from New York City, where influenza was raging in September 1789. The infectious disease moved northward, reaching Hartford, Connecticut, in mid-October, where noted lexicographer Noah Webster was one of many stricken with the flu that month. From Connecticut, it spread to Rhode Island and Massachusetts, where many residents of Boston became infected in early November. It continued to travel northward that month, striking New Hampshire and later Maine and Nova Scotia in December before waning.

Males and females of all ages and socioeconomic classes were attacked by the epidemic, which lasted in each locality for about four to six weeks and was particularly harsh on the elderly and the chronically ill. Many of the deaths were from secondary pneuemonia, and case-mortality is believed to have been less than 50 percent during the epidemic.

In the spring of 1790 many New Englanders contracted influenza anew, and in the fall parts of the northeastern United States were again fighting the flu virus.

Further reading: Duffy, *A History of Public Health in New York City;* Patterson, *Pandemic Influenza.*

New England Scarlet Fever Epidemic of 1793–95 Serious outbreak of scarlet fever or scarlatina (sometimes called angina maligna in early days) that occurred in various parts of New England and killed several hundred men, women, and children. Caused by streptococcal bacteria, the disease is characterized by fever, a sore throat, and a red rash, and it is transmitted by coughing and sneezing (droplets in the air).

In August 1792 the town of Bethlehem in eastern Pennsylvania endured a mild form of scarlet fever; nearly every family and child was affected there. Then a severe outbreak occurred from February to May 1793 in Bethlehem; 19 children died from "angina maligna." By November the disease had disappeared, but returned in January 1794 to claim the lives of 14 children and leave others deaf or blind in Bethlehem. Some speculate that scarlet fever advanced from there northeastward into coastal Connecticut (see NEW ENGLAND DIPHTHERIA AND SCARLET FEVER EPIDEMICS OF 1735–40); others say it came from

Vermont south into Connecticut, where many persons succumbed to this contagious disease, notably in the towns of New Fairfield and Litchfield, in 1793 and 1794 (in late winter and spring, when the illness most commonly strikes).

Hartford, Connecticut, suffered many human deaths from the epidemic, first in May 1793 and again in February 1794, when a second wave of scarlet fever claimed more lives than the first. New Haven, on the coast, was struck severely as well, beginning in January 1794. Within the next six months, more than 700 cases of scarlet fever were reported, along with 52 children's deaths, in this area of Connecticut. The epidemic reached Boston the following year, where it culminated and ended. Because human beings communicate the disease, it was not able to spread much in the sparsely populated areas to the north and west of Boston.

Further reading: Winslow, *The Conquest of Epidemic Disease;* Duffy, *Epidemics in Colonial America;* Webster, *A Brief History of Epidemic and Pestilential Diseases.*

New Haven Yellow Fever Epidemic of 1794   Severe outbreak of yellow fever (also called yellow jack) that reportedly killed 64 persons out of 160 who were infected in New Haven, Connecticut, between June and November 1794. Most residents stayed in New Haven and only a few fled, after the sudden onset of yellow fever (which received its name because of the jaundice accompanying the high fever, hemorrhaging, and vomiting that are symptoms of this viral disease, which is transmitted by the bite of a specific mosquito).

In June 1794 a sloop from Martinique in the West Indies arrived in the Long Wharf area of New Haven harbor. According to some local physicians at the time, a chest of clothes belonging to a recently diseased sailor on the ship was the culprit for bringing yellow fever to New Haven. Within days after the arrival of the sloop, members of the family of Isaac Gorham, a local fisherman living in the Long Wharf area, came down with the dreaded disease; they reportedly had been in direct contact with the sailor's chest. Mrs. Isaac Gorham died from yellow fever on June 14, becoming the first fatality of the epidemic. As the disease spread in New Haven, some local doctors said that only those persons who had been in contact with the Gorham family contracted yellow fever, because it was "propagated only by contagion."

American lexicographer Noah Webster, who observed and wrote about this epidemic, did not subscribe to the contagionists' theory and tried to dispel the belief that yellow fever came to New Haven on board the sloop. He claimed there had not been any cases of yellow fever on the sloop while in transit to New Haven and suggested there may not have been any clothing in the chest.

Furthermore, Webster attempted to prove that Mrs. Gorham did not contract the disease from any one identifiable source; he also declared that she may have been nowhere near the sloop, for a child was the only witness of her visit to the ship. Webster believed that certain atmospheric conditions, notably the cleanliness of the air, determined whether or not the disease would spread in a certain geographical area. In this case, he hypothesized that some fish that Mr. Gorham cleaned near his house may have contributed to filthy air; consequently his wife would have been more susceptible to yellow fever. In addition, Webster had observed a case of yellow fever in March 1794, accompanied by a multitude of caterpillars; he asserted that somehow the caterpillars caused the atmosphere to be conducive to the disease. Not until the late nineteenth century was the discovery made that the *Stegiomyia fasciata* (later called *Aëdes aegypti*) mosquito transmits the yellow fever virus.

Further reading: Top, *The History of American Epidemiology;* Webster, *A Brief History of Epidemic and Pestilential Diseases;* Winslow, *The Conquest of Epidemic Disease.*

New Mexico Plague of 1965   Outbreak of mainly bubonic plague. It was distinguished by the fact that plague has occurred in the United States every year following, that the case average for each year between 1965 and 1977 was almost ten times greater than that for each year since a 1924–25 outbreak in Los Angeles, and that this epidemic's circumstances could have led to a major outbreak in the United States.

The 1965 New Mexico epidemic ended with five confirmed and two probable cases, with at least one confirmed death. Epizootics had swept through an area the size of Massachusetts, New Jersey, Rhode Island, Connecticut, and Delaware combined— 23,000 square miles. In addition, over 100,000 prairie dogs had been poisoned to control the spread of the disease. (Chinese immigrants had brought the plague to the United States at San Francisco in 1900. Since 1907, plague had been endemic to the western United States, moving eastward from California.)

The rodent bacterium *Yersinia pestis (Pasteurella pestis),* which causes plague, became a threat to human beings only when it became epizootic among nearby rats or rodents. Primary among the 200 fleas (not the human flea) that transmitted plague was the rat flea *Xenopsylla cheopis.*

Symptoms of plague include stupor, high fever and chills, aching head, back and limbs, memory failure, uncontrolled staggering and hand motions, flushed face, and hot, dry lips and skin. Most important, a swelling (bubo) as large as an egg in the groin, throat, or armpit gave the disease its name of bubonic. Symptoms develop fully within one day. Untreated, the disease kills 60 to 90 percent of its victims within five days. Modern antidotes include streptomycin, tetracyclines, and chloraphenicals.

In 1965 New Mexico, two events preceded the discovery of plague. First, multitudes of prairie dogs had died in the spring. Second, a young Navajo girl from Red Rock was treated for a respiratory infection accompanied by a fever and sore throat on June 21. Two weeks later, this little girl took ill again and was diagnosed with pneumonic plague. A little boy also contracted the disease. The infection occurred in a vast Indian reservation just before some major Navajo tribal affairs that, in toto, would have drawn together crowds of nearly 70,000 persons. Thus, a major epidemic could have erupted due to the territory's immensity, poor roads and communications, diverse non-English speaking populations, and, most important, the difficulty of developing an effective organization to control a pestilence in diversely owned lands, i.e., federal, private, and Indian.

By August 1965, radio warnings about plague were broadcast in English and Navajo. By August 15, the army, Fish and Wildlife Service, and Centers for Disease Control (CDC) had begun massive emergency measures to control the disease. Information was disseminated by television, radio, and newspapers. "Plague" booths went up at all large Indian gatherings. Insecticides were sprayed and prairie dogs were poisoned. Cold weather also halted the spread of the disease. See also LOS ANGELES PLAGUE OF 1924–25.

Further reading: Collins et al., "Plague Epidemic in New Mexico, 1965"; Gregg, *Plague: An Ancient Disease in the Twentieth Century*; Rail, *Plague Ecotoxicology*.

New Orleans Yellow Fever Epidemics of 1878–79
See U.S. YELLOW FEVER EPIDEMICS OF 1878–79.

New York Poliomyelitis Epidemic of 1907
Outbreak of poliomyelitis (or infantile paralysis or Heine-Medin disease) in the New York City area. There were at least 750 polio cases (probably as many as 1,200), and the disease was edging toward becoming a national problem (see U.S. POLIOMYELITIS EPIDEMIC OF 1916).

The chairman of the New York Neurological Society, Dr. Bernard Sachs, appointed a committee or board of 12 members (including neurological experts) to oversee the 1907 epidemic; this was the last time that neurologists (physicians concerned with the nervous system and its disorders) would have a domi-

nant influence in the study and treatment of poliomyelitis. Virologists, pediatricians, public health officers, physical medicine specialists, internists, and orthopedists eventually gained predominance, using neurologists as consultants. A prominent committee member, Dr. Simon Flexner, who was director of the Rockefeller Institute for Medical Research, carried on a careful study into the disease.

Sachs' committee did not issue a formal report on the epidemic until 1910. The report significantly included the recent discovery of a poliovirus by Austrian-born pathologist Dr. Karl Landsteiner, who taught at the University of Vienna and later (1922) came to the United States to join the staff of the Rockefeller Institute. The report also included experiments by Dr. Flexner and other Rockefeller researchers that for the first time in the United States isolated the poliovirus; their experiments succeeded in transmitting polio to monkeys and from one monkey to another.

Despite scientific discoveries about polio, proper treatment of victims and prevention and cure of the disease remained a mystery, and a preventive vaccine would not be discovered until mid-century. In 1907 doctors had no idea how to help their patients and lacked even a written description of the disease. Paralysis was still thought to be a primary characteristic, thus polio's familiar but not very accurate alternate name "infantile paralysis" (the infection attacks nerve cells controlling muscles but infrequently causes paralysis). Furthermore, there was no notion how the disease was spread (by direct contact with pharyngeal secretions or feces of infected persons), although it was known to be contagious by 1907. New York had another similar polio outbreak in 1911.

Further reading: McGrew, *Encyclopedia of Medical History*; Paul, *A History of Poliomyelitis*.

New York Smallpox Epidemics of 1868–75
Series of smallpox outbreaks that affected New York City. The contagious viral disease, which occurred almost simultaneously in many other American cities (notably Philadelphia), was associated partly with an influx of European immigrants following the end of the Franco-Prussian War (1870–71) (see EUROPEAN SMALLPOX EPIDEMIC OF 1870–75).

In the winter of 1868–69, a severe outbreak of smallpox erupted in New York, where inspectors found that nearly half of the children in some city schools had not been vaccinated. The Board of Health in May 1869 appointed 60 inspectors to go door-to-door and ensure that all residents were vaccinated. Over a six-week period, some 700,000 people were reportedly offered the vaccination (they could not be coerced into taking it), and the epidemic soon ended.

Early in 1870, New York City's Board of Health suggested that all residents be vaccinated in view of a possible smallpox outbreak. This idea was promptly lambasted by the press for creating an atmosphere of panic and allowing doctors to profit. Throughout 1870, the disease was rampant in New York even as the free vaccination program was being carried out. The School Board cooperated by appointing a special medical inspector and declaring vaccination mandatory for admission into its schools. The Board of Health established another temporary vaccination unit. However, the inspection units were underfunded and had to contend with a rapidly strengthening anti-vaccination movement and a steady influx of rural and foreign immigrants (many reluctant to be vaccinated) swelling the non-immune population. Also, free vaccination for the poor was an unpopular notion in certain parts of the city, where, despite these efforts, smallpox erupted again in 1871. Doctors and landlords were required to report cases but did not always do so. Many families hid their patients for fear that they would be moved into an isolation hospital where the conditions were apparently horrid. As a result, many patients died without receiving any medical treatment, and 101 of the reported 805 deaths occurred at home. Another intensive vaccination campaign (using human lymph fluid, since bovine lymph was not available) was conducted and helped end the epidemic, but not before 3,084 cases had occurred. The Board of Health spent $75,000 on its vaccination and treatment programs that year.

Another year brought yet another outbreak of smallpox in New York City. The vaccination unit was reactivated in the spring of 1872, disbanded on July 1 when the outbreak seemed to be under control, and reactivated again in the winter of 1872–73 when the disease flared up once more. Despite door-to-door checks in apartment buildings (where mobility was very high) and free vaccination, the inspectors could not insist that people be vaccinated unless they had been around smallpox patients. Smallpox deaths numbered 929 in 1872. The disease was prevalent again in 1874, leading the city to establish a permanent 12-man vaccination bureau with access to extra staff should the need arise. That year, 484 deaths were recorded from smallpox.

During the summer of 1875, smallpox became epidemic again. The city's Board of Health publicized the importance and free availability of vaccination in every tenement area and urged the Board of Education to strictly enforce its vaccination policy. The latter supplemented this by enacting legislation (December 15, 1875) requiring school janitors and their families to be vaccinated as well. Reporting of smallpox cases improved when the city's isolation hospital was revamped and put under the jurisdiction of the Board of Health, which reported 1875's mortality from smallpox at 1,280 deaths. The next year, the city opened its own vaccine production unit in Lakeview, New Jersey. When the epidemics subsided, so did the intensity and fervor of the vaccination campaigns. Given the constraints faced by the Board of Health, it was not surprising that smallpox, though declining, remained a threat through the rest of the century.

Further reading: Duffy, *A History of Public Health in New York City;* Duffy, *The Sanitarians: A History of American Public Health.*

New York Smallpox Epidemic of 1901–03   See

U.S. SMALLPOX EPIDEMIC OF 1901–03.

New York Yellow Fever Epidemic of 1668   One

of the earliest recorded epidemics of yellow fever in colonial America, killing many inhabitants of New York City in the late summer and early fall of 1668. This epidemic occurred before physicians consistently identified yellow fever correctly and well before they were aware that the *Aëdes aegypti* (first named *Stegomyia fasciata*) mosquito carried the disease.

Later, American lexicographer Noah Webster described this 1668 epidemic as a "autumnal bilious fever in infectious form" in his book *A Brief History of Epidemic and Pestilential Diseases* (1799); he rejected the idea that "invisible animalcules" caused infection and that contagion could be carried in clothing. Webster attributed epidemics to great natural phenomena (electrical, underground, and miasmatic disturbances, indicated by thunderstorms, earthquakes, floods, and droughts, as well as "sickly and tasteless" oysters and prodigious catches of shad). Though most historians today state that the 1668 epidemic was yellow fever, some doubt it, claiming that if it were yellow fever, observers certainly would have noticed and commented on the characteristic or symptom of black vomit, while the severe fever observed in patients could have resulted from malaria, typhoid, or dysentery—diseases characterized by high fever.

In September 1668 Governor Francis Lovelace of New York proclaimed a "General Day of Humiliation" because of the "unusual sickness." He noted that many persons died each day and that many more were sick with the fever. Displaying his Puritan views, Governor Lovelace declared that the sickness resulted from people's improvident living, intemperance, and impiety in New York (an English colony since the Dutch surrendered it in 1664). For the next

200 years or so, observers of yellow fever would have various imaginative yet incorrect explanations for the origin of the disease and how it spread. Scientists did not hypothesize until 1881 that yellow fever was transmitted by a mosquito.

Further reading: Duffy, *A History of Public Health in New York City*; Duffy, *Epidemics in Colonial America*; Webster, *A Brief History of Epidemic and Pestilential Diseases*.

New York Yellow Fever Epidemic of 1702   U.S. epidemic of yellow fever, then also known as the "American Plague." Yellow fever attacked New York City in the summer of 1702, three years after the first outbreaks in the United States occurred in Charleston, South Carolina, and Philadelphia. Twenty people died daily during this 1702 outbreak, and according to a missionary who visited New York, 500 people died within a three-month period. The final death toll reached about 570 persons. The population of New York City was estimated to be 8,000 by the year 1730, and it was believed to have been much lower in 1702. Thus, it is estimated that the yellow fever outbreak of 1702 probably killed between one ninth and one tenth of the town's inhabitants. This siege of yellow fever killed a much higher percentage of people than the earlier Charleston Yellow Fever Epidemic of 1699 (q.v.).

New York City authorities spread quicklime and coal dust in the streets and lit bonfires in order to cleanse the air. These methods, however, posed an equal if not greater threat of death to the inhabitants than the yellow fever. The New York epidemic, which lasted until October, was predominantly centered in the city, although one nearby town also reported an outbreak. It is believed, however, that those victims were infected with yellow fever while visiting New York City. Yellow fever usually was contained to the port city, as the *Stegomyia fasciata* (*Aëdes aegypti*) mosquito that carries the disease cannot fly long distances to spread the pestilence. Physicians in the 1700s did not realize that yellow fever was linked to the mosquito, and the origin of yellow fever remained a mystery until the late 1800s.

The symptoms of yellow fever were yellow-tinted skin, accompanied by severe vomiting, usually black, which was the result of internal hemorrhages. Before yellow fever was positively identified as such in 1699, it was also known as the "Barbados Fever" or the "black vomit." Another characteristic of yellow fever was that it occurred only during the summer and fall months. This was due to the fact that the mosquito that carries the yellow fever can not live during the cold winter months. Thus, cities that were affected by the yellow fever were relieved once the winter weather killed the mosquitos.

Further reading: Duffy, *Epidemics in Colonial America*; Kammen, *Colonial New York: A History*; Lockwood, *Manhattan Moves Uptown: An Illustrated History*.

New York Yellow Fever Epidemics of 1743 and 1745   Two outbreaks of yellow fever—an acute, intestinal infection—the first of which ravaged New York City between July and October of 1743. A total of 217 people died form July 25 to September 25; this figure represented only about two percent of New York's 11,000 inhabitants. Thus, this outbreak was fairly insignificant when compared with other colonial outbreaks of yellow fever, where the disease killed up to ten percent of the population.

Yellow fever struck New York again in 1745. The "bilious plague," as it was then also called, broke out in June. Physicians recognized the symptoms of the disease, which were yellow-tinted skin, accompanied by severe vomiting, usually black, which was the result of internal hemorrhages. Doctors began to investigate the causes of the disease, and Dr. Cadwallader Colden, a member of the Governor's Council of New York, diagnosed the yellow fever and noted that the fever always developed in June and in the dock areas. He attributed the yellow fever's origin in the docks to the filthy conditions there. New York City officials spread quicklime and coal dust in the streets and lit bonfires in order to cleanse the air. These methods, however, posed an equal if not greater threat of death to the inhabitants than the yellow fever.

It was not until the late nineteenth century that physicians and scientists understood the causes of yellow fever. The discovery that the *Stegomyia fasciata* (*Aëdes aegypti*) mosquito carries the disease explained why the disease was centered around a port and why it ran its course during the summer and fall. The mosquito's flying range limited the spread of the disease, and its inability to live during the cold winter months limited the duration of any epidemic.

Further reading: Duffy, *Epidemics in Colonial America*; Lockwood, *Manhattan Moves Uptown: An Illustrated History*; Marks and Beatty, *Epidemics*.

New York Yellow Fever Epidemic of 1795   Outbreak of yellow fever in New York City killing 732 persons out of an estimated population of about 50,000. The cause of this epidemic was disputed to a great extent, but most observers then believed that the disease arrived aboard the brigantine *Zephyr*, which landed at the port of New York in late July 1795. A health officer stationed at the port, Dr. Treat, soon died from yellow fever on July 29. However, according to one source, a case of yellow fever had been observed in New York two weeks before the docking of the *Zephyr*.

Because physicians and scientists in the eighteenth century did not know how yellow fever was transmitted (by the bite of a certain mosquito), various reasons were postulated for the 1795 outbreak: Yellow fever was contagious or lack of hygiene by persons in a certain place were commonly believed to be the origin of the disease. Because one frequent symptom of the disease is black or bloody vomit, physicians may have interpreted it as a sign of filth by human beings. In addition, American lexicographer Noah Webster, who wrote extensively about epidemics at that time, carried on a revealing correspondence with his New York friend Elihu Smith. Both men disputed that disease contagion carried in clothes could cause epidemics; they believed that certain external (or natural) circumstances or conditions had to exist for a disease to rise to epidemic proportions. Webster also credulously believed that the cleanliness of the air would determine if a disease would take hold, not whether there were mosquitoes present to transmit it.

In 1795 most citizens did not flee as yellow fever spread throughout New York City, where a relatively large number of foreigners (almost 500 immigrants) died from the fever. In 1798 the disease again erupted severely in the city, causing more than 2,000 deaths, many of them countrymen and -women this time.

Further reading: Duffy, *A History of Public Health in New York City*; Top, *The History of American Epidemiology*; Webster, *A Brief History of Epidemic and Pestilential Diseases*; Winslow, *The Conquest of Epidemic Disease*.

New Zealand Epidemics of the 1790s

Outbreaks of various unidentified diseases. In or around 1790, a serious dysentery-like disease broke out among the native New Zealanders and was linked to the arrival of an English ship at Mercury Bay. Generally fatal, it was called *tikotiko toto* (literally, bloody feces). Also, small outbreaks of influenza were reported in various parts of New Zealand during 1791.

Another epidemic attacked the Bay of Islands region (on North Island) sometime in 1795. Again, the precise nature of the disease, which the natives called *Tingara* (perhaps *Te Ngarara*, an illness caused by the lizard god), is not known. However, records indicate that it suddenly turned fatal. Apparently the bay area was devastated by this outbreak.

Sometime between 1790 and 1800, a virulent epidemic of yet another unspecified disease ripped through New Zealand's North Island. Christened *rewararewa (rewharewha)*, which means "foreign disease" according to some historians, it was described as a cutaneous affliction that left small spots all over the body. Some sources believe that it may have been a severe, influenza-like illness. The epidemic

was both widespread (native sources indicate its prevalence in Taranaki, Mercury Bay, and Tuhoe) and devastating. Apparently, so many people died that there were not enough left behind to bury the dead.

Further reading: Wright, *New Zealand, 1769–1840*; Gluckman, *Tangiwai: A Medical History of 19th Century New Zealand*.

New Zealand Epidemics of 1820–40

Several serious outbreaks of disease that decimated New Zealand's native Maori population (see NEW ZEALAND MEASLES EPIDEMICS OF 1835 AND 1854). Localized outbreaks of influenza had been reported from New Zealand in 1791 (see NEW ZEALAND EPIDEMICS OF THE 1790s). There was also mention of an unidentified epidemic in the North Auckland area around 1810.

A severe epidemic broke out in the Thames area about 1820, consequent upon the arrival of a European ship. Maori tribes engaged in warfare carried the disease southward. According to a missionary's account, it killed almost three fifths of the Maori population in the southern sections of North Island. Some villages were left with only one or two survivors.

The first major epidemic of influenza apparently struck the Bay of Islands in 1826, not long after the arrival of the H.M.S. *Coromandel* from Sydney, Australia. By all accounts it was a serious outbreak among the Maoris, who had had no previous contact with the disease. The Maori custom of jumping into cold water during a fever only exacerbated the situation. Since the advent of the white Christian missionaries, many Maoris wrapped or covered themselves in their newly donated clothes, often to disastrous results.

Whooping cough arrived in New Zealand in September–October 1828 on a ship that entered the Bay of Islands. It spread like wildfire among the children of both Maoris and Europeans. Many Maori children died during this epidemic, which faded away early in 1829.

There was a noticeable increase in influenza cases in 1837 (see ASIATIC AND EUROPEAN INFLUENZA PANDEMIC OF 1836–37). A British doctor who arrived in the middle of this epidemic lost his own children to it and treated over 800 Maori patients during a six-week period. Early in 1838, a streptococcus-type infection erupted in the Bay of Islands and spread north to the North Cape and into the interior of North Island. It reportedly caused painful symptoms such as swollen jaws and arrived at the Matamata mission in July 1838. Later in the year, a serious epidemic of influenza began in the Bay of Islands. Eyewitness accounts testify to the virulence of this outbreak, which apparently infected everyone, young and old, in the northern part of North Island. The epidemic rendered most Maori natives prostrate for quite some time. Many of the weak and elderly succumbed to the illness. About 200 natives were attacked by influenza in the Karikari region.

Influenza became epidemic in New Zealand again in 1844 and in 1852–53, but because the native population had developed some immunity, the mortality was not as high.

Further reading: Marks and Beatty, *Epidemics;* Wright, *New Zealand, 1769–1840.*

New Zealand Influenza Epidemic of 1918–19

Part of a worldwide pandemic of influenza (see SPAN-ISH INFLUENZA EPIDEMIC OF 1917–19; INDIAN INFLU-ENZA EPIDEMIC OF 1918–19; INDONESIAN INFLUENZA EPIDEMIC OF 1918). Even before the first onslaught of July 1918 was over, a second wave burst upon the scene in late October 1918. Unlike in Australia (see AUSTRALIAN INFLUENZA EPIDEMIC OF 1918–19), this attack was very severe and the death toll very high. Among the Europeans 5,559 deaths were reported, a fatality rate of 500 per 100,000 persons, while among the Maoris (aboriginal people of New Zealand) there were 1,130 deaths, the fatality rate a staggering 2,260 per 100,000 persons.

From the city of Auckland, New Zealand, in early November 1918, the trading vessel *Talune* transported the infection to Fiji, Samoa (see SOUTH PACIFIC ISLANDS INFLUENZA EPIDEMIC OF 1918–19), and Tonga, where it literally decimated the local populations.

In early 1919, the mortality rate from influenza was significantly lower in New Zealand, but later that year the country was once again attacked by influenza. The first wave peaked in August–September 1919. The second wave, which struck in November 1919, was extremely severe. The natives generally seemed to be more susceptible to the infection than the Europeans.

Influenza outbreaks were again reported in February 1920 (from Auckland), October 1922 (with pneumonic complications), June 1923, and July 1926.

Further reading: Jordan, *Epidemic Influenza;* Mackenzie, ed., *Viral Diseases in South-East Asia and the Western Pacific.*

New Zealand Measles Epidemics of 1835 and 1854

Virgin-soil epidemics of measles, representing New Zealand's first contact with the disease during the nineteenth century.

Measles was apparently first imported into New Zealand in March 1835 by a Maori native returning home from Sydney on the sailing vessel *Children.* The infection did not spread beyond New Zealand's South Island but had a devastating impact on the Maoris, many of whom died from their first exposure to the disease. Unaware of how to cope with a foreign disease, entire Maori communities apparently resorted to bathing in streams in order to rid themselves of the spots. Measles was reportedly prevalent in 1838 on South Island's Otago Peninsula.

The country's next measles epidemic occurred in 1854, courtesy of a Tasmanian ship that arrived in North Island. The epidemic spread concurrently with a scarlet fever epidemic. Together, they claimed about 4,000 Maori lives.

Further reading: Marks and Beatty, *Epidemics;* Gluckman, *Tangiwai: A Medical History of 19th Century New Zealand.*

New Zealand Measles Epidemics of 1915–16 and 1938

Two of the more severe epidemics of measles (rubeola) that attacked New Zealand early in the twentieth century. Relatively milder outbreaks were recorded in 1902–03 (277 human deaths), 1907 (101 deaths) and 1920–21 (122 deaths in 1920).

The epidemic of 1915–16 began in November 1914 at the newly established Trentham Camp, which was built to accommodate 2,000 soldiers-in-training; the number quickly swelled to 7,000, with new recruits arriving at regular intervals. Here were ideal crowded conditions for the spread of respiratory ailments. Fourteen people came down with measles in November, 16 in December, 23 in January, 24 in February, and 59 in March. The camp's medical staff tried to isolate the patients and impose quarantine on those who had been in contact with them, but the outbreak continued to spread, so in mid-May 1915 the authorities gave up the fight. As cooler weather set in, the virulence increased; 95 cases were reported in April, 180 in May, 492 in June, and 132 in July, after which the camp was closed. Overall, 1,035 measles cases were registered in the camp by July 1915.

The Wellington Hospital could not admit any more measles patients after the beginning of April so the army housed the rest of the patients in premises built in 1900 as a plague hospital. The conditions here were so primitive that it came to be known as "Behrampore" (alluding to a squalid town in India), where 104 measles cases were housed by June 2, 1915. Measles mortality among Europeans during the epidemic was considerable: 33 deaths in 1914, 64 in 1915, and 93 in 1916. A high proportion of deaths occurred in young men 20 to 35 years of age; most of them had escaped the disease during the previous four outbreaks.

In 1938, measles resurfaced in unexpectedly virulent form and was particularly devastating among New Zealand's native Maoris. The outbreak began in November 1937 in the North Auckland Health District and spread rapidly across the country. According to the district medical officer's conservative estimate, between 3,000 and 4,000 people were infected in the area. Of them, 60 Maoris and 16 Europeans died of the disease and its complications. The latter were apparently very severe, including heart problems, broncho-pneumonia, hemorrhages (mouth, nose, bowel), complications of the nervous system, and reactivation of latent tuberculosis.

The epidemic was also very virulent among the Maoris on the east coast, where at least 50 percent of the children contracted the disease. Once again, the complications were many and serious. More than 100 patients developed pneumonia and 24 died of it. Four cases of encephalitis and one death from it were recorded. Nearly half of the patients in some districts had severe conjunctivitis; other complications included otitis media, pleurisy, jaundice, strabismus, and nephritis.

The epidemic caused 212 deaths representing ten percent of all deaths that year among the Maoris (death rate 24.32 per 10,000 people) and 163 deaths among the Europeans (death rate 1.07 per 10,000 people). Eighty-four percent of the Maori deaths were in children under five and eight percent in persons age ten or over. On the other hand, 45 percent of the European deaths were in children under five years of age and 33 percent in people over ten years of age. A higher proportion of adult Europeans was attacked this time. This disrupted normal community life and caused economic losses. Government records indicate that 2,909 people were treated for measles in hospitals during 1938. On the positive side, the epidemic helped break down the Maori reluctance to accept Western medical treatment; soon they began to welcome the district nurses into their homes, which led to improved hygiene and sanitation and therefore a reduced threat of disease.

Further reading: Maclean, *Challenge for Health: A History of Public Health in New Zealand*; Donovan, "A Study in New Zealand Mortality: 6, Epidemic Diseases."

New Zealand Poliomyelitis Epidemics Six major epidemics of poliomyelitis, or polio, that occurred in New Zealand after 1914, when it was declared a notifiable disease (also called infantile paralysis). A "notifiable disease" must be reported to official health authorities.

A mild polio outbreak in 1914 killed 25 people and apparently infected over 200. However, it barely received casual mention in New Zealand's Health Department annual report for 1915. The short, intense epidemic that followed began in December 1915, when a few polio cases were reported in Auckland province. By mid-January 1916 the epidemic

was already under way; in February, it spread to the southern part of North Island. South Island, which had been affected by the 1914 outbreak, reported only 76 of the 1,018 European cases that occurred overall. Most of the cases (960) occurred between January and June, 61 percent in children below five years of age; morbidity and mortality rates were highest in children less than nine years old. There were 123 deaths (76 males, 47 females). Basic preventive measures were recommended; the authorities barred child contacts from attending school and adult contacts from handling food.

Another polio epidemic, considered the most severe, broke out in Wellington in December 1924 and spread across the country, infecting 1,185 Europeans by the end of June 1925 but bypassing the Maori natives. The provinces of Taranaki, Wellington, and Canterbury suffered the most. Once again, young children were the primary victims; more than 50 percent of the cases occurred in children below five years of age; 79 percent of the cases and 74 percent of the 173 deaths (91 males, 82 females) occurred in children under ten years of age. The notification rate for this epidemic was 87.3 per 100,000 people. To prevent children from gathering together and spreading the infection, schools remained closed for the summer vacation until mid-April.

The epidemic of 1937, milder than its predecessors, began in the city of Dunedin in November 1936. Over the next three months, it spread across the Otago health district. From April to July 1937, it raged in the province of Canterbury and most of North Island. Between December 1936 and November 1937, 896 cases—656 with some degree of paralysis—had been reported among Europeans and Maoris. Forty-six people died. Incidence was highest in those aged five to nine, but the paralytic rate was highest in children under five. Attack rates were almost equal for Maoris and Europeans. The case-fatality rate for people over 25 years of age was highest during this epidemic. When it began, all schools were closed until early February. When it continued to spread nonetheless, only the affected schools were closed for three weeks.

Unlike the previous polio outbreak, the epidemic of 1947–49 (caused by the type 1 poliovirus) began late in the spring of 1947. It continued to rage through 1948 and ended officially in August 1949. The Auckland health district reported its first cases in mid-November 1947, and a week later cases occurred in the Hamilton and New Plymouth districts. Cases were reported across North Island by April 1948 but only four occurred in South Island. During June–October 1948, the emphasis shifted from the northern to the southern districts of North Island, the Wellington area in particular. By the end of that year, the Wellington outbreak was over and the disease had moved to South Island, especially Dunedin, where it prevailed until late July 1949, with only sporadic cases occurring after that. From November 1947 to July 1949, 1,406 confirmed polio cases (805 paralytic to varying degrees) and 77 deaths (including six Maoris) were reported. During this slow-moving epidemic, the highest attack rates were in children five to nine years of age, although many more older people were also involved. Incidence was noticeably higher in some rural areas and twice as high in the Plymouth health district as anywhere else. Overall incidence was higher on North Island. Initially, all schools were closed and all congregations of children were banned. Parental pressure later led to the lifting of these restrictions.

During the second quarter of 1952, poliomyelitis was on the rise again; in June, the epidemic (caused by the type 2 poliovirus) began in Auckland. Throughout the winter and spring of 1952, the epidemic moved rapidly across most of North Island. Three months later, it reached South Island. Of the 1,298 confirmed cases reported during 1952–53, 1,205 occurred between June 1952 and March 1953. Attack rates were uniformly high in people under 20 years of age. Rural areas recorded disproportionately higher morbidity, paralysis, and mortality rates. Actual cases and their contacts were isolated, and parents were urged to watch out for signs of illness and report them immediately. The importance of general hygiene was stressed.

Two years later, in August–September 1955, poliomyelitis (mainly the type 1 poliovirus) broke out again (this time in the Hamilton and New Plymouth areas) and quickly spread across North Island, peaking there in November. South Island was infected two months later, most of the cases occurring there after January 1956. Dunedin was attacked in October 1955, but the epidemic began to subside there even before it peaked over the rest of the island. Of the 1,485 cases reported during 1955–56, 925 were paralytic and 73 people died. The paralytic rate per 10,000 people was higher on South Island (5.9) than on North Island (3.5) as were the death rates (0.6 per 10,000 versus 0.2 per 10,000). Cases occurred through the end of 1956, even though the worst of the epidemic was over by July 1956.

The Salk polio vaccine was first made available in New Zealand in September 1956, and by the end of 1959, more than 80 percent of school and preschool children were immunized. In April 1962, the Sabin oral polio vaccine was introduced and taken by 95 percent of school and preschool children.

Further reading: Maclean, *Challenge for Health: A History of Public Health in New Zealand*; Donovan, "A Study in New Zealand Mortality: 6, Epidemic Diseases."

New Zealand Scarlet Fever Epidemics

Several epidemics of scarlet fever during the nineteenth and twentieth centuries. An infectious disease caused by streptococcal bacteria, scarlet fever was introduced into New Zealand sometime during the late 1840s or mid-1850s. The first really severe outbreak occurred in Dunedin during 1863–64; this South Island town of some 15,000 people reported 119 deaths from scarlet fever between November 1863 and October 1864, a fatality rate of 79.3 per 10,000 people. That year, diarrhea, dysentery, and typhoid had already wrought havoc upon the citizens of Dunedin.

The next major epidemic of scarlet fever, apparently an importation from Australia (see AUSTRALIAN SCARLET FEVER EPIDEMIC OF 1875–76), occurred during 1876–77. It spread quite extensively across the country during these two years, but its effects were by no means uniform everywhere. For instance, in 1876, the city of Christchurch escaped with only a mild outbreak, but the district of Otago suffered a death rate (79 deaths, 7.0 per 10,000 people) double that of the rest of the country (136 deaths overall, 3.51 per 10,000 people). During this epidemic, Dunedin's local board of health enforced a strict quarantine of infected families and established a fever hospital. In 1877, New Zealand reported 195 scarlet fever deaths (4.83 per 10,000 people). That year, the outbreak was most virulent in Westland province (42 deaths, 24 per 10,000); in particular, the borough of Hokitika (2,738 persons) had 40 deaths, a rate of 146 per 10,000 people. Otago's death rate was still high—10.25 per 10,000 people (121 deaths). It is not clear whether the high case fatality rate was due to the exceptional virulence of the virus or its extensive spread.

Scarlet fever struck again in epidemic form during 1881–82. In the first year, 104 deaths (2.11 per 10,000) occurred—73 in Auckland (7.29 per 10,000 people) and 24 in Otago. There were many more deaths (153) in 1882; once again, Auckland was hit hardest (98 deaths, 9.46 per 10,000 people), followed by Nelson (19 deaths, 7.08 per 10,000 people) and Otago (21 deaths, 1.5 per 10,000 people). The disease was widespread in Christchurch too, but was reportedly quite mild there and did not cause any deaths. Overall, scarlet fever's very inconsistency and unpredictability made it a dreaded disease. Ships arriving in the country with scarlet fever on board were subject to the strictest quarantine laws.

Incidence of scarlet fever declined gradually until 1903 when it erupted again to cause 131 deaths (1.6

per 10,000 people). Case mortality, however, was low. For instance, in the Wellington health district, there were 2,014 reported cases and 32 deaths in the two years ending March 31, 1904.

During the first few decades of the twentieth century, hundreds of cases occurred each year, but death rates remained low. The next outbreak of the disease occurred in 1944–45; there were 7,622 cases with 27 deaths in 1944 and 5,033 cases (4,101 in children below 15 years of age and the rest mainly below 25 years of age) with 13 deaths in 1945. After this outburst, the disease reverted to its generally mild form. Most patients were successfully treated at home, and doctors did not bother notifying cases because of the resulting inconvenience (isolation and quarantine); in addition they found that the imposition of established control procedures did not necessarily prevent epidemics. New Zealand's Health Act of 1956 declared that scarlet fever was no longer a notifiable disease.

Further reading: Maclean, *Challenge for Health: A History of Public Health in New Zealand*; Donovan, "A Study in New Zealand Mortality: 6, Epidemic Diseases."

New Zealand Troops Poliomyelitis Epidemic of 1940–41 (Egyptian Poliomyelitis Epidemic of 1940–41)

Probably the first sizable military outbreak of poliomyelitis or polio ever recorded struck New Zealand troops sent to the Middle East during World War II. Not expecting to see polio cases among the soldiers, the attending physicians were surprised when the epidemic appeared exclusively within an adult male population, especially since other features of the outbreak were exceptional as well. The epidemic, for instance, came in two distinct waves, but was marked by a low mortality rate (only four fatal cases out of a total of 40) and a below-average degree of paralysis (19 patients, or less than half).

In retrospect, it is easy to say that the doctors should have been prepared for adult polio cases. During the two decades prior to World War II, the age distribution of the disease had shifted in the United States, Britain, New Zealand, and other Westernized countries. Until 1920 poliomyelitis had been predominantly a disease of childhood, but soon afterward larger numbers of adolescents and young adults began to succumb. During an outbreak in New Zealand in 1937, for example, 20.4 percent of victims were over 15 years of age, compared to 13.3 percent in a 1916 outbreak. Although the New Zealand soldiers, who were between 20 and 40 years old, would likely have lived through one or more of their country's polio epidemics (another one had taken place in 1925), some of them had apparently not acquired immunity before they went to the Middle East.

Starting in November 1940, doctors with the New Zealand Expeditionary Force observed two clusters of polio patients. Fourteen cases were reported before March 1, 1941, then eight weeks went by with no newly diagnosed patients, and finally, a second, more intense wave of cases began in April. In just two weeks 16 new patients were admitted to the hospital, with the remainder falling ill over the next few weeks (until July). The seasonal nature of the epidemic corresponded not to the pattern usually seen in the Northern Hemisphere (where polio outbreaks are most common from May to December), but to that found in New Zealand. In other respects, however, the epidemic in Egypt differed from earlier ones in New Zealand, both in its higher incidence (2.2 cases per 1,000 population based on the estimate of 18,000 troops present during the nine months) and in its low mortality and paralysis rates. These unusual figures may be explained by the fact that in a military camp, mild cases were more likely to be admitted for medical observation than in a civilian setting.

The military doctors could provide no definitive explanation for the spread of the disease. Contact between patients was difficult to establish: Cases were found in 16 widely separated units at two different base camps, as well as in hospitals at some distance away. Poliovirus was endemic in Egypt, however, although polio incidence among native Egyptians did not increase during the years 1940–41, as compared with the two preceding years. Throughout 1941 and 1942 two U.K. army physicians had observed more than 100 poliomyelitis or encephalitis cases among troops in Egypt, and had even isolated six different strains from seven fatal cases. While their experimental findings were published in 1943, wartime censorship held back detailed reports of the epidemic among the New Zealand soldiers for several more years.

Further reading: Caughey and Porteous, "An Epidemic of Poliomyelitis Occurring among Troops in the Middle East"; Paul, *A History of Poliomyelitis*.

New Zealand Whooping Cough Epidemics of 1873 and 1907

Two of the most severe epidemics of whooping cough ever to strike New Zealand. This contagious, bacterial respiratory disease, the medical term for which is pertusis, chiefly affects infants and children.

Whooping cough first attacked New Zealand in epidemic form in 1828 (see NEW ZEALAND EPIDEMICS OF 1820–40) and again in 1847. However, since most of the victims were children under five years of age and the disease was not notifiable, outbreaks generally went unreported. The epidemic of 1873, considered the most severe of them all, also met the same fate; the local authorities did not even record its existence.

The outbreak was widespread but some areas suffered more than others; for instance, the provinces of Auckland (119 deaths, 17.4 per 10,000 people), Wellington (mortality 13.0 per 10,000 people), Nelson (13.8 deaths per 10,000 people), and Marlborough (14.2 deaths per 10,000 people) were especially hard hit. That year (1873), there were 356 deaths (159 males, 197 females) from whooping cough among the white population. Of these, 221 occurred among children below one year of age and 340 of the victims were less than five years old. Its severity is evident from the fact that 20 infants died from the disease for every 1,000 live births that year. The overall death rate was 12.33 per 10,000 people.

Serious local epidemics of whooping cough occurred in 1877. The region of Taranaki reported 12.9 deaths per 10,000 people and Wellington province had 8.6 deaths per 10,000 and a similar outbreak in 1878. In 1882 Hawke's Bay recorded 13.9 deaths per 10,000 people. Whooping cough outbreaks occurred in 1883 in Canterbury and Otago, in 1884 in Auckland city, in 1891 in Wellington city and Marlborough province, and in 1903 in Westland and Marlborough provinces.

The epidemic of 1907 is considered the last major outbreak of the disease in New Zealand. It began in Otago in 1906 and ended in Auckland in 1908. Only Westland and Marlborough provinces escaped infection. The 307 deaths (3.34 per 10,000 people) recorded among the country's white population in 1907 were evenly spread out across the four main provinces (Auckland, Canterbury, Otago, and Wellington). Of these, 207 (67.4 percent) were among children less than one year old and 304 (99.0 percent) among children below five years of age. Infant mortality that year was 8.3 per 1,000 live births.

Immunization against whooping cough became widespread after 1946 and, together with the general improvement in infant health, helped reduce mortality from the disease.

Further reading: Maclean, *Challenge for Health: A History of Public Health in New Zealand*; Donovan, "A Study in New Zealand Mortality: 6, Epidemic Diseases."

Nicobar Islands Poliomyelitis Epidemic of 1947
Severe epidemic of poliomyelitis on one of the Nicobar Islands, situated several hundred miles off the eastern coast of India in the Bay of Bengal.

The end of World War II in 1945 and the subsequent movement of soldiers across many different areas of the world led to a rash of poliomyelitis outbreaks in many places. The virus is believed to have entered one of the Nicobar Islands of India in this manner, through the agency of British troops. From that island it spread to another where, during November and December 1947, 800 cases of poliomyelitis were reported in a population of 9,000. Of these, 566 were paralytic (see VIETNAMESE POLIOMYELITIS EPIDEMICS OF 1958–60). During these two months there were 118 fatal cases in the Nicobars.

Unlike poliomyelitis outbreaks on many other islands (Malta and Mauritius, for instance), this one in the Nicobars mainly affected individuals between age six and twenty-five. Most of the fatalities were reported in this age group as well. Clearly, this was an intense epidemic representing the islands' first contact with the disease. See also TAHITIAN POLIOMYELITIS EPIDEMIC OF 1951.

Further reading: World Health Organization, *Poliomyelitis*; Hobson, *World Health and History*.

Nigerian Influenza Epidemic of 1918–19 Offshoot of the worldwide Spanish Influenza Epidemic of 1917–19 (q.v.), striking Nigeria in west-central Africa and resulting in the deaths of at least 512,000 people. Afterward influenza broke out almost annually in isolated regions, such as the towns of Ibi and Kano, in the country's north.

In September 1918 the viral infection first occurred in Lagos, Nigeria's capital, largest city, and chief port, where it was brought by sick oceanliner passengers and servicemen returning from Europe. Advanced medical facilities helped reduce fatalities from the Spanish flu in Lagos. However, it spread quickly into the neighboring southern provinces, where about 250,000 human deaths were eventually recorded; in a great many cases of flu, complications such as pneumonia, bronchitis, and heart problems occurred, along with the usual symptoms of head colds, high fevers, chills, and aching bones and muscles.

In Benin province, where many fled from the disease into the bush, there were sometimes not enough men to bury the dead. Their flight also helped spread the flu to the bush, where many stricken natives died along roadsides or in canoes found drifting at sea. Camphor and Islamic amulets were often worn to ward off the disease. Sacrifices were offered in the town of Abaja to ward off the spirits thought to carry the flu to the Igbo natives there, where nine out of ten villagers were stricken. Many Igbo children born during that time were named "Ogbe Infelunze."

After flourishing about four to six weeks in each particular Nigerian village or town, influenza subsided and then vanished. Authorities have estimated that probably 32 per 1,000 Nigerians perished from flu during the epidemic, which is considered one of Nigeria's worst disasters.

Further reading: Isichei, *A History of Nigeria*.

Nigerian Meningitis Epidemics of 1949 and 1950

Severe epidemics of cerebrospinal meningitis (CSM) that killed 16,055 persons out of 98,458 who were infected in Nigeria in western Africa.

The disease was endemic in Nigerian areas before 1905, when the first serious outbreak was reported; CSM cases occurred annually until 1921, when 45,900 Nigerians died from the disease in one district alone. It did not reach epidemic proportions again until 1937, when it entered Nigeria from Chad in the east; major outbreaks happened every year thereafter, with those in 1949 and 1950 being the most devastating.

In 1949 CSM first broke out in the semi-arid grassland areas around the northern Nigeria towns of Katsina, Sokoto, and Kano during the long dry season when the cold evenings brought more people indoors to sleep. Infection of CSM is by direct contact, including by droplets and discharges from the nose and throat of infected persons. Nigerians sleeping in poorly ventilated and overcrowded mud houses easily spread this acute bacterial disease. At first, some 9,000 persons in Katsina became sick with fevers, violent headaches, dizziness, delirium, rashes, and stiff necks. Then the Kano district was struck, and the disease moved eastward, helped by a dense and mobile populace. Before the rainy season came in 1949, the mortality rate from CSM was over 20 percent, with 8,732 human deaths reported for the year.

In 1950 infections from CSM increased to 57,549 reported cases, and once again the epidemic was centered in the northern regions of Nigeria (the northwest was hardest hit). Better medical treatment kept the mortality rate at 12 percent, with 7,323 deaths. There was a higher proportion of deaths among young children and the elderly in both 1949 and 1950.

British health officials in Nigeria frequently removed the sick from their homes (despite family opposition in many cases) and isolated them in special huts. In addition, government authorities closed border areas, cordoned off roads, suspended school and market (trade) activities, banned all funerals, and confined troops to their barracks. However, these precautionary measures were hampered by native African resistance.

Annual outbreaks of CSM occurred in Nigeria from 1951 to 1960; they were of varying intensity. Between 1960 and 1962, more than 72,000 cases of CSM were reported, with more than 5,000 deaths. Afterward there was a substantial decrease in the number of CSM cases. Preventive measures were introduced: avoiding direct contact with the infected; preventing overcrowding in all areas if possible; and vaccinating as a general measure (a polysaccharide vaccine).

Further reading: Hartwig and Patterson, *Cerebrospinal Meningitis in West Africa and Sudan in the Twentieth Century;* Waddy, "African Epidemic Cerebro-Spinal Meningitis."

Nigerian Smallpox Epidemic of 1930–35

Outbreak of smallpox in Nigeria in western Africa (north of the Gulf of Guinea), killing 10,438 persons out of 45,386 who were infected. Nigerians had suffered from the disease in sporadic outbreaks during the nineteenth and early twentieth centuries.

In 1930 the viral disease erupted during the hot, dry season (November to February), when the variola virus survives better because of lack of humidity and when Nigerians' greater mobility and social activities help spread the infection. (Transmission occurs through close contact with patients, through respiratory discharges, or through contact with contaminated clothing or other articles touched by victims of the disease.) In 1930 numerous regions in Nigeria became infected, including Lagos (the capital), Bauchi, Sokoto, Enugu (inhabited by many Ibo black natives), and Ogbomosho (inhabited by many Yoruba black natives). By the end of the year, most age groups had been infected with smallpox, and 5,119 infections and 1,038 deaths had been reported from the disease.

The incidence of smallpox declined in Nigeria in 1931; there were 2,315 persons infected, 568 of whom died. A radical increase of the disease occurred in 1932 and 1933, and it claimed 4,891 human lives out of 22,065 reported cases. In the country's more populated regions, the grim effects of smallpox (which blinded or disfigured many) were worsened by the sleeping sickness that also attacked much of the population at the time. Smallpox cases numbered 10,389 (out of which 2,538 were fatal) in 1934.

A smallpox vaccine had been available for use in Nigeria since 1918 and had been effectively administered in the large coastal cities of Lagos and Port Harcourt. However, vaccination had been (and was in the 1930s) strongly resisted by the Yorubas in southwestern Nigeria. In Ogbomosho, Oyo, Ilesha, and other Yoruba-dominated towns and cities, smallpox was thought to be an indication or sign of divine displeasure and supposedly infected those being punished for some wrongdoing. The Yorubas, who had suffered for many years from smallpox, had developed a culture worshipping a smallpox deity called Shapona or Soponna. Every Yoruban village and town had a shrine erected to Shapona, to whom festivals were held every September during an epidemic period. Smallpox declined to 5,498 reported infections (with 1,403 fatalities) in 1935. It remained a serious health problem in Nigeria into the early 1950s, when newly developed, highly stable, freeze-dried vaccines contributed to a decreasing incidence of the disease in the country. The global smallpox eradication efforts of the World Health Organization (beginning in 1967) contributed to making Nigeria smallpox-free by the early 1970s.

Further reading: Dixon, *Smallpox;* Isichei, *A History of Nigeria.*

Nigerian Yellow Fever Epidemic of 1986–90

Worst and longest recorded outbreak of yellow fever ever to strike the African country of Nigeria, where it spread to 19 out of 22 states, raged for five years, and killed a reported 3,633 persons out of 16,230 who were infected by the virus that is transmitted by the bite of infective *Aëdes aegypti* mosquitoes. All of Africa during this period reported a total of 16,782 yellow fever cases with 3,919 deaths, and thus most of the cases occurred in Nigeria; this was also the highest number of African cases in any five-year period since 1948.

In June 1986 the mosquito-borne disease broke out in the Benue state in southeast Nigeria; more than a third of the 559 persons infected perished. The disease then spread southwestward into the Cross River area, killing 222 out of 697 persons infected, and by the end of 1986 the epidemic had moved farther to the southwest, infecting (but less severely) six other Nigerian states.

Nigeria was struck by both urban and jungle yellow fever. In urban areas, the reservoir of infection is human beings and the female *Aëdes aegypti* mosquitoes; monkeys are the main reservoir for jungle yellow fever. In Nigeria's non-urban areas, human beings contract jungle yellow fever through the bite of forest mosquitoes that have bitten infected jungle animals, like monkeys or apes.

In 1987 the epidemic's epicenter became Ogbomosho, a city of some 600,000 people in Oyo state in southwestern Nigeria, where there were 905 cases and 482 deaths from the fever. From Ogbomosho it spread to six other southwestern states, including the capital city Lagos, before dying out in September. However, a month earlier, in August 1987, a new focus of yellow fever had been established in several northwestern states in the country; the areas around Sokoto and Kaduna were affected until early 1988. Nigeria then remained free of the disease for several months until early June 1988, when the states of Kaduna, Katsina, Kano, and Bauchi (in the north-central region) reported cases. That year there were 4,920 yellow fever cases with 1,502 fatalities, com-

pared to the year before (1987) when total infections were 2,676 with 866 fatalities.

In 1989 Nigeria was the only African country reporting yellow fever; it had 3,270 cases and 618 fatalities. The disease escalated in Nigeria the following year—4,075 cases—but because of effective mass immunization, fatalities dropped to 223. The countries of Cameroon and Niger, Nigeria's neighbors to the east and north respectively, also reported cases of yellow fever in 1990. (Throughout the rest of the world in 1990, there were only 90 cases of the sickness, with 69 fatalities—all coming from six South American countries.)

During the five-year epidemic in Nigeria, children and teenagers were the large majority of the cases and deaths from the fever, according to hospital records. A number of epidemiological investigations were carried out that suggested that the actual number of cases was four to perhaps 90 times higher than officially reported figures. Consequently, the Nigerian government decided to include yellow fever vaccination routinely in its national child-immunization program.

Further reading: Howe, ed., *A World Geography of Human Diseases;* World Health Organization, "Yellow Fever in 1989 and 1990," *Weekly Epidemiological Record.*

Northern Rhodesian (Zambian) Plague of 1917–18

Unexpected outbreak of plague in the northeastern district of Northern Rhodesia (Zambia), killing 177 out of 184 persons infected. The disease, carried by rats with plague-infected fleas, entered British East Africa about 1912 (see PLAGUE PANDEMIC, THIRD) and later reached the Luangwa River valley in Northern Rhodesia in late January 1917. Within two months, plague had spread to seven villages along the Lumenzi River, killing 90 African natives.

Smallpox was first thought to have killed 25 natives in the village of Tembwe in the Luangwa Valley. An investigation by the area's magistrate found victims suffering with buboes (swellings in the groin and armpit) and chest pains, and the discovery of bubonic-diseased rats in Tembwe. In nearby villages along the Lumenzi River, the natives contracted bubonic, pneumonic, and septicemic plague (the three clinical forms), and often those infected with the latter two forms die before developing buboes and coughing out infectious microorganisms. By April 1917 plague had moved eastward from Northern Rhodesia to Karonga in northern Nyasaland (another British protectorate, the present Malawi).

Another outbreak of "rat" plague (bubonic) in the Luangwa Valley occurred between September and December 1917, and authorities, hoping to prevent the spread of the disease, offered a reward of one penny for each rat killed. All 30 plague cases were fatal. Another plague outbreak, centered in the village of Chimbirima in March 1918, took the lives of 56 out of 59 stricken; about 30 more died before the epidemic ceased and more than a million and a half rats were eradicated in the area.

Further reading: Gelfand, *Northern Rhodesia in the Days of the Charter*; Shattuck, *Diseases of the Tropics.*

Northern Rhodesian Smallpox Epidemic of 1955

See ZAMBIAN SMALLPOX EPIDEMIC OF 1955.

O

Oberammergau Plague of 1634 See THIRTY YEARS' WAR EPIDEMICS.

Omaha Indian Smallpox Epidemic of 1802 Outbreak of smallpox that killed about two thirds of the Omaha, a Siouan tribe of North American Indians living in the Missouri River valley of present-day northeast Nebraska.

Increasing trade and contact between the Plains Indians and Europeans resulted in the former being more and more infected by smallpox and other "foreign" communicable diseases in the late eighteenth century; smallpox seriously attacked the Mandan, Shoshone, and Blackfoot tribes in the upper and middle Missouri River regions after 1780 (see MANDAN INDIAN SMALLPOX EPIDEMIC OF 1837; BLACKFOOT INDIAN SMALLPOX EPIDEMIC OF 1837–38). It is most likely that the smallpox (variola) virus also reached the Omaha Indians in the lower Missouri region, for explorers had observed pockmarked Omahas (the disease leaves pockmarks on the skin of survivors).

The Omaha, who had actively engaged in trade with white Europeans, were severely infected by smallpox in 1802. The systemic infection was acute and spread rapidly through the Omaha villages, some of whose members became desperate and crazed and burned their houses to try to stop the spread of the lethal disease. Some Indians put their wives and children to death so that they might be spared the agonies of smallpox, frequently including blindness and, usually, disfigurement. At the time the mortality rate was higher among the Omaha than it was among Europeans, of whom 15 percent to 40 percent usually died.

At the height of the 1802 epidemic, the Omaha chief Wash-guh-sah-ba, better known as Blackbird, who had been one of the first Indians in the Missouri Valley to trade with the white man, was stricken by smallpox. His loyal people did not desert him, but instead they drew around his bedside and unwittingly became infected themselves. (It is one of the most communicable of diseases, requiring only a breath to blow the variola virus from one mouth to another.) Honoring Blackbird's dying request, the surviving Omahas buried him astride his favorite horse on the summit of a bluff overlooking the Missouri Valley, so that he could observe the white man's boats coming up the river to trade with his people.

In 1803 Meriwether Lewis and William Clark were sent to explore the vast Louisiana Territory and later reported the Omaha smallpox epidemic and catastrophe (the tribe was sizably depopulated) to U.S. President Thomas Jefferson, who in turn directed Lewis and Clark to promote vaccination among the Indians in this new territory of the United States. The Indians, despite their sufferings, remained wary of vaccination.

Further reading: Heagerty, *Four Centuries of Medical History in Canada;* Hopkins, *Princes and Peasants: Smallpox in History.*

Ontong Java Island Influenza Epidemics During the twentieth century, a series of influenza epidemics of varying intensity in the southwest Pacific coral island group Ontong Java (or Lord Howe), a dependency of New South Wales. Its native inhabitants are Polynesians.

Ontong Java, one of the largest atolls in the group, had an estimated population between 3,000 and 4,000 in 1900. It was struck by a severe influenza epidemic in 1906. At its height, the epidemic claimed 30 to 40 victims every day. Many of Ontong Java's smaller settlements were abandoned, and the population of the two main villages (Luanguia and Pelau) substantially reduced.

Influenza struck again in 1926 (33 deaths) and in 1928 (several deaths), killing many infants. In most cases, mortality resulted from pneumonia complications following the influenza infection.

In 1935 and 1936, influenza outbreaks killed 50 people. Luanguia village was more severely affected (7.2 percent mortality) than Pelau (3.4 percent mortality), perhaps because the infection was first brought into port by a trading ship, the *Southern Cross.*

The district officer, named Brownlees, was convinced that the infections were brought into Ontong Java by outside ships. He suggested that these ships should not be granted entry except on presentation of a medical clearance certificate. He also recommended restrictions on emigration by native islanders. After another bout of influenza in 1939 (eight deaths), Brownlees reiterated his suggestions. He argued that Luanguia, which had more outside contact than Pelau, had suffered a 17 percent decline in its population since 1928 against an eight percent decline in Pelau for the same period.

Later in 1939, the Closed District Regulations were enacted. Thereby, foreign ships were denied entry unless a certificate of medical clearance was produced. The regulations remained in effect until 1970 but were not strictly enforced as time went on. When World War II began, trading and missionary activities came to a grinding halt, and the Luanguia trading station was permanently closed. Even government shipping was sharply limited. Ontong Java remained quite isolated until the early 1950s.

Further reading: Carroll, ed., *Pacific Atoll Populations.*

Oporto Plague of 1899   See SPANISH PLAGUES OF 1905–06 AND 1923.

Oregon Malaria Epidemic of 1829–33   Catastrophic outbreak of malaria that killed an estimated 150,000 Native Americans (Indians) residing in what is now Oregon, Washington, and California. Because the mortality rate appeared to be overmuch for malaria, some have argued that the disease depopulating the various Indian tribes during these years was either influenza, scarlet fever, typhoid, or typhus. Also, malaria exists more in tropical or subtropical areas. However, accounts of the epidemic by white settlers and Indians have stressed malarial symptoms: high fever, aching, nausea, shaking chills, shock, delirium, and coma. They also referred to the disease as "ague" (a fever of malarial character). In addition, the infection occurred only during the warm weather in the valleys and along the coast of America's West.

In February 1829 the brigantine *Owhyhee* unknowingly brought malaria into the Columbia River region. This trading vessel from Boston had made a port of call for peach trees at the Juan Fernández Islands, off the coast of Chile, before proceeding north to Oregon. Infective Chilean mosquitoes, which easily bred in water tanks on board ships, transmitted malaria to human beings through their bites, and another vessel a month later arrived with more disease-carrying mosquitoes. By spring, the Columbia River had overflowed its banks, creating ideal breeding spots (stagnant water bodies and swamps) for malarial mosquitoes.

The Multnomah Indians on Sauvie Island at the mouth of the Willamette River (which flows into the Columbia) were the first to be struck by malaria, which wiped out the entire tribe in three weeks in the summer of 1829. Nearly 1,000 members of another tribe at nearby Fort Vancouver (Vancouver, Washington) also contracted the disease and died that summer.

Similar devastating malaria outbreaks in the summers of 1830, 1831, and 1832 struck the Kutenai (or Kootenai) and Thompson Indian tribes in the Willamette Valley and the Nootka and Salish tribes along the Pacific coast. Other valley and coastal Indians were attacked, too. In Fort Vancouver and other places, the mortality rate (deaths per thousand population) went as high as 95 percent at times. Each outbreak came to a close with the arrival of winter. Before the summer of 1829, the Indian population in this region (now parts of Oregon and Washington) totaled about 100,000 natives; at the end of the epidemic in 1833, their number had been reduced to about 20,000.

Indians who fled in terror from their villages carried the protozoan (miasmodium malaria) and infective mosquitoes with them into California, where eventually some 70,000 Indians fell victim to malaria. White settlers also contracted it, but the death rate among them was far lower. Some authorities have claimed that the deaths of some 150,000 natives in these regions made the settlement of white emigrants easier there in the succeeding years.

Further reading: Harrison, *Mosquitoes, Malaria and Man*; Simpson, *Invisible Armies.*

Oxford Typhus Epidemic of 1577 (Black Assize)   Sudden outbreak of typhus fever among the jury, presiding officials, and courtroom spectators at the county court, or assize, held at Oxford, England, on July 5 and 6, 1577.

An English Catholic bookbinder called Rowland Jencks was then being tried for various offenses against the government and Anglican Church, and the trial occasioned considerable interest among the Oxford citizenry. The crowded courtroom was an ideal place for typhus fever to spread, as the largely unwashed spectators undoubtedly were full of lice, the vectors of this highly infectious and often fatal disease. The fever killed over 500 people, all of whom had attended the assizes; no women were reported to have died in this epidemic, although there is no evidence that none were present in the courtroom. Among the fatal cases were approximately 100 men associated with Oxford University. The more reliable contemporary accounts state that symptoms began appearing around the middle of July and that the disease ran its course in about one month. Jencks, the man on trial, was found guilty and had his ears cut off, but escaped infection and lived another 33 years.

This deadly and seemingly mysterious epidemic caused much alarm and curiosity. The English philosopher-scientist Francis Bacon investigated the evidence and concluded that corrupted air, or miasma, caused the disease. This idea was believed by many men of science and medicine until the late nineteenth century. Washing the body and changing into clean clothes regularly, the simple means by which lice would have been eliminated and typhus fever avoided, would not become common practice among either the lower or the higher classes in Great Britain for another 300 years.

Further reading: Creighton, *A History of Epidemics in Britain*; Zinsser, *Rats, Lice and History*.

Oxford Typhus Epidemic of 1643

Widespread epidemic of lice-borne typhus fever that erupted among Royalist army troops at Oxford, England, in the spring of 1643 during the English Civil Wars.

An eyewitness who wrote a detailed account of the epidemic observed that the "disease became so epidemical that a great part of the people was killed by it; and as soon as it had entered a house it ran through the same, that there was scarce one left well to administer to the sick." This statement attests to the rapidity with which the human body-louse transmitted typhus fever from person to person, especially in crowded living quarters and among people whose lack of personal hygiene encouraged the breeding of these parasitic vectors. The author also provides a detailed description of the symptoms and course of the disease that identifies it unmistakably as typhus fever. The infection spread quickly through the town and surrounding countryside. Mortality was especially high among old men, but also among "not a few children, young men, and those of a more mature and robust age." So devastating was the epidemic to both the Royalist and Parliamentary forces, who were suffering from the disease at Reading (see READING TYPHUS EPIDEMIC OF 1643), that war hostilities were interrupted for many months.

The two opposing armies spread epidemic typhus fever far and wide throughout England as they moved from place to place during the English Civil Wars of the 1640s. So commonplace did the infection become during these years that few accounts of individual outbreaks were recorded. An exception is the devastating attack suffered by the town of Tiverton, England (see TIVERTON TYPHUS EPIDEMIC OF 1644).

Further reading: Creighton, *A History of Epidemics in Britain*; Zinsser, *Rats, Lice and History*.

P

Pakistani Malaria Epidemic of 1929 Severe but localized outbreak of malaria that ravaged the northern part of the province of Sind in present-day Pakistan. Extremely drought-ridden for several years, the province was deluged by torrential rains during July and August 1929. This caused extensive flooding that, in addition to destroying crops, homes, and trade, extended the lifespan of the adult anopheline mosquitoes and created more breeding places for their larvae. These were ideal conditions for the spread of malaria, which is caused by a tiny parasite in the human bloodstream and transmitted from person to person by the bite of an infective female anopheline mosquito.

During the autumn of 1929, malaria spread throughout northern Sind; *Plasmodium falciparum* was discovered to be the main parasite involved. In the initial phase, many people acquired benign tertian infections, some of which developed into full-blown attacks of malaria in the spring of 1920. Complications of the spleen were found to be exceptionally high (near 90 percent in some affected areas) following the epidemic. The Larkana district, among others, suffered severely. It was apparently a devastating outbreak that killed about 40,000 people in Sind province. Most of the victims were children born since the previous epidemic 12 years earlier.

Further reading: Covell and Baily, "The Study of a Regional Epidemic of Malaria in Northern Sind"; Harrison, *Mosquitoes, Malaria and Man.*

Panamanian Yellow Fever Epidemics of 1880–1904 Outbreaks of yellow fever during the building of the Panama Canal, attacking French laborers at first and U.S. and other workers later. Panama, during the canal years, was referred to as a "white man's graveyard" because the disease would break out in groups of non-immune whites arriving daily for work on the project and kill off many of them.

In 1879, French engineer Ferdinand de Lesseps was put in charge of construction of a Panama Canal, but in 1889 the project was abandoned when the French company failed, partly from financial mismanagement and partly from the ravages of yellow fever among the laborers.

During the time the French were in Panama, yellow fever, transmitted by the *Aëdes aegypti* mosquito, never died out, and outbreaks usually occurred every two to three years. In 1882, 125 people died of yellow fever; the number doubled the following year; and in 1885, about 1,300 people perished. The mortality rate from yellow fever in Panama fluctuated from 12 percent to 70 percent. With 20,000 laborers digging the canal in 1884, one third of them were sick or dying of disease. In 1886, 30 French engineers arrived and, within a month, 13 of them had died. The death rate was then estimated at 176 per 1,000 workers.

A new director general for the French, Jules Dingler, arrived in Panama in 1883 and proclaimed that only drunkards and the dissipated died from yellow fever. Dingler's daughter and son soon died of the disease and his wife died in 1884. He soon returned to France, a broken man.

As early as 1854, the theory that mosquitoes transmitted yellow fever had been put forth by Carlos Finlay, a Havana physician. It was largely ignored due to the conviction of the medical community that yellow fever was caused by filth and poisonous gases arising from marshes, and could be contracted only by touching soiled clothing and bedding of a patient.

The *Aëdes aegypti* mosquito breeds in domestic water containers and survives in close contact with humans. The conditions in Panama were ideal for the mosquito; at the time, bowls of still water were scattered throughout buildings to keep ants off beds and flowers, and rainwater was gathered in large barrels, and doors and windows were kept wide open, letting in mosquitoes.

The digging of the canal was taken over by the United States in 1904, and American military doctor William C. Gorgas was sent to the canal area, where yellow fever and malaria, which is also carried by mosquitoes, were hindering the excavation work. Gorgas had previously worked with Dr. Walter Reed on the 1898 campaign to rid Havana of yellow fever; Reed had proved that yellow fever was transmitted by the *Aëdes aegypti* mosquito. Gorgas isolated all yellow fever patients in mosquito-proof rooms, and sanitary brigades were organized to drain off stagnant water and fill in pools. Clogged drainage channels were sprayed with weed killer to eliminate stagnant water places where adult mosquitoes could breed. By 1907 yellow fever had been eradicated, and the completion of the Panama Canal (in 1914) was made possible. Gorgas had persisted despite the belief of the canal's chief engineer George W. Goethels that the sanitary measures were a waste of time and energy.

Further reading: McCullough, *The Path Between the Seas: The Creation of the Panama Canal;* McNeill, *Plagues and Peoples;* Bassett, "Yellow Fever"; Williams, *The Plague Killers.*

Papua New Guinea Influenza Epidemics of 1969–70

Two influenza epidemics, offshoots of the Hong Kong Influenza Pandemic of 1968 (q.v.).

Both epidemics were caused by the same virus strain, later identified as the 1969 Hong Kong (A/New Guinea/1/69H$_3$N$_2$), but the attack rate and other features varied dramatically from area to area. According to one estimate, the 1969 epidemic was neither as widespread nor as serious as most contemporary accounts said it was. Nevertheless, influenza and complications arising from it claimed over 3,000 human lives between July and October 1969. The town of Mendi, in the southern highlands of Papua New Guinea, suffered a very high attack rate and the mortality ranged between three percent and five percent. Many of the deaths were not even reported until an official investigation into the mortality began. Strangely, the adjoining Tari Valley region reported a low attack rate and no deaths.

A similar situation prevailed in the country's eastern highlands. In some villages, nearly every person came down with the clinical symptoms and the morbidity was nearly 100 percent. Other villages in the same region escaped relatively lightly, with a five percent to ten percent attack rate despite an equally susceptible population and close and constant contact with affected persons. Prompt reporting of outbreaks, the establishment of properly equipped medical centers, and the drafting of a plan of action in the event of an outbreak, it was recommended, would substantially reduce mortality in future epidemics.

In 1970, the same virus strain reappeared to cause another influenza outbreak. Some of those who had escaped the previous infection were attacked this time, but not everybody. Many of the island groups in the Pacific Ocean experienced influenza outbreaks in 1969–70.

Further reading: Mackenzie, ed., *Viral Diseases in South-East Asia and the Western Pacific; Health and Disease in Tribal Societies.*

Paris Cholera Epidemic of 1832 See FRENCH CHOLERA EPIDEMIC OF 1832–33.

Paris Diphtheria Epidemic of 1576

Outbreak recorded by the contemporary physician Guillaume de Baillou (1538–1616). Although fatal illnesses involving sore throat, difficulty in breathing, and paralysis of the soft palate had been noted throughout late classical and medieval times, it is only from the 1500s that detailed records of possible diphtheria epidemics exist. In Holland and Basel in 1517, for instance, many people died of suffocation, often within a day, their throats inflamed and the tongue and pharynx covered with a whitish membrane. Baillou's accurate account of the 1576 epidemic reflects the increasing differentiation among diseases in the sixteenth century, as do his vivid descriptions of other infections in Paris, France (see PARIS WHOOPING COUGH EPIDEMIC OF 1578).

Born and educated in Paris, Baillou stayed there to practice medicine, becoming a champion of the methods of Hippocrates (an ancient Greek physician). Baillou's writings, none of which were published in his lifetime, emulate the great Greek doctor by describing various diseases that ran their course during a given year. In 1576 Baillou observed a number of patients stricken with rapid, shallow breathing—though without a cough, phlegm, or marked fever—that continued until they died. Disagreeing with other physicians who believed it was a lung disease, Baillou claimed the cause was in the lower abdomen. His suspicions were confirmed when an autopsy revealed a purulent kidney in one of his patients.

Another autopsy on a seven-year-old boy, whose pharynx was slightly swollen before he died, found the false membrane characteristic of the disease. As Baillou put it, "sluggish resisting phlegm was found which covered the trachea like a membrane and the entry and exit of air to the exterior was not free." In describing a similar epidemic two years later, Baillou wonders whether "an opening in the larynx" might work to restore complete breathing; however, he does not seem to have performed a tracheotomy himself.

Parisians in the 1500s were highly susceptible to infectious diseases; epidemics of one sort or another were an almost annual occurrence. Students, merchants, and ambassadors to the French court came and went in the city, adding to the already large population. (One of Baillou's diphtheria victims was a Spaniard.) The residents of Paris had to put up with houses crowded close together, an inadequate water supply, unpaved roads, and poor sanitation. On top of unhealthy living conditions, Parisians also suffered disproportionately during the Wars of Religion then ravaging France. The French kings—first Charles IX and then his brother Henry III—had struggled to maintain their power against many contenders, including their own relatives, factions in the nobility, French Protestants, and the rulers of England and Spain. To support their battles the kings had taxed Paris, the seat of their court, for millions of francs by 1576, while the lawless troops quartered in the city had pillaged so many supplies that poorer people were without food. The weakened city was especially vulnerable to contagious disease.

Further reading: Baillou's account in Ralph Major's *Classic Descriptions of Disease*; Sutherland, "Parisian Life in the Sixteenth Century"; Thompson, *The Wars of Religion in France, 1559–1576*.

Paris Influenza Epidemic of 1918–19 Unprecedented epidemic of influenza that killed approximately 11,500 Parisians in the last six months of 1918 and the early part of 1919, nearly one third of them in the five weeks from October 5 to November 2. *Le grippe* ("Spanish Flu" in English-speaking countries) first appeared among French soldiers in April 1918 and was transmitted by them to Paris, where unusually high numbers of influenza deaths were recorded in July. The epidemic escalated through the next two months and reached its peak in the second half of October.

Paris experienced the usual conditions of an unexpected and deadly epidemic: overcrowded and understaffed hospitals, lack of adequate medical supplies, shortage of coffins, hasty nocturnal burials. Although newspapers gave the epidemic some coverage, France's government chose to deflect attention from it in an effort to minimize alarm among a public already wearied from the stresses of World War I (1914–18). Accordingly, standard measures of public health control such as the closing of schools and theaters and restriction of public transportation were not immediately imposed. As the epidemic exploded in mid-October, however, disinfection of private homes and public places was ordered, and schools were closed from October 26 to November 4.

Prescribed medicines, those hawked by unscrupulous pharmacists but also those recommended by medical practitioners, were marginally effective at best. The onion cure, popularized by New York businesswoman Mrs. Hetty Green, was taken quite seriously. The medically sanctioned treatments included quinine powder mixed with coffee; aspirin; stimulants such as acetate of ammonia, caffeine, alcohol, camphor, strychnine, and arsenic administered orally or intravenously; various antiseptics; and newly developed vaccines and antipneumonic serums. Even bleeding and scarification (whereby turpentine was injected subcutaneously into the thigh to provoke an abscess) were employed.

The epidemic at Paris was part of a global pandemic that killed millions of people throughout the world (see SPANISH INFLUENZA EPIDEMIC OF 1917–19). Influenza is usually fatal mainly among elderly people, who die from pneumonic complications; this time, the flu killed not only in huge numbers, but also an abnormally high proportion of healthy young adults (a phenomenon shared with plague). The extraordinary mortality of the influenza of 1918–19 has never been explained.

Further reading: Delumeau and Lequin, *Les malheurs des temps*; van Hartesveldt, *The 1918–1919 Pandemic of Influenza*.

Paris Plague of 1466 Large-scale epidemic of plague that killed an estimated 40,000 people, according to contemporary chronicles. Climatic factors (along with astronomical phenomena, connivance of lepers or Jews, sorcery, etc.) were often cited as explanations for outbreaks of plague; Parisians attributed the onslaught of plague in August 1466 to a series of summer heat waves. Throughout the plague centuries, in addition to seeking causes for its arrival in their towns, people also attempted to bring epidemics to an end through religious supplication. The citizens of Paris made a grand and solemn procession through the streets in hopes of alleviating their misery in 1466, but the plague only increased in violence and shortly thereafter spread to the outer environs of the city.

Further reading: Biraben, *Les hommes et la peste en France*; Nohl, *The Black Death*.

Paris Whooping Cough Epidemic of 1578 First definite outbreak of whooping cough, described by the noted French physician Guillaume de Baillou, who claimed that he had read of no similar illness in the writings of any other author. The disease, however, may have existed for years before, since nearly a century later one writer says that "old women and empirics" treated it. A disease handled mostly by midwives and other unofficial healers would be unlikely to attract attention from doctors and learned writers.

The victims Baillou saw tended to be young children and infants of four months, ten months, and a little older; though some of them recovered, many others died. Their principal symptom was a violent cough, which sometimes abated for four or five hours at a time (perhaps the reason, Baillou suggests, for the disease's common name "quinta," from the Latin for "five"). Many patients also suffered from fever and vomiting. They breathed with such difficulty that it seemed they were being strangled; they expelled blood from the nose and mouth after a coughing attack. Relying like the ancient Greek physician Hippocrates on close observation of his patients, Baillou believed that an irritation of the lung was at fault, since he noticed that many victims coughed up "putrid phlegm."

Baillou also followed Hippocrates in noting climate conditions, like the "burning and hot" summer that preceded the epidemic. Other contemporary records indicate that no rain fell for months in much of France that year; because of the widespread drought food was scarce. Excessive heat and famine could only add to the misery of Parisians, who already endured unhealthy living conditions. As a university city, an important trading center, and the seat of the French court, Paris drew many travelers both from France and from other countries. In the crowded city many of them moved from one lodging to the next, renting space in the attics or spare rooms of other people's homes. With its dense population and poor sanitation, Paris was hit by numerous epidemics throughout the sixteenth century, including another one described by Baillou, the Paris Diphtheria Epidemic of 1576 (q.v.).

Further reading: Baillou's account in Ralph Major's *Classic Descriptions of Disease*; Mahoney, *Madame Catherine*; Rosen, "Acute Communicable Diseases"; Sutherland, "Parisian Life in the Sixteenth Century."

Peking Pneumonia Epidemics of 1949, 1952–53, and 1958–59

Three epidemics of bronchopneumonia in Peking (Peiping, now Beijing), the capital of the communist People's Republic of China. The common feature of the three outbreaks was that they predominantly attacked preschoolers and young children.

The first epidemic struck Peking during the winter of 1949, affecting mainly preschoolers and young children in schools. Infants apparently did not suffer to the same extent. By all accounts, the disease was clinically mild and mortality very low; this has been attributed to the efficacy of aureomycin treatment. The southern Chinese city of Shanghai was concurrently attacked by a similar outbreak.

The next epidemic was closely associated with an outbreak of influenza in Peking just before and during the winter of 1952. In January 1953, the incidence of juvenile bronchopneumonia began to climb dramatically. During the next four months, 3,148 cases (87.7 percent of them infants less than two years old) were treated at Peking's Second Children's Hospital.

Influenza virus type A was isolated from a couple of patients. Most (66.6 percent) of the cases occurred during January and February, and the fatality rate was reportedly a staggering 52.6 percent. The illness lasted about three weeks and was often complicated by neurological symptoms such as convulsions and coma; pleurisy was also noted in some cases. The generally prescribed treatment of antibiotics and sulfa drugs did not prove efficacious. Autopsies revealed that death was caused by interstitial pneumonia, necrosis of the bronchial and alveolar walls, and hemorrhages in the alveoli. The northern Chinese city of Tientsin was also infected during this period.

The third pneumonia epidemic, perhaps the worst and certainly the most extensive, struck Peking during the winter of 1958. Starting in October 1958, 3,398 cases were treated at one of the city's pediatric hospitals over the next five months. Clearly, this was a very severe epidemic, with many patients not responding to aureomycin or other antibiotic therapy. Mortality was exceptionally high; 528 of the 3,398 patients mentioned above died, a mortality rate of 15.5 percent. On the basis of statistics compiled from eight hospitals, of 535 critically ill patients 180 died, a 33.6 percent fatality rate. As in the previous epidemic, most of the patients were infants less than two years of age; the majority of those were in the six-months to one-year-old category.

The epidemic began in October 1958, peaked in mid-December and began subsiding after the middle of January 1959. Cases continued to be observed after February and even into May, but these later cases were much milder and had noticeably lower mortality. During the height of the epidemic, most of the patients suffered a very severe form of the disease involving the respiratory, cardiovascular, gastrointestinal, and neurological systems. The main causative agent was identified as a type 7 adenovirus, which had apparently also infected most of the cities north of the Yellow River, including Harbin (Pinkiang), Changchun, Shenyang (Mukden), Huhehot (Kweisui), Changchiakou, and Tientsin, but had spared most areas south of it. Around the same time, most of the country was ravaged by a serious outbreak of measles wherein the fatality rate was unusually high because of complications such as pneumonia.

Further reading: Chin-Hsien, "Adenovirus Pneumonia Epidemic Among Peking Infants and Preschool Children in 1958"; Evans, ed., *Viral Infections of Humans.*

"Perinthus, Cough of"

See "COUGH OF PERINTHUS."

Persian Cholera Epidemics of 1821–22

Series of cholera epidemics, resulting from the Asiatic Cholera

Pandemic of 1817–23 (q.v.), that struck Persia (Iran) and other countries around and near the Persian Gulf in 1821 and 1822.

Cholera was introduced into southeastern Arabia in 1821 by British troops arriving in Muscat, Oman, from Bombay (see INDIAN CHOLERA EPIDEMIC OF 1817–18). When the disease first attacked the unsuspecting population with vomiting and severe diarrhea, they were not even sure what to call it. Among those who were infected, some died within hours, others within two to three days; very few actually survived. The epidemic claimed more than 10,000 lives in Muscat alone.

From Muscat, it spread along the coast to Bahrein and the Persian port of Bandar Abbas (at the mouth of the Persian Gulf). In August 1821, cholera entered Bushire on the northeastern coast of the Persian Gulf. Within a week, the Persian (Iranian) towns of Kazerun and Shiraz reported outbreaks. In Shiraz, the prince's camp was struck with great severity. From Shiraz, the disease traveled north to Jedz and Tehran; in 1822–23 it spread to Resht on the south shore of the Caspian Sea and then across the waters to Astrakhan (see ASTRAKHAN CHOLERA EPIDEMIC OF 1823).

Meanwhile, in 1821 cholera had invaded Basra, the most important port of the Persian Gulf region, with tremendous virulence. About 15,000 to 18,000 people died there within a three-week period. Caravan and water traffic carried the infection up the Tigris River to the city of Baghdad and the surrounding areas. A Persian Army that had besieged the city at this time was engulfed by the epidemic. Its commander, Muhammad Ali Mirza, succumbed to it, as did many of his soldiers. With the onset of winter, cholera subsided in the area.

However, in the spring of 1822, cholera erupted once again along the Tigris and Euphrates rivers. The Persian Army, having defeated the Turks at Erivan (Yerevan), had pursued them westward and was once again attacked, this time viciously, by cholera. Panic-stricken troops retreated to Khoi (in northwestern Iran) and dispersed from there in various directions, thereby spreading the disease across all of Persia. Tabriz was among the towns hard hit by the epidemic, as was Tauris, where nearly 5,000 people died within a few weeks (see PERSIAN CHOLERA EPIDEMIC OF 1829–30). From Tauris, cholera was transported to Tiflis (Tbilisi, Georgia) and then to Astrakhan, which had already been invaded across the Caspian Sea from Resht. In 1822, the disease struck Syria (see SYRIAN CHOLERA EPIDEMIC OF 1822–23). Sometime in 1821, cholera was also reported from Zanzibar on the east coast of Africa.

Further reading: Pollitzer, *Cholera*; Macnamara, *A History of Asiatic Cholera*.

Persian Cholera Epidemic of 1829–30   Part of the Asiatic Cholera Pandemic of 1826–37 (q.v.), invading the city of Tehran (Teheran) in the fall of 1829 en route from its origin in India to Russia and Europe (see INDIAN CHOLERA EPIDEMIC OF 1826–27). The infection is believed to have been imported from the city of Herat in Afghanistan, where two Afghan princes were among its victims.

In 1830, cholera attacked the Persian city of Tabriz and the territories across the Russian frontier. Tehran was again infected during that year and the infection spread to the cities of Kazvin, Kashan, and Isfahan. In the same year, Tabriz was also invaded by a severe plague epidemic (see PERSIAN PLAGUE OF 1830).

Efforts to contain the spread of this cholera epidemic by introducing sanitary and quarantine measures did not yield results since most of the water supply sources were already contaminated. Persia (Iran) suffered other devastating cholera epidemics in 1846 and 1852–53 during the Asiatic Cholera Pandemic of 1846–63 (q.v.).

Further reading: Elgood, *A Medical History of Persia and the Eastern Caliphate*.

Persian Cholera Epidemics of 1846–63   Outbreaks connected with the Asiatic Cholera Pandemic of 1846–63 (q.v.).

According to C. Macnamara in *A History of Asiatic Cholera* and R. Pollitzer in *Cholera*, the epidemic invaded Meshed (Mashhad) via Afghanistan (see PERSIAN CHOLERA EPIDEMIC OF 1829–30) at the end of 1845. However, the Persian epidemic is generally considered to have begun in Tehran in the summer of 1846. The infection was carried from Bombay to the countries of the Arabian Peninsula, from where it spread to Iran, Iraq, and southern Russia.

Tehran's first case was reported on July 23, 1846. The Persian shah, who was at his summer retreat a few miles from Tehran, panicked at the mere mention of the disease and fled with his entourage to a village 20 miles away in the hills. The shah's hasty flight scared his subjects in the city, even though the mortality was still no more than 15 people a day. Following his lead, they too fled Tehran in panic.

By then, the epidemic had intensified and even the shah's camp was not spared. He lost four of his immediate family members—a seven-year-old son, a daughter, and two wives—to cholera. His minister for foreign affairs met with the same fate. Cholera also made inroads into the British mission, killing one person there. In fact, almost every infected person died. The European doctors were unable to treat cholera patients, and the estimated death toll in Tehran rose sharply to 12,000, nearly one quarter of its population. Meshed, Tabriz, and all of Ghilan province were affected too. By the end of 1846, cholera had penetrated as far north as Derbent on the Caspian Sea. The epidemic did not spread beyond Qazvin (Kazvin) in the west and subsided as rapidly as it had started.

However, in 1852, cholera reappeared in Tehran, spreading from its focus in India. Once again, the shah and his entourage left the city for the hills; some four fifths of the city's residents left their homes as well. Those left behind were already severely afflicted by the disease. Apparently, more than 100 people died every day. The shah's camp was affected too but no one died. This time, the epidemic spread west up to Zenjan, south to Shiraz and Hamadan, and east up to Shahrud and Mazanderan. Thus, by 1853, it had devastated the entire central part of the country. In Mazanderan, for instance, the mortality rate was so high in some villages that no one escaped.

In 1861, severe cholera broke out again in Tehran, just as the famine situation there was improving. Again, the source of the original epidemic was in India. Cholera struck Meshed in 1862, killing 100 to 120 people daily. One of the shah's sons died in the epidemic, and the shah once again fled to the country with his camp. Tehran's public health authorities did nothing to curb the epidemic. Rather, they were careless in allowing entry to a large contingent of 5,000 pilgrims from Meshed (where cholera raged in full fury) without taking any precautions either before or immediately following their arrival. Two days later, on August 7, 1862, cholera began spreading rapidly through Tehran's poorer sections. Mortality was not high. The epidemic then traveled to Iraq, the Saudi Arabian region, and then into southern Russia.

Further reading: Elgood, *A Medical History of Persia and the Eastern Caliphate*; Pollitzer, *Cholera*; Macnamara, *A History of Asiatic Cholera.*

Persian Cholera Epidemics of 1866–70

Annual outbreaks of cholera, recrudescences of the Asiatic Cholera Pandemic of 1865–75 (q.v.).

In 1866, cholera traveled from Mecca into Mesopotamia (Iraq) and then north along the Tigris and Euphrates rivers, attacking Tabriz, the Caspian Sea coast, and the Caucasus region with tremendous virulence. The British consul based in the city of Tehran promptly alerted the government of India about cholera's arrival in Persia via Kurdistan. The disease was rampant in western India then and may have been spread by Indian merchants from Afghanistan to Kurdistan.

Tehran was severely infected early in the summer of 1867, presumably a continuation of the 1866 outbreak. Later in the summer, cholera spread along the route from Tehran to Meshed (Mashhad) and as far

south as Kashan, and then through the provinces of Amul, Balfurush, and Sari into the Astrabad (Asterabad) district, from where it posed a direct threat to Europe. Most of Persia was overrun by cholera during 1868. In February, for instance, 1,868 cases were reported from Mazanderan province. Cholera was particularly severe along the Meshed-Astrabad route and also along the routes from Herat to the extreme northwest of the country. The outbreak in Meshed occurred in July at the height of the pilgrimage season; every day 100 to 120 pilgrims died of the disease. Among the dead was Jalal-ul-Dowla, son of the shah and prince governor of Khorasan (Khurasan) province. The panic-stricken shah fled the country with his entourage. A large band of 5,000 Muslim pilgrims returned to Tehran from Meshed on August 5. Despite being forewarned about the arrival of this group, the Tehran officials did not introduce any preventive measures. Two days later, cholera spread among Tehran's poorer sections but did not cause heavy mortality. Other bands of homeward-bound pilgrims transported the disease to the towns of Khat, Birjand, Yezd, Kirman (Kerman), and west to the cities of Hamadan and Isfahan and north to the Atrak River.

In 1869, cholera revisited most of the same areas, even extending farther south from Isfahan to Shiraz (2,000 deaths) and the Persian Gulf and farther west through Kirmanshah (Kermanshah) into the Turkish district of Khalis. The cities of Kashan and Tabriz in the northwest were also affected; from there, cholera spread to Kiev in Russia during July and August 1869 (the start of a long and devastating invasion of much of European Russia). Simultaneously, cholera also spread into the Central Asia region and into the Arabian Peninsula. The disease subsided in Persia during the winter of 1869–70. See also PERSIAN CHOLERA EPIDEMICS OF 1846–63.

Further reading: Elgood, *A Medical History of Persia and the Eastern Caliphate*; Macnamara, *A History of Asiatic Cholera.*

Persian Influenza Epidemic of 1833

Probably part of the influenza epidemic occurring then at several places throughout the world and attacking thousands of people.

The epidemic is believed to have arrived in Persia (Iran) via Syria and Constantinople (Istanbul). It erupted with great virulence in Tehran (the capital) in the summer of 1833 and left scarcely anyone untouched. In fact, numerous employees at the government of India's mission at the summer resort of Shemiran (10 miles to the north) were attacked and their chief, Sir Robert Campbell, was forced to vacate and take refuge in Tehran! The shah of Iran did not escape either. Tehran was badly hit; the epidemic claimed dozens of human lives every day and caused widespread morbidity. Quantitative morbidity and mortality data are not available.

A serious shortage of bread and other food supplies left people even more helpless. Meanwhile, the shah's condition was rumored to have worsened—apparently because of improper medical treatment. He subsequently recovered, but a general state of confusion prevailed in the country. It was exacerbated by the announcement of the death of the ailing prince royal (eldest son of the shah) late in 1833.

Further reading: Elgood, *A Medical History of Persia and the Eastern Caliphate*; Patterson, *Pandemic Influenza, 1700–1900.*

Persian Influenza Epidemic of 1918
Severe epidemic of influenza—part of the worldwide Spanish Influenza Epidemic of 1917–19 (q.v.)—that simultaneously invaded Persia (Iran) from several directions during the latter half of 1918.

The epidemic was first reported in early August with invasions from the north and west. From southern Russia, influenza traveled to the cities of Ashkhabad (on the Persian border) and Meshed (arriving August 3), west along the Teheran (Tehran) highway, and south to Birjand (August 4). On the same day, a flu offshoot from Baku entered Enzeli. Meanwhile, influenza was also creeping in from neighboring Mesopotamia (Iraq) in the west, which suffered two rounds of infection (June–August and September–November). From Baghdad, the infection traveled eastward along the motorways to arrive in the city of Kermanshah in August, and Hamadan, Qazvin (Kazvin), and Teheran in September.

On September 2, the city of Tabriz was invaded via the rail route from Tbilisi, and the province of Seistan by road from Birjand. Highway traffic carried the virus from Teheran south to Isfahan (mid-October) and on to Yezd. Following yet another route of infection, influenza crossed the Indian Ocean from India (see INDIAN INFLUENZA EPIDEMIC OF 1918–19) to various Persian Gulf cities. Both Bandar Abbas (which suffered an epidemic lasting three months) and Mohammerah (Khorramshahr, via Basra) were attacked on October 1. From the latter, influenza spread to the towns of Ahwaz, Shushtar, and Dizful, causing two outbreaks. The first, a mild one, occurred among civilians in August. The second, a more severe outbreak, attacked British forces in Ahwaz. From the Persian Gulf port of Bushire (September 4), the epidemic spread inland to Shiraz (October 3) and Kerman (November 2).

The epidemic was very uneven in its impact across the country. Mortality was generally much higher in rural areas and among the native population. Death was most commonly caused by thoracic complications following the influenza.

The epidemic broke out rather suddenly in the capital of Teheran (250,000 population) on September 22, 1918. It is believed to have been introduced by visitors from Qazvin. The attack rate was very high, as were the casualties among the poor. Two thousand deaths reportedly occurred, but this is considered an understatement.

The city of Shiraz (50,000 population) suffered intensely. Normal life was disrupted as the epidemic spread rapidly across Fars province, killing over 2,000 people. Some of the Indian and Persian troops were severely depleted. Young males were more susceptible than any other segment of the population.

Bushire (population 30,000) reported some 15,000 cases and about 1,500 deaths. Thousands fled the city in panic. Seventy thousand of Meshed's 100,000 residents were infected; 3,500 died. Influenza attacked the entire province of Khorassan (Khurasan) before proceeding to Seistan, which suffered three separate outbreaks, the last in January 1919.

In Tabriz (200,000 inhabitants), half the population took ill with a relatively mild flu attack. Isfahan (80,000 residents) also reported a fairly mild outbreak with 300 deaths. The infection was widespread in Hamadan (30,000 population), claiming 1,000 lives.

Clearly, the epidemic had a devastating effect on a Persian populace only recently recovered from the ravages of famine (1916–17) and from outbreaks of typhus and relapsing fever in 1917–18. A British traveler visiting northern Persia in 1919 observed that the epidemic had left many villages almost completely without human inhabitants. See also PERSIAN INFLUENZA EPIDEMIC OF 1833.

Further reading: Jordan, *Epidemic Influenza: A Survey; Reports on Public Health and Medical Subjects, No. 4.*

Persian Plague of 1772–73
Perhaps one of the most severe recorded epidemics of bubonic plague, killing an estimated two million people in Persia (Iran) and Persian-controlled lands to the west.

It began in Baghdad in the winter of 1772 and by April 1773 had reached the city of Basra. Here, the agent and senior staff of the British East India Company promptly quarantined themselves in a house far from the city, while the rest of the company staff remained locked up in the factory in order to avoid being infected. All contact with the locals (natives) was strictly forbidden. These preventive measures plus the expected summer heat, it was hoped, would allow the epidemic to subside. However, the heat only exacerbated the disease. More than a thousand deaths were recorded daily. Frustrated, the agent fled to Bombay, India.

Meanwhile, the epidemic traveled southward along the Persian coast of the Gulf to Bushire and, subsequently, extended over most of Persia, except the extreme interior. The epidemic moved south down the Arabian shore of the Gulf coast to Bahrain (Bahrein). Persian officials declared the town of Shiraz out of bounds for all travelers. Despite many precautionary measures, the plague claimed 250,000 victims in Basra alone. Several prominent European residents were among those killed.

Toward the end of 1773, the epidemic began to subside. There was a small outbreak of plague in 1798, followed by another severe epidemic in 1800 (see PERSIAN PLAGUE OF 1800).

Further reading: Elgood, *A Medical History of Persia and the Eastern Caliphate.*

Persian Plague of 1800   As virulent as the Persian Plague of 1772–73 (q.v.), though not as widespread, forcing the introduction of quarantine practices in the Persian Gulf region.

The city of Mosul was the site of the first major outbreak. From there, it spread west and south, invading all the villages between Baghdad and Constantinople (Istanbul). Baghdad was the next to be invaded. Frequent epidemics had already interrupted trade and caused the road between Baghdad and Constantinople to be sealed off. Fearing that this bubonic plague epidemic would soon reach India, in the opposite direction, if unchecked, the authorities introduced emergency quarantine measures.

Workers of the British East India Company were moved to Maghil, a village outside the port of Basra, and denied any contact with the local population. The company's factory quarters at Maghil and all ships bearing the British flag in the Shatt-al-Arab were cordoned off. Crews were not allowed offshore and ship-to-shore contact was severely curtailed. To ensure enforcement of these orders and to evacuate the staff in an emergency, a cruiser lay anchored off the Maghil facility. Finally, the Indian government sent a physician to Basra. His job was to prevent any non-British subject from traveling through the affected areas and the Persian Gulf to India.

In Baghdad, Britishers and their belongings underwent fumigation. They could not travel anywhere unless they produced a certificate of immunity countersigned by the chief surgeon and the resident (diplomatic envoy). In Mosul, Catholic missionaries were asked to ensure and supervise the fumigation of houses and furniture. These quarantine measures were effective in that the plague did not claim any European victims this time.

Further reading: Elgood, *A Medical History of Persia and the Eastern Caliphate.*

Persian Plague of 1830   Virulent epidemic of plague, reminiscent of the severe Persian Plagues of 1772–73 and 1800 (qq.v.). It quickly infected the entire Persian Gulf region in 1830.

The epidemic began in the fall of 1830 with an outbreak in the city of Tabriz, where nearly 30,000 people reportedly died from it. Fearing infection, Prince Abbas Mirza of Persia shifted his entire court to Ardebil in the northwest during the winter. The panic-stricken lower classes fled their homes in search of refuge from the dreaded scourge but, in doing so, spread the infection to outlying villages. By 1831, all of Gilan (province) on the Caspian Sea was reeling under the viciousness of the disease.

The Turkish-held cities of Baghdad and Basra were already engulfed by severe outbreaks of plague. From Baghdad it reached Kermanshah in western Persia. Baghdad's pasha (Turkish governor) isolated himself in his house; he caught the disease anyway and was lucky to recover from it. Two of his seven wives died of plague, as did the area's Roman Catholic bishop (of Babylon). The death toll in Baghdad climbed to 30,000 people. Baghdad and Basra were contested by the Persians and Turks.

Basra (a port near the Persian Gulf) was hit hard, losing almost 100 residents to the disease every day. The local Turkish government did little to arrest the spread of the plague epidemic. In fact, the governor quarantined himself in his house, and when some of its inhabitants succumbed to the disease, he merely threw the corpses out on the street across his garden wall. So many people were dying of the disease that many traders were forced to supply free cloth to cover the corpses. Once again, the poorer people tried to escape the epidemic by fleeing into the countryside but succeeded only in spreading it farther so that most of the Persian Gulf region was affected. The epidemic left Basra desolate and empty and seriously disrupted trade in the region.

Further reading: Elgood, *A Medical History of Persia and the Eastern Caliphate.*

Persian Typhus Epidemic of 1942–44   See IRANIAN (PERSIAN) TYPHUS EPIDEMIC OF 1942–44.

Peruvian Cholera Epidemic of 1991–92   Severe outbreak of cholera, infecting an estimated 426,000 persons and killing about 3,300 of them during 15 months in 1991–92. The acute, bacterial intestinal disease also spread north into Ecuador and Colombia (February–March 1991), south into Chile, and east into Brazil (April 1991). It continued to diffuse through these countries and was transmitted to 16 other Latin American countries, bringing the total number of cholera cases to about 533,000 and human fatalities to about 4,700 in the Western Hemisphere by April 1992. At the time, more than 100 associated cases of the *el tor* biotype of cholera that infected Peru were reported in the United States; the cholera bacterium *(Vibrio comma)* was found in oyster beds in Alabama's Mobile Bay in the summer of 1991.

The epidemic's first cases were reported in the Peruvian seaport of Chimbote (January 23, 1991), whose harbor waters were supposedly infected by contaminated ballast dumped from a ship from Southeast Asia. Fish and shellfish were contaminated by cholera bacteria, which soon spread to Chimbote's inhabitants via their eating of seviche (ceviche), an uncooked seafood dish. The disease spread quickly from Chimbote to several other coastal cities, and by mid-February there were at least 14,000 infections and 90 deaths in Peru. The country's capital, Lima (about 5,257,000 people), was infected through streams that serve both as drinking water supplies and open sewers, mainly for the poor in the slums. They ingested water and food contaminated with fecal matter containing the *Vibrio comma;* the poor, who had inadequate water systems, were the most susceptible to cholera.

By early February 1991 Peru's Ministry of Health was advising the population to boil all drinking water, to wash all fruits and vegetables with boiled water, and to avoid eating raw fish. But the epidemic continued to spread in Lima, peaking in the spring of 1991 when the city's hospitals were crowded with thousands of people suffering from diarrhea, colicky abdominal pains, dehydration, and vomiting. In untreated cases, death occurred within a day or two; infections and fatalities were particularly high among Lima's elderly.

The coastal city of Trujillo (about 323,000 people) was struck by the epidemic in early February 1991, when health facilities mainly in the poorer sections reported treating several hundred cholera cases daily. By mid-March the disease was especially severe in Victor Lacco, a new section of Trujillo containing about 32,000 inhabitants; Trujillo's largest hospital (Belen Hospital) was then admitting 20 to 30 cholera patients a day. The infection spread in the city with contaminated, unchlorinated municipal water; in many neighborhoods, running water was available for only one to two hours a day, thus forcing families to store water in containers. Drinking unboiled, polluted water accounted for most cases in Trujillo. Attending fiestas, where food and beverages were more likely to be contaminated, and eating uncooked cabbage even at home, were also associated with the spread of cholera in the city.

The epidemic diffused into the province of Trujillo, which recorded some 16,400 cases by March 31, 1991 (a disease attack rate of 2.6 percent in the provincial population of about 626,500 people). There were 6,623 hospital admissions for cholera (with 71 deaths) in the province in two months; the 0.4 percent fatality rate was low due to the availability of health care and the people's health education and effective employment of oral rehydration and antibiotics.

Controlling the diffusion of cholera in Latin America is almost impossible, according to epidemiologists, who cite poverty, isolation of many towns and jungle villages, easy movement of infected persons across largely unpatrolled borders, and lack of education about how to guard against illness. Furthermore, combating the disease might further impoverish some Latin American countries because of extra medical costs, canceled tourist trips, and lost exports.

Further reading: Suro, "The Cholera Watch"; Swerdlow et al., "Waterborne Transmission of Epidemic Cholera in Trujillo, Peru: Lessons for a Continent at Risk."

Peruvian Smallpox Epidemic of 1525–27

Widespread epidemic that killed Huayna Capac, the Inca ruler of Peru, and approximately 200,000 of his subjects. Smallpox, once one of the world's most deadly diseases, was not known in South America before 1492; yet in the ensuing years it would take its toll and become a major contributor to the Spanish Conquest there.

Smallpox is thought to have been brought to the New World via slave ships from Africa. These ships with their cramped quarters and unsanitary conditions made an ideal breeding ground for smallpox. By 1510, slave ships were making regular runs from Africa to the New World.

In 1520, when Hernando Cortes was in the midst of his conquest of the Aztecs in Mexico, he inadvertently embarked on biological warfare: His Spanish soldiers infected the Aztecs with smallpox. An epidemic that began with the Aztecs ran rampant, spreading into Central America. Tribe after tribe was stricken, and in just two years, several million Indians perished from smallpox (see MEXICAN SMALLPOX EPIDEMIC OF 1520–21). It spread southward into Peru, where the Inca Empire was at the zenith of its Golden Age.

Huayna Capac, the most revered of Inca rulers, had built a mighty empire. He ruled most of the Andean mountain chain, from southern Colombia all the way to central Chile. Huayna Capac first heard of the arrival of the Spaniards in 1524, but soon his most immediate danger was smallpox. The virus had crossed the foothills to devastate and lay waste his empire. The epidemic raged from 1524 to 1527, killing Huayna Capac and his wife, and precipitated the downfall of the Inca Empire. With Huayna Capac's death, civil war erupted between his two living sons and thus paved the way for conquest by the Spaniard Francisco Pizarro, who landed in the heart of the empire in 1532.

Smallpox moved swiftly and struck with deadly force at the Indian population. The Indians had a greater susceptibility to the disease; even into the nineteenth century, their mortality rate was 50 percent to 90 percent. The Indian population lacked the natural defenses needed to ward off the disease, and their living conditions contributed to the high death rate. Since they were quartered many to a hut and in close proximity, the disease could easily spread. The Indians were also nomadic, which helped spread the disease from tribe to tribe.

Smallpox is associated with three main viruses called variola viruses. The most deadly is the classic smallpox or *variola major*; another name associated with smallpox is *viruelas*. The disease has an incubation period of 12 days and its assault is quick; its first symptoms are a splitting headache, a knifing sensation in the back, and a high fever. These symptoms abate and a rash appears, pustulating sores quickly cover the body, and the temperature rises again. The course of the disease runs approximately two weeks. Also, smallpox is a highly contagious disease that is spread by direct or indirect contact; it has no natural animal carriers and does not live long outside the human body. It is contracted by inhalation of particles bearing the virus. Today, vaccination has virtually eliminated the disease, but there is no specific treatment. Isolation and vaccination are the means of prevention.

For Peru's Indian population in the sixteenth century, smallpox was an enemy for which they had no defense. The Incas' most common way to deal with an epidemic was an offering or sacrifice that usually consisted of textiles, guinea pigs, llamas, and, more rarely, human sacrifice. One treatment used by Indians was to put the infected person in a sweatbox and then into cold water; this served only to hasten death.

Quarantine proved the most effective weapon; yet it was not attempted until 1730. Although smallpox was among the most deadly of diseases to be imported into the New World, it was not alone. In 1585, Sir Francis Drake and the English arrived with typhus and soon to follow was influenza. Each new disease brought large death tolls and provided no immunity to its successor.

Translated by Christopher Dilke, "Letter to a King," published in 1978, is a firsthand account by an Inca, Huaman Poma, of the conquest of Peru by the Spaniards and was written sometime between 1567 and 1615.

Further reading: Hadingham, *Lines to the Mountain Gods;* Shurkin, *The Invisible Fire.*

Peruvian Smallpox Epidemic of 1585 *Variola major* smallpox epidemic that struck northern Peru. Epidemics had periodically been introduced to northern Peru in 1533, 1535, and 1558, and South America had experienced several smallpox epidemics since Christopher Columbus first made contact with the New World in 1492. These epidemics spread from Indian village to village through trade routes, migrating tribes, or sailing vessels coming into harbors and ports.

Smallpox is an acute infectious disease characterized by a high fever and back pain. A rash soon develops that goes through the stages of papule to vesicle to pustule. It is only at the pustule stage that the disease is contagious. It requires large pools of people to survive. The disease in Peru thrived when it encountered the native Indians, who lacked immunity to the virus, while their life-style of living in crowded huts was ideal for the disease to spread.

When smallpox struck northern Peru in 1585, the Indians died by the hundreds every week. Villages were extinguished, and the dead were left scattered over the fields or piled in houses. All trading activity came to a halt. The fields were left unharvested and there were no laborers to work the mines. Food prices rose so high that if a person did survive, he or she would usually die of starvation. Smallpox would continue to strike Peru and all of South America in the following centuries until it was eradicated in the 1970s.

Further reading: Hopkins, *Princes and Peasants: Smallpox in History;* Cartwright, *Disease and History;* World Health Organization, *The Global Eradication of Smallpox.*

Philadelphia "Legionnaires' Disease" Epidemic Alarming outbreak of a mysterious flu-like illness that killed 26 out of 260 persons who attended an American Legion state convention at the Bellevue Stratford Hotel in Philadelphia in July 1976. Called "the greatest medical mystery of the century," the disease's causative agent was later identified as a previously unknown bacterium, which was named *Legionella pneumophila.*

On July 20, 1976, the eve of the American Legion convention, the air conditioner repairman at the Bellevue Stratford Hotel became ill with flu-like symptoms; he was never hospitalized and recovered. On July 24, the last day of the convention, a number of legionnaires suffered the same symptoms, and three of them were hospitalized as supposed typhoid cases by July 30. Meanwhile 14 other legionnaires, who had returned to their hometowns in Pennsylvania, became ill with the same symptoms; swine flu was first suspected. During the first week of August, epidemiologists at the U.S. Centers for Disease Control (CDC), U.S. Public Health Service, and the Pennsylvania State Health Department began studying the baffling ailment, which had alarmed inhabitants of the Philadelphia area, fearful of contagion. At first the CDC suspected the disease to be lassa fever (an acute viral illness first described in Nigeria in 1969) or pneumonic plague. In addition, the disease was even linked to theories of conspiracy by various militant groups and germ warfare, further alarming the public.

One hundred and seventy-nine cases of so-called "legionnaires' disease" or "legion fever" were reported by August 31, 1976, and 28 of them had been fatal (two of the deaths were a nun and a priest, members of a Eucharistic Congress at the Bellevue Stratford Hotel on August 1–8). None of the hotel staff (with the exception of the air conditioner repairman), who dealt directly with the legionnaires, had become infected. A prostitute at the hotel during the convention became infected but recovered; later a researcher non-fatally contracted the disease in October while examining tissue specimens from victims.

Health officials first thought pigeon droppings might have spread the infection through the hotel's air-conditioning system and might have fouled the water supply; this was never proven. The CDC finally concluded that the disease was airborne transmitted, and the causative agent's most likely habitat was the hotel's rooftop water tower, which fed the air-conditioning system. The agent was thought to have emerged into the Bellevue through the vent above the registration desk; lobby employees may have become immune to its effect over a period of time.

Due to bad publicity, many bookings for the Bellevue were cancelled, and on November 18, 1976, the hotel closed. Scientists finally announced (January 19, 1977) the cause of the mysterious disease and later said that erythromycin, an antibiotic, was effective in treating it. Twenty-nine persons (26 American Legion members and three others) perished from legionnaires' disease before the discovery of *Legionella pneumophilia*, which proved to be the same bacterium responsible for an earlier strange outbreak of fatal pneumonia at St. Elizabeth's Hospital, a federal mental institution in Washington, D.C. The new bacterium was also found in water from a cooling tower at a hospital in Vermont in May 1977 and was the

cause of an outbreak there. Since then, cases of legionnaires' disease have occurred in the United States, Canada, and Europe.

Further reading: Thomas and Morgan-Witts, *Anatomy of an Epidemic*; Fraser et al., "Legionnaires' Disease: Description of an Epidemic of Pneumonia."

Philadelphia Yellow Fever Epidemic of 1793   Legendary epidemic that spread infection to 17,000 people, leaving 5,000 dead (10 percent of the population) and paralyzing local, state, and national government. While the city of Washington was under construction, Philadelphia took over as the country's capital. Philadelphia's renewed role as a trade center in the 1790s brought with it this virulent outbreak of yellow fever (also called black vomit, and over 150 other names throughout history). In the summer of 1793, thousands of French refugees from Santo Domingo poured into Philadelphia with talk of the French Revolution and a pestilence that raged in the Caribbean islands. Other circumstances perpetuated the spread of the infection: a hot, damp atmosphere, low ground level, and, because of a protracted drought, much standing water in waterways and marshes. The water ebbed so low that rotting animals and fish washed up, causing further stagnation. The shallow sewer canal collected rotting debris. All this resulted in a ubiquity of mosquitoes and stench.

The disease was carried by the female of the *Aëdes aegypti* mosquito, which bred in still water, including water supplies aboard ships. By sucking and incubating (for 12 days) infected human blood, a mosquito carried the infection for life (terminated by cold weather). A human infected with the virus showed symptoms within five days. At the onset, the disease caused a high temperature, chills, pains, and near cessation of abdominal purging. Afterward, the victim might appear to recover, but high fever returned, skin yellowed, and partially digested blood in the stomach caused black vomit. Of course, eighteenth-century physicians knew the cause neither of the disease nor its symptoms.

Noting the virulent symptoms and increasing frequency of deaths, doctors and government officials of Philadelphia began conferring in August 1793. Rotting coffee beans long since dumped on a wharf by the ship *Amelia* from Santo Domingo were postulated to be the cause of yellow fever. On August 25, Mayor Clarkson of Philadelphia convened the College of Physicians. Unaware of already existing West Indian cases, the college at first deduced that hygiene and climate, not contagion, caused the disease. By September, doctors realized that all attempts to stop the disease had failed. A controversy about the cause of the disease split the medical community, adding to the city's general panic and anarchy. Two groups emerged: the contagionists, who believed the pestilence passed from person to person, and the climatists, who insisted cleaning up the city would help clear the air of impurities.

On the day the College of Physicians met, fear gripped the city. Many interpreted the plague as a judgment of providence. A general exodus began. In September, everyone left who could, including George Washington, cabinet members and other officials, business and tradespeople, families and individuals. In all, some 12,000 people decamped to escape the dreaded pestilence. However, news of the Philadelphia plague preceded the refugees. Some were robbed, brutalized, and ostracized. Others were quarantined at isolated locations. In Philadelphia, the plague asserted itself. Victims were often turned out by their own families. People, especially the poor, were dying in the streets. Yellow fever deaths in the second half of September averaged 70 per day. Not knowing the cause of the disease, people tried all manner of preventive devices. Many antidotes appeared in newspapers, like setting bonfires, floating oil on water supplies, sprinkling vinegar on clothing and throughout the house, and firing guns so that the smell of gunpowder permeated the air. The epidemic peaked when 111 people died on October 12.

Despite awareness of the disease, many businesses kept up their normal pace until routines broke down because of illness. Many ships docked daily. Those remaining in business prospered: doctors, coffin makers, apothecaries, and a few storekeepers. Once the pestilence took hold, the delivery of mail ceased, most newspapers suspended operations, and meetings were postponed. Once a quarantine went into effect, all trade, cash flow, and news stopped. Mayor Clarkson's government collapsed for lack of personnel: Those not ill had fled. People normally independent were starving.

As chaos began to envelope Philadelphia in September, Mayor Clarkson laid the groundwork that eventually led to the city's recovery. He asked for and got volunteers to help him run the government and control the disease. Most were common people who simply stepped into the breach. Because of previous exposure to yellow fever, French refugees were able to work with the stricken. Some of the committee's most important tasks were to help improve the hospital so that people actually recovered, establish an orphanage, dispose of the dead, and provide relief for the poor. Their work went so well that by September 16, donations of money, food, supplies, and livestock started flowing in from Pennsylvania and other states.

An old mansion called Bush Hill served as the hospital for yellow fever victims. The hospital's doctor, Jean Duvèze, had survived yellow fever twice, and had previously run a hospital. Dr. Duvèze and others successfully refuted the disease treatment developed by the established Dr. Benjamin Rush who, despite the best intentions and his effectiveness in a fearful time, had probably killed many people who might otherwise have recovered. Most of the hospital staff were also French refugees. Records showing admissions, departures, results, and dates most clearly exemplified the new hospital organization.

By October 26, the disease began to abate. Only 20 people died daily. The committee attributed the easing of the disease to divine providence. By November, trade, the Philadelphian refugees, the president's cabinet, and the traditional norms had returned. Charles Brockden Brown dramatized the 1793 yellow fever epidemic in *Arthur Mervyn* and two other novels.

Further reading: Ackerknecht, *A Short History of Medicine* and *History and Geography of the Most Important Diseases;* McGrew, *Encyclopedia of Medical History;* Powell, *Bring Out Your Dead.*

Philippine Beriberi Epidemics of 1901–02 and 1909

Three epidemics of beriberi, the first two occurring in prisons in 1901 and 1902, the third in a leper colony in 1909.

The first epidemic broke out in Bilibid Prison in Manila in December 1901, immediately following a change in food rations. In that month, 52 cases of beriberi and two human deaths were reported. Over the next few months, the epidemic quickly worsened. For instance, in February 1902, 1,087 beriberi cases and 16 deaths were recorded. Until October 1, 1902, a staggering 4,300 cases occurred in this prison. Then, on October 20, another major change in rations was effected; the quantity of bread and potatoes was increased while the rice portion was reduced almost in half. In December 1902, the incidence of beriberi among the prisoners declined noticeably: Only 89 cases and three deaths were reported. Overall, 5,448 beriberi cases with 229 deaths were reported during this epidemic, which subsided by early January 1903.

The second epidemic, relatively minor, broke out in the Lingayen Prison in 1902. In this case, the Chinese white rice being supplied to the prisoners was found to be the culprit. Every month, 20 new beriberi cases and an average of five deaths were reported from the prison. The patients were transported to a nearby hospital, where their diet remained unchanged. Many died while others continued to suffer endlessly. At another prison in the vicinity there was no beriberi, since the rice was purchased from the local market. In February 1902, the prison surgeon ordered that locally purchased rice be used instead of the Chinese white rice. Once again, there was a dramatic improvement, and no new cases of beriberi were reported in subsequent months.

In 1909, an outbreak of beriberi occurred in the Culion leper colony, causing 329 deaths among an inmate population estimated at between 1,500 and 1,900 persons. Following the introduction, in February 1910, of unpolished rice in the rations at the leper colony (also introduced at other Philippine charitable institutions, jails, and lighthouse stations), there were no deaths from beriberi that year. The incidence of beriberi in the country's institutions declined sharply after this change, and the disease subsequently disappeared from these places. Around this time, infantile beriberi became recognized as a form of beriberi, and infant deaths from the disease, recorded for the first time, were consistently high (see JAPANESE ARMY BERIBERI EPIDEMIC OF 1904–05).

During 1902–10, the Philippine Scouts (a unit of local soldiers led by American officers) recorded a total of 3,233 cases of beriberi among its soldiers. Also during this period, 313 to 1,478 beriberi deaths were recorded annually in Manila. See also THAI BERIBERI EPIDEMICS OF 1890–1910; SINGAPORE BERIBERI EPIDEMICS OF 1942–45.

Further reading: Williams, *Toward the Conquest of Beriberi*.

Philippine Cholera Epidemic of 1820–21

Devastating epidemic that killed thousands of people. The cholera infection was apparently introduced into the country via the port of Manila in 1820, no doubt an offshoot of the Asiatic Cholera Pandemic of 1817–23 (q.v.), which began in India (see INDIAN CHOLERA EPIDEMIC OF 1817–18) and left a trail of destruction in many Asian countries (see THAI CHOLERA EPIDEMIC OF 1820; INDONESIAN CHOLERA EPIDEMIC OF 1821; CHINESE CHOLERA EPIDEMIC OF 1820–22; JAPANESE CHOLERA EPIDEMIC OF 1822).

Dr. Carlos Luis Benoit of the Philippine Medical Corps, who was himself struck during the epidemic, said that it first erupted in September 1820 and subsided by April 1821. According to Dr. Benito Francia, the Philippines' last Spanish Inspector-General of Health and Charity, the first case of cholera was observed along the Pasig River on October 4, 1820. By all accounts it was an extremely severe epidemic, though approximate mortality figures are not available. Another physician who witnessed the epidemic's destruction said that people with carts carrying the dead hurried through Manila's streets day and night. A month later, there were not enough people left to tend the sick or to bury the dead.

Rumors spread in the terrified communities that foreigners were contaminating the drinking water supplies with the intention of killing the natives and assuming control of the Philippines. Frenzied mobs attacked foreigners in Manila, Cavite, Tondo, and Binondo. Twenty-eight Europeans and several Chinese were killed over two days. A frantic appeal from the governor finally calmed the mob.

Major cholera epidemics were recorded in 1842–43, 1862, 1882–83, and 1902–04.

Further reading: Bantug, *A Short History of Medicine in the Philippines during the Spanish Regime*.

Philippine Cholera Epidemics of 1882–83 and 1888–89

Major outbreaks of cholera (offshoots of another widespread Asiatic cholera epidemic) that swept through the Philippines in 1882–83 and 1888–89.

By all accounts, the epidemic of 1882–83 was devastating. An imported epidemic, it began in the Philippine capital of Manila on August 20, 1882, and caused widespread havoc in the city during the next few months. Eyewitnesses have left behind varying estimates of mortality during the great epidemic. According to one, at its peak, 1,300 people died of cholera every day in Manila; the German consul stationed there estimated total casualties between 15,000 and 20,000. Another chronicler wrote that cholera had carried away 30,000 people in Manila and the surrounding area in less than three months. For days, dead bodies littered the streets around the San Lazaro hospital and corpse-laden vehicles blocked access to cemeteries, further compounding the health hazards. The government was finally forced to organize mass burials. Most of the victims were natives, but some foreigners living in Manila were also infected

Available records indicate that when the epidemic ended in Manila (December 5, 1882), the city-wide death toll was 5,413 persons. However, cholera also spread to some of the surrounding provinces during 1883, although figures are not available to bolster that. It is known that the epidemic ended in Bulacan province on January 29, 1883, and in Pampanga province on February 2, 1883.

The cholera epidemic of 1888–89 would have been just as lethal as its predecessor, but for the construction of the Mariquina River project (Manila's main water source) during the intervening period. Some believe that this epidemic began in Taytay, Rizal province. Others have argued that cholera was present in the Philippines consistently since 1882 and that the epidemic represented merely a change in its status. Many of the early cases, it is now believed, were deliberately not diagnosed as cholera in order to avoid creating panic among the public and to allow the government to introduce emergency measures to deal with the outbreak. In some districts, people reportedly did not want to believe that cholera was in their midst. In some instances, cholera patients were apparently transported in a comatose state and buried alive. The government consequently ordered that dead bodies be kept in a shelter for a few hours before internment. Mortality statistics for this epidemic are not available. See also PHILIPPINE CHOLERA EPIDEMIC OF 1902–04.

Further reading: MacLeod and Lewis, eds., *Disease, Medicine, and Empire*; Bantug, *A Short History of Medicine in the Philippines during the Spanish Regime*.

Philippine Cholera Epidemic of 1902–04

Severe cholera epidemic, killing about 109,461 persons, over 4,000 of them in Manila, the capital, alone. However, eyewitnesses to the disaster, particularly in the provinces, reported that more than 200,000 people died during the epidemic.

First noticed in Manila in March 1902, cholera may have been imported from Canton or Hong Kong, where it had been raging intermittently. Manila's vegetable markets were stocked with produce grown by Chinese farmers who, it was reported, used infected human waste as fertilizer. The cholera epidemic in the Philippines was thus attributed to the consumption of these contaminated vegetables. Imports of all green vegetables from Hong Kong were promptly banned, but by then the disease was well-entrenched.

The third cholera epidemic (see PHILIPPINE CHOLERA EPIDEMICS OF 1882–83 AND 1888–89) to hit the Philippines in two decades, its virulence quickly became apparent. In the early stages of the epidemic, many victims died within hours of suffering the first symptoms—cramping and severe fluid loss. Hospitals reported mortality rates of 80 percent to 90 percent. Even the American community on the islands, which had believed itself to be immune from such tropical ailments, was affected. By July 1902, at least 50 American soldiers were said to have died of the disease. The death rate was 31.51 per 1,000 for Americans, 21.74 per 1,000 for the Chinese inhabitants and 108.29 per 1,000 for the local population. Public health authorities were urged to exert great vigilance, particularly in the face of perceived apathy or resistance on the part of the Filipinos.

In 1901, the American authorities in the Philippines had established an Insular Board of Health to regulate and control health services in the country. When the epidemic struck, the then commissioner of the Philippines launched a radical anti-cholera strategy, similar to the measures launched during the Philippine Plague of 1899–1903 (q.v.). Among these measures were isolation of the sick, safe disposal of the bodies of cholera victims, and strict surveillance of people and their homes. Homes where infection was suspected were disinfected; a few were even burned.

The commissioner then ordered the quarantining of Manila's water supply source—the Mariquina River—to prevent the epidemic from worsening and claiming more lives. This strategy was not effective and, in fact, backfired. He also established—on the grounds of the San Lazaro detention camp—a cholera hospital, a morgue where postmortems could be done on cholera suspects, and a crematorium for victims. The association of these facilities with the frightening images of the detention camp could hardly have been reassuring for patients and their families, many of whom, in any case, believed that disease was a spiritual affliction that could not be cured by Western scientific medicine. This feeling was further exacerbated by the inefficacy of the cholera hospitals. The epidemic began to subside early in 1904, by which time Filipino resistance to the American anti-cholera measures had already peaked.

Further reading: MacLeod and Lewis, eds., *Disease, Medicine, and Empire*.

Philippine Cholera Epidemic of 1961–62

Extensive epidemic of cholera that ripped through the Philippine Islands. It was an early offshoot of the Asiatic Cholera Pandemic of 1961–75 (q.v.) caused by the *Vibrio el tor* bacterium.

The outbreak began late in September 1961 when several cases were noted among adults in a poorer section of the city of Manila. Most of the early patients had close contacts with Manila's northern port district, where the disease may have initially arrived on foreign ships. Its later epidemic diffusion along the coast and inland waterways has been linked to people's consumption of raw and contaminated seafood. The disease spread rapidly in the city and adjacent provinces and then moved south to infect many of the main islands in the country. The Bikol Peninsula and jungle areas inland were spared.

In Manila, during an eight-week period (October 7 to November 30, 1961), 423 cholera patients were admitted to the San Lazaro hospital, then the main facility for the treatment of infectious diseases in the metropolitan area and the only one to admit cholera patients. In the province of Negros Occidental, for instance, the epidemic began explosively in November 1961 with 333 cases reported in the first week alone. Until September 15, 1962, a total of 2,756 confirmed cases and 106 deaths (3.9 percent mortality) were reported from the entire province. The epidemic peaked in December 1961 when 1,452 patients were treated during one week, and by April 1962 the numbers had dwindled to less than 100 per week. Nationally, statistics indicate that of the 15,000 people attacked by cholera between September 22, 1961, and March 1, 1962, 2,005 (approximately 13 percent) died. Most of the deaths were among the very young or the very old.

The infection caused by the *Vibrio el tor* is sometimes called paracholera to distinguish it from classical cholera, but may experts believe that the two infections are identical in their clinical and epidemiological manifestations. The Chinese Red Cross responded promptly to this crisis by presenting the Red Cross in the Philippines with 300,000 doses of the cholera vaccine. The usual quarantine and sanitary measures were implemented in most of the affected areas.

Further reading: Felsenfeld, "Some Observations on the Cholera (El Tor) Epidemic in 1961–62"; Barua and Burrows, eds., *Cholera*.

Philippine Dengue Epidemics of the 1950s and 1960s

Several outbreaks of dengue hemorrhagic fever (DHF). In the Philippines during 1953, DHF was first identified and designated as a clinical entity separate from the classical form of dengue. DHF, marked by fever, hemorrhaging, and sometimes shock, primarily infects young children and can be fatal. Sporadic cases of DHF were reported in the country after 1950. There was a small outbreak in the port city of Manila in 1954 when pediatricians reported several serious cases of DHF among their patients and called it Philippine hemorrhagic fever.

The first large outbreak of the disease occurred during the 1956 rainy season (July–October) in Manila. A total of 1,207 cases were treated, most of them in children below six years of age, and some six percent of these died. All the reported cases occurred in native Filipino children living in areas where the *Aëdes aegypti* mosquito was abundantly present. Although similar in some ways to the epidemic hemorrhagic fevers in Manchuria and Korea, the Philippine hemorrhagic fever could be clinically differentiated. Studies conducted during this epidemic led to an understanding of dengue's relationship with hemorrhagic fever and to a recognition of dengue viruses type 3 and 4. The dengue virus type 2 was also implicated in this outbreak.

Hemorrhagic fever became entrenched in the Philippines after this outbreak, with about 100 to 500 cases treated annually at the country's hospitals. The next outbreak occurred on the Philippine island of Luzon during March–June 1961. The Isabella region was hardest hit, reporting 1,160 clinically confirmed cases during that three-month period. Overall, 1,459 cases and 33 deaths were reported that year.

In the ensuing years, incidence fell off slightly, but in 1966, the Philippines suffered a severe hemorrhagic fever epidemic. Over four months, 7,794 cases and 63 deaths occurred. The total for the year was 9,384 cases and 250 deaths. Throughout the remainder of the 1960s, more than a thousand cases of hemorrhagic fever were reported each year.

Further reading: Halstead, "Mosquito-borne Haemorrhagic Fevers of South and South-East Asia"; World Health Organization, *Dengue Haemorrhagic Fever: Diagnosis, Treatment and Control*.

Philippine Influenza Epidemic of 1918–19

Offshoot of the devastating worldwide Spanish Influenza Epidemic of 1917–19 (q.v.) affecting the Philippine Islands in two separate waves.

The first wave of influenza was mild and lasted through May and June 1918. The disease was initially observed in mid-April 1918 among the city of Manila's waterfront laborers and became more widespread in late May and early June. However, the epidemic could not be traced to the recent arrival of a flu-infected vessel in Manila's harbor. It was a mild outbreak, as reflected in a low case fatality rate, and did not spread very rapidly.

The second visitation, in the autumn of 1918, was more severe. In October 1918, 1,908 deaths from influenza were reported. During the next two months, the epidemic exploded; data from 26 provinces yielded a death rate of 890 per 100,000 people, with 36,884 deaths in November and 26,652 deaths in December. Overall, there probably were nearly 100,000 deaths on Luzon Island alone. Among pregnant women in Manila's Philippine General Hospital, deaths from influenza (48 percent) exceeded deaths from eclampsia (41 percent) or from typhoid (16 percent). (Eclampsia is a convulsive state or coma.) Influenza claimed the lives of 4,675 people in the Philippines in 1925.

Further reading: Jordan, *Epidemic Influenza*.

Philippine Plague of 1899–1903

Epidemic of bubonic plague, offshoot of the Third Plague Pandemic (q.v.), (see HONG KONG PLAGUE OF 1894; INDIAN PLAGUE OF 1904–07; SYDNEY PLAGUE OF 1900).

The disease first erupted in Manila in December 1899, just months after the American occupation of this port city. It then spread to Cavite and other towns in the vicinity and then to Cebu, the Philippines' most important port after Manila. The outbreak continued to spread and presented the first major challenge for the newly created board of health, which soon launched an intensive campaign (that many found repressive) aimed at eradicating the disease. A huge disinfecting plant was built at Mariveles; infected ships could also use the smaller disinfecting facilities at Cebu and Iloilo. The United States public health and marine hospital service devised an effective quarantine system all around the Philippine archipelago to prevent those with a contagious disease from entering the country.

According to the official figures, there were 427 plague deaths in 1901, 10 in 1902, and 174 in 1903. Manila was reportedly declared plague-free in January 1902. *The Manila Times* praised the health authorities for their efforts at civic cleanliness, which helped keep sickness at bay. However, the Philippine Cholera Epidemic of 1902–04 (q.v.) diverted many of the health board's resources to combating that new scourge. Plague prevention thus became a second priority, as proved by the higher incidence of plague deaths in 1903. After that, plague incidence gradually declined (78 deaths in 1904, 43 in 1905, seven in 1906, and none in 1907) until 1912, when it began to increase again.

Further reading: Worcester, *The Philippines: Past and Present*; MacLeod and Lewis, eds., *Disease, Medicine, and Empire.*

Philippine Poliomyelitis Epidemic of 1944–45 Epidemic that invaded the American troops on the island of Leyte during World War II.

The epidemic struck rather suddenly in November 1944. Within 16 days of the landing of troops on Leyte (see PHILIPPINE SCHISTOSOMIASIS EPIDEMIC OF 1944–45), 47 polio cases (37 paralytic and 10 nonparalytic) were reported among the American military. British and American forces serving in the Middle East during World War II had faced a similar invasion from the polio virus, but this news apparently had not reached the American medical staff in the Philippines. The authorities believed that the virus had been imported into the country by the troops, particularly since no recent cases were reported among the native population. Moreover, the first case had occurred a mere five days after the troops landed at Leyte. This theory was later disproved by the renowned Dr. Albert Sabin, who showed that the virus had its source in the local population.

American troops in the China-Burma-India theater of war operations and in Japan and Korea also showed a high incidence of poliomyelitis. See also NICOBAR ISLANDS POLIOMYELITIS EPIDEMIC OF 1947.

Further reading: Paul, *A History of Poliomyelitis*; World Health Organization, *Poliomyelitis.*

Philippine Schistosomiasis Epidemic of 1944–45
Epidemic of schistosomiasis or bilharziasis that struck American troops when they landed at Leyte in the Philippine Islands during World War II.

Schistosomiasis favors warm, humid climates. In the Philippines, it is caused by the parasitic worm *Schistosoma japonicum*, which is transmitted to man through an intermediate host, the snail. It is endemic on the islands of Leyte, Samar, and Mindanao. The American troops landed on Leyte on October 20, 1944. The first cases of schistosomiasis were noticed in December 1944 among the soldiers being treated at the 118th Field Hospital.

Eighty cases were reported in December, 155 cases in January 1945, over 1,000 cases by May 1945, and 1,300 by 1946. Most of the soldiers had caught the infection through the water (diseased larvae emerge from snails and penetrate human skin, usually while a person is working or swimming in water). The manpower situation in the U.S. Army was becoming critical, and the disease was beginning to attract much medical attention within the army. This was the army's first major contact with schistosomiasis, and its medical department rose admirably to meet the challenge. The main foci of the disease were identified and troops moved to a safer location. Infected persons were given prompt medical treatment, thus ensuring complete recovery.

The medical department also launched an extensive educational campaign consisting of mobile demonstration labs, posters, and cartoons. In February, the 5th Malarial Survey Unit and a medical research unit became part of the 118th Field Hospital, in order to facilitate study of the disease in all its aspects. The Washington-based Army Epidemiological Board dispatched a sub-commission on schistosomiasis to Leyte in April. This group was joined in May by a three-member team from the Naval Research Unit. Together they began an exhaustive study of the disease. Their work, published after the end of the war in reputed medical journals, greatly advanced the cause of research in tropical diseases. It brought schistosomiasis to international attention.

Further reading: Howe, ed., *A World Geography of Human Diseases*; Arnold, ed., *Imperial Medicine and Indigenous Societies.*

Philippine Smallpox Epidemic of 1591 First recorded epidemic of smallpox to invade the Philippines. It was one of the early outbreaks and linked to the arrival of a Spanish ship from Mexico. According to an eyewitness account by Father Chirino, a Jesuit priest, the epidemic was vicious, affecting both young and old. Manila and its environs and the Batangas province were apparently hard hit. One third of the population of Batangas was bedridden with hardly anyone, including children, spared the infection. Mortality was high among the adults and the elderly.

Further reading: Bantug, *A Short History of Medicine in the Philippines during the Spanish Regime.*

Philistine Plague (Plague of Ashdod) Epidemic that struck the Philistines when they tried unsuccessfully to conquer the Hebrews in the second half of the eleventh century B.C. The disease has been identified by some as bubonic plague, but another suggested diagnosis is hemorrhoids accompanying dysentery. According to the account in book I Samuel of the Old Testament, the Philistine Army succumbed to the disease after capturing the ark of the covenant from the Hebrews. The pestilence followed the Philistines wherever they carried the ark, first to Ashdod, then to Gath, and finally to Ekron. In each city the people were afflicted with what the Bible calls "emerods"—literally, swellings or tumors—"in their secret parts." After seven months in which many of them died, the Philistines returned the ark to the Hebrews, sending along a gift of five golden emerods and five golden mice.

The association of rodents with the disease, the location of the swellings (which could have been buboes), and the rapid spread and high mortality have led some scholars to identify the epidemic as bubonic plague. Historian J. F. D. Shrewsbury argues, however, that mice do not generally carry bubonic plague; he believes that the biblical account records two distinct epidemics, one of field mice that destroyed the crops of the Philistines, and one of disease that afflicted the people themselves. Noting that bacillary dysentery often strikes mobile armies, he concludes that the emerods affecting the Philistines were actually hemorrhoids, a complication of dysentery.

Further reading: I Samuel 5:6–6:18; Shrewsbury, "The Plague of the Philistines"; Castiglioni, *A History of Medicine;* Zinsser, *Rats, Lice and History.*

Picardy Sweat Sudden outbreak of an inflammatory disease of profuse sweating that first appeared in 1718 in France's northern province of Picardy, whence the French name of *Suette des Picards* for the strange disease and epidemic. Victims of the disease, which resembled the English Sweat of the sixteenth century (see ENGLISH SWEATING SICKNESS EPIDEMICS), complained of chills, severe headache, high fever, violent and frequent nosebleeds, excessive perspiration and itching (beginning within 12 to 24 hours), a reddish rash (beginning within 48 hours), and sometimes delirium. There were many victims who died within two days; however, the mortality rate was lower for the Picardy Sweat than for the English Sweat. The main difference between these two diseases seemed to be the eruption and mental anguish associated with the Picardy Sweat.

The startling onset and rapidity of the 1718 *suette* terrorized the French living in various parts of Picardy, especially in the towns of Abbeville, Amiens, and St. Quentin. The neighboring province of Normandy (particularly the Orne area) was soon struck by a *suette* epidemic (which usually remained limited to one region and lasted only a few months). Next the French provinces of Poitou, Île de France (where Paris lies), Burgundy, and Flanders (notably the Nord area) were struck. At the time (1718), physicians seeking the cause of this unknown illness blamed outside or foreign influences; some ascribed the infection to noxious or toxic air blown over northern France from the Netherlands; others asserted that it came into France from abroad, arriving in the port of St. Valéry, near Abbeville. There were still others who attributed it to dirt and filth.

At times the *suette* was identified by various authorities as perhaps a form of measles or scarlet fever or typhus or influenza or relapsing fever. But the absence and mismatch of important symptoms of these diseases makes such an identification erroneous or highly unlikely. There has been stronger evidence that the *suette* resembles a fulminating meningococcus infection sometimes seen during a meningitis outbreak in a military camp. In addition, physicians have identified and linked it with miliary fever (miliaria), a disease of the sweat glands characterized by the eruption of small, isolated red spots or vesicles resembling millet seeds in form or size. It is also accompanied by excessive sweating and itching. Miliary fever was prevalent in numerous provinces of France, especially in the northeast part of the country, from the time of the Picardy Sweat until about 1880. Notable French outbreaks of miliary fever include those recorded in the districts of Oise in 1832, 1849, and 1854; Calvados in 1737 and 1763; Seine-et-Marne in 1783, 1839, and 1853; Somme in 1849; Haute-Marne in 1854; Bas-Rhin in 1849 and 1853–54; Vosges in 1854; Puy-de-Dôme in 1757–62; Jura in 1842 and 1854–55; Haute-Saône in 1832, 1842, and 1849; and Dordogne in 1832 and 1841. The learned medical historian Dr. August Hirsch (see below) listed 194 epidemics of miliary fever in France from 1718 to 1879.

Further reading: Hirsch, *Handbook on Geographical and Historical Pathology;* Zinsser, *Rats, Lice and History.*

Plague of Antoninius See ANTONINE PLAGUE.

Plague of Ashdod See PHILISTINE PLAGUE.

Plague of Athens, Great (Plague of Thucydides)
Epidemic that struck Athens early in the summer of 430 B.C. and continued through the following year; after subsiding greatly, the disease broke out again in 427 B.C. Described in vivid detail by the Greek historian Thucydides, himself a victim, the initial outbreak was devastating. Crowded within the city walls while their enemies, the Spartans, attacked the countryside, the Athenians were easy targets for a contagious disease; about one third of them died, including many soldiers. The resulting loss of manpower and morale hurt Athens just when its conflict with Sparta was entering a new stage. By preventing an immediate Athenian victory, the plague may have helped to prolong the Great Peloponnesian War (431–404 B.C.).

Thucydides' account provides much of our information for the epidemic. At the time, people believed that the plague had originated in Ethiopia and traveled through Egypt and the eastern Mediterranean before reaching Athens. The first cases appeared in Peiraeus, the Athenian port city and base for many travelers and merchants, who undoubtedly contracted the disease in their journeys abroad.

People were stricken suddenly with severe headaches, inflamed eyes, and bleeding in their mouths and throats. The next symptoms were coughing, sneezing, and chest pains; when the illness descended to the digestive tract, it brought stomach cramps, intense vomiting and diarrhea, and unquenchable thirst. Sufferers broke out in a rash and many became delirious. Death usually came on the seventh or eighth day of the illness, although those who survived the first phase often died from the weakness brought on by constant diarrhea. Many who recovered lost their eyesight, their memory, or the use of their extremities.

The Athenians tried to avoid infection by not caring for the sick and not observing proper burial rites for friends and family. Thucydides tells of whole households perishing with no one to help them, and of dead bodies lying in the streets and temples, untouched even by animals and birds of prey. Such attempts mattered little, however, as people of all ages, incomes, and levels of general health succumbed. Those who were lucky enough to recover had a partial immunity: If by chance they got the disease again, the second attack was never fatal.

Despite the detailed eyewitness observations of Thucydides, modern scholars cannot pinpoint the nature of the epidemic. According to one expert, the sudden onset, the seasonal occurrence, and the raised rash all indicate a variety of smallpox; other less plausible suggestions include typhus fever or bubonic plague. The epidemic was unlike anything the Athenians had seen before, says Thucydides, and its true nature will likely remain unknown to us as well.

The conditions leading to the plague's spread are easier to determine. Fearful of the Spartan attack, the Athenian leader Pericles had ordered the inhabitants of the surrounding countryside to move inside the city, where they could be protected by the army and the fortified walls. Many country dwellers, coming to an already overpopulated city, had no place to live except in poorly ventilated shacks and tents. This mass of people, crowded together in the hot summer, created a situation ideal for rapid transmission of the disease.

Approximately one third of them died, including 300 out of 1,000 cavalry and about a quarter of the land army. Even an expedition sent in late June of 430 B.C., before the plague reached its height, was not immune. On their way to Epidaurus in the Peloponnese (the Spartan sphere of influence), many of the soldiers fell ill and could not take the city by siege. The weakened Athenian force then traveled north, near Macedonia, to help fellow soldiers already stationed there, but succeeded only in infecting them. Otherwise the plague remained confined almost entirely to Athens.

Seeing the other Greek cities untouched by the plague, the demoralized Athenians became convinced they had been singled out by the gods, Thucydides claims. Spending money extravagantly, ignoring the rules of gods and of humans, the people turned to lawlessness and pleasure-seeking.

Although the Athenians went back to more virtuous behavior when the plague subsided, lasting damage had been done to their military might. In the first summer of the epidemic, their army stayed inside the city, unable to force a showdown with the Spartans. The Athenian forces were also diminished for years to come, which may have been one reason the war dragged on for nearly a decade, with the upper hand switching between Athens and Sparta. When a peace treaty (unenduring) was finally signed in 421 B.C., the Athenians searched for more effective gods to replace those who had failed them during the plague. The cult of the healing deity Asklepios, introduced in Athens in 420 B.C., included Sophocles and Socrates among its devotees.

Further reading: Thucydides, *History of the Peloponnesian War; Cambridge Ancient History;* McNeill, *Plagues and Peoples;* Zinsser, *Rats, Lice and History.*

Plague of Cyprian Epidemic, possibly of measles or smallpox, that began in A.D. 251 and raged throughout the Mediterranean basin for at least 15 years. Although most sources say the plague ended in 266, the Roman emperor Claudius is known to have died from it in early 270. The epidemic added to the misery of the third century A.D., a time when barbarian peoples kept attacking the frontiers of the Roman Empire, when numerous military usurpers claimed the position of emperor, and when citizens were burdened with heavy taxes intended to maintain the imperial army. The sufferings to which the epidemic contributed also encouraged mass conversions to Christianity, a fact celebrated in the writings of Saint Cyprian, bishop of Carthage, whose name is used to identify the pestilence.

His tract *De Mortalitate* lists the various symptoms of the disease, from the red eyes and inflamed throat that came first, to the gangrene of the feet and the continual vomiting and diarrhea that followed, and finally the loss of hearing and eyesight that afflicted many who recovered. Most victims also suffered from burning fever and unquenchable thirst, according to other ancient writers, one of whom says that the disease could be spread indirectly through the clothing of an infected person.

Because no accounts mention buboes or swellings, most modern scholars believe that the epidemic was not bubonic plague. But its effects were just as devastating: Moving through Africa, the Near East, and much of Europe, the disease at its height claimed 5,000 deaths a day in Rome alone. Such widespread mortality may indicate the introduction of a disease previously unknown in the classical world, whose inhabitants had no immunity to it. U.S. history professor William McNeill therefore identifies the epidemic as one of either smallpox or measles, whichever one had not struck already, during the Antonine Plague of A.D. 165–180 (q.v.).

Several decades of incursions on all fronts of the empire—by Goths and other Germanic peoples into the Balkans and Asia Minor and by the newly powerful Sassanids in the Near East—had already stretched the Roman imperial army to its limits. The many dissatisfied army legions repeatedly put forward their own candidates for emperor, only to turn against them when adequate pay and rewards were not forthcoming. By killing large numbers of soldiers and by disrupting supply lines and tax collection, the disease further heightened the instability of the army and the imperial leadership.

If the epidemic weakened the forces of war, it strengthened those of Christianity. Attracted by the message of a rewarding afterlife, many people turned to the new religion, especially when they noticed how Christians tended to all who were sick, even the pagans. If one ancient writer is correct, the epidemic also brought a change in fashion, as Christians began to wear black as a sign of mourning.

Further reading: *Cambridge Ancient History;* Grant, *History of Rome;* McNeill, *Plagues and Peoples;* Zinsser, *Rats, Lice and History.*

Plague of England, Great

Plague of England, Great   Terrifying epidemic of bubonic plague in 1348–50 that destroyed much of England's population and caused lasting social and economic disruption. Part of the pandemic of bubonic plague called the Black Death (q.v.) on continental Europe, the Great Plague or Pestilence (or the Great Mortality) most probably entered England at the southern coastal port of Melcombe Regis (modern Weymouth) in late June or early August 1348, possibly direct from the French seaport of Calais, then an English possession, or from the Channel Islands. The disease subsided in 1350 and intermittently returned, although not as drastically, during the next three centuries.

Bubonic plague is a rodent disease and is transmitted to man by infected fleas that, after sucking the bacilli *Pasteurella pestis* into their stomachs along with their blood meal from the rodent host, dump the deadly bacilli into the bloodstream of any human being the flea then bites. Appreciation of the rodent-flea-man chain of infection is essential for a proper understanding of the cause and spread of bubonic plague. Except in the case of the pneumonic type, which attacks the lungs and can be transmitted from man to man through bacilli exhaled in droplets, a human being contracts plague only by flea-bite; and since pneumonic plague, because of its virulence, kills its victims quickly, the spreading of plague through huge areas is attributed to the bubonic type.

Thus, wherever there were large numbers of plague victims, there necessarily were large numbers of epizootic rats. Because these black rats were house-dwellers (as opposed, for example, to brown field rats) they infested closely-packed wood and thatch houses occupied almost exclusively by the poor. The plague has been labeled a poor man's disease simply because the house-rat found the poor's thatched roofs, earthen floors, and straw bedding such inviting habitats. The houses of the privileged, built of stone with roofs of slate or tile, were not sought out by the house-burrowing rat with its attendant disease-carrying fleas, and thus, as contemporary chronicler Robert of Avesbury attests, the plague attacked "few among the wealthy." The high mortality among the well-housed clergy—ecclesiastic records were carefully kept and most statistical assessments are based on them—is accounted for, among other factors, by their visits to the flea-infested dwellings of suffering parishioners. Bubonic plague attacked adolescents and young adults more than any other age group, a phenomenon that remains unexplained.

Town authorities ordered clearance of filth from streets and rivers, but since plague and dirty conditions have little connection, these admirable measures of public health did not help. Some relief was experienced during the winter months, as rat-fleas hibernate in frosty weather.

Of the plague's symptoms, a contemporary chronicler called Le Baker wrote that victims were "afflicted by swellings which appeared suddenly in various parts of the body . . . Others had small black blisters scattered over the whole body." The swellings were the buboes, found in the groin, armpits, and neck, from which bubonic plague gets its name. Severe headache, violent chest pains, swelling of the tongue, and subcutaneous hemorrhages were other outstanding symptoms. The sufferer often became distracted and staggered about, and if the attack was fatal would normally die within three days.

Chronicles of the time show general agreement about the course the plague took through the British Isles but vary so much in statistics that definitive statements regarding mortality figures are not possible. Estimates range from one twentieth to two thirds of the total population. It can be stated with certainty, however, that the more densely populated areas in eastern, central, and southeastern England suffered the most. Coastal areas and inland river towns, such as London, were most susceptible to plague because ship rats (house-dwellers on land) and fleas imbedded in cargo were constantly unloaded at these places.

Assessing the effects of plague is greatly hampered by the confusion of one disease with another in extant records, due to the medieval tendency to lump different diseases under a few generic names. A variety of distinct diseases, therefore, were labelled plague, leprosy, or fever, making it impossible for scholars to differentiate among deaths caused by plague or the many other diseases then prevalent, including typhus, smallpox, dysentery, diphtheria, cholera, typhoid, and scarlet fever.

Medieval people were accustomed to recurrent epidemics. The Great Pestilence, however, was unlike any other sickness they had experienced and its psychological effects went deep. Its mysterious appearance (the connection between plague and rats was not even guessed); its high case-mortality rate (nine out of ten who contracted it died); its concentration on young men and women; and the apparent lack of contagion from other men, which had been observed in other diseases, combined to make bubonic plague especially terrifying. Although hysteria evidently was not as great in the British Isles as it was in Europe, many people believed the plague was visited upon them by an angry God. Those physicians and other learned men who disregarded divine involvement suggested causes and recommended remedies that were ineffectual at best.

Extensive social and economic unrest marked the period following the Great Pestilence. Agriculture suffered through lack of laborers; workers demanded higher wages; corruption among the clergy grew. Worst of all, perhaps, was the disruption of family life and the abandonment by family members of those in the throes of this "Great Mortality."

Further reading: McNeill, *Plagues and Peoples;* Mullet, *The Bubonic Plague and England;* Smith, *Plague on Us;* Shrewsbury, *A History of Bubonic Plague in the British Isles;* Winslow, *The Conquest of Epidemic Disease.*

Plague of Florence (Black Vomit) Devastating epidemic of bubonic plague, often called the Black Vomit, that hit Florence, Italy, during the winter of 1347 and again in the spring of 1348. Florence was already weakened by a famine in 1347. Estimates vary, but possibly between 45 percent and 75 percent of the city's citizens died during the six months in which the plague raged. Shops and factories closed, and prices soared. Many doctors charged extraordinary prices for their services, and many Florentines died from malnutrition before the plague could claim them. The Florence plague was a severe offshoot of the Black Death (q.v.), which was then sweeping through Europe.

Those who were stricken with the illness developed black swellings on the groin or under the arms. The swellings were followed by boils and black blotches on the skin. Sometimes the victims spit foul-smelling blood. Some people died 24 hours after the first symptoms appeared, and almost all who were stricken died within three days. The epidemic spread quickly, and was highly contagious. Even contact with the clothing of a sick person was dangerous. People reacted with fear, and the fear gave way to terrible callousness. The sick were often ignored and left to die; husbands and wives deserted each other, and parents deserted children. People fled the city and tried to escape the disease by hiding in the country. Unfortunately, there was little guaranty of immunity. Conditions in the country were often as bad as they were in the city.

The Black Death, which had come from Asia and entered Western Europe with ships and travelers, spread to many countries. To some historians, this plague is more closely linked to Florence than to any other city or locality. There are several reasons for this: The plague raged in Florence with exceptional intensity, and at the time Florence was one of the most splendid and richest cities in Europe. The city was hit so severely that the Black Death is often thought of and referred to as the Plague of Florence.

Another reason why the Black Death is so closely associated with Florence is that the epidemic was chronicled by Italian writer Giovanni Boccaccio in his book, *The Decameron* (1353). His is the best-known eyewitness account of the bubonic plague, and he provides a horrible, somber description of the epidemic. Boccaccio, whose father died of the plague, wrote about the large number of quacks who emerged during the crisis, and how they took advantage of the sick. He criticized the medical profession, and maintained that they were no help at all. Some of his descriptions are probably accurate: the way the rich fled the city, how the sick were deserted, the rushed burials in large communal pits, crops wasting in the fields, and animals wandering untended over the countryside. It is possible, however, that Boccaccio portrayed the Black Death in Florence in bleaker terms than it actually was. He made no mention, for example, of the nuns and doctors who devoted themselves to healing plague victims, and no mention was made of the efforts the Florentine government made to control the plague.

A committee of eight was set up by the city government to maintain order in Florence. The men were chosen from among the wisest and most respected citizens, and were given almost total power to organize the city. The committee concerned itself with the removal of decaying matter and disposal of the dead from the streets. Ultimately, there was not much that the committee could do to stop the destruction of the plague.

Some Florentines responded to the strain by giving in to hedonistic desires. They drank and spent money with reckless abandon, trying to enjoy themselves before falling victim to illness. Others took advantage of the crisis. In particular, a group called the becchini often behaved in a horrible manner; they were men, often of lower social rank and usually themselves afflicted with the plague, who carried the dead away and performed other tasks that no one else would do. Some of them raped, assaulted, and even murdered their fellow citizens. Perhaps the most heartless act that some performed was bribing family members before carrying their dead members away. See also PLAGUE OF ENGLAND, GREAT.

Further reading: Gottfried, *The Black Death*; Zeigler, *The Black Death*; Tuchman, *A Distant Mirror*.

Plague of Florence in 1417   Outbreak of mainly bubonic plague that killed about ten percent of the population of approximately 40,000. The Italian city's Grain Office kept a series of particular "Books of the Dead" that recorded the number of human deaths from epidemics. The 1417 epidemic evidently had four times as many victims as plague outbreaks in 1411 and 1424 did. An earlier epidemic in 1400 purportedly killed about 12,000 Florentines, and possibly as many as that may have perished in the "major" 1417 plague epidemic, the eighth visitation of this highly contagious, bacterial disease in Florence since the Plague of Florence (Black Vomit) (q.v.) in 1347–48.

In May 1417 numerous Florentines became infected with plague through intimate contact with the commensal black rat (the rodent host of the disease) and its infected fleas (infection is generally contracted by a flea bite). During the early weeks of the epidemic, wagons collected as many as 500 poor people daily for transport to hospitals. Florence's densely populated working-class sections were chiefly affected, and the Tuscan countryside was spared, unlike plague outbreaks in the previous century, which killed many country folk. By October about 6,000 Florentines had contracted plague, which caused painful swellings (buboes) in their groins, armpits, or neck areas; the buboes varied in size from a walnut to a grapefruit, according to Italian chroniclers of plague. In 1417 physicians did not segregate or isolate the sick in Florence, despite having experienced plague problems before.

By the end of the epidemic in late 1417, approximately 4,000 people had died (probably more). The patients with pneumonic plague coughed up blood and frequently died within hours of their infection; about 65 percent of the bubonic patients perished within one to five days after being infected. There were many incidences of multiple deaths in a household (where an infection can be transmitted person-to-person by airborne droplets); often entire families were wiped out in the poorer sections. A number of important, wealthy citizens fell victim, but the disease was less severe in the prosperous districts of Florence. See also ITALIAN PLAGUES OF 1477–79.

Further reading: Carmichael, *Plague and the Poor in Renaissance Florence*; Cloudsley-Thompson, *Insects and History*.

Plague of Florence in 1630–33   Epidemic that claimed the lives of about ten percent of the population. In the winter of 1630 and the spring of 1631, the bubonic plague hit the Italian city of Florence, which previously had suffered from several cold and wet winters that had led to a disastrous crop failure and a shortage of food when the 1630 epidemic began. Although mortality was less than it had been during the 1348 Plague of Florence (Black Vomit) (q.v.), an estimated 7,000 persons perished during the three years that this plague epidemic raged.

Victims of the plague suffered a sudden and high fever; they often had large and foul-smelling boils on their bodies; they were sometimes delirious; and a terrible headache was usually the prelude to death. Those who did not die from the disease were terrorized by it and lived in fear of catching it. Many people starved themselves, purged themselves, sprayed themselves with acid and snake poison, or paid shop clerks for vats of vinegar to protect themselves. Those who died from plague were often the more productive members of Florence's society; a large percentage of the roughly ten percent who died were artisans and Capuchins (a Franciscan order) or those who performed much of Florence's custodial work during the epidemic.

In some ways, the plague was considered beneficial, for it mitigated the problem of overpopulation and allowed the rations of food to spread to more people. In addition, the plague epidemic contributed to greater enthusiasm for religion; people felt that the disaster was a result of God's wrath, and they responded by making efforts to correct their behavior. Large Christian masses were celebrated in the streets, and some special fasts were instituted. In that way, Florence was transformed into an extremely moral city for the three years of the epidemic.

The Florentine people responded well to the crisis. No one broke the 40-day quarantine, and no one apparently touched the property of the helpless. People appointed by the Office of Public Health dedicated themselves to their tasks of fumigating the homes of those stricken with disease—scrubbing floors, burning mattresses and clothes, and carrying away the dead to be buried. The grand duke of Florence made a daily round to ensure that citizens were receiving food and were well cared for.

Unfortunately, the economic effects of the epidemic were bad; for six months in 1631 and for four months in 1633, all business and trade in Florence came to a nearly complete standstill. Many people were unemployed; Florence had become a city of industrial workers without industry. The only way to avoid mass starvation was the distribution of public charity, which was very expensive and was paid for by drawing on the Florentine state bank, the *Monte Comune*.

Like the earlier Florentine plague in 1348, mass graves were dug; however, dead human bodies were perceived as degrading, and people wanted to dispose of them as quickly as possible. Anyone hoping for a church burial, rather than suffering the humiliation of anonymity in a mass grave, needed a signed certificate from a physician guaranteeing the "nonsuspect" nature of the illness.

Some historians believe that the plague epidemic started in Florence with an invasion of Milanese mercenaries after the war of succession over Mantua (1628–31). Numerous plague-infected goods had been exchanged, and people most likely had contracted the disease from some of them. Public health officials in Florence imposed strict regulations, most of which were followed by the citizens. Despite the efforts of guards to keep everyone within the city boundaries, some people did leave, and the disease moved from Florence north to Milan, as well as to Bologna and Trespiano.

Further reading: Cochrane, *Florence in the Forgotten Centuries*; Symonds, *Renaissance in Italy*.

Plague of Galen   See ANTONINE PLAGUE.

Plague of Iceland, Great   Devastating epidemic of bubonic plague in 1402–04 that affected Iceland's population, economy, and social structure for centuries to come.

Although Iceland had not been hit by bubonic plague before, the country had suffered indirectly from the European pandemic 50 years earlier (see BLACK DEATH). With few natural resources of its own, Iceland relied exclusively on Norway for a wide variety of import goods. When Norway lost about one third of its population in the pandemic, its foreign trade ceased almost completely, leaving Iceland without many needed products. Earthquakes, volcanic eruptions, famines, and diseases that killed people and livestock had also taken their toll on Iceland during the fourteenth century.

Coming after so many natural disasters, the "Great Plague" (also named the Black Death) further dislocated Icelandic society. Whole families died out, and many of those who attended funerals did not return, struck down by the same disease that had killed their relatives. An estimated 40 percent to 50 percent of the people succumbed; later annals suggest that the population may not have grown significantly again until the early nineteenth century. Widespread mortality also changed social relations: Nuns at one convent had to milk their cows themselves, since all their servants died.

Worse still was the depopulation of many Icelandic farms. A 1404 law that required fishermen to work on farms testifies to the decreased number of farmers. The plague therefore encouraged a shift in Iceland's export goods from homespun cloth to fish and fish products—a shift begun in the previous century in response to changes in foreign markets. Because the plague killed not only many individual owners of small farms (who combined held about one half of all land in Iceland), but also their children, traditional inheritance patterns were changed. Farmland became concentrated in the hands of a few wealthy owners, the most important of which was the Catholic Church, to which many people donated their property in hopes of staving off death from the plague.

Further reading: Gjerset, *History of Iceland*; Hastrup, *Nature and Policy in Iceland*; Magnusson, *Northern Sphinx: Iceland and the Icelanders from the Settlement to the Present*.

Plague of Ireland, Great

Severe offshoot epidemic of the bubonic plague in the British Isles, which reached Ireland in late June or early August 1348, probably via ships from the English port of Bristol, into which it had been recently imported through ship-borne plague-infected rats and their disease-transmitting fleas. Attacking towns along the eastern and southeastern coasts of Ireland first, the plague appeared in Dublin and Drogheda (a port north of Dublin) later in August of the same year, and continued its course, although diminished in force, until at least early in 1351.

Extant Irish annals attest to the high mortality rates occurring in coastal areas, but because they do not record death figures, except estimates based on hearsay, it is difficult to assess the effects of this epidemic in Ireland accurately. It is certain, however, that the plague caused much distress. Friar John Clyn, who died in 1349 possibly from plague, wrote that "In scarcely any house did only one die but all together, man and wife with their children and household, traversed the same road, the road of death." Among other contemporary documents is a moving prayer left by a young man called Hugh MacEagen: "This is Christmas night, and I place myself under the protection of the King of heaven and earth, beseeching that He will bring me and my friends safe through this plague." See also PLAGUE OF ENGLAND, GREAT.

Further reading: Mullet, *The Bubonic Plague and England*; Shrewsbury, *A History of Bubonic Plague in the British Isles*.

Plague of Justinian (First Plague Pandemic)

Pandemic of bubonic plague that swept Asia Minor, Africa, and Europe and arrived in Constantinople (Istanbul), the capital of the Eastern Roman (Byzantine) Empire, in the late spring and summer of A.D. 542. After the plague started in Egypt the previous year, merchant ships and troops carried it throughout the Western world, enabling it to flare up repeatedly over the next 50 or so years. Decades of wars, famines, and natural disasters in the Mediterranean lands may have helped the plague take its enormous toll; about 300,000 people were said to have died in Constantinople alone during the first year. Even the Eastern Roman (Byzantine) emperor Justinian fell ill; though he recovered, his imperial ambitions did not. The mortality and disruption caused by the plague prevented him from recapturing the western provinces and restoring the former extent of the Roman Empire.

According to Procopius, the Greek historian and court insider who is our primary source, the epidemic started near Ethiopia. Although ancient tradition held that diseases came from Africa, there may be some truth to Procopius's account. The plague bacillus appears to have originated in both central Africa and India, the latter also the probable home for the species of black rat that carried the plague. Ships plying the Indian Ocean and the Red Sea on their way to Egypt could have brought rat and bacillus together in a deadly combination.

Knowing only that they could be struck without warning at any time, people were terrified, Procopius tells us. Many attributed their illness to the touch of a supernatural being who appeared in dreams or waking apparitions. To prevent such demons from slipping into their homes, people barred their doors against all visitors, family and friends alike. The mild fever that was the plague's first symptom did not seem alarming, however, and many people did not worry until they developed bubonic swellings within the next few days.

Once the swellings appeared, most sufferers either went into a deep coma or became violently delirious, sometimes paranoid and suicidal. In either case it was difficult to feed and care for them properly, although mere contact with the sick did not seem to increase one's chances of falling ill. Most victims died within a few days, but recovery seemed certain for those whose buboes filled with pus. Black blisters taken by one modern scholar to indicate a co-infection of smallpox, were a sure sign of immediate death. Otherwise, doctors often could not predict the course of the disease or the success of various treatments. Even autopsies, which revealed unusual carbuncles inside the swellings, did not provide much help.

For four months the plague raged in Constantinople, with the death toll climbing from 5,000 a day to 10,000 and even higher during the three most virulent months. Justinian appointed a court detail to dispose of dead bodies when relatives would not or could not bury them, but even the officials were overwhelmed by their task. When all the tombs became filled, they placed corpses on boats set adrift or in towers on the fortifications, which were then roofed over. All other work ceased, including that of supplying the city with food; the resulting shortages may have hastened the deaths of many plague victims.

The epidemic could not have come at a worse time. Justinian's court was already riddled with corruption and intrigue; the deaths of many officials—not to mention the illness and long recuperation of the emperor himself—threw the administration into chaos. At the same time, crises throughout the empire and on its borders demanded a capable central government. Recent famines, floods, and earthquakes in Asia Minor and Europe had forced many people to leave their homes and stop all agricultural production. Despite imperial success in turning back a Persian invasion into Syria earlier in the year, the Near East remained a volatile region. The Goths in Italy and the Vandals in North Africa continued to occupy lands that had once been part of the Roman Empire.

As they traveled to all frontiers to deal with these ever-restless barbarian tribes, Justinian's troops helped spread the plague, even as they themselves succumbed. With his army diminished and his fiscal resources drained, Justinian saw his dream of unifying the Mediterranean basin crumble before it became a reality.

Further reading: Procopius, *History of the Wars*; Browning, *Justinian and Theodora*; McNeill, *Plagues and Peoples*.

Plague of London, Great

Fearful pestilence that ravaged London in 1664–65 and killed some 75,000 (perhaps 100,000) inhabitants, at least 20 percent of the city's population. The plague, an acute infectious disease caused by a bacterium (*Pasteurella pestis*), was thought to have been introduced into England by some Dutch merchants, who apparently brought it into London in bales of cotton. The disease had been intermittently in Holland since 1654. In the Dutch city of Leiden 13,000 persons died; in Amsterdam over 13,250 died in 1655. Those attacked by the plague became suddenly delirious, rolling around as if intoxicated and then perspiring profusely. The poor in London, in their crowded, ill-kempt, wooden houses, were especially threatened by contagion.

Ancient fears and superstitions resurfaced in London when, in late December 1663 and then again in March 1664, bright comets appeared in the sky. There were accounts of people seeing fire and coffins in the heavens and hearing sounds of cannon. Londoners believed these were signs from God of an imminent punishment for their immorality. During the winter of 1664–65 there were reports of several deaths from plague, a periodic invader of London since the Black Death (q.v.) of the mid-fourteenth century; the deaths were attributed to God's wrath. Because the winter was extremely cold and icy, the disease was checked from spreading rapidly; but the spring and summer months were unusually sunny, warm, and dry, and the plague ran rampant.

It supposedly began in the slums of St. Giles-in-the-Fields, a London outer parish (though it lies near the British Museum today). The disease then spread to Westminster and moved from the western parishes to the eastern and southern parishes; by early July 1665 it was in the city of London; King Charles II of England and his court then left the city for Oxford, as did many wealthy merchants, lawyers, and professors. Only a small number of apothecaries, physicians, and clergymen remained to treat the sick. All shops and businesses in London closed up, as the plague raged all summer (1665). Newspapers advertised old plague remedies, giving information about the disease and printing weekly accounts of the mounting death toll. Deaths crept up to 1,000 persons a week, then 2,000 a week, and in September (1665) went over 7,000 a week. Afterward the deaths began to lessen. Whole families perished at the time.

Both night and day the dead were carted off to churchyards for burial, and when the churchyards were completely filled, huge pits were dug for the corpses. Publicly appointed physicians, along with persons who volunteered to care for the sick without pay, issued as preventive medicine pungent smells—burnt brimstone, pepper, hops, or frankincense. Poor people burned old shoes and horn. When the plague persisted and seemed to grow, the authorities ordered fires to be kept burning day and night in the streets, to purify the air. In addition, tobacco smoking was recommended (even mandated in some places) as protection against the plague; even children were forced to smoke at times. Quarantines were put into effect; new pesthouses were built to take in some of the plague victims; national money collections were established.

By late fall (1665) the situation had improved, and by February 1666 King Charles II returned to London. (The Lord Mayor and aldermen had stayed at their posts and had not sought safety in flight.) The plague finally ended after the Great Fire in London (September 2–5, 1666); by then it had spread to France, where it died out the following winter. After the Great Fire, London was rebuilt with wider streets (thus less congestion) and with improved sewer drainage; thatch for the roofs of houses was forbidden. The English novelist Daniel Defoe wrote *A Journal of the Plague in London*, published in 1722, which is a fictional narrative telling about the 1665 plague through the eyes of a citizen who stayed in London.

Further reading: Bell, *The Great Plague in London in 1665*; Slack, *The Impact of Plague in Tudor and Stuart England*.

Plague of Lyon in 1564

Outbreak of bubonic plague that spread throughout Lyon and southeast France during the spring, summer, and autumn months of 1564. The young French king Charles IX and his mother, Catherine de Medici, had just begun a two-year tour of the provinces, hoping to consolidate royal power after a bloody civil war. Continual recurrences of the plague, however, kept the court moving from town to town, sometimes forcing it to bypass intended stops or change its route.

Wealthy and populous Lyon was especially hardhit. Its silk weaving, printing, and other industries supported a population estimated at around 60,000 in the mid-sixteenth century. At the confluence of the Rhône and Saône rivers, Lyon attracted many foreign merchants with its four annual fairs. Travelers and traders could easily have brought plague with them, and the large population of the city would have been an easy target. In fact, people in Lyon had complained several decades earlier that plague outbreaks occurred almost annually.

The 1564 epidemic seems to have been exceptionally deadly. By the time Charles's entourage arrived in mid-June, Lyon was almost paralyzed after two months of plague. According to the then-English ambassador Sir Thomas Smith, nearly one house out of three was closed up because its inhabitants were stricken, while other victims were sent to tents around the town, presumably to remain in isolation. On their way out to buy food, Smith's servants sometimes saw ten or 12 corpses lying in the streets until the authorities came to cart them away. Such measures were of little avail, since there was no place to put so many dead bodies, nor enough money to pay gravediggers. Many corpses were simply thrown in the river, and the fishing industry was thereby shut down. Although some victims recovered from the plague, Smith claimed they were not necessarily fortunate. They were likely to die of hunger, since healthy people were afraid to care for them and food was in short supply.

Few other towns in the regions of Provence and Languedoc were spared. Vienne saw its first cases at the beginning of June. A month later the government of Chambery recorded the appearance of plague in its suburbs; by mid-July the epidemic began to claim victims in Nimes. Though autumn brought a lull, local outbreaks were reported as late as mid-December at places like Lunel, from which the French king had to be turned away. A severe winter finally ended the epidemic.

Although exact numbers are not available, the mortality must have been high. For the past few years the region had been devastated by inflation and civil war. Upheaval at the court and the increasingly intense conflict between Huguenots (French Protestants) and Catholics had combined to ruin many areas of France. Staunch Catholics circulated rumors blaming the Huguenots for bringing the plague to Lyon as a means to kill the king. Such rumors may have begun when several members of the royal entourage, including an attendant to the queen, died of plague. Yet Catherine, who had hoped that the tour would calm the troubled provinces, could not be dissuaded from her plans. Despite leaving Lyon on July 9, the court traveled throughout the plague-stricken region for months to come.

Further reading: Baird, *The Huguenots and Henry of Navarre*; Boutier et al., *Un Tour de France Royal*; Davis, *Society and Culture in Early Modern France*; Thompson, *The Wars of Religion in France*.

Plague of Lyon in 1628–29   Deadliest large-scale epidemic of bubonic plague experienced by a French city in the seventeenth century. Unemployment, especially among workers in Lyon's silk industry, excessive taxes imposed by noblemen to raise armies, and high food prices were already burdening the city when the plague struck in the summer of 1628. Soldiers passing through Lyon were accused of having carried the plague with them "as their baggage," perhaps because one of the first reported deaths was that of a soldier lodging in a nearby village, whose corpse, buried in a garden and exposed from its shallow grave by heavy rains, was said to have infected surrounding households and thence spread to the city. In a panicked attempt to assess blame, Catholics claimed that Huguenots (Protestants) had spread a poisonous plague-producing ointment through the streets and churches. A more considered opinion was offered by members of the Collège de Lyon, who announced that plague appeared wherever there was "deep putrefaction of nature," a reference to the idea that disease arose from contaminated air or soil.

Plague had not appeared in Lyon for 50 years, but anti-plague regulations established in previous epidemics were put into effect immediately by the city's 13 commissioners of health. Guards were posted at city gates, health certificates were required from travelers, and a 40-day quarantine was imposed on goods and people entering the city. Rioting commonly broke out during serious epidemics, and the commissioners were invested with authority to execute violators of plague restrictions to help suppress public disorder. The usual pillaging of vacated houses took place. Many families buried their dead themselves in gardens or caves to avoid the *corbeaux*, the men who collected the dead and who routinely stripped both the homes and corpses of plague victims.

Lyon's hospital of Saint-Laurent, run down from disuse, was hurriedly prepared. Lack of space forced many patients to construct huts on the grounds of the hospital; others piled up corpses for shelter against the cold autumn winds. According to the Abbé Cahour, who wrote an account of the epidemic, 4,000 patients crowded the halls and precincts of the hospital at any given time. Abbé Cahour's chronicle depicts the horrors that were typical of many epidemics, especially the French Plagues of 1625–40 (q.v.), France's worst plague years since the Black Death (q.v.):

> the city was nothing but a vast hospital; the streets as well as the houses were strewn with corpses; they were buried hastily in gardens and even in cellars. Monks and nuns were often obliged to pass among the dead stretched out in rooms or staircases to bring help to those who were still breathing. Entire families succumbed at once and no one was there to give them medicines and burial. Abandoned corpses were discovered after more than eight days in deserted houses.

Many of Lyon's government officials and wealthy citizens left the city for their houses in the countryside, and many people found refuge on islands in the Saône and Rhône rivers. Laborers and others of Lyon's poorer classes who had no second homes or means to sustain themselves, but who nonetheless also sought safety in the countryside, "were chased away with stones by the peasants, the wiser ones returned to Lyon, others died of hunger or were eaten by wolves in the forest."

The epidemic abated somewhat at the end of December, but broke out again with great force in early 1629, gradually diminishing from March through the summer months. Perhaps as many as 35,000 people died in Lyon during the 12-month epidemic, but this figure is an estimate only. Plague was also active at this time in dozens of towns and villages in the surrounding area.

Further reading: Canard, *Les pestes en Beaujolais, Forez, Jarez, Lyonnais du XIVème au XVIIIème siècle;* Lucenet, *Lyon: malade de la peste.*

Plague of Marseilles

Plague of Marseilles Devastating epidemic of bubonic plague that struck the French city in 1720. It lasted until 1722 and killed approximately a third to a half of the population of Marseilles and the surrounding areas (maybe 80,000 people). The plague bacillus, which was spread by certain fleas, was identified by black spots and buboes (swellings of the lymph glands) found on the groin, the neck, and under the arms. Generally, the fatal illness lasted only a few days and was extremely contagious.

The plague of 1720 was most likely introduced in Marseilles by a merchant ship that had sailed from Syria, where the plague was raging. When the *Grand St. Antoine* arrived in Marseilles on May 25, 1720, the health commissioners at the port of Marseilles impounded the merchandise on the ship and quarantined the passengers and crew for several weeks. When the sailors were released, however, they came into contact with the people of Marseilles and sold contraband lengths of contaminated cloth. The street porters who carried the cloth and several of the sailors became sick. The merchandise was confiscated and burned, but most of the people who had bought the cloth became sick and died quickly.

At first, authorities did not want to admit that the plague had entered Marseilles. Local doctors who tended the victims were convinced that their patients were suffering from the bubonic plague, and one doctor alerted the aldermen of Marseilles. The aldermen asked another doctor, Dr. Bauzon, for his expert opinion. Dr. Bauzon said that the people were probably suffering from a fever that was caused by intestinal worms. New cases were discovered in July, but the aldermen still did not want to take extreme measures. They were probably afraid to alarm the people and injure the commerce of the city by reporting that the infection had entered Marseilles.

By the end of July, the number of deaths had increased. In August, the disease had spread to all sections of the city. Finally, a decree of the parliament of Aix put Marseilles under an interdict, and the chamber of commerce forbade all commerce between the city and the province. Tragically, it was too late to stop the epidemic. Nearly 10,000 citizens had already fled and brought the plague to numerous other localities, such as Toulon, Aix, and Arles.

In the beginning of August, a blockade of Marseilles was instituted. People were not supposed to cross the barriers, and merchandise was allowed to pass only at specified points. Unfortunately, the blockade was inefficient because the necessary troops could not be assembled quickly enough to stop the people from fleeing. The plague spread quickly and ravaged Provence, Venaissin, and part of Languedoc (three neighboring provinces in southern France).

The epidemic brought economic disaster, administrative disorganization, and social disintegration. Initially, city officials were afraid to close the city, as there was a shortage of food and no stock of provisions in Marseilles. By the end of the summer of 1720, when the plague had reached its maximum deadliness, it was no longer possible to bury all the dead. Bodies were put in the vaults of neighborhood churchyards, and quicklime and water were thrown on them. Many physicians and surgeons fled Marseilles, and the very people who had been posted to prevent the flight of others fled themselves. Shopkeepers locked their doors and people could not buy supplies. Even commands by the board of trade for all tradesmen and shopkeepers to open their doors had no effect. When a person became infected, he or she was often deserted or driven out of the house. Hospitals were not able to contain the numbers of sick people, many of whom lay on pavements around them. Public services were virtually nonexistent as policemen, public servants, tradesmen, and doctors either fled the city or died.

One man, Bishop Henri François de Belsunce (a French Jesuit), demonstrated extreme bravery during the epidemic. He remained at his post in Marseilles and went into the homes of the sick to provide food, comfort, and friendship. As a result of his heroic care of plague victims, he earned the title "Good Bishop."

The epidemic continued for two years, although it gradually became less violent. There were a few cases recorded in Marseilles between April 18, 1721, and August 19, 1721. On February 3, 1722, approximately 260 people became sick, 194 of whom died. Severe quarantines followed these outbreaks, and no new cases were discovered after that. Slowly, the city began to restore itself and recover from the epidemic. However, people lived in fear of another epidemic for a long time.

Further reading: Biraben, "Certain Demographic Characteristics of the Plague Epidemic in France, 1720–1722"; Carey, *A Short Account of the Malignant Fever*; Rail, *Plague Ecotoxicology*.

Plague of Milan, Great   See ITALIAN PLAGUES OF 1629–31.

Plague of Scotland, Great

Another devastating visitation of bubonic plague (called the Black Death [q.v.] in continental Europe) in the British Isles; first entered England in the summer of 1348 at Melcombe Regis (modern Weymouth), a port town on the southern coast. Although Scots chroniclers of the time did not attempt to explain how the plague reached their country, English writers asserted that it simply traveled north through England till it crossed the Scottish border. Modern historians consider it far more likely that it entered Scotland by sea, in ships carrying large numbers of epizootic, house-dwelling rats and their plague-ridden fleas. Once these rats infested the thatch and wood houses of the poor, it was not long before their infected fleas began biting human hosts and, in so doing, transmitting to them the deadly plague-causing bacillus *Pasteurella pestis*. Like the English chroniclers, Scots observers noted that the plague attacked "especially the meaner sort and common people;—seldome the magnates." This is because the homes of the wealthy were usually built of materials—mostly stone—into which these diseased black rats could not burrow.

The violence of the symptoms, which included painful swellings or "buboes," severe headache, and spitting of blood, and the rapidity with which it killed its victims—patients usually died within three days—invoked much dread. According to the contemporary Scots writer Fordun, "Men shrank from it so much that, through fear of contagion, sons, fleeing as . . . from an adder, durst not go and see their parents in the throes of death." As in other countries afflicted with plague, Scots writers emphasized the disruptive effect on family bonds that the plague engendered.

Perhaps the most famous instance of plague in Scotland was suffered by the Scots Army. Gathering at Selkirk Forest, they planned to take advantage of the havoc and death the plague was causing their hated English neighbors. The army itself was stricken, however, and reportedly 5,000 men died, putting an end to their military hopes.

Mortality rates, as in other parts of Britain, are difficult to determine with accuracy. It can be stated with some certainty, however, that deaths in the barren Highlands, which comprise much of Scotland, were relatively few, due to low population density and the consequent small numbers of plague-bearing rats. According to the poet Andrew of Wyntoun and others, the plague first entered Scotland in 1349, was at its height in 1350, and lasted more than a year.

Little information is available to scholars regarding the presence of bubonic plague in Wales during this first outbreak of 1348–50. It is likely that towns and villages contiguous with the English border were somewhat affected. Less population density and the absence of extensive sea or river shipping left Wales largely untouched. See also PLAGUE OF ENGLAND, GREAT.

Further reading: Mullet, *The Bubonic Plague and England*; Shrewsbury, *A History of Bubonic Plague in the British Isles*.

Plague of Thucydides   See PLAGUE OF ATHENS, GREAT.

Plague of Vienna, Great

Devastating outbreak of mainly bubonic plague that killed thousands of inhabitants of Vienna, the imperial residence of the Austrian Habsburg rulers, in 1679. The city was crippled by the lingering epidemic, which continued fitfully into the early 1680s; the exact number of plague cases and fatalities for these years cannot be determined.

In 1679 plague evidently spread from the Ottoman Empire (Turkey and much of the Balkans) into Austria, from where it moved into Bohemia (western Czechoslovakia) and Saxony (a state in southeastern Germany) and other German areas. Vienna, located on the Danube River, was a major trading crossroads and center between east and west; it had suffered from plague outbreaks since the Black Death (q.v.) of the mid-fourteenth century (see VIENNA PLAGUE OF 1349). There were no sewers in the crowded city, where conditions were so unhealthy and filthy, with stinking domestic garbage and refuse littering the streets, that "Viennese death" was a moniker used to describe plague in other parts of Europe. Hordes of plague-infected rats flourished in the homes of the poor and the rich, and diseased rat fleas easily lodged in clothing, carpets, rags, grain, and other goods, surviving from six weeks up to a year. When the rats (primary hosts of plague) died, their fleas sought out the closest host, human beings, who become infected initially from the bite of diseased fleas. Painful swellings (buboes) develop in victims' groins, armpits, or necks, and the mortality can range between 30 percent and 50 percent for bubonic plague and higher for victims of pneumonic and septicemic plague.

During the 1679 epidemic, the Brotherhood of the Holy Trinity (a religious order operating in Vienna) ministered to many sick children and adults, who were also treated in special hospitals. Knowing no cure for the disease, doctors treated their patients by bloodletting and using emetics (agents that induce vomiting), ointments, and other methods. Superstitions were bolstered, such as the belief that plague was carried by a *Pest Jungfrau* (Plague Maiden). In addition, an amusing anecdote survived the 1679 epidemic that concerned a Viennese street-singer named Augustin, who reportedly fell totally inebriated to the ground, was mistaken for a plague victim, carted away as dead, and thrown into a plague-pit; however, he awoke before being burned to death.

In the aftermath of the epidemic, the Viennese erected monuments, like the famous Karlskirche and Baroque Pestsäule (baroque plague columns, 69 feet high), to commemorate the city's deliverance from the dreaded plague.

Further reading: Ackerknecht, *History and Geography of the Most Important Diseases;* Gregg, *Plague: An Ancient Disease in the Twentieth Century.*

Plague of Xerxes   Outbreak of dysentery that, according to ancient Greek historian Herodotus, hit the Persian Army in late 480 B.C. on its retreat from Greece into Asia Minor. After winning at Thermopylae (August) and even occupying Athens, the Persian general Xerxes was soon stopped in his attempt to conquer Greece. Tricked into fighting in the narrow waters near Salamis, the Persian fleet could gain no advantage from its overwhelming numbers and was easily defeated by the Greek Navy (September).

Most of the Persian soldiers remained in Thessaly, where they prepared for another attack on Greece in the spring. Xerxes, though, wanted to secure a line of retreat into Asia Minor and guard against possible uprisings by the Asiatic Greeks. After sending his defeated navy home, he marched northward with a contingent of soldiers, many of whom suffered undernourishment, hunger, and disease (dysentery and/or plague).

Unreliable in detail and biased toward the Athenians, Herodotus's account exaggerates both the initial size of Xerxes's forces and the extent of their losses on the retreat. With his flair for the dramatic, Herodotus tells of the Persians eating grass, leaves, and tree bark for want of supplies, and of the sick being left behind as Xerxes rushed home. By painting such a vivid picture, Herodotus undoubtedly wanted to instill in his Greek readers a sense of pride at turning back the Persians, who represented barbarism and decadence—a theme present also in Greek dramatist Aeschylus's play *The Persians.*

Further reading: Herodotus, *The Histories;* How and Wells, *A Commentary on Herodotus;* Bury and Meiggs, *A History of Greece;* Zinsser, *Rats, Lice and History.*

Plague Pandemic, Third   One of the three great plague epidemics that ravaged most of the inhabited world, lasting from the 1850s to about 1959 (see PLAGUE OF JUSTINIAN; BLACK DEATH). Since at least 1800 the plague disease had been festering almost solely among wild rodents in China's Yünnan province. With the outbreak of a Muslim rebellion in Yünnan in the 1850s and the subsequent human deaths and fleeing refugees, the plague began spreading slowly southward and throughout China. Chinese seaports such as Pakhoi (Pei-hai) in 1882, Canton in early 1894, and Hong Kong several months later suffered brief plague epidemics. Bombay, which had not had a plague outbreak since the seventeenth century, was hit in the summer of 1896 and suffered more than 30,000 deaths by the end of 1898. The plague outbreak then spread to Calcutta and other cities in India, which were reporting more than 80 percent death rates, most often from the plague hospitals that most victims tried to avoid unless they were too ill to resist. This death rate ignored the great number of victims who were stricken but eventually recovered without entering the hospitals.

Symptoms of the plague included fever, bronchitis, swollen glands or buboes (especially in the groin and armpit), and intestinal problems. Until the late 1800s plague had been thought to be caused by such things as the poisoning of wells by Jews or lepers, arrows from angry angels, clouds coming from corpses in the ground, and the devil smearing poison on homes. These long-time superstitions were only gradually being overcome when Dr. Paul Louis Simond, a Frenchman studying plague in Indochina in the 1890s, discovered a connection between human and rat plague and postulated about the role of the flea in transmitting the plague bacillus between them. His work met initially with hostility but was eventually accepted after a Swiss doctor, Alexandre E. J. Yersin, isolated the *Bacterium pestis* in 1894. It was renamed *Bacillus pestis* in 1900, *Pasteurella pestis* in 1923, and is today commonly known as *Yersinia pestis*.

The plague epidemic meanwhile began a rapid journey around the world. It struck Egypt in 1899 and Madagascar, which had till then never had a case of plague, in November 1898, by way of an Indian ship carrying rice (and plague). Ever since then, Madagascar has been a current plague focus in the world. The disease was then transmitted to Thailand in 1904 through another plague-carrying ship, to Burma in 1905, and to Tunisia, which had been safe from the disease for nearly a century, in 1907. From China the disease had also spread eastward, arriving in Honolulu, Hawaii, in early June 1899 on board nine ships from Hong Kong and moving subsequently throughout the Hawaiian Islands. The fact that most early victims were Asian prompted a series of quarantines of Asians and some burnings of Chinatown homes and a number of restrictions on Asian passenger and freight travel. Nevertheless, because of the arrival in Hawaii of two other plague-infected ships in November 1899 and the plague's rapid transmission by rats and fleas, the epidemic continued in the islands until the end of March 1900.

The disease had already reached South America by April 1899, at Asunción, Paraguay, and began moving down to Argentina by way of the Parana River. Ships arriving in Trinidad, Venezuela, Peru, and Ecuador in 1908 brought the disease to these areas and, a while later, it spread to Bolivia and Brazil. During the Boer War of 1899–1902 ships from plague-stricken ports in South America carried the disease into South Africa, where it spread northward by railroad and the cargo carried. Australia experienced plague outbreaks from 1900 to 1905 along its eastern coast after plague-infested rats arrived in Sydney by ship. In late June 1899 the disease reached San Francisco on board one of the Hong Kong ships that had previously infected Hawaii. Thus began an epidemic in the United States that lasted several decades and has traces even today.

The plague continued to spread through the rest of the world, killing millions of persons. By 1918

India reported 10,000,000 human deaths, and between 1920 and 1927 there were an average of 9,000 plague deaths each year in Asia. Egypt, Morocco, and Australia were again visited by plague epidemics, as were central Africa, South Africa, and Madagascar. By 1927 the Soviet Union alone had had 73 separate outbreaks of plague in various places and a total of nearly 4,500 cases. Great Britain and France were hit briefly. Cuba and Puerto Rico had plague epidemics in 1912. Argentina and Peru had repeated outbreaks of the disease, one of which occurred in Peru in 1945 but was halted after four days of intensive DDT insecticide application or spraying.

Major outbreaks of plague occurred in Indonesia, Africa, South America, and Vietnam in the 1960s and 1970s. Since then, isolated cases continue to be reported and minor outbreaks continue periodically. However, because of the development of plague vaccines, antibiotics such as streptomycin and tetracycline, and DDT and other rodenticides, the number of plague cases and the mortality rate due to plague have declined drastically. According to the World Health Organization, the Third Plague Pandemic ended officially in 1959, when only about 200 cases were reported worldwide.

Further reading: Hirst, *The Conquest of Plague*; Gregg, *Plague: An Ancient Disease in the Twentieth Century*.

Portuguese Plagues of the 1400s

Period of several large-scale, destructive epidemics of bubonic plague that invaded Portugal. The first great outbreak, which affected most areas of the country, occurred in 1415. An epidemic of three years' duration broke out in 1435; in 1438 Portugal's King Duarte (Edward) died of plague, transmitted to him, it was believed, through a contaminated letter. Another widespread three-year epidemic occurred from 1479 to 1481. Plague invaded several of Portugal's northern towns in a somewhat less extensive outbreak in 1484. In 1486 the northern coastal city of Oporto, as well as many other localities, suffered the last major epidemic to afflict Portugal until well into the next century. See also SPANISH PLAGUES OF THE 1400S.

Further reading: Ballesteros Rodríguez, *La peste en Córdoba*; de Barcelona, *Datos históricos sobre las epidemias de peste ocurridas en Barcelona*.

Portuguese Plagues of the 1500s

Series of plague epidemics that spanned about 80 years of the sixteenth century and mainly affected Portugal's more populated coastal regions, beginning with a terrible outbreak in 1521, when the seaport city of Oporto was scourged by what was possibly the fulminating type of the disease, the most deadly, horrible, and rare manifestation of plague. As was usual in Portugal and Spain (and elsewhere in Europe) during epidemics of any kind, people who could do so fled the city, an action recognized as the only effective way to avoid the plague. The port city of Lisbon and many other localities were invaded by a deadly outbreak in 1531, which left them depopulated both by death and desertion of their inhabitants; from March to August of 1568 Lisbon suffered a second major epidemic. Oporto again experienced extremely high mortality during a six-month epidemic that started at the end of 1569, and once more in 1581–82, when the city was struck so lethally that King Philip II of Spain sent money to succor its residents. See also SPANISH PLAGUES OF THE 1500s.

Further reading: Ballesteros Rodríguez, *La peste en Córdoba*; Ayuntamiento de Barcelona, *Datos históricos sobre las epidemias de peste ocurridas en Barcelona*.

Príncipe Sleeping Sickness Epidemic of 1898–1913

Alarming outbreak of African sleeping sickness (African trypanosomiasis) on the small, Portuguese-ruled island of Príncipe in the Gulf of Guinea, off the west coast of Africa. More than 3,500 people on Príncipe died during a 15-year epidemic from the tropical disease, which is transmitted to human beings by the bite of the tsetse fly (genus *Glossina*).

During the 1800s Príncipe served as a stopover for African slaves being transported to the Americas. The infective tsetse fly species known as *Glossina palpalis* (called Mosca do Gabão by the Portuguese) arrived in Príncipe with slaves and cattle from Portuguese West Africa (Angola), the Gold Coast (Ghana), and Gabon, all regions where sleeping sickness was endemic. In 1893 and 1894 about 600 black laborers were conscripted from Cassinga (Kassinga), Portuguese West Africa, to work on the cocoa estates in northern Príncipe. Some of the workers arrived already infected; others contracted the disease locally. In 1898 sleeping sickness was killing them sometimes at the rate of ten persons a day; poor working conditions were also taking a toll of lives. In 1901 a fifth of the total fatalities among the workers and others on the estates throughout Príncipe were attributed to sleeping sickness, whose main symptoms include lesions and rashes, chills, severe headache, insomnia, lymph node enlargement, and anemia (leading after about two weeks to body wasting, somnolence, and, frequently, death). The total labor force on the estates fell from about 3,000 persons in 1885 to 800 in 1900 to 350 by 1907, and from 1902 to 1907 sleeping sickness killed a recorded 2,095 people (more than 35 percent of the population, which consisted of Europeans, natives, and conscripted African workers).

The dire loss of African laborers became an economic disaster for the island and forced the Portuguese government to take specific steps to improve the poor working conditions and rid the island of the infectious tsetse fly. Earlier, in 1901, a Portuguese commission (the first ever to deal with sleeping sickness) officially announced the presence of the disease on Príncipe; a second sleeping sickness commission studied the epidemic in 1907 and 1908 and planned a strategy for tsetse fly and disease control. But the Portuguese government did not enforce these two commissions' recommendations until a third commission in 1911 had looked into the epidemic. The recommendations included trapping tsetse flies on sticky clothes (smeared with "rat varnish") and requiring laborers to wear a light hood over their head (with a flap to cover the nape of the neck to ward off the flies). Sanitary brigades were eventually formed (at first made up of 43 war prisoners from the nearby Portuguese island of São Tome); they wore sticky protective clothing, went into the bush, and snared flies while clearing trees and draining swamps. Portuguese doctors relied on inoculations of arsenic in the form of atoxyl to kill the disease's trypanosomes (infectious protozoan agents).

The wild pigs on Príncipe were also responsible for spreading the infection; they were immune to the sting of the tsetse fly and harbored the parasites of the disease. The raising of pigs was forbidden, and pig owners were instructed to destroy their animals. Also, stray dogs and civet cats, hosts to the tsetse flies as well, were ordered destroyed. The tsetse fly population soon petered out, and by 1914 few flies could be found on Príncipe. From 1908 to 1913 there had been 1,255 reported human deaths on the island; in 1913 there were only 136, the lowest annual number of fatalities in 15 years. Príncipe remained free of the disease until 1956, when the tsetse fly reinvaded the island without serious effect.

Further reading: McKelvey Jr., *Man Against Tsetse*; Scott, *A History of Tropical Medicine*.

Prussian Army Dysentery Epidemic of 1792

Dysentery outbreak that struck the 42,000-man army of Prussia's King Frederick William II during its incursion into northeastern France in August 1792. Dysentery spread violently among the Prussian troops, killing or weakening some 12,000 (typhus fever accounted for some of these deaths). After their depleted forces were defeated by the French in the Battle of Valmy on September 20, the sick and demoralized Prussians, led by the Duke of Brunswick (Charles William Ferdinand), gave up the campaign and retreated across the Rhine River into Germany.

More losses were incurred on the march back, as men fought incessant rain, mud, hunger, cold, and lingering illness; corpses and dead horses lined the roads. Brunswick arrived in Germany with less than half his original army, the vast majority dead not from fighting—just 484 died or were wounded at Valmy—but from disease and exposure. Ailing soldiers were left behind, so pursuing French troops and inhabitants of towns through which the armies passed also became infected with dysentery. In the towns of Verdun and Longwy, both of which had been occupied by the Prussians, hospitals were scenes of incredible filth, refuse filled the streets, and dead bodies lay scattered about.

Further reading: Prinzing, *Epidemics Resulting from Wars;* Tranié, *La patrie en danger 1792–1793: Les campagnes de la révolution.*

Prussian Plague of 1602 Devastating outbreak of plague in the Baltic port city of Danzig (Gdańsk, Poland). The epidemic killed some 18,700 people, an enormous number relative to the city's total population, which in 1601 was about 49,000. Some 12,000 human deaths reportedly occurred in just one week; however, this is probably an exaggeration. (Plague was also present in Danzig, although in a less virulent form, in 1601 and 1603.) Königsberg (Kaliningrad), another east Prussian port city, as well as other places in the surrounding region including Riga (in Latvia) and Vilna (Vilnius, Lithuania), also experienced outbreaks of plague during these years (1601 through 1603). Danzig would not see plague again in serious form until 1653 and 1709 (see DANZIG PLAGUE OF 1709).

Further reading: Siegler, *Danzig, Chronik eines Jahrtausends;* Biraben, *Les hommes et la peste en France.*

Prussian Plague of 1709 See DANZIG PLAGUE OF 1709.

Prussian Typhus Epidemics of 1812–14 Virulent outbreaks of epidemic typhus fever in the German provinces of Prussia and Silesia, caused by infected French and Russian forces moving through these areas immediately after Napoleon's campaign in Russia in 1812. Transmitted by the human body louse, typhus spread quickly among unwashed ranks huddled together, first in camps and later in hospitals, while inhabitants quartering troops and working as attendants in hospitals contracted the disease immediately upon contact with the lice-infested soldiers.

French forces in Russia had been decimated by epidemic typhus fever (see NAPOLEON'S ARMY EPIDEMICS IN RUSSIA). Tens of thousands died, abandoned in Moscow and other places along the terrible return march toward Germany. The pursuing Russian Army was ravaged by typhus as well: It killed an estimated 60,000 men. The first eruptions of the disease among the civilian populations in German territory were caused by contact with remnants of the French Army moving through towns and cities of eastern Prussia (present-day Poland). French soldiers who survived the scourge of typhus at the Lithuanian city of Vilnius (Vilna)—where thousands of troops and civilians died—crossed into Prussia at the end of 1812 on their homeward journey, carrying the dreaded fever with them:

> [typhus] fever spread also among the civilians, who were not only afflicted by the terrible scourge of our passing armies, but also became the victims of a murderous contagion. It was a fatal present which we gave them, and which caused such a high mortality among the inhabitants of the country through which we passed. Wherever we went, the inhabitants were filled with terror and refused to quarter the soldiers.

Where people refused to house soldiers they were forced to do so anyway. In the small town of Gumbinnen in eastern Prussia, typhus killed as many as 40 residents per day in January and February 1813, and in Königsberg, annual burials rose 60 percent that year. Altogether, an estimated 20,000 civilians died from typhus fever in eastern Prussia in 1813.

Farther west, the Baltic port of Danzig (Gdańsk, Poland) which was besieged by the Russians from January 11 to November 29, 1813, lost 5,592 citizens to typhus fever, while 11,400 soldiers, one third of the French forces staying there, died in hospitals from January through May. To the south, many places in Silesia were seriously afflicted by typhus from the last months of 1812 until the spring of 1814, mostly due to infected Russian prisoners cared for in military lazarets or lazarettes (provisional hospitals) throughout the region. Breslau's overcrowded hospitals accommodated thousands of soldiers, 1,800 of whom died from typhus from mid-September 1813 to February 1814.

Further reading: Prinzing, *Epidemics Resulting from Wars;* Cloudsley-Thompson, *Insects and History.*

Punjab Malaria Epidemics of 1878–79 Serious epidemics of malaria that hit India's province of Punjab on the heels of a widespread famine in the region. This historic province had enjoyed several years of average and above-average harvests, and the year 1877 began on an upbeat note. However, that year the rainfall was very poor, and the little that fell was unevenly distributed. This in turn destroyed the fall harvest of 1877 and greatly depleted 1878's spring harvest. What began as an acute shortage of food for people and livestock soon worsened into famine. Officially, though, it was still referred to as a minor scarcity. Then the crisis was further compounded when an epidemic of malaria broke out in the region in 1878.

In the first year, the epidemic remained concentrated around the Sutlej River and the towns of Batala, Ludhiana, Jullundur, and Hoshiarpur. Small outbursts of malaria also occurred in the Gurgaon, Delhi, and Rohtak areas. Intensity was highest in October–November 1878 when, according to one source, 180,356 deaths occurred in Punjab province. The city of Amritsar recorded 1,690 human deaths in 1878.

The epidemic of 1879 affected mainly the southern districts of the province, which were deluged that year by extremely heavy rains. Its focus was the town of Hissar and parts of the Gurgaon district, from where it also penetrated western Uttar Pradesh (then the United Provinces). It is estimated that 103,000 people, roughly a seventh of Gurgaon district's population, were killed during 1878–79 (more than 14,000 persons in the month of October 1879 alone). The annual death rate per 1,000 people was 68 in 1878 and 18 in 1879. The excess mortality over normal years was reportedly more than 60,000. In 1879, localized outbreaks also occurred in Ellenabad, Rania, Sirsa, Indri, Butana, and Nisang. One source put the province's registered deaths for October–November 1879 at 141,996.

During the remaining decades of the nineteenth century, epidemic malaria was recurrent in the Punjab. One of the worst was the Punjab Malaria Epidemic of 1908 (q.v.).

Further reading: Christophers, *Malaria in the Punjab*; Hehir, *Malaria in India*.

Punjab Malaria Epidemic of 1908 Devastating and widespread epidemic of malaria in India's northwest province of Punjab. (Punjab means "five rivers" and is so-called from the five tributaries of the Indus flowing through much of it.)

The first inkling of the epidemic's presence came from Lahore, a major city and Punjab's capital, in the fall of 1908. Train services at this junction were seriously hampered when a large number of employees failed to report for work because of fever. Almost simultaneously, the entire central and eastern areas of the province were overrun by malaria; some 50,000 square miles were apparently infected. More than the rural areas, the towns and cities bore the brunt of its impact. In some communities, malaria seemed to have struck almost everyone. Such was the case in Amritsar (population 160,000), where normal activities came to a grinding halt.

Though most of the province came under attack, there were two areas of special intensity—one including Gujarat, Gujranwala, and Shahpur in the north and the other covering Gurgaon, Delhi, and parts of Rohtak in the southeast (see PUNJAB MALARIA EPIDEMICS OF 1878–79). In fact, through the Gurgaon district, the epidemic penetrated into the western part of present-day Uttar Pradesh. Two smaller foci were also noted in Ludhiana and Jullundur. Throughout the province, the mortality figures were staggering especially in October–November 1908. Infant mortality was exceptionally high. Normal mortality in the Punjab for those two months was about 50,000 human deaths; in 1908, 307,316 deaths were recorded for the same period. The Gurgaon district also reported 15,740 deaths in October 1908. The mortality rates for this period varied from district to district: Delhi (149 per 1,000 people), Amritsar (over 200 per 1,000), Gurgaon district (267 per 1,000), Palwal (420 per 1,000), and Bhera (493 per 1,000).

In Amritsar, there was a noticeable increase in malaria admissions late in August 1908, but the seriousness became obvious in mid- to late September when the numbers kept escalating. During the third week of October, for instance, 566 people were treated for malaria at the city hospital. Malaria killed an estimated 7,000 to 10,000 people in the city, a significant proportion of them children under five years of age. Everywhere, though, children below ten years of age figured prominently in the death registers.

Generally, it was observed that areas of highest epidemic intensity coincided with areas of unusually heavy rainfall or flooding. Also, malarial infections were usually more virulent during epidemics, when the risk of contracting malignant tertian malaria increased.

Further reading: Christophers, *Malaria in the Punjab*; Hehir, *Malaria in India*.

Q

Quebec Smallpox Epidemic of 1776

Outbreak of smallpox that badly disrupted American colonial forces assaulting Quebec, Canada, at the start of the American Revolution.

Colonel Benedict Arnold and a force of about 700 rebel New Englanders marched north through the Maine wilderness in the fall of 1775, encamped below Quebec City, and rendezvoused with a second force of some 300 men under General Richard Montgomery, who had advanced from Ticonderoga, seizing Montreal en route (November 12, 1775). On a snowy New Year's Eve 1775 the combined American colonial force attacked Quebec, was repulsed, and Montgomery was killed. Arnold, severely wounded, began a vain siege until spring. Major General John Thomas was sent to Quebec to command the American forces, which had begun to be struck by the smallpox disease in March 1776. At the time nearly a third of the 2,500 American soldiers in Quebec were unfit for duty because of smallpox, which reduced them to 1,900 men (of whom 900 were sick with smallpox) by May. General Thomas, who was a physician, had prohibited self-inoculation because most men who tried it to produce immunity contracted smallpox; yet more than 200 soldiers disregarded Thomas's order in a desperate attempt to avoid the deadly disease. Sadly and ironically, Thomas himself died from smallpox on June 2, 1776.

No one is certain exactly how the smallpox virus came to infect the American troops in Quebec. One theory is that Montgomery's troops brought the disease with them; another is that the British intentionally sent young women from Quebec City who were infected with smallpox to seduce the American soldiers. Regardless, the disease had a profound effect on the soldiers and the outcome of the campaign. At the peak of the epidemic in June and July 1776, reportedly 50 to 60 men died each day. In all, at least 30 army captains perished; one American officer said that he could not look into a tent without seeing at least one dead or dying man. Arnold managed to escape the smallpox, as did Brigadier General John Sullivan, who took over as American commander in Quebec after Thomas died. The British troops were generally immune as a result of having had mild bouts with smallpox in childhood or, in some cases, by having been inoculated. About one third of the American forces succumbed to the disease and, in July 1776, the remaining troops retreated from Quebec and Canada. This meant that the British could now use Canada as a base, march into New York, and isolate New England. A number of historians believe that Quebec certainly would have fallen to the Americans had smallpox not decimated them; the war would likely have ended sooner as a result.

In January 1777 General George Washington procured the approval of Congress to inoculate his entire Continental Army against smallpox.

Further reading: Burt, *The Old Province of Quebec*; Hopkins, *Princes and Peasants: Smallpox in History*; Shurkin, *The Invisible Fire*.

Quebec Yellow Fever Epidemic of 1710

Outbreak of yellow fever, a mosquito-borne disease, that killed untold numbers of people.

This acute, infectious intestinal disease was unknown to Canada until the summer of 1710, when a ship from the West Indies, the *Belle Brune*, arrived at the port of Quebec along the St. Lawrence River with a number of passengers and crew sick with yellow fever. Several of the crew had died of it during the trip from the Caribbean, where the disease was then prevalent. The mosquito vector easily propagated in ship water tanks and bilges. Though the natural habitat of the vector is usually warmer climates in the south, it was able to breed in Quebec's northerly latitude during the intensely hot summer of 1710; because the disease is spread person-to-person by the bite of the mosquito, a large susceptible population is also needed for it to become epidemic. In 1710 the bulk of Quebec's provincial population of about 12,000 people lived in the lower region, close to the port.

At first the disease aboard the *Belle Brune* was thought to be plague, especially when four or five of the men on board died within 24 hours after becoming sick. Furthermore, surgeons, enlisted to examine the sick on the ship, assured Quebec authorities there was no danger to the community; sick men were allowed to disembark for admittance to Quebec's hospital, the Hôtel-Dieu. A male nurse was the first city inhabitant to contract yellow fever; he became fatally ill while wrapping the bodies of the victims from the ship in burial shrouds. His symptoms were the same as all the patients in Quebec who contracted the disease: high fever, delirium, jaundice, and vomiting. At the Hôtel-Dieu, six out of 24 nursing sisters who contracted the disease perished, but outside the facility all of the 12 priests who visited the sick in their own dwellings died from yellow fever. The epidemic raged widely throughout this colony of New France in the summer and fall and ended with the winter frost, by which time Quebec physicians had finally diagnosed the infection as "Mal de Siam," a term given to yellow fever at that time.

Further reading: Cartwright, *Disease and History;* Heagerty, *Four Centuries of Medical History in Canada.*

R

Reading Typhus Epidemic of 1643 Destructive epidemic of lice-borne typhus fever that scourged the Parliamentary army at Reading, to the east of London, in the spring of 1643 during the English Civil Wars. The Earl of Essex besieged Reading with his Parliamentary troops, numbering about 18,000, on April 15 and entered the town upon its surrender on April 26. He found the townspeople suffering from an illness that quickly infected his men, so badly that in June he removed them north to the border of Buckinghamshire, where the disease persisted and grew much worse. Because epidemic typhus fever is transmitted by the human body-louse, the disease was a constant threat to army troops forced to live for long periods of time without washing or changing clothes. Once infected by the inhabitants of Reading, it was inevitable that the fever would spread rapidly through the garrisoned troops. Although mortality figures were not recorded, so many of the Earl of Essex's men died as a result of the fever that he was forced to abandon his plans to attack Oxford, England, where the enemy Royalist troops were stationed (see OXFORD TYPHUS EPIDEMIC OF 1643).

Further reading: Creighton, *A History of Epidemics in Britain*; Zinsser, *Rats, Lice and History*.

Red Influenza Epidemic of 1977–78 See RUSSIAN (RED) INFLUENZA PANDEMIC OF 1977–78.

Rhodesian Smallpox Epidemic of 1946–48 Outbreak of smallpox (variola) that infected a reported 2,689 persons following a country-wide vaccination program in the British colony of Southern Rhodesia (the nation of Rhodesia after 1965, renamed Zimbabwe in 1980). After a grave outburst in 1938, the variola virus continued to be a health problem, and a smallpox vaccination program was undertaken in 1941 that included vaccinating migratory laborers from other African territories; this resulted in Southern Rhodesia being smallpox-free from 1942 to 1945, except for 33 mild cases discovered at Bulawayo

among immigrant workers from Northern Rhodesia (Zambia).

In Southern Rhodesia's sparsely settled western area of Wankie in 1946, smallpox-infected African laborers from neighboring British-ruled Bechuanaland (Botswana) transmitted the very contagious disease to 148 natives, and 33 others in the area caught it that year too. A mass vaccination program did not prevent the disease from spreading to Southern Rhodesia's Matabeleland in the west and south, where 102 persons out of 568 who were infected in 1947 perished. In 1947 there were also 117 smallpox cases reported from localized foci in Mashonaland in the north.

The epidemic persisted in Metabeleland in 1948, with a mortality rate of 35 percent (1,181 cases, of which 413 were fatal), almost double that of the previous year. Most of the 1948 cases occurred in remote areas between Wankie and the Zambezi River, where natives for more than 20 years had been untouched by smallpox and most had little or no immunity. (Probably the natives in the remote regions had not been inoculated with the smallpox vaccine during the 1941 campaign.) The mortality rate overall for the 1946–48 epidemic was 23 percent (at least 614 infected people died). Although widespread vaccination was carried out among the native population in 1948, smallpox continued to break out epidemically in localities throughout Southern Rhodesia in the 1950s, infecting an estimated 3,000 to 7,000 persons each year.

Further reading: Dixon, *Smallpox*; Simmons et al., *Global Epidemiology*.

Rio de Janeiro Smallpox Epidemics of 1904 and 1908 Two severe epidemics responsible for the deaths of over 13,000 persons in Brazil's then capital city of Rio de Janeiro. The deaths were particularly ironic since smallpox (*variola major*) was at the time wholly preventable by inoculation, and smallpox vaccine was widely available in the city. The epidemics took place during the great public health campaign of the reformer President Francisco Rodriguez Alves and his director of public health, Oswaldo Cruz. Cruz sought to transform Rio de Janeiro from an inhospitable backwater perpetually plagued by smallpox and other endemic diseases to a healthful modern metropolis on the European model. Along with the cessation of outbreaks of bubonic plague and yellow fever, Cruz's health campaign sought to eradicate smallpox from the capital city by mass inoculation.

Smallpox arrived in Brazil in 1555 and reached Rio de Janeiro by 1568, where the first epidemics occurred in the late seventeenth century. Thereafter, the disease was considered endemic to Brazil and was present to some extent until wiped out by World Health Organization efforts in 1973. Edward Jenner's vaccine against smallpox was available from 1810 on, and after the creation of a Vaccination Institute in 1846, locally produced (and therefore more potent) vaccine became accessible. In 1904, the first cases of epidemic smallpox were seen in early March. By May, the epidemic had reached alarming proportions; prominently, 31 victims died of smallpox in one day at the Saint Sebastian Hospital. During the last week of July, 309 cases were treated there, 92 of them resulting in death. The number of victims and the number of deaths increased every week thereafter until the last week of August, when 408 smallpox cases were hospitalized at Saint Sebastian, and 137 persons died there of the malady.

Despite the strong efforts of Cruz and other governmental officials to encourage mass inoculation, resistance to the vaccination program was fierce. The press derided Cruz and questioned the wisdom of vaccination. Followers of the positivist movement also rallied against the notion of obligatory vaccination, which they contended violated personal liberty. Along with this formidable organized opposition, wild rumors circulated among the population, which had never been accustomed to taking vaccination seriously, that the vaccine itself was responsible for septicemia and death. Despite these considerable obstacles, the government successfully vaccinated 8,200 persons in May 1904. As the epidemic worsened, more people willingly came forth to be inoculated; there were 18,266 vaccinations in June and 23,021 in July.

In August, however, the fervent anti-vaccination propaganda took its toll, resulting in a sudden drop in vaccinations to only 6,036. The decrease in August was not due to any diminution of immigration by unvaccinated foreigners, who streamed into Rio in search of work. The presence of these foreigners among a largely unvaccinated population of approximately 800,000 created a condition ripe for an epidemic that would take 3,566 lives by the end of 1904. Since smallpox had long been endemic to Rio de Janeiro, that was not an unusually high number of victims (3,944 died of the disease in 1891, and there were over 1,000 victims in both 1895 and 1899). However, in the face of the vigorous anti-variola campaign, the number of smallpox deaths in 1904 was remarkable.

By October, Cruz and his supporters were able to push successfully for passage of a mandatory smallpox vaccination law. The law was widely flouted. There were street riots in opposition to it, and members of the military revolted, leading to the near collapse of the Alves administration. A large part of the city remained unvaccinated at year's end. The residents of Rio de Janeiro would pay dearly for their reticence. After a decrease in smallpox incidence during the years 1905–1907, death rates from smallpox were again high in April of 1908. Two hundred thirty-one perished in that month. At one point, the Saint Sebastian Hospital treated 600 smallpox cases. The government stepped up its anti-smallpox propaganda. Much of the anti-inoculation sentiment of the Brazilian press had been quelled by 1908 in light of the high number of deaths, although agitation against the public health campaign continued among certain extremists. Religious and social customs of some of the populace may have been responsible for spreading the disease. Reports of a funeral for one victim indicate that the corpse was carried through the streets among a throng of unvaccinated positivists. Smallpox, which can be transmitted through contact with corpses, quickly spread through the district. There was great difficulty in convincing the poorer classes of the worth of vaccination. As a result, they suffered greatly during the outbreak.

Traditionally, smallpox in Brazil had been known to affect the black population at a greater rate than the white population (while the reverse was true for yellow fever). However, no district and no class was spared during the 1908 outbreak. Even members of the business class, accustomed to taking modern, hygienic precautions, were not immune. Vaccination gradually became more acceptable as the populace saw that only the unvaccinated were succumbing. By September, the epidemic began to subside. By the end of 1908, over 9,000 had been killed in the outbreak, which then spread from Rio along the central railway line to São Paulo and Santos.

Further reading: Cruls, *Aparência do Rio de Janeiro*; Rosa, *Rio de Janeiro*; Hopkins, *Princes and Peasants: Smallpox in History*; Maul, *O Rio da Bela época*; Guerra, *Osvaldo Cruz*; Stepan, *Beginnings of Brazilian Science*.

Rio de Janeiro Yellow Fever Epidemics of 1849–1902 Yellow fever (*febre amarela*, *bicha* or black vomit), a virus spread by the *Aëdes aegypti* mosquito, was endemic in the city of Rio de Janeiro in the last half of the nineteenth century, taking 70,000 human lives before being brought under control by a successful public health campaign.

While yellow fever had existed in Brazil in epidemic form during the seventeenth century (especially severe in northeastern Brazil in 1660–1694), thereafter it was confined to local outbreaks and was not responsible for large numbers of deaths until November 1849. It is possible that the disease was reintroduced by the crew of an American vessel that docked in New Orleans and Havana, both focal points of the malady, before arriving in Bahia. In any event, a Danish ship with a sick crew sailed from Bahia in late November and set anchor in Rio de Janeiro, at that time Brazil's capital, in early December. The sailors dispersed, some spreading the disease to guests at an inn. By January 4, 1850, medical officials were aware of the presence of yellow fever. The epidemic then spread progressively from one street to the next. By March 1850, the entire city was affected. More than 100 deaths were recorded on a single day in March alone; 4,160 out of 90,658 yellow fever sufferers succumbed to the disease in 1850.

For the remainder of the nineteenth century, yellow fever would plague Rio de Janeiro's populace; in some years the situation would improve, only to return with a vengeance a few years later. Mortality figures for those decades, grouped in five-year periods, indicate the following numbers of yellow fever deaths: 1850–1854—7,448; 1855–1859—2,725; 1860–1864—1,523; 1865–1869—292; 1870–1874—5,922; 1875–1879—7,218; 1880–1884—4,628; 1885–1889—4,935; 1890–1894—14,944; 1895–1899—5,722; and at the turn of the century, 344 deaths in 1900 and 299 in 1901. So frightening were the symptoms of the virus—abrupt onset of headache, backache, fever, commonly jaundice (whence the disease's name), and in the worst cases, the dreaded black vomit (caused by hemorrhaging into mucous membranes), convulsions, coma and death—and so mysterious were its causes, that Rio achieved a reputation as an inhospitable, dangerous city unfit for modern settlement and industrialization by Europeans. The greater propensity of young, white settlers to contract the disease over that of both the older plantation owners and blacks, both of whom had developed immunity due to childhood exposure to the virus, may have slowed the pace of the transfer of economic power from the rural landowning class to the urban capitalists. A cholera epidemic among the black population occurred simultaneously in 1850–70, with its own political ramifications (see ASIATIC CHOLERA PANDEMIC OF 1846–63).

Late-nineteenth-century Rio de Janeiro was a dirty, crowded, and unsanitary city. In 1889, Rio suffered an exceptional summer, with blazing heat and drought. Funerals for the many victims of yellow fever reportedly took place in the cemeteries until all hours of the night, and corpses lay at home for days while awaiting burial. Doctors were among those who succumbed to the virus; 2,115 deaths from yellow fever were reported in that year. This figure was dwarfed by the deaths from the virus in 1891, 1892 and 1894, in each of which years over 4,000 persons were felled.

Among the various theories put forth as to the causes of yellow fever, acceptability was achieved for the mistaken notion that fomites, i.e., infected bed clothes and personal belongings of infected persons, were the primary source of the contagion. The possibility that yellow fever is mosquito-borne was first proposed in 1881 by the Cuban doctor Carlos Finlay. This notion did not gain primacy until U.S. Army studies in Cuba, headed by Walter Reed, proved that the *Aëdes aegypti* mosquito carried the illness. A campaign to eradicate yellow fever in Rio de Janeiro began in 1903 under the leadership of Dr. Oswaldo Cruz. This effort was met with great distrust by the populace, particularly the lower classes, and with fanatical derision in the press. The federal legislature agreed to finance Cruz's Yellow Fever Service (which sought to police suspected zones of infestation, wipe out the foci of mosquitoes, and identify and isolate infected patients) for only three years. The success of the program was swift and complete. In 1902 there had been 984 cases of yellow fever in the city. By 1906, yellow fever officially no longer existed in epidemic form. In 1908 there were only four deaths from the disease, and in 1909 there were none. Although there was a small epidemic in 1928, yellow fever was virtually eradicated from Rio de Janeiro by 1908.

Further reading: Da Silva Araújo, *Fatos e personagens da historia da medicina e da farmacia no Brasil*; Bacellar, *Brazil's Contribution to Tropical Medicine and Malaria*; Freyre, *The Mansions and the Shanties*; Moll, *Aesculapius in Latin America*; Santos, *Chorographia do Districto Federal*; Parahym, *Endemias Brasileiras*; Poppino, *Brazil, the Land and People*; Stepan, *Beginnings of Brazilian Science*.

Roman Pestilence of 451 B.C. Severe outbreak of an unidentified infectious disease that struck the city of Rome and its surrounding countryside. The ancient historians Livy and Dionysius of Halicarnassus describe the devastation of the epidemic, if not its symptoms. Nearly all the slaves died, but other social classes were not immune: The victims included one of the Roman consuls, four tribunes, and numerous senators. Fearful of catching such a contagious disease, people did not want to attend the sick or observe proper burial practices. Instead, they merely threw corpses in the sewers or the river, thereby polluting the supply of drinking water. Food was scarce as well, since the disease attacked animals (cows and sheep) and farmers throughout rural areas.

Without any information on symptoms, modern scholars cannot identify the pestilence with any certainty. It is known, however, that by the middle of the first millennium B.C. both tuberculosis and anthrax were established among domesticated animals and the humans who tended and used them. Either disease is a likely cause of the outbreak of 451 B.C.

Romans in the fifth and fourth centuries B.C. suffered many similar epidemics, ones that hit both humans and their farm herds and that were accompanied by famine. Social unrest often increased during an epidemic, and military campaigns were delayed or abandoned. For instance, the Aequians of Latium had to forgo their plans to attack nearby Rome in 451 B.C. when they, too, succumbed to the disease that had weakened their enemies.

Further reading: Dionysius of Halicarnassus, *Roman Antiquities*; Livy, *History of Rome*; Hare, "The Antiquity of Diseases Caused by Bacteria and Viruses."

Roman Pestilence of 212 B.C. Outbreak of infectious disease, possibly influenza, that struck both the Roman Army as it besieged Syracuse on Sicily, and the city's Carthaginian defenders. The siege was only one battleground of the Second Punic War (218–202 B.C.), in which Rome had been fighting Carthage in Italy and Spain as well. On the Sicilian front the disease may have spread rapidly because of when and where it hit: during an extremely warm autumn, and in a swampy area around the Roman camp. Sick men were left to fend for themselves and dead bodies lay strewn about, since no one wanted to risk catching the disease. Some soldiers even dashed into enemy lines, preferring to die honorably by the sword rather than from illness.

An epic poem by the first-century A.D. Latin writer Silius Italicus describes the disease that brought such fear in the Roman camp. Its victims suffered from shivering and sweating, dry tongue and throat, harsh coughs that often brought up blood, sensitivity to light, extreme thirst, and finally wasting. The symptoms remind one modern scholar of influenza, but any diagnosis based on a literary work can be only speculation. The Roman historian Livy provides no details of the epidemic's nature, but tells us that it

was not always fatal. When the Roman general Marcus Claudius Marcellus took soldiers out of the camp and into the city, relief from the heat revived many of them.

Despite their high mortality, the Romans were at a military advantage after the epidemic. Many Sicilians with the opposing forces fled to their hometowns to avoid the plague, while the Carthaginians perished in greater numbers, even losing their generals to the disease. Until the epidemic, Syracuse had withstood the siege by using artillery and other devices designed by the Greek mathematician Archimedes. But heavy losses on the Syracusan side enabled the Romans to take the city.

Further reading: Livy, *History of Rome*; Silius Italicus, *Punica*; Goodall, *A Short History of the Epidemic Infectious Diseases*; Heichelheim et al., *A History of the Roman People*.

Roman Plague of c. A.D. 165–180 See ANTONINE PLAGUE.

Roman Plague of c. A.D. 251–266 See PLAGUE OF CYPRIAN.

Roman Plague of A.D. 542 See PLAGUE OF JUSTINIAN.

Roman Plague of A.D. 590 Outbreak, almost certainly of bubonic plague, that indirectly changed the course of the medieval papacy. Pope Pelagius II, one of the epidemic's first victims, was succeeded by Gregory the Great, whose accomplishments were considerable: reform of the Catholic liturgy, establishment of the new literary genre of saints' lives, defense of Italy against incursions by the Lombards, and efficient administration of the papacy's vast territorial holdings.

The late sixth-century chronicle by Gregory of Tours includes an account of the epidemic given him by his deacon, who was in Rome at the time. In November 589 the Tiber River overflowed its banks, destroying many granaries. People claimed they saw serpents and dragons floating on the flood waters down to the sea. The pestilence that Gregory of Tours calls "the plague of the groin" (*lues inguinaria*) began a few months later. Although he outlines no specific symptoms, the other information he gives— that the disease killed its victims rapidly and affected all classes and households—also points to bubonic plague. At about the same time similar epidemics raged at Viviers and Avignon in Frankish Gaul (see FRANKISH PLAGUES OF THE SIXTH CENTURY A.D.).

After Pelagius died in February 590, the clergy and the people of Rome unanimously chose the deacon Gregory (Saint Gregory I) as his successor. He had served as prefect of Rome before becoming a church official and a monk—a role he much preferred to that of pope. Gregory was sympathetic, however, to the plight of his fellow Romans. Several days after an impassioned sermon in which he urged them to repent of their sins, he led them in prayers and procession around the churches of Rome. So swift was the plague's attack that 80 marchers died en route.

A later legend has it that as the procession neared Hadrian's Mausoleum, Gregory had a vision: Michael the Archangel sheathed his sword, symbolizing that the plague was over. Gregory's procession became a popular theme in later medieval art.

Further reading: Gregory of Tours, *The History of the Franks*; Paul the Deacon, *History of the Langobards*; Crawfurd, *Plague and Pestilence in Literature and Art*.

Roman Plague of A.D. 680

Severe epidemic, perhaps of bubonic plague, that struck Rome and much of Italy in the summer of A.D. 680; it may have given rise to a new saint's cult. Although Paul the Deacon, Italian Benedictine monk and a primary source, provides no details on symptoms, he does note the widespread mortality: parents were placed on the same bier with their children, and brothers with their sisters. People knew how many in each household would die, he claims, after they saw an angel knocking on the door of the house a certain number of times.

The inhabitants of Pavia in northern Italy went to the mountains to flee the plague; grass and bushes grew in the abandoned streets of their city. Such mass escape, however, would have been difficult in Rome itself, at the time a center for pilgrims, travelers, and religious refugees from East and West. For over a century the Byzantine Empire had been steadily shrinking, because of Lombard campaigns in Italy and Muslim conquests in the Near East and Africa. As these political and military conflicts rocked the Mediterranean world, Rome assumed greater importance as a holy city—the arbiter of Christian dogma and ritual and the home of churches, shrines, and cults. In the sixth and seventh centuries A.D. evergrowing numbers of pilgrims came to Rome, often from the newly converted lands of modern-day France and Great Britain. Once the Muslims took over their lands, Easterners flocked to Rome as well, bringing their religious and iconographic traditions. In the crossroads that Rome was in the late seventh century A.D. a plague epidemic could easily spread, especially since sanitation in the damp, low-lying city was poor and food supplies had dwindled after the Muslims disrupted Mediterranean trade.

It was probably around this time that Sebastian, a martyr from the late third century A.D., became celebrated as a protector against pestilence. According to Paul, the epidemic stopped only after the saint's bones were moved from Rome and set up in the church of San Pietro in Vincoli in Pavia. The Roman church of the same name still contains a mosaic icon of St. Sebastian, perhaps also from this time period, that reflects the artistic influences brought by settlers from the East.

Further reading: Paul the Deacon, *History of the Langobards*; Crawford, *Plague and Pestilence in Literature and Art*; Krautheimer, *Rome: Profile of a City, 312–1308*.

Rome and Naples Plagues of 1656–57

See ITALIAN PLAGUES OF 1656–57.

Russian Cholera Epidemic of 1829–31

Massive epidemic of cholera that invaded much of Russia. It was part of the Asiatic Cholera Pandemic of 1826–37 (q.v.) which, like its predecessor (see ASIATIC CHOLERA PANDEMIC OF 1817–23), originated in India (see INDIAN CHOLERA EPIDEMIC OF 1826–27). More importantly, it marked the beginning of cholera's first and most devastating attack on Europe.

The first case was reported from Orenburg (Chkalov, Russia) on August 26, 1829, followed by several more over the next two weeks. The local medical board took a fortnight to diagnose the disease as cholera and to announce that preventive measures were necessary. According to one account, 747 cases were reported by the end of October and, by November 20, the epidemic had subsided in the city. The infection was apparently carried into Orenburg by caravans from Bukhara or Khiva, where cholera was prevalent among the Kirghiz tribes. In fact, a local commission charged with investigating cholera in Central Asia had confirmed its existence but also rejected the possibility that it might pose a threat because of the vast distances in between. Its report reached St. Petersburg just as Orenburg's first case erupted. This was not surprising since both Bukhara and Khiva carried on a flourishing trade with Orenburg, an important commercial center on the Ural River, which divides European Russia from Central Asia.

Any hopes that the epidemic would remain localized, as did the Astrakhan Cholera Epidemic of 1823 (q.v.), were dashed when cholera was reported from Rasypna on September 28, from Iletsk on October 8, and from Bugulma (nearly 200 miles away) in early November. Cholera also spread 200 miles north and northwest and 60 miles west of Orenburg before disappearing from the region at the end of February 1830. From August 1829 to February 1830, 3,590 cases and 865 deaths (mortality rate was 32 percent) were reported. The military governor of Orenburg ordered a quarantine on October 9. The city was cordoned off and only vendors allowed to continue trading at the barriers. These regulations were not as strict as those for plague and were more loosely enforced. Cholera patients were sequestered, their personal belongings washed separately, and their living quarters fumigated. At first, many fled the city, but otherwise the disease did not cause any undue alarm. The Central Medical Council urged immediate treatment for patients and a longer quarantine period.

Even though the epidemic was far more serious than the Astrakhan outbreak, it did not get any national coverage until August–September 1830, when it had already penetrated the heart of Russia. Preoccupied with political upheavals in Europe and tension in Poland, Czar Nicholas I of Russia delayed any preventive action until August 29, 1830, when his government assumed charge of all cholera regulations and appointed a special cholera commission to spearhead the fight against the disease. Stricter regulations were introduced, but the annual Nizhny Fair was allowed to proceed as usual since the government believed that cholera was not spread by direct contact or through goods. Besides, restrictive quarantine rules against bubonic plague had led to riots at Sevastopol in May 1830 and prompted a more moderate official stance.

Cholera outbreaks were reported from Tbilisi, Tauris (Tabriz), and Elisavetpol (Kirovabad). On July 3, 1830, a military camp outside Astrakhan was struck by virulent cholera that intensified very rapidly and entered the city on July 20. Two hundred people, including the civil governor and the director of police, died within the first 24 hours. Local administration collapsed, leading initially to mass panic and later flight. The epidemic peaked between July 20 and August 15, recording the highest mortality rate of any city in Russia or Europe during the pandemic. The city of Astrakhan (population 37,320) reported 3,633 cases with 2,935 deaths, a 90.8 percent mortality rate. In Astrakhan province (population 328,776), 4,856 out of the 5,912 people affected died (an 82 percent fatality rate) between July 4 and August 27.

Tbilisi suffered a similar devastating attack, and nearly two thirds of its inhabitants fled in panic. Many died within hours of the attack. Baku and Elisavetpol were attacked by a cholera strain from Persia (see PERSIAN CHOLERA EPIDEMIC OF 1829–30) that later merged with the Orenburg strain, reporting 4,557 cases with 1,655 deaths by July 21. Transcaucasia, Kizlian, Katchalinskaia, Guryev, and Uralsk were also invaded. From Astrakhan, the epidemic traveled north to engulf Tzaritzin and Saratov on August 4, 1830 (70 percent mortality), Kazan (60

percent mortality), Nizhny Novgorod (Gorky) (1,887 cases and 1,105 deaths), Moscow (50 percent mortality), Novgorod (30 percent mortality), and eventually the Baltic provinces and Archangel (Arkhangelsk). Another strain spread westward from Saratov and Kazan into Tambov, Voronezh, Poltava, Kursk, Kiev, Podolia, and Kherson—intensifying as it moved west. Between August and November 1830, much of European Russia was affected. In the provinces of Tambov and Kursk, riots broke out and military intervention was needed. Everywhere, cholera caused a major disruption of normal life.

In Moscow, the epidemic apparently began on September 10–11, 1830; official confirmation came three days later. There had been panic in the city weeks prior to the actual outbreak, and thousands of its wealthy citizens had fled. The government announced a series of private and public preventive measures. The citizens joined forces with each other and with the newly created Moscow Cholera Council to combat the disease. A practical and comprehensive quarantine was established for the city and its environs. All frontiers and roads leading from Moscow were sealed and four observation points set up. All merchandise, including the mail, was inspected and fumigated, and any suspected case of cholera was to be reported immediately.

In October, 5,532 cases with 3,102 deaths were reported in Moscow. During this very early phase, very few survived the cholera attack. Even the military garrison there was hard hit, suffering 25 percent of the city's cholera casualties. The Moscow outbreak marked the culmination of the epidemic in 1830. The military cordons were withdrawn on December 6, even though scattered outbreaks continued to occur in the provinces and along Russia's European frontiers during the winter. From September 15, 1830, to January 20, 1831, Moscow recorded 8,431 cholera cases with 4,588 deaths. The Moscow epidemic officially ended in mid-March 1831.

Overall, in 1830, the epidemic affected 68,091 people and killed 37,595 in 31 provinces. In 1831, the situation was far more serious: Cholera raged in 48 provinces, where a total of 466,457 cases and 197,069 deaths were reported. In the spring of 1831, cholera reemerged with greater intensity and was particularly severe in the provinces of Volhynia, Podolia, Grodno, and Vilna. In Moldavia (Moldova) and Wallachia, it merged with an outbreak of plague and was deadly. Podolia became the center of the 1831 epidemic. From Volhynia, cholera was carried by the Russian troops into Poland. Warsaw was attacked on April 14 and Riga in Latvia was hit very violently soon afterward. Russia's ongoing fighting in Poland was considered by many to be the catalyst that sped the entry of cholera into the rest of Europe. Others believed that cholera had entered Poland before the Russian troops did (to quell eventually the Polish Rebellion of 1830–31).

St. Petersburg, which escaped the disease in 1830, was struck in June 1831, despite the strict sanitary cordon and imperial orders banning infected people from entering or leaving the city. Moscow, St. Petersburg, and their surroundings recorded 250,000 cases and over 100,000 deaths in 1831. In St. Petersburg, the anti-cholera commission's brutal policing tactics led to widespread rioting, followed by the most intense phase of the epidemic. Riots also disrupted life in the town of Staraya Russa and in the Novgorod military camps.

During the fall of 1831, cholera generally subsided except for minor outbreaks during the winter and spring of 1831–32. It then moved westward, leaving behind a trail of destruction. Perhaps the only positive aspect of the epidemic was that it spurred the development of Russian medicine and led to the publication of a significant body of cholera studies that helped broaden the general understanding of the disease.

Further reading: McGrew, *Russia and the Cholera, 1823–1832.*

Russian Cholera Epidemic of 1892–93

Major and devastating epidemic of cholera, part of the Asiatic Cholera Pandemic of 1881–96 (q.v.).

Once again, Astrakhan (see ASTRAKHAN CHOLERA EPIDEMIC OF 1823) on the Caspian Sea was the port of entry for the disease that had recently caused much havoc in Afghanistan and Persia (Iran). According to R. Pollitzer (see below), cholera's invasion of Russia began at Baku, also a Caspian port. The populace, already weakened by a severe famine (1891–92), fell an easy prey to the dreaded disease, which spread rapidly across Astrakhan province. Heavy mortality was recorded here; 3,151 (70 percent) of the 4,499 cholera patients who registered between June 14 and July 31, 1892, died. The poor, it seemed, suffered the most, and mobs petrified with fear vented their frustrations by destroying and burning the cholera quarantine barracks, freeing the patients inside, and attacking the medical staff. Troops were dispatched to enforce law and order and quarantine regulations. Strict naval quarantine was imposed on all ships arriving at Astrakhan harbor. Hundreds of migrant workers fled north along the Volga River, spreading the news and the disease as they did so.

As cholera spread upstream along the Volga, it was greeted with more violence and wanton destruction. In Saratov city and province, cholera barracks

and patients met with the same fate. The homes of doctors and prominent police and city leaders were raided by frenzied mobs and a temporarily assigned cholera doctor bludgeoned to death.

Singled out by the disease, the lower classes became convinced that the epidemic had been created by the government in order to destroy certain sections of the population. Thus, government actions intended to alleviate the hardships caused by the epidemic were routinely misinterpreted. However, some of the actions of the administration also fostered this mood of terror and anarchy. Cholera patients were forcibly hospitalized in the barracks, their belongings confiscated, and their homes disinfected. Rioting mobs faced mass arrest, flogging, and death sentences, or they were forced to do hard labor. The ban on large religious meetings and the strict rules regarding funerals (no church services allowed for cholera victims) and burials (ritual bathing of the body not permitted) were unfavorably received. Mass hysteria was thus exacerbated by the government's response to the crisis.

A dedicated group of Russian volunteers, including the famous writer Anton Chekhov, assisted the medical staff by recommending sanitary improvements in factories and villages and urging local authorities to adopt precautions against the advancing epidemic. Their service was generally appreciated both by the masses and by the administration. Although doctors were sometimes regarded with deep suspicion because they were government employees, in many provinces where the physicians were given greater powers, they were successful in gaining the confidence of the people by relaxing key government strictures with regard to hospital admissions, funeral services, and burial rites. This was the case in provinces like Moscow, Simbirsk, Kazan, and Nizhny Novgorod, where the violence that accompanied the epidemic in Astrakhan and Saratov provinces was largely averted.

Though cholera spread to Moscow and St. Petersburg and along the country's western frontiers, mortality was highest in the lower Volga region. Morbidity estimates for 1892 vary greatly (from 433,643 cases to 648,000 cases). Apparently, Moscow's contribution to this figure was a mere 654 cases against 29,332 cases recorded in neighboring Tver (Kalinin). The death toll was 300,321 for the year, officially.

The epidemic of 1892 waned with the advance of winter, but as with previous epidemics, the Russian authorities expected a stronger backlash in 1893 and began preparations to deal with it. When it struck again in 1893, however, cholera was not the force it had been in 1892. A total of 106,600 cases and 42,250 cholera deaths were recorded in 1893, when serious outbreaks of the disease were reported from the Volhynia-Podolsk area.

Famine and cholera, both of which devastated Russia during 1891–93, prompted major reforms in disaster management.

Further reading: Frieden, *Russian Physicians in an Era of Reform and Revolution;* Pollitzer, *Cholera.*

Russian Cholera Epidemic of 1910

Severe epidemic of cholera that struck several provinces in southern Russia.

The outbreak began in June 1910 in the Donets Basin, a major coal production center in Russia (in the eastern Ukraine). It quickly intensified over the following month. More than 200,000 cases of cholera were reported from four Ukrainian districts (Kharkov, Jekaterinoslav, Kherson, and Taurida) and from the Don River army camps. Overall, more than 230,000 cases and 110,000 deaths occurred during this epidemic. Jekaterinoslav (18,894 cases), St. Petersburg (4,591 cases), Kiev (4,077 cases), and Orenburg or Chkalov (3,355 cases) were among those severely hit. The case fatality rate was a staggering 45 percent.

The epidemic's intensity alarmed and stirred into action the Congress of Mining Industrialists of South Russia, the mineowners' organization. Fearing a shortfall in production levels, further spread of the epidemic, and the possibility of popular uprisings, the organization petitioned the Russian government to employ drastic measures to contain it. The Council of Ministers responded to this appeal by passing a resolution at its meeting on July 20, 1910. Thereby, it urged the International Red Cross to urgently dispatch medical teams to the affected area and to appoint a field commander to coordinate the efforts.

Dr. G. E. Rein, appointed to that post, left immediately for the disaster area, accompanied by a battery of various professionals. He soon found that the local authorities did not want to take the initiative and favored stopgap and piecemeal measures. Also, resources were not allocated equally nor were there sufficient trained personnel. The sanitary facilities in most of the mines, Rein found, were grossly inadequate. He requested financial support to fight the epidemic from the mineowners as well as the local authorities. Also, he urged the mineowners to employ emergency sanitary officers and to initiate a campaign to educate their employees regarding basic cleanliness. Rein predicted that epidemic cholera would strike again in the spring of 1911 and urged the continuation of the preventive measures until the summer of that year. Finally, he pleaded with Russia's Czar Nicholas II to establish a separate ministry of public health to deal with the planning and implementation of public health issues nationwide.

From southern Russia the infection was carried, apparently by gypsies, to southern Italy.

Further reading: Hutchinson, *Politics and Public Health in Revolutionary Russia;* Pollitzer, *Cholera.*

Russian Cholera Epidemics of 1915–22

Cholera epidemics that ravaged various parts of Russia during 1915–22 and considered offshoots of pandemic cholera that began about 1899.

Cholera had been particularly unkind to Russia ever since its first entry in 1823 (see ASTRAKHAN CHOLERA EPIDEMIC OF 1823; RUSSIAN CHOLERA EPIDEMIC OF 1910). It broke out again in July–August 1915, as the Russian troops beat a forced retreat from Poland and Galicia, and thousands of them fleeing the danger zones were stranded in hot weather, amid inadequate sanitary conditions in the heart of Russia. Typhus (see RUSSIAN TYPHUS EPIDEMICS OF 1914–22) had already established a strong presence in the camps when cholera struck. Together, the two epidemics coursed through the provinces of Volhynia, Minsk, Mogilev, and Grodno.

The arrival of cholera pressured thousands more into fleeing north toward the Baltic area, south into the Ukraine and New Russia, and east into Central Russia and even Siberia. Cholera traveled with them all across European Russia and beyond the Ural Mountains. The towns lining the main refugee routes suffered severe outbreaks in August–September 1915. More than 66,000 cases of cholera were reported in 1915. The epidemic subsided with the onset of winter.

Then, in April 1918, the Russian regions of Astrakhan and Saratov were visited by an epidemic of cholera. Instead of spreading along the waterways as it had been wont to do, it spread along the rail routes. At its peak in July and August 1918, the epidemic had affected about 30 provinces. A relatively mild outbreak, it ended before the beginning of winter. Overall, 41,586 cases of cholera were reported in the country in 1918. Cholera was fairly quiescent in 1919, when only 5,119 cases were registered.

In 1920, cholera broke out very severely in southern Russia's Rostov area. Almost 30,000 people were affected in that year. The outbreak peaked in July 1921 in the lower Volga River region; 207,389 cases were registered in that year. In 1922, the incidence was lower (86,178 cases), perhaps because by then the cholera vaccine had been administered to over ten million Russians, including everyone in the Red Army. Also, a concerted effort was made to improve the water and sewage systems. Cholera disappeared from Russia (by then, the Soviet Union) after 1927.

Further reading: Sigerist, *Medicine and Health in the Soviet Union;* Pollitzer, *Cholera.*

Russian Diphtheria Epidemic of 1992–93 Severe outbreak of diphtheria that forced the authorities to issue a travel alert for incoming tourists and to launch a massive two-year immunization campaign at home.

Diphtheria is a highly infectious, airborne disease of the upper respiratory system caused by the bacillus *Corynebacterium diphtheriae.* In its more serious manifestations, it can affect the cardiac muscle and the peripheral nervous system, leading to paralysis. Death, particularly in young children, is caused by suffocation due to blocked airways. During the 1960s and 1970s, Russia conducted an effective immunization campaign against the disease that lowered its incidence (morbidity) and removed much of the fear associated with it. Subsequently, however, some parents neglected to have their children vaccinated. Even in 1991, according to the World Health Organization, barely 47 percent of Russian infants below one year of age had been immunized against diphtheria. Adults often avoided vaccination because of rumors of contaminated needles and vaccines.

During the 1980s, diphtheria was once again on the increase in Russia. More than a thousand cases were reported each year from 1983 to 1985 and in 1990. In 1991, there were 1,876 cases and 80 deaths reported throughout the country. The following year, however, it became clear that an epidemic was underway in most of the Russian *oblasts* (administrative regions). Incidence rates were particularly high (ranging between 8.7 and 17 per 100,000 people) in the Moscow, St. Petersburg, Kaliningrad, and Orlov *oblasts.* In 20 regions, incidence among children (7–14 years of age) was far higher than the average for the entire country. For instance, 25 percent of the diphtheria cases reported in Moscow occurred in children below 14 years of age. Outbreaks also occurred among adults working at hospitals, railway stations, and airports. Overall, 3,897 cases (2.6 per 100,000 people) and 125 deaths (0.07 per 100,000 people) were reported in 1992. Forty-seven percent of the deaths were in adults over 40 years of age. The epidemic also spread to the Ukraine (1,553 cases in 1992), Latvia, Belarus, Lithuania, and Norway.

That year, immunization of infants against diphtheria was quite low in Moscow, St. Petersburg and elsewhere. Eighty percent of the country's 16-year-olds—against only 66 percent of Moscow's—were protected with a booster dose of the vaccine. However, no concerted effort was made to immunize adolescents and adults in high-risk groups.

Then, in 1993, the diphtheria epidemic began to intensify, and by September of that year, more than 4,000 cases and 106 deaths (70 percent in adults) had been reported, and the disease was still spreading. Something had to be done. Prior to this epidemic, barely two million of Moscow's 7.5 million adults and a mere 15 percent of the adults nationwide had been immunized. In mid-August, the Russian government announced a two-year national immunization campaign that would ensure the protection of 90 percent of the children and 75 percent of the adults in the country against diphtheria by 1995. The two-year delay was dictated by vaccine shortages. The epidemic caused alarm among many foreigners in Russia; Moscow's two main private health clinics were inundated with foreigners seeking protection against the disease, which had already killed a Belgian woman. The Russian authorities issued a travel advisory urging all tourists to secure vaccination against diphtheria before entering the country (a single booster dose, if their last vaccination was more than ten years old or, for first-timers, two doses at four-week intervals followed by a third dose after six months).

Further reading: Erlanger, "Diphtheria in Russia Worsens, Killing 100 in '93," *New York Times; Weekly Epidemiological Record.*

Russian Epidemics of 1854–56 See CRIMEAN WAR EPIDEMICS.

Russian Ergotism Epidemic of 1722 Epidemic of ergotism in Russia in 1722 that forced Czar Peter the Great (Peter I) to call off a proposed military campaign against the Caucasus chiefs and Persia during the Russo-Persian War of 1722–23.

Ergotism is a disease of the central nervous system caused by eating cereal grains (primarily rye) infected with the ergot fungus (*Claviceps purpurea*). Rye grown on newly cultivated, shady, moist land is particularly vulnerable to the infection. Ergotism can be convulsive (also called spasmodic or creeping) or gangrenous in form, the latter generally known as Saint Anthony's Fire or Holy Fire after the monastic order of Saint Anthony, founded in 1089 by Pope Urban II, that gained repute in treating it. Convulsive ergotism affects the spinal cord; other symptoms include numbness of the extremities, vomiting, diarrhea, headache, vertigo, noises in the ear, lassitude, insomnia, extreme hunger, delusions, and convulsions. Gangrenous ergotism is characterized by itchy, burning feet, blisters, and loss of sensation in the affected part, followed by recovery in mild cases and by dry gangrene in severe cases. Low-grade fever is a persistent feature. Death results from sheer exhaustion or septicemia.

The Russian epidemic, caused by the ingestion of bread made from ergot-infested rye, unexpectedly affected thousands of people. The death toll was reportedly around 20,000. Among these were thousands of soldiers from the Russian Army who were stationed in camps along the Volga River en route to the Caucasus and Persia. The strength of the troops was so greatly depleted and the survivors so severely weakened that the czar had no choice but to abort his proposed campaign.

Further reading: Cornell Jr., *The Great International Disaster Book;* Kiple ed., *The Cambridge World History of Human Disease.*

Russian Influenza Epidemic of 1918–19

Russian Influenza Epidemic of 1918–19   Severe and widespread outbreak of influenza, part of the Spanish Influenza Epidemic of 1917–19 (q.v.).

Despite the apparent severity and penetration of the epidemic in Russia, little is known about it. No doubt the Russian Revolution (1917) and the chaotic and crisis-ridden political climate made official records of the epidemic hard to keep and harder to obtain. Prisoners returning from Germany are believed to have introduced the disease into the country sometime during the third quarter of 1918 because, by the end of that year, it was very widespread across the country. It is one of the few epidemics that invaded Russia from the west, instead of the east.

The epidemic was particularly intense in the Ukraine. About 70,000 people were reportedly affected in Odessa (population 500,000) around mid-October 1918. The city of Archangel (Arkhangelsk, near the Arctic Circle, on the northern Dvina River) and its suburbs were also infected this time; the outbreak persisted there until December. Although precise mortality statistics are not available, V. M. Zhdanov (see below) has reported some figures for four major cities for 1918–19. According to him, the mortality rate per 100,000 people during 1918 was 35.7 in Moscow, 67.3 in Saratov, 94.2 in Petrograd (St. Petersburg), and 100.7 in Odessa. The corresponding figures for 1919 were: Moscow (39.9), Saratov (33.7), Petrograd (57.9), and Odessa (66.0). These figures indicate an overall mortality considerably lower than that experienced by many European cities.

Further reading: Zhdanov et al., *The Study of Influenza; Reports on Public Health and Medical Subjects.*

Russian Influenza Epidemics of 1925–50

Russian Influenza Epidemics of 1925–50   Periodic outbreaks of influenza (flu) in Russia.

The first of these epidemics began in July 1925, when there was a noticeable rise in influenza cases. Morbidity (disease incidence) increased very gradually through the rest of the year and did not pick up momentum until late January 1926. Over the next few months, flu spread across the country. Attack rates were high, but the disease was very mild and mortality was low, except among the very young and the elderly. The attack rate in the city of Moscow and its *oblast* (region) ranged between 58.6 to 246.4 per 10,000 people. The epidemic subsided briefly during the summer, but incidence began increasing again during the fall and winter of 1926–27 and was quite high between February and April 1927. After that, it began to decline. Influenza was prevalent over much of Europe during this period.

Russians again suffered a flu epidemic in 1936–37. (Flu was previously observed in New York in December 1936 and affected the North American and European continents, China, and Japan.) It is not known when the epidemic began in Russia, but it peaked in Moscow at the end of February 1937 and in Leningrad (St. Petersburg) early in March 1937. These type A flu outbreaks lasted about 45 days in each of the cities; the attacks were not severe and mortality was not high. It was during this epidemic that researchers discovered the ability of the influenza virus to alter its antigenic properties, giving rise to several new strains.

During 1943, when flu was once again breaking out in England and the United States, an epidemic reportedly began in Moscow at the end of November and peaked in mid-December. Nearly 18 percent of the city's inhabitants were infected over the course (40 days) of the epidemic. In Leningrad, then under the most prolonged military siege of World War II, an epidemic began on December 9 or 10 and peaked early in January 1944. It lingered for about 55 days in Leningrad; while the attack rate was high, mortality was lower than in the epidemic of 1936–37.

From December 1946 to March 1947, Russia was again invaded by flu, this time caused by the variant type B virus, which affected many. In the winter of 1949–50, another epidemic of type B flu broke out in several major Russian cities. In Krasnodar, it peaked during November and December 1949, and many other cities were affected before the epidemic peaked in Moscow between December 1949 and January 1950. Generally, though, it was a prolonged but mild outbreak. See also RUSSIAN INFLUENZA EPIDEMIC OF 1918–19; RUSSIAN INFLUENZA EPIDEMIC OF 1964–65.

Further reading: Zhdanov et al., *The Study of Influenza.*

Russian Influenza Epidemic of 1964–65

Russian Influenza Epidemic of 1964–65   Widespread epidemic of influenza affecting most regions of the former Soviet Union (commonly called Russia). Influenza, caused by a variant of the second A-strain virus, arrived in Leningrad (St. Petersburg) from eastern Germany between December 28 and 30, 1964, and was first observed in Moscow on January 18, 1965. During February, most of the major cities in

Russia, Ukraine, and Byelorussia, and in the Central Asian republics recorded influenza outbreaks. In most towns, the epidemic peaked between nine and 17 days after onset and was over within 25 to 30 days on average. Most of the country was invaded between January and March 1965. Its rise and decline was not as rapid and steep as that of the Russian Influenza Epidemic of 1968–69 (q.v.).

It also differed from the later epidemic in that the attack rate among children below 15 years of age was extremely high, especially during the early stages. In the Russian city of Sverdlovsk, for instance, morbidity among children in this group was two to two-and-a-half times greater than among adults. In the country of Latvia (then a Russian satellite), 50 percent to 54 percent of the children under 14 years of age were infected. In Erivan, Kiev, Kazan, and some other cities, the situation was similar. Overall morbidity during this epidemic was 11.2 percent. The highest attack rates were reported in Moscow (36.9 percent) and Leningrad (35.7 percent), the lowest in Vladivostok (13.8 percent), where the epidemic's intensity was somewhat diluted. From Russia, the flu traveled to Finland, Sweden, Poland, Hungary, and Rumania.

Further reading: Zhdanov and Antonova, "The Hong Kong Influenza Virus Epidemic in the USSR."

Russian Influenza Epidemic of 1968–69

Prolonged outbreak of influenza in many countries of the former Soviet Union (commonly called Russia), part of the Hong Kong Influenza Pandemic of 1968 (q.v.).

The epidemic's presence was first noted in groups of adults and in a school in Moscow in mid-December 1968. Around the same time, influenza was also on the increase in the cities of Frunze and Dushanbe (formerly Stalinabad), peaking there late in December. The culprit was discovered to be the "Hong Kong" flu virus, which spread in January 1969 to parts of the Central Asian and Transcaucasian regions of the vast Soviet Union. From the central area of European Russia, the epidemic once again headed toward Moscow, Leningrad (St. Petersburg), and Tallinn. In February, the disease invaded the Baltic areas, Byelorussia, Ukraine, and Moldavia (Moldova), and then traveled east on the main railway line. Over a two-month period, the whole country was infected.

On January 6, 1969, there was a dramatic rise in influenza cases in both Moscow and Leningrad, almost double that of January 3, 1969. On January 13, the incidence was double that of January 6. In both cities, the epidemic continued to rise until the end of the month. By the end of January, about 77,500

clinically confirmed influenza cases had been reported in Moscow and 39,500 in Leningrad. The infection hovered around Moscow, Riga, Kharkov, Alma Ata, and other cities for more than a month. In April, influenza cases began declining, but the incidence of acute respiratory disease (ARD) increased appreciably. During May–June, numbers dropped to pre-epidemic levels in both categories.

Widely dispersed and slow moving (it lasted four months), the epidemic was of moderate intensity. Most of the complications were pulmonary in character. Children under seven years of age (particularly those below two years) suffered a 14 percent to 25 percent attack rate during the first quarter of 1969 and a 30 percent to 45 percent attack rate (especially in Archangel, Kazan, and Dushanbe) during the second quarter of 1969. Some 30 million people (then 12.4 percent of the population) were infected during this epidemic, compared to 11.2 percent during the Russian Influenza Epidemic of 1964–65 (q.v.). The average duration in most towns was 50 to 80 days and, at its height, the recorded incidence was lower than that of the epidemic of 1964–65. A number of anti-epidemic measures introduced by the public health authorities may have robbed the epidemic of some of its intensity and greatly reduced the number of fatalities.

Further reading: Zhdanov and Antonova, "The Hong Kong Influenza Virus Epidemic in the USSR."

Russian (Red) Influenza Pandemic of 1977–78

Major epidemic of influenza that actually began in China but did not receive attention until outbreaks were reported from Russia in November 1977.

The first "flu" outbreaks occurred in Tientsin (Tianjin) and in Liaoning province in northeastern China in May 1977. Most of those attacked were children in the 7 to 12 year age-group. The attack rate for this group ranged between 25 percent and 50 percent. The infectious agent was later discovered to be a subtype of the H1N1 influenza virus, which had been dominant during 1947–57 but disappeared thereafter (see ASIAN INFLUENZA PANDEMIC OF 1957–58; HONG KONG INFLUENZA PANDEMIC OF 1968). The epidemic spread south across China between June and October. By November 1977, it had reached Hong Kong, the Philippines, Singapore, and Vladivostok, to the north. Russian virologists drew the attention of the international community to this outbreak in Vladivostok. Meanwhile, within Russia, the virus traveled west to arrive in Moscow in December 1977. Even here, it mainly attacked children and young adults in the 10 to 20 year age-group.

From Moscow, the epidemic spread to Europe. In Britain and most of western Europe, the outbreaks began in January 1978. During the same month, outbreaks were reported from Japan, Indochina, and Indonesia in the east. Across the Atlantic Ocean, outbreaks also occurred in the United States in January. In February, the virus was associated with causing influenza epidemics in the Scandinavian countries, southern France, Italy, Greece, Israel, and in more cities in the United States and Canada. In March 1978, influenza broke out in Panama, Denmark, and southeastern Australia, and in April in Argentina and the Pacific Islands. Chile and Brazil were infected in May and New Zealand in June 1978. Thus, over a one-year period, the epidemic had spread over many continents. More countries in the southern hemisphere came under attack from this virus in March and April 1979.

In the United States, this virus (A/USSR/77) raged concurrently (the first time this has ever happened) with the Victoria and Texas strains of the H3N2 subtype, which affected people of all ages. Mortality in that country during this epidemic was higher than elsewhere because of the different subtypes involved. Elsewhere in the world, people above 21 years of age who had presumably been exposed to this virus during its previous appearance in 1947–57, remained immune to it.

Further reading: Pyle, *The Diffusion of Influenza;* Beveridge, *Influenza: The Last Great Plague.*

Russian Malaria Epidemic of 1922–23

Perhaps Europe's most devastating malaria epidemic of the modern era, killing millions of people. It is sometimes referred to as a pandemic because of its extent and intensity.

It began in the central Volga River basin—one of Russia's three main malaria centers—and spread north, even penetrating the Arctic region for the first time. The Volga basin had received no rain for two years in a row. Crops failed, livestock perished, and thousands of people were forced out of the area in search of greener pastures, where they became acquainted with new types of malaria. Those who remained behind were considerably weakened by scarcity of food and water and fell easy prey to disease. Eventually rain fell and the Volga flooded vast areas of plain along its left bank. When summer came the floods receded, leaving behind marshy tracts, ideal breeding grounds for malaria-carrying anopheles mosquitoes. New parasites were also brought in by the masses who returned home.

More than 2.4 million people (186 per 10,000 people) were infected in 1922, while the morbidity for 1923 was in excess of five million (415 per 10,000 people). According to another estimate, at least 12 million people were infected during these two years.

In some areas of the Volga basin, the Caucasus, and central Asia, the attack rate ranged between 75 percent and 100 percent. Sixty thousand people died of malaria in Russia during each of those years. The country's meager quinine supplies—a mere 8,000 to 10,000 kilograms at the peak of the epidemic—could not possibly be sufficient to treat the millions who were suffering, and a blockade ensured that no new supplies could come in. Despite heroic efforts by the Soviet authorities, cases of malaria remained in the millions through the remainder of this decade and part of the next.

Early in the 1920s, the Institute of Malaria, Medical Parasitology, and Helminthology was established in Moscow. Also, the number of rural anti-malaria stations (each equipped with a dispensary, hospital, and laboratory) was expanded from eight in 1921 to 33 in 1922 to 139 in 1924. The first All-Union Malaria Conference met in 1923 and regularly thereafter, and Soviet physicians were given special training in malarial work. With the active cooperation of the relevant government departments, swamps were drained, water sheds treated with petroleum, and public education campaigns carried out. In the infected areas, quinine was distributed more efficiently and people examined for signs of the disease. Between 1925 and 1927, antimalaria laws were enacted and a malaria control fund established from the proceeds of a special tax levied on peat sales. All these efforts bore fruit more than a decade later, when malaria incidence in Russia finally began to decline.

Further reading: Bruce-Chwatt, "Malaria Research and Eradication in the USSR"; Sigerist, *Medicine and Health in the Soviet Union.*

Russian Plague of 1738–39

Epidemic of bubonic plague that invaded the south-central region of the Russian empire and accelerated the end of the Russo-Turkish War of 1736–39.

The plague outbreak occurred in the spring of 1738 among the Russian troops at newly captured Ochakov, formerly a Turkish fortress on the Black Sea. Plague had reappeared at Ochakov almost every summer, but it is not known whether this outbreak began locally or was the result of importation from the Balkans or the Kuban (southeast Russia), where plague had raged during the previous year. At any rate, the presence of thousands of soldiers in an area known to be plague-infested, and the mild winter of 1737–38, combined to create conditions ideal for the outbreak of the disease.

Already, during the fall and winter of 1737–38, Russian soldiers in the unit commanded by General Stoffeln at Ochakov were falling ill and dying by the hundreds. More than 1,000 soldiers died in January 1738 alone—a fact that Field Marshal Münnich attributed to scurvy, caused by poor and inadequate rations, impure water, and cramped living quarters. Thus, when plague broke out among these troops in the spring of 1738, it was hardly noticed at first. Then, in mid-June, General Stoffeln reported the loss of 1,722 soldiers over a six-week period, and it became clear that the presence of the deadly disease among them could no longer be ignored. Along with other diseases, plague plowed through entire units at Ochakov and the nearby garrison at Kinburn (in Moldova), killing hundreds. When General Stoffeln returned to the Ukraine in September 1738, less than one third of his soldiers returned with him. Overall, Russia lost 30,000 soldiers that year—many of them to plague.

The epidemic did not spare civilians either. In the Ukraine, garrison towns and the capital of the Zaporozhian cossacks were severely attacked. At Izium, crowds gathered for the annual summer fair were struck by plague in mid-June 1738. For over two months, the entire area was terrorized by the disease, which reportedly killed thousands. Many fled in panic and the streets were littered with human corpses and animal carcasses. In Kharkov, a town in southern Ukraine, 800 people succumbed to the plague, 500 of them in October alone. By December, with the onset of cold weather, the epidemic had left the area.

In 1739, plague invaded the Russian town of Azov and nearby settlements along the Don River. Small outbreaks were reported as far north as the city of Kursk. However, the winter of 1739–40 was unusually severe in southern Russia and the spread of the epidemic was arrested.

This epidemic did not invade any major cities (see ASTRAKHAN PLAGUE OF 1727–28) and remained confined to the huge, sparsely populated region of south-central Russia. Nevertheless, it caused a disproportionate hysteria and prompted the Russian imperial government to introduce rigid quarantine measures. A cordon was drawn up along the Dnieper River and, when the epidemic entered the Russian Ukraine, also between Ukraine and Russia and between southern and central Russia. An ad hoc committee (including many doctors) assumed charge of all administrative and medical activities relating to plague prevention. Special precautions were taken to prevent plague from reaching Moscow. Checkpoints were set up 100 miles south of the city and medical supplies for 100,000 people kept in readiness. Also, dispatches from the south were rewritten at a special office established in the suburbs by the post office. The cordon around Moscow was not withdrawn until

mid-1739, while restrictions in Azov were lifted only in July 1740.

Further reading: Alexander, *Bubonic Plague in Early Modern Russia.*

Russian Typhus Epidemics of 1914–22

Massive epidemics of louse-borne typhus that devastated Russia (the Soviet Union) during and after World War I.

Morbidity from typhus fever had been consistently high in Russia for many years before the war began. When war erupted, the mobilization of troops and the exodus of refugees fleeing the combat zones for the interior regions of the country, created ideal conditions for the spread of this disease. In fact, by the end of 1914, epidemic typhus was raging in the provinces of Kaluga, Voronezh, Riazan (Ryazan), and the Povol'zhe. The authorities acted promptly to set up isolation hospitals and improve sanitary facilities. Even as their efforts were in progress, the already overburdened hospitals received a constant influx of war prisoners transferred by train from the battlefronts into the heart of Russia. Many of the Turkish prisoners, for instance, were brought in from the Caucasus region, where typhus was rampant. They later carried the infection to Samara in northern Iraq. By January 1915, the typhus epidemic had spread to Tambov, Iaroslavl, and other Russian provinces.

The forced retreat of Russian troops from Poland and Galicia in July–August 1915 led to another exodus of refugees into central Russia, further straining the grossly inadequate sanitary facilities. Very soon, cholera broke out in the typhus-ridden camps (see RUSSIAN CHOLERA EPIDEMICS OF 1915–22). Epidemics of both diseases raged concurrently in Volhynia, Minsk, Mogilev, and Grodno provinces. Cholera subsided with the onset of cooler weather, but by then the refugees had already carried it across the country. At the end of 1915, 154,800 cases of typhus had been officially registered; the epidemic had apparently affected more than 30 Russian provinces.

In the winter of 1917–18, there was a localized outbreak of typhus in Petrograd (St. Petersburg). It was, however, contained within a relatively short period.

Then, in the autumn of 1918, typhus fever attacked Russia from three sides—from Petrograd, from across the Rumanian border, and from the Volga River basin. It eventually spread over much of the country and lingered for several years. According to one estimate, five million people were infected during 1919–22 alone. A Russian epidemiologist, Tarassevitch, estimated there were a staggering 30 million cases, but this is generally believed to be too high.

By the end of 1918, official statistics recorded 130,164 cases (21.9 per 10,000 people), in 1919 over two million cases (265.3 per 10,000), and in 1920 over three million cases. The country was in the midst of a civil war and the constant movement of civilians and soldiers aided the rapid spread of the disease. Also, the Allied blockade meant that the country was denied access to even basic medical supplies. A tremendous scarcity of soap and fuel (for disinfectant use) exacerbated the situation. The epidemic (or pandemic, as it has been called) peaked in 1920, subsided briefly in 1921 (633,250 cases, 54.0 per 10,000), but reappeared in 1922 to infect more than one million people, mainly in the famine-threatened Volga region.

Clearly, it was one of the worst and most extensive disasters of all time. Mortality reached ten percent. Russian authorities were completely overpowered in their efforts to fight the disease. Quarantine stations were established at various railway junctions, where patients arriving by train were isolated. Two hundred and fifty thousand beds were set aside to treat patients suffering from typhus and other infectious diseases. Other passengers were bathed and disinfected. In some towns, entire areas were disinfected. An extensive educational campaign alerted people to the dangers of the disease. These efforts were spearheaded by the newly formed Central Epidemics Commission.

The epidemic subsided after 1923, but typhus continued to infect thousands of Russians until late into the decade.

Further reading: Hutchinson, *Politics and Public Health in Revolutionary Russia;* Sigerist, *Medicine and Health in the Soviet Union.*

Rwandan Cholera Epidemic of 1994   Sudden cata-

strophic outbreak of cholera in central Africa, among an estimated 1.2 million Rwandan refugees encamped on the outskirts of Goma in eastern Zaire, on the border of Rwanda. In mid-July 1994 the refugees (virtually all Hutus, the ethnic majority of Rwanda's population) fled into Zaire from advancing Tutsi rebel forces, who had recently overthrown Rwanda's Hutu-based government during a three-month-long civil war. After the death of Rwanda's president (a Hutu) in a mysterious plane crash on April 6, 1994, the Hutu leaders and army had waged a brutal genocidal campaign against the minority Tutsi people

(blamed for the president's death). However, the Tutsi-led Rwandan Patriotic Front seized control of most of the country and then began a retaliatory slaughter of the Hutus, many of whom fled into Zaire, Tanzania, and other lands. Out of the 7.5 million people who lived in Rwanda (about the size of Maryland) before the civil war, some 500,000 died, 2.5 million were displaced inside the country, and 2.4 million became refugees in neighboring countries.

In the teeming refugee camps around Goma, living conditions were filthy, with lack of clean water and sanitation facilities. Men, women, and children wandered in search of fresh water and food only to find some slimy, befouled sustenance that did more to spread cholera and other diseases than allay thirst and hunger. Within 24 hours after the first confirmed cases of cholera (July 20), more than a thousand persons were dead from this fiercely contagious intestinal disease, which causes diarrhea, vomiting, dehydration, acidosis, and circulatory collapse.

During the following days, dead bodies of cholera victims lined the dusty roadways and littered the fields, and relief workers began to pile up hundreds of corpses, which they doused in chlorine for disinfection and to speed the decomposition of the bodies. Refugees and relief workers wore handkerchiefs, scarves, and surgical masks to try to block the acrid stench of rotting bodies, which were buried in hastily dug mass graves. French Army soldiers helped supervise the burials as quickly as possible and helped the Red Cross and volunteer physicians treat the sick and survivors amid the squalor and filth. The deteriorating conditions in the camps drove many refugees into despairing passivity or crazed terror. During July and August 1994 in Goma, more than 50,000 men, women, and children died of malnutrition, cholera, dysentery, and other diseases in the fetid, crowded camps, overwhelmed in mud, human waste, piles of garbage, and swarms of flies.

The Rwandan mass exodus and subsequent epidemic prompted a vast and sustained international relief effort to speed the flow of medical supplies and clean water and food to the refugee camps in eastern Zaire (Goma, Bukavu, and Uvira), western Tanzania (Benaco and Ngara), and Burundi (Ngozi, Kirundo, and Muyinga).

Further reading: *The New York Times,* July and August 1994 (numerous articles).

S

St. John's Dance   See DANCING MANIA.

St. Louis Yellow Fever Epidemic of 1778   See SENEGALESE YELLOW FEVER EPIDEMIC OF 1778.

St. Vitus's Dance   See DANCING MANIA.

Samoan Influenza Epidemics of the 1800s   Successive influenza outbreaks that occurred in the Samoa Islands in the southwest Pacific Ocean. Influenza was apparently introduced into the Samoan island of Savaii by the English missionary John Williams when he arrived with his group on the *Messenger of Peace* in 1830. Subsequently, the disease erupted to cause major and minor outbreaks almost on an annual basis. According to some, the first major epidemic struck in May 1837, but no details are available to substantiate this claim.

Two years later, there was another outbreak whose presence was well documented by missionaries on the various islands. According to a missionary at the village of Pago Pago on Tutuila, influenza gripped this island during April 1839, and 30 to 40 human deaths occurred. Around the same time, the disease was also widespread on the island of Upolu. Apparently, it was quite mild to start with but rapidly turned serious when secondary complications, mainly pulmonary, set in. These killed many people long after the actual epidemic had subsided.

The next epidemic struck in November 1846 and persisted through January 1847. Judging by contemporary accounts, it was an extremely severe and fatal outbreak. According to one report, 60 deaths occurred in one district with a population of 2,500, and many more in the humid and damp areas.

No further outbreaks of influenza were reported until 1891, but in the interim dysentery, mumps, and whooping cough infected the Samoans. The influenza epidemic of 1891 was quite extensive and reportedly killed many people on the larger, more populous islands (Savaii, Tutuila, and Upolu).

Together, all these epidemics had a marked impact on the strength and endurance of the Samoans. But the most devastating influenza epidemic was still to come (see SOUTH PACIFIC ISLANDS INFLUENZA EPIDEMIC OF 1918–19).

Further reading: McArthur, *Island Populations of the Pacific.*

Samoan Influenza Epidemic of 1918–19   See SOUTH PACIFIC ISLANDS INFLUENZA EPIDEMIC OF 1918–19.

Samoan Whooping Cough Epidemics   Outbreaks of whooping cough (pertussis) that ripped through the Samoan Islands in the South Pacific several times during the nineteenth and twentieth centuries.

Whooping cough was introduced into Samoa in 1849 by a shipping vessel from Tahiti. It quickly spread over these islands, affecting many people. At the same time, civil war had been raging in several parts of Samoa since 1848. Together, these two events (war and disease) had a disastrous effect on the country; over an 18-month period, at least five percent of the Samoan population became a casualty of one or the other. On Upolu, it appears, many children died of whooping cough. Also, it is recorded that the epidemic claimed 150 lives on the northern coast of Savaii (Samoa's largest island) over a few months.

In 1907, the islands of Western Samoa suffered an epidemic of whooping cough in which many children died. There were further epidemics in 1926, 1936–37 (in which about 400 children died), and 1950.

Whooping cough is an acute bacterial infection of the trachea, bronchi, and bronchioles caused by the bacterium *Haemophilus pertussis* or *Bordetella pertussis*. Mainly a childhood disease, it spreads through direct contact with an infected patient or articles. While the overall fatality rate is low, nearly 70 percent of the deaths occur in children less than one year old. The typical "whooping" sound—a loud, spasmodic cough with difficulty in catching the breath—occurs when a child or adult inhales between coughs; vomiting may result after coughing spells. The infection is contagious while the cough lasts (up to a month). Immunization is recommended for all infants at an early age.

Further reading: McArthur, *Island Populations of the Pacific;* Simmons et al. *Global Epidemiology.*

San Francisco Plague of 1900–04   First known epidemic of bubonic plague in continental North America, resulting in 122 cases and 121 fatalities. In San Francisco, those who died ranged in age between four and 62 years old. The majority were between the ages of 20 and 50, which reflected the population distribution in San Francisco's Chinatown, where the disease hit the hardest; 27 plague victims were women.

The *S.S. Nippon Maru* arrived in San Francisco from China via Hawaii. In 1899, it had carried the plague disease into Honolulu, so in San Francisco the ship was quarantined, despite the absence of any cases on board. It is possible that rats from the ship carried infection ashore. A Chinese man in San Francisco's Chinatown died of plague on March 6, 1900, the 35th day of the Chinese Year of the Rat (see HAWAIIAN PLAGUE OF 1899–1900).

This San Francisco epidemic was one of the most notorious scandals in the annals of U.S. public health. San Francisco's quarantine officer performed the necessary clinical tests to prove the disease was bubonic plague. The city Board of Health chairman, Dr. J. M. Williamson, placed Chinatown under quarantine and conducted a search for more human plague victims; two were found. However, conservative business people of San Francisco, fearing that news of plague would destroy commerce, fought every effort to control or even acknowledge the presence of plague. The quarantine was canceled, but inspectors examined everyone (especially the Chinese) trying to leave the city, which split the quarantine effort into two factions. One faction advocated controlling the disease and included the city government and public health board, many California physicians, the San Francisco Medical Society, the U.S. Marine Hospital, and the *Occidental Medical Journal.* The other faction, which attempted to suppress news of the disease, included the business community, Governor Henry T. Gage of California, Chinese who bristled at the seeming racist enforcement of the quarantine, most other residents, newspapers, *Pacific Medical and Surgical Journal,* and a medical society that had backed the governor politically.

On March 21, 1900, the Associated Press announced that San Francisco was the host of a plague outbreak. The state of Texas barred entry to all people or goods from California on April 1. San Francisco's Board of Health officially recognized the plague in an announcement on May 17, 1900. Although measures against the disease in Chinatown were attempted by the Board of Health, the Chinese were granted a restraining order because of the racial overtones of the quarantine, which was to affect only the Chinese. Later, city supervisors placed Chinatown in quarantine; the California State Board of Health agreed with the decision. Meanwhile, Colorado also refused entry to people or goods from California.

But Governor Gage refused to entertain any notion of plague in San Francisco and replaced the members of the state's Board of Health with his own people. At the same time, he cut funds to the San Francisco Board of Health, and his new state health board issued a 1900–1902 report that did not mention the 61 known deaths from plague or the disease itself. Before this, Governor Gage had denounced the plague as a fraud, brought in from the outside. The governor's faction argued that no human being had carried the plague into San Francisco, and therefore, it could not exist. They chose to ignore the *S.S. Nippon Maru*'s past history.

Federal officials then stepped in to investigate the matter, despite interference from state officers, and confirmed the plague one year after the first plague death had been discovered. The California governor had fought the federal officials every step of the way, even objecting to the U.S. president and shutting down University of California research facilities used by the federal investigators. Despite Governor Gage, the business community and others had come to recognize that the notoriety created by the plague had to be resolved by eliminating the disease threat. Business had been disrupted, and California had become completely isolated and quarantined by other states and countries internationally.

In April 1901, a cleanup of Chinatown left every house hygienically scoured. After cleaning, each house was treated with mercuric chloride; furnishings were aired outdoors, and stuffy rooms and basements were whitewashed. Houses that had held plague victims were fumigated with sulfur dioxide.

Governor Gage continued to deny publicly a plague epidemic, blaming the deaths on syphilis among the Chinese. (This aspersion became typical in America when plague afflicted minorities.) Although Governor Gage bragged that he had saved the state money by scrimping on spending the funds allotted for the epidemic, the threat of plague had totally disrupted mercantilism because no person or company would do business with California. George C. Pardee, M.D., Ph.D., was elected California governor at the end of Gage's term, and instituted good public health practices, soundly upheld the plague findings, and reinstituted the original state public health board. The last San Francisco plague victim died on February 29, 1904, in Concord, California. See also SAN FRANCISCO PLAGUE OF 1907–09.

Further reading: Gregg, *Plague: An Ancient Disease in the Twentieth Century;* McGrew, *Encyclopedia of Medical History.*

San Francisco Plague of 1907–09

Severe epidemic of bubonic plague that infected 205 inhabitants of San Francisco and killed 103 of them. The San Francisco Earthquake (April 18, 1906) had shattered the city, which even a year later remained a refugee camp (without proper water, sanitation, or housing). The 1906–09 plague's fatality rate was 51 percent, which is typical for this highly contagious disease, against which sulfa drugs and some antibiotics are effective.

The San Francisco Earthquake, the most destructive to hit the North American Continent, destroyed about 28,000 buildings, reducing many people to living in filthy, squalid conditions. Many primitively kept stables and chicken yards had plague-carrying rats, on whom fleas lived and flourished; the fleas transmitted the plague bacillus (*Yersinia pestis*) through their bite. Refugee camps were built by the Red Cross and contractors, some of whom (unlike the Red Cross) took advantage of the refugees by padding bills; providing a primitive sewer system consisting of latrines that were only holes in the ground, without waste removal; and failing to provide trash removal.

The plague epidemic got underway within a year. Although the first suspected case, a 14-year-old boy from Oakland, occurred at the same time as the earthquake, it was never fully diagnosed as plague. A year later, a 24-year-old sailor from an oceangoing tugboat entered the U.S. Marine Hospital in San Francisco only to die later of the plague. A 50-year-old man who became ill with plague on August 1, 1907, died by October. Shortly after this man took ill, a sailor from the S.S. *Samoa* died of plague in the Marine Hospital; no other cases developed on the ship, which was quarantined. Eventually, plague cases were reported in different places throughout the city; 25 cases developed from August 1 to September 4, 1907.

Major Edward Taylor of San Francisco requested federal assistance from U.S. President Theodore Roosevelt, who commissioned Dr. Rupert Blue, a retired assistant surgeon of the Marine Hospital and Public Health Service as well as a prominent figure in the 1900–04 epidemic, to take charge. Clinical tests performed on samplings of rats revealed a dangerously high level of plague at the end of 1907; by then, 190 persons had been reported with plague and 96 of them died.

In contrast to the San Francisco Plague of 1900–04 (q.v.), there was widespread cooperation and an extensive control program during this epidemic. Infection had begun to abate by the time preventive measures went into effect. The measures taken had a lasting impact on the quality of public sanitation and safety in the Bay area. A Citizens' Health Committee, made up of many doctors and other prominent citizens, sought the implementation of solid public sanitation regulations and raised money. Laws were passed requiring private and public sanitation measures, such as covered garbage cans, rat trapping, and concrete floors for stables and chicken yards. A new sewer system was built for the city, and a plague hospital was established. By June 1908, some 1,700 people suspected of carrying plague had been examined, and some 100,000 rats had been trapped. By April 1909, the plague had ended (Seattle had also had a similar epidemic during this time). See also LOS ANGELES PLAGUE OF 1924–25.

Further reading: Ackerknecht, *History and Geography of the Most Important Diseases;* Gregg, *Plague: An Ancient Disease in the Twentieth Century.*

Santiago Meningitis Epidemic of 1941–43

Outbreak of cerebrospinal meningitis (CSM), also called meningococcal meningitis, that killed 971 persons out of 5,885 who were infected in Santiago, Chile. The disease's morbidity rate may have been the highest recorded among a large urban population.

In the winter of 1941, this acute bacterial inflammation of the meninges (membranes) surrounding the brain and spinal cord unexpectedly erupted in the most crowded sections of Santiago, Chile's capital and largest city, located on the Mapocho River. About 60 percent of the country's inhabitants live in this central valley area, where the poor were sometimes known to lodge seven persons per room and sleep three in a bed. CSM is transmitted by direct contact, by droplets and mucus through sneezing and coughing; the infection usually takes place indoors in overcrowded sleeping conditions in poorly ventilated accommodations. Most of the Chileans contracted CSM from asymptomatic carriers, who had no symptoms except for perhaps a sore throat, and yet harbored the pathogen in their noses and throats; few Chileans caught the infection from being exposed to sick patients.

CSM spread rapidly in Santiago, infecting about one in every 300 inhabitants of the city; a large number of the infected were children under 15 years of age. Patients were ill from one to three weeks with symptoms of high fever, violent headache, dizziness, vomiting, stiff neck, and a rash; some became delirious and went into a coma (the onset of CSM is usually sudden, with acute fulminating attacks causing death within 24 hours).

The epidemic continued into 1942, concentrated in the same urban area of Santiago where it had originated. CSM cases rose again in the spring of 1942, and the epidemic finally concluded in 1943. Although the overall mortality rate for the epidemic was 16.5 percent, the fatality rate among afflicted children under four years old was 38 percent, strikingly high.

Further reading: Evans and Brachman, eds., *Bacterial Infections of Humans*; Marks and Beatty, *Epidemics.*

Saudi Arabian Malaria Epidemic of 1950–51

Severe epidemic of malaria concentrated in the Jedda (Jidda) region of Saudi Arabia.

Malaria, endemic in certain areas of the Saudi Arabian peninsula, sometimes assumed epidemic strength, as it did in 1950–51. While Jedda and its vicinity bore the brunt of the attack, the epidemic also traveled inland, affecting villages in the Wadi Fatima en route to Mecca. It was particularly severe from October 1950 to January 1951, with November and December being the peak months. Jedda reported more than 4,000 cases in November alone, compared to the estimated 16,000 to 32,000 cases recorded for that year in all of Saudi Arabia.

The *Anopheles gambiae* mosquito, a long-lived vector that breeds in small, sunlit pools of water, was found to be the transmitter of malaria. (The mosquito bites a person with the disease, sucks in blood containing the parasite [plasmodium in human blood], and then bites a healthy person, infecting him or her.) The Saudi Arabian government, with the active cooperation of the Egyptian Health Ministry and skilled personnel of the Arabian American Oil Company, launched a campaign aimed at destroying the *Anopheles gambiae*. Together they were able to control the spread of the epidemic.

Further reading: Simmons et al., *Global Epidemiology.*

Saudi Arabian Smallpox Epidemic of A.D. 569–71

Epidemic that forced an Ethiopian army to retreat in haste from Mecca in A.D. 570, thus ending Ethiopian rule in Arabia.

Hoping to convert the Arabs to Christianity, Abraha (a ruling Christian prince) ordered them to make a pilgrimage to a new cathedral he had specially built in the city of Sana'a. Angered by this order, an Arab desecrated the cathedral. In retaliation, Abraha led his Ethiopian troops into Mecca.

Vastly outnumbered, the Arabian soldiers faced certain defeat but were saved by a severe illness that struck the Ethiopian army and almost completely destroyed it. The "Elephant War epidemic," named for the majestic white elephant on which Abraha rode into Mecca, was later allegorically described in Chapter 105 of the *Koran,* the Muslim holy book compiled about A.D. 651. Citing divine intervention, the *Koran* states that birds armed with stones were dispatched to destroy the army from above. Other writings mention that pustules (blister-like swellings) broke out on soldiers' skin, leading many to conclude that this was a destructive epidemic of smallpox. Hardly a soldier in the army camp escaped infection, and Abraha himself fled to Sana'a, where he too succumbed to the disease.

Smallpox was believed to have been imported into Mecca either from Syria or by sea from India. Some scholars say that it was introduced into Arabia by Abraha's troops. What is certain, though, is that it was one of the earliest known epidemics of smallpox.

Further reading: Hopkins, *Princes and Peasants: Smallpox in History*; Brothwell and Sandison, eds., *Diseases in Antiquity*; Haj, *Disability in Antiquity.*

Scandinavian Epidemics of 1736–39

Several outbreaks of influenza, dysentery, and smallpox in Sweden, Denmark, and Iceland (as well as Finland) in the late 1730s (see EUROPEAN INFLUENZA EPIDEMICS OF 1708–09, 1712, 1729–30, AND 1732–33). In April 1737, after months during which medical officers had been reporting increasing morbidity and mortality in their districts, the government established a special commission to monitor diseases both inside and outside Sweden. As envoys abroad sent back word of widespread infections in north Germany, Prussia, and Poland, Swedish provincial governors were ordered to check the crews of ships from foreign ports in which deadly diseases were known to be prevalent.

The Swedish medical reports are supplemented by fairly comprehensive population statistics for all of Scandinavia. From 1736 on, the annual number of births and deaths had been recorded in each of the 43 provinces of Denmark, Finland, Iceland, Norway, and Sweden, and some information, though not as complete, had been kept in the previous decades. From 1720 to 1735, the population in Sweden had greatly increased, primarily because the death rate was abnormally low, but infections soon brought an end to this growth. In 1736 deaths exceeded births in Stockholm and Copenhagen and in their surrounding areas. During 1737 the seaports of Göteborg in Sweden and Turku (Abo) in Finland and the island of Gotland in the Baltic Sea all experienced similar population deficits. The mortality wave came to Scandinavia from the south, probably originating in countries such as Germany, along the Baltic coast;

after diseases gained a foothold in the ports of Scandinavia, they traveled inland through Sweden, Denmark, and Finland, but left Norway untouched.

Determining what diseases were involved in the epidemics is more difficult than tracking the epidemics' diffusion. It is certain that smallpox played a role; the first known outbreak of it in Sweden occurred in Malmo in 1736. By the following year dysentery was claiming many victims in western Sweden, though it had been uncommon since the 1690s, a decade of food shortages and high mortality throughout Europe. During 1736 and 1737 influenza swept over parts of Scandinavia: Swedish doctors described cases of fever, shivering, headache, chest pain, and cough, as well as the extreme dizziness that suggests relapsing fever.

During the seventeenth and eighteenth centuries, troop movements and famines often exacerbated epidemics, but both factors were missing in the outbreaks of the late 1730s. Scandinavia enjoyed both peace and good to abundant harvests from 1735 to 1738 (with the exception of a deficient yield in Denmark in 1736). Instead, lowered resistance to disease can explain why an epidemic spread so rapidly, at least in Sweden. In the 15 or so years prior to 1736, Sweden had been largely free of the scourge of infections, as the unusually low death rate proves. When the diseases arrived in 1736, they attacked a population with little immunity to them; some doctors noted that pregnant women and old people were especially vulnerable.

These epidemics abated almost as quickly as they arose; by 1738 they had passed their peaks and by the following year had almost entirely disappeared. The overall Scandinavian mortality rate in 1739 dropped back to 29.1 per 1,000 people, and would not rise again until the far more lethal Swedish Epidemics of the Early 1740s (q.v.). The only areas that still suffered high mortality were Iceland in 1739 (whose trade with Denmark represented its sole contact with the rest of Europe), and Finland, where 52 out of every 1,000 inhabitants died in 1740.

Further reading: Utterstrom, "Some Population Problems in Pre-Industrial Sweden"; Imhof and Lindskog, "Les causes de mortalité en Suède et en Finlande entre 1749 et 1773"; Post, *Food Shortages, Climatic Variability, and Epidemic Disease in Preindustrial Europe.*

Scottish Plague of 1349–51 See PLAGUE OF SCOTLAND, GREAT.

Scottish Plague of 1585 See EDINBURGH PLAGUE OF 1585.

Scottish Plague of 1597 See EDINBURGH PLAGUE OF 1597.

Scottish Plague of 1600–1608 Violent outbreak of bubonic plague that persisted in various parts of Scotland from 1600 through 1608, first appearing in Edinburgh in the spring of 1604 and disappearing at the end of November 1607 (including the usual subsidence of the disease during the winter months). Mortality figures are not known, but the large sums of public money spent on the maintenance of the sick indicates a high incidence of the disease, especially among the poor, who had little means to care for themselves or to move to safer areas. Food and domestic supplies were provided to plague victims, who were segregated in huts outside the city. Workers were hired to cleanse the houses and belongings of infected persons. Grave diggers and people to supervise the isolation site also had to be paid.

Stiff penalties were inflicted for violating the many regulations instituted to control the plague, including heavy fines and even execution. Court sessions and meetings of parliament were suspended, trade fairs were canceled, and people from other towns had to produce proof that they had come from a place where the plague was absent.

The extent of the epidemic during these years is evidenced by a report written in October 1606 by the Lord Chancellor of Scotland, who declared, "The onlie truble we haiff is this contagious sickness of peste, whilk [which] is spread marvelouslie in the best townes off this realme." Many of the wealthier citizens were unaffected because they were able to flee the towns to escape infection.

The origin of this visitation of plague in Scotland is not recorded. Its most likely cause was the importation to a coastal port of house-dwelling rats infected with a particularly virulent strain of the plague bacillus (see EDINBURGH PLAGUE OF 1530).

Further reading: Creighton, *A History of Epidemics in Britain;* Shrewsbury, *A History of Bubonic Plague in the British Isles.*

Scottish Plague of 1644–48 Second major epidemic of bubonic plague, with the exception of a brief outbreak in 1636, to afflict Edinburgh and other parts of Scotland in the seventeenth century. The death toll for Edinburgh is unknown, but this visitation was certainly one of the most destructive in Scotland's history, severely affecting many places throughout the country, as evidenced by the antiplague measures taken by civic authorities everywhere.

The disease erupted in Edinburgh in the fall of 1644, possibly introduced into the city by Scottish soldiers returning from a battle with the English Army at the city of Newcastle-upon-Tyne in northern

England, where plague was reportedly present in the surrounding area. Records show, however, that city officials, always alert to the danger of importation of plague into Scotland by foreign ships, focused their efforts at this time on preventing its arrival by this route. Whatever the origin, the extent of this epidemic is revealed in Edinburgh's financial accounts, where the high cost of maintaining the sick and paying personnel to carry out plague duties is carefully recorded. Its virulence is also demonstrated by the unwillingness of the commander of the English Army in August 1645 to enter and take possession of Edinbrugh after he had defeated the Scots in battle. The movements of the Scots and English armies accelerated the spread of disease.

Some historians believe that typhus fever, which spreads more easily than bubonic plague, as its transmission depends on the human body louse rather than the rat flea, which has a limited range, was responsible for many of the deaths ascribed to plague. The epidemic of these years was very likely a combination of both diseases.

Although some devoted officials remained to help the sick and administer the city of Edinburgh, a majority of the nobility and other wealthy citizens fled to safer places. In February 1646, city councillors who had left Edinburgh were ordered to return and resume their duties.

An interesting feature of this epidemic is the miraculous cure concocted by a Dr. Burgess, who guaranteed it would work "not only for the common plague which is called the Sickness, but also the smallpox, missles, surfeat [abdominal disorders] and divers other diseases." The remedy was totally useless, as were all such medicines of the centuries before modern medical science, but Dr. Burgess's claim shows that many other diseases were prevalent in Scotland besides bubonic plague.

In 1646 the plague's virulence began to subside, although some cities suffered severe outbreaks, notably Glasgow in the west of Scotland, which was scourged for several years, especially in 1647 and 1648. Although it reappeared briefly in Glasgow in August 1900 and caused 16 deaths, 1648 marks the virtual end of plague in Scotland.

Further reading: Creighton, *A History of Epidemics in Britain*; Shrewsbury, *A History of Bubonic Plague in the British Isles*; Smout, *A History of the Scottish People*.

Scottish Smallpox Epidemics of 1823–31 Outbreaks of smallpox with many fatalities in Scotland between 1823 and 1831. Because statistics on causes of death were not kept in Scotland until 1835, the extent and virulence of the infection during these years can only be estimated from contemporary observations. The city of Glasgow experienced high mortality during the entire period, while the worst years for the nearby towns of Stranaer and Ayr were 1829 and 1830, respectively. Fatalities were greatest in Edinburgh (Scotland's capital) during the winter of 1830–31. Articles written for medical journals and private communications by physicians attending the poor attest to the appalling conditions of crowding in the slum areas of Glasgow, which accelerated the spread of contagion. As was the case in the British Isles until the latter half of the nineteenth century, the vast majority of deaths from smallpox in this period were among infants and young children. This partially explains the lack of information about these epidemic years, as infantile diseases were generally considered a fact of ordinary life and thus not especially worthy of mention.

Further reading: Creighton, *A History of Epidemics in Britain*.

Scottish Typhus Epidemic of 1836–40 Major outbreak of epidemic, louse-borne typhus fever that spread to many parts of Scotland, including the main cities of Dundee, Aberdeen, Glasgow, and Edinburgh. An economic depression in 1836 may have precipitated the rapid increase in human deaths from typhus fever, a disease that thrives in conditions of poverty and overcrowding when standards of personal and domestic hygiene decline. Data on numbers of cases and fatalities for Scottish cities are not available, but the rise in cases admitted to various city hospitals indicates a higher than usual incidence of typhus fever among the population of any given urban center in the period 1836–1840. For example, admissions for fever to the Edinburgh Infirmary almost doubled from 1836 (about 650) to 1837 (about 1225), then jumped to about 2,250 in 1838. Cases in the Royal Infirmary and special fever hospitals in Glasgow rose from about 1,360 in 1835 to 3,125 in 1836, to the peak number of 5,390 in 1837. In Dundee, fever admissions to the town infirmary greatly increased during the 12-month period from mid-June 1836 to mid-June 1837. The worst year for the northeastern town of Aberdeen, where the disease appeared later than in the rest of Scotland, was 1840, when about 535 cases were admitted to its two fever wards.

Scotland's visitation of typhus fever from 1836 to 1840 was part of the larger epidemic that affected many parts of the British Isles during these years (see ENGLISH TYPHUS EPIDEMIC OF 1835–38; IRISH TYPHUS EPIDEMIC OF 1836–40).

Further reading: Creighton, *A History of Epidemics in Britain*; Wohl, *Endangered Lives: Public Health in Victorian Britain*.

Seneca Indian Measles Epidemic of 1592–96

Evidently one of the earliest outbreaks of measles (rubeola) among Native Americans, striking the Seneca Indians' Cameron village in what is now western New York state. Indian fear, panic, and inability to cope with the very contagious, viral disease contributed to hundreds, possibly thousands, of deaths between 1592 and 1596.

Although there is a lack of hard evidence about specific and identifiable diseases among the Indians, historical researchers strongly support the belief that numerous measles outbreaks occurred in the entire Atlantic coastal region from Florida to the Great Lakes and New England from 1528 to 1596. Enough human skeletal evidence at the site of the Cameron village confirms the measles epidemic there of 1592–96.

At various times during the sixteenth century, Spanish ships' crews and troops carried the measles virus (transmitted by direct contact or airborne droplets) to the West Indies and Florida, infecting the native peoples. Also, French fur traders who traveled up the St. Lawrence River might have carried the infection. However, the Seneca Indians most likely contracted measles through their trading and social interaction with the southeastern Indian tribes of what is now the United States.

Sometime in 1592 the virus was transmitted to the Cameron village, where it was especially fatal among Seneca infants and children (who accounted for nearly half the death toll). Mortality among adults was less grave, undoubtedly because some older Seneca were immune, having apparently survived earlier exposure to the virus from 1564 to 1570.

Further reading: Dobyns, *Their Number Becomes Thinned: Native American Dynamics in Eastern North America;* Ramenofsky, *Vectors of Death: The Archaeology of European Contact.*

Senegalese Plague of 1942–44

Epidemic of plague (mainly in the bubonic form) that killed almost 700 persons in Senegal (then part of French West Africa).

Minor outbreaks of plague had occurred at irregular intervals in Dakar (the capital of Senegal and of French West Africa) and other coastal areas of Senegal since 1912, when the disease was first officially recognized in French West Africa. It had been dormant from 1936 to 1942, when in June several natives in Dakar developed painful golf-ball size buboes (swellings) in their groins or armpits. At the time Dakar's coastal region had an abundance of rats and other wild rodents; an epizootic (temporary prevalence of a disease among animals) existed in which wild rats died from the plague bacillus and their fleas then transmitted it either to other rodents or to human beings. Dakar's first plague victims ran high fevers, became sick with splitting headaches, and suffered bouts of diarrhea and vomiting. In 1943 there were reportedly 207 human deaths from plague in Dakar and the surrounding villages. The epidemic escalated in June 1944, when about 570 Senegalese were reported infected in Dakar; by the end of the year, 448 persons had died of plague.

Although most of the plague infections in the city (Dakar) and the rural areas were bubonic, a number of cases were septicemic in form (contracted also by a flea bite), which saw victims dying sometimes hours after contracting the disease, before buboes had time to develop. Few of the cases were pneumonic plague, the most serious and highly infectious form, spread via the airborne route by inhalation of exhaled droplets from victims.

Without doubt, overcrowding and poor sanitation were largely responsible for the abundance of plague-infected rodents in Dakar and the native villages. A comprehensive DDT-spraying program was introduced in late 1944 to rid the infected areas of rodents; also, anti-plague immunization was made compulsory and certificates of vaccination were required of all persons entering or leaving certain districts. This resulted in extinguishing the focus of the disease in rural Senegal. In 1945 there were 58 reported cases of plague in the country; only four persons died of it in Dakar. The disease seemed absent from Senegal in the years following.

Further reading: Pollitzer, *Plague;* Simmons et al., *Global Epidemiology.*

Senegalese Yellow Fever Epidemic of 1778

Outbreak of yellow fever among the British troops occupying the French fort of St. Louis on an island at the mouth of the Senegal River in West Africa. At the time (1778) the British and French were vying for control of coastal Senegal, which became a recognized French possession in 1814.

At St. Louis, the onset of the epidemic was sudden among the troops, who had chills, fever, headache, general pains, and nausea. A survivor of the epidemic, John Peter Schotte described the acute infectious disease in detail, mentioning the jaundice and black vomit that appeared in severe cases as well as the hemorrhages that caused numerous deaths. The number of infections and fatalities remains unclear at St. Louis, but that same year (1778) yellow fever spread to the Senegalese island and town of Gorée to the south, infecting 93 white Europeans there (60 of them died). Only much later was yellow fever discovered to be caused by a virus transmitted from person to person, or by an infected jungle animal, through the bite of the *Aëdes aegypti* mosquito.

For a long time the Senegalese epidemic was considered the first recorded African epidemic of yellow fever until the writings of a Jamaican surgeon, John Williams, were discovered. Williams, who worked on a transatlantic slave trading ship that plied the waters between Guinea and the West Indies in 1740–41, described yellow fever (also called yellow jack) as endemic in parts of West Africa. The fever in Senegal was evidently imported from Sierra Leone (bordering Guinea), lying some 500 miles south of Gorée (a major slave trading center, along with the Cape Verde Islands to the west).

In the seventeenth and eighteenth centuries, many black West Africans who were transported as slaves to the West Indies had a relative immunity (recovery from yellow fever is followed by lasting immunity). This fact later convinced some epidemiologists that the original habitat of the fever was West Africa; others contended that the disease originated in Central America and was introduced to Africa. Wherever it originated, the disease remained prevalent in Senegal during the rest of the 1700s and into the 1800s, notably striking Europeans and their military forces.

Further reading: Cartwright, *Disease and History*; Scott, *A History of Tropical Medicine*.

Senegalese Yellow Fever Epidemic of 1965

Outbreak of yellow fever that may have infected as many as 20,000 people in the West African nation of Senegal. However, only 2,000 cases and 140 deaths were officially reported, because of Senegalese reluctance to publish exact figures in order to minimize the epidemic publicly.

After Senegal gained its independence from France in 1960, it could not afford to continue its former mass vaccination programs against yellow fever (undertaken since the 1930s) and to maintain special officials to report new outbreaks of the disease. As a result, in 1965 the regions around Diourbel and Mbacke (east of Dakar, Senegal's capital) were severely struck by yellow fever, a viral infection transmitted mainly by the bite of the *Aëdes aegypti* mosquito; it may also be transmitted from person to person or by a monkey, ape, opossum, or other infected jungle animal.

In this former French colony, African natives in the past had built up a high resistance to the yellow fever, which had always provided a massive reservoir of infection there and thus ensured that most everyone living in an endemic area became infected as children, acquiring permanent immunity after a mild illness.

During the 1965 epidemic, about 130,000 small children were inoculated with the then new 17D vaccine, which was fired (injected) through the skin

without breaking it by a new jet-pressure gun; this new method with the neurotropic strain of virus was effectively used in the place of the customary syringe and needle. However, some complications occurred when the older inoculation method using the Dakar vaccine was administered to about 90,000 other Senegalese children, 240 of whom were hospitalized with encephalitis, 25 of them dying from this brain infection.

Because of successful eradication of the mosquito vector and its breeding places in Senegal, large numbers of Africans have escaped contracting yellow fever during childhood; they may be at risk if mosquito control is relaxed and new outbreaks occur.

Further reading: Ransford, *"Bid the Sickness Cease": Disease in the History of Black Africa*; Williams, *The Plague Killers*.

Serbian Typhus Epidemic of 1914–15

Epidemic of typhus fever that raged among Serbian troops and civilians during the first winter and spring of World War I (1914–18). The fear of catching the disease kept the Central Powers (Austria-Hungary and Germany) from renewing attacks on a vulnerable Serbia. Claiming about 150,000 human lives in six months, the epidemic became one of the worst typhus outbreaks of modern times.

World War I began with the assassination on June 28, 1914, of Austrian Archduke Francis Ferdinand, the heir to the Austro-Hungarian throne. Convinced that the Serbian government had been involved, Austria-Hungary declared war on July 28. Weakened by the Balkan Wars against the Ottoman Empire (Turkey), which ended in August 1913, the small country of Serbia seemed no match for the united forces of Austria-Hungary. Yet the Serbs twice pushed the invaders back across the border, first in August and then again four months later, when they recaptured Belgrade, their capital. The Serbian victory there cost the Austrians tens of thousands of soldiers, including 60,000 to 70,000 whom the Serbs took prisoner.

At the time of their great military success, however, another enemy began to strike at the Serbs. A few typhus cases had appeared among their troops in November 1914, although it was not until the following month that the disease broke out extensively. Its spread was aided not just by moving troops and by trains of enemy prisoners, but by a civilian population that had been fleeing the Austro-Hungarian attacks in northern Serbia. Food, shelter, clothing, and medical care were insufficient for the large numbers of troops and prisoners, let alone for the refugees, many of whom were barefoot and ill-clothed. The few hospitals that existed were short on beds, supplies, and medicines. There were only a few hundred doctors in the entire country, and over 100 of them died from typhus themselves. During the height of the epidemic in April 1915, over 2,500 cases were admitted each day to the military hospitals alone; the incidence among civilians was approximately three times that. Before ending in the summer of 1915, the epidemic hit nearly half a million people and killed about 150,000 of them, including half of the Austrian prisoners of war.

While it contended with the epidemic, the Serbian Army would have been an easy target for the Central Powers. The Austro-Hungarians, however, stayed beyond the border, afraid to contract typhus themselves and content instead to allow the disease to kill their enemies. At the same time, the Germans were occupied with fighting in Poland, where they did not succeed in pushing back the Russians (allies of Serbia) until April 1915. Once the epidemic subsided, however, action resumed on the Serbian front; in the fall of 1915 the Central Powers decided to attempt direct communications with their ally the Ottoman Empire by driving through Serbia.

Further reading: Dedijer et al., *History of Yugoslavia;* Heppell and Singleton, *Yugoslavia;* Petrovich, *A History of Modern Serbia, 1804–1918;* Zinsser, *Rats, Lice and History.*

Shanghai Hepatitis Epidemic of 1988
Massive food-borne outbreak of hepatitis A that affected Shanghai, China, in the spring of 1988 (see XINJIANG [SINKIANG] HEPATITIS EPIDEMIC OF 1986–88).

Late in December 1987, about 2,000 tons of clams made their way into the Shanghai markets, where almost one third of the city's residents consumed them. From February to April 1988, 320,746 cases of clinical acute hepatitis (4,082 per 100,000 people) reportedly occurred in the city. This outbreak was linked to consumption of raw or half-cooked clams harvested from sewage-contaminated water. Analysis of clams from the market and the seabed revealed a high concentration of the causative virus. Also, the attack rate among susceptible persons who had eaten the clams was 32.4 percent compared to 1.82 percent among those who had not. It must be remembered that not everyone infected with the virus actually experienced the clinical symptoms of hepatitis A; these were classified as inapparent infections. Forty-seven deaths—mainly from complications—were recorded during this outbreak.

Hepatitis A, one of the most widespread of the infectious diseases in China, is transmitted from person to person mainly through the fecal-oral route and, less frequently, through the ingestion of contaminated food or water. It can also be transmitted, albeit rarely, through the blood (particularly among drug users). The disease, however, generally occurs in acute form only, and mortality is often less than 0.1 percent.

Thanks to improved living conditions and better sanitation, the annual risk of hepatitis A infections has declined from 20 percent to between one and three percent in the Shanghai region of eastern China. In addition, the disease has shifted from being primarily a childhood infection in the 1950s to one that favors young adults in the 1990s. In the near future, the development and use of a vaccine is expected to play an important role in controlling the incidence of hepatitis A wherever it is a public health menace.

Further reading: Wen et al., eds., *Viral Hepatitis in China;* Szmuness et al., eds., *Viral Hepatitis: 1981 International Symposium.*

Sierra Leonean Influenza Epidemic of 1918
Severe outbreak of virulent influenza in the then British colony in West Africa, killing 1,072 people in five weeks in August–September 1918.

The Spanish Influenza Epidemic of 1917–19 (q.v.) had stricken many parts of the world by mid-August 1918, when a British ship, the *H.M.S. Mantua*, with 200 influenza-infected mariners, arrived in Freetown, Sierra Leone's seaport capital. Freetown was an important coaling station for ships plying the waters between Europe, South Africa, and the Far East. Nine days after black African colliers of the Sierra Leone Coaling Company fueled the *Mantua*, the "flu" broke out throughout Freetown. Four days later (August 27, 1918) about 500 of the company's 600 workers failed to come to work, and consequently sailors from the ships in Freetown had to help in refueling their own vessels (to keep wartime schedules on track). One of those vessels, the *H.M.S. Africa*, suffered an acute flu outbreak on its voyage to England; 75 percent of the crew and passengers became sick, and 51 persons died. A New Zealand transport vessel, the *Crepstow Castle*, suffered similarly after refueling in Freetown on August 26–27; on the high seas after leaving port, it had 900 flu-infected people on board, with 83 fatalities.

A false theory developed that the influenza's virulence for Europeans had greatly increased after a milder strain had passed through susceptible black Sierra Leoneans; it was also falsely speculated that the imported Sierra Leonean strain was responsible for initiating severe outbreaks in Europe about that time (however, similar mutations of the flu virus occurred in England, France, and America in late summer 1918).

In Freetown, about two thirds of the native population contracted the flu. Though most of the sick suffered from the ordinary symptoms of headaches, severe colds, fevers, and aching bones and muscles, 75 patients perished from complications such as pneumonia, purulent bronchitis, mastoid abscess, and heart problems. Influenza soon spread to other areas in Sierra Leone and took the lives of over a thousand inhabitants before the end of September 1918. At the same time the disease moved northward, hitting Gambia and Senegal and other West African colonies, and southward into Ashanti (part of Ghana), where some 9,000 people died, and into Nigeria, where apparently 512,000 died from the virus (see ASHANTI INFLUENZA EPIDEMIC OF 1918; NIGERIAN INFLUENZA EPIDEMIC OF 1918–19). The epidemics in Ashanti and Nigeria, evidently introduced from Sierra Leone, have also been said to have come from Europe, according to some sources. In addition, a serious flu epidemic erupted in South Africa in September 1918, claiming nearly 140,000 human lives; it apparently originated in Sierra Leone or another colony in West Africa.

Further reading: Clarke, *Influenza*; Crosby, *America's Forgotten Pandemic: The Influenza of 1918*.

Sierra Leonean Yellow Fever Epidemics of 1815–85

Series of 15 epidemics of yellow fever that devastated the Europeans living in Sierra Leone, West Africa. The disease hardly touched the native Africans there but hindered the development of this small country (then a British colony); it was difficult at times for an effective and stable government to take hold while these epidemics occurred generally within two to eight years of each other (in three continuous years in one period).

The earliest evidence of yellow fever in West Africa was recorded in Sierra Leone in 1764. African slaves from Sierra Leone, who were transported to the Caribbean area, retained a relative immunity to the devastating effects of yellow fever, in contrast to American Indians and Europeans, who suffered severely from outbreaks of the disease in the Caribbean. It is sometimes thought that yellow fever was present in Sierra Leone long before 1764; it may even have originated in West Africa, an area sometimes called the "white man's grave." (Some epidemiologists contend that the disease's origin was in Central America.)

In Sierra Leone, malaria and yellow fever were often confused for many years; both mosquito-borne diseases were fatal for European settlers and travelers in the port city of Freetown. During the rainy season, settlers frequently contracted malaria, which they called "bilious remittant fever"; those who survived managed to build up an immunity. On the other hand, yellow fever (called "malignant remittant fever") attacked the settlers more unpredictably, although usually in the dry season. The medical authorities in the colony monitored the frequency of the outbursts and observed the differences in the two diseases. They were helpless, however, in combating the yellow fever epidemics of 1815 and 1823. There is much uncertainty about the exact number of people afflicted and the fatalities; the 1823 epidemic reportedly ravaged Freetown in only a few days and caused the death of the chief superintendent of the liberated Africans, a Reverend Johnson.

Some physicians noted that yellow fever (like malaria) was more destructive in the low-lying sections of Freetown and seldom infected those living in the outer villages. By July 1823, 89 out of the 150 Europeans in Freetown had perished during that year's epidemic; most died from yellow fever, including four of the five Christian missionaries sent to the city in 1823. Freetown, the capital of the colony, suffered the loss of numerous administrators, including the chief justice, a lawyer, and the chaplain; government was nearly helpless in dealing with the epidemic. The local Temne natives were not seriously attacked by the disease, as the newcomer Europeans were. Three years later, in 1826, the next yellow fever epidemic struck Sierra Leone; 115 of the 535 soldiers assigned to the British garrison there fell victim to the disease between June 14 and August 24.

Some attributed the cause of yellow fever to the "bad air" from heavy rainfall, tornadoes, and hot sun; others were convinced that the malignant fever was brought by infected travelers on ships coming to Freetown. Common breeding grounds for the female *Aëdes aegypti* mosquitoes, which carry the yellow fever virus, were water supplies (tin cans, barrels, gutters) on ships. During the next yellow fever epidemic in Sierra Leone in 1837, the ship H.M.S. *Curlew* was badly infected while staying a week in Freetown harbor and then carried the disease up the coast to Gambia. Authorities remain uncertain whether the ship had brought the disease to Freetown or had picked it up in port. The latter contention, however, seems the case for the ship H.M.S. *Eclair* in 1845, when yellow fever seemed endemic in Sierra Leone. The ship's log recorded no illness among the crew from departing Plymouth, England, to entering Freetown three weeks later, on February 22, 1845. Some crewmembers spent time in the port city before leaving with their ship on March 16. The first case of yellow fever on board the *Eclair* occurred on April 3, followed by 12 additional cases on June 15 (seven were fatal). The *Eclair* returned to Freetown on July 4, and the crew went ashore during a two-week stopover. On the ship's journey north to Gambia, 14 of the crew contracted yellow fever (half of them died). Then on the journey west to Boa Vista on the Cape Verde Islands, 39 more seamen perished; the fever spread to the inhabitants of Boa Vista, which had been free of it until the *Eclair* arrived there on August 21, 1845. (It should be noted that the disease was also referred to as "yellow jack" and that a vessel flying a yellow flag warned of infectious disease aboard or of quarantine.)

The 1884 yellow fever epidemic killed 20 people in Freetown, and the European population there understood more about the disease and was able to take precautions. After the discovery that the female *Aëdes aegypti* mosquito carried the virus (1900), Sierra Leone was made safe for Europeans by the 1930s, with help from the Rockefeller Yellow Fever Commission, working then in West Africa.

Further reading: Peterson, *Province of Freedom: A History of Sierra Leone*; Scott, *A History of Tropical Medicine*.

Singapore Beriberi Epidemics of 1942–45 Series of outbreaks of beriberi among British, Australian, and Eurasian prisoners being held by the Japanese at the Changi Prison in Singapore during World War II. They are generally considered the last of the major beriberi epidemics.

Changi Prison was home to somewhere between 20,000 and 30,000 prisoners of war during this three-and-a-half-year period. The turnover among the prisoners was high. Large groups of them were transferred to Japanese prison camps elsewhere in Asia, such as in Thailand, Japan, and French Indochina, and they were replaced by other groups from Java, Sumatra, and other Indonesian islands. At any given time, there were never less than 12,000 prisoners at Changi Prison.

The first cases of beriberi broke out less than a month after prisoners were first brought to Changi in February 1942. Between May and June 1942, more than 1,000 cases were recorded among a prison population ranging between 40,000 and 50,000. No doubt many more cases went undiagnosed and unreported.

There were actually two major outbreaks. The first, occurring from April to October 1942, registered 206 cases in the initial phase and 54 cases during a rather spotty second phase. A high proportion of these beriberi patients also suffered from dysentery and malaria. During the second outbreak (May 1944–August 1945), 140 cases (many complicated by protein and calorie deficiencies) were recorded. Patients suffering from a severe form of acute cardiac beriberi were admitted into the hospital. See also THAI BERIBERI EPIDEMICS OF 1890–1910; PHILIPPINE BERIBERI EPIDEMICS OF 1901–02 AND 1909.

Further reading: Williams, *Toward the Conquest of Beriberi*.

Singapore Bornholm Disease Epidemic of 1946 Outbreak of Bornholm disease (pleurodynia) at the Singapore Naval Base. The uncommon Bornholm disease, named for a Danish island in the Baltic on which it was first studied, begins as a sudden but severe pain in the lower chest and upper abdomen area, accompanied by fever of a short duration. Infectious but benign, this viral disease has also been known as epidemic myositis, epidemic myalgia, or epidemic pleurodynia. Each of these names refers to an important clinical manifestation of the disease.

The epidemic in Singapore (an island off the southern tip of the Malay Peninsula) began on June 8, 1946, when 42 men stationed at the naval base complained of fever, chest pain, and the inability to move around. Expecting the situation to escalate into an outbreak, the British authorities and others promptly set up an emergency ward and prepared one of the barracks to receive patients. Twenty-eight new patients checked in on June 9 and 23 more on June 10. The food-borne epidemic subsided by June 21, having infected 125 people in all.

Further reading: Cope, ed., *History of the Second World War: Medicine and Pathology*.

Singapore Conjunctivitis Epidemics of 1970–80 Series of outbreaks of severe viral conjunctivitis (a disease of the conjunctiva and cornea) in the small island nation of Singapore.

In 1970, an acute and extensive epidemic of viral conjunctivitis invaded Singapore, where from September to December, 60,118 patients reportedly received treatment at government clinics. The illness began rather suddenly with the patients developing mild to severe conjunctivitis, including teary eyes and a feeling that they were invaded by a foreign body. In six percent to 11 percent of the cases, subconjunctival hemorrhage was also observed. Some patients also developed respiratory symptoms. Most recovered completely within two weeks. The causative virus of this epidemic was discovered to be a new variant of Coxsackie virus A24. It is considered to be the first human enterovirus that caused an epidemic disease with conjunctivitis as its main feature.

Two years later, a second epidemic struck. It was similar in its manifestations but caused by a new enterovirus (Type 70). From June to December 1971, government-sponsored clinics treated 38,156 patients.

Viral conjunctivitis invaded Singapore for the third consecutive year in 1972. During June to November 1972, a reported 29,989 patients sought treatment at clinics. Once again, the symptoms were similar to those seen in previous years. However, the majority of the cases, it was later discovered, were caused by an adenovirus (AV11). The enterovirus 70 was also isolated in a few cases. Another epidemic occurred in 1975, and about 60,000 cases were reported between June and December of that year. The culprit was the Coxsackie virus A24. In 1980, the enterovirus 70 was responsible for another outbreak. A total of 48,915 people were affected from July to December.

Doctors observed that epidemics caused by the Coxsackie virus A24 were generally more extensive than the ones caused by enterovirus 70. Ophthalmologists in Singapore found that clinical differentiation on the basis of causative virus was not possible. The disease, which is spread by close contact, seemed to cut across all ethnic and socioeconomic barriers. However, in these epidemics males, older children, and young adults were found to be more susceptible than other groups.

In the interepidemic period, several minor outbreaks of viral conjunctivitis were reported in which all of the above viruses plus four more adenovirus types were involved.

Further reading: Mackenzie, ed., *Viral Diseases in South-East Asia and the Western Pacific.*

Singapore Dengue Hemorrhagic Fever Epidemics

Series of epidemics that struck Singapore during the 1960s and 1970s.

In Singapore, the disease was first identified during an epidemic of dengue in 1960, when many patients were also found to be suffering from mild hemorrhages. Subsequent tests revealed the presence of dengue virus types 1 and 2. In 1961, cases of DHF were noticed among children. Thereafter, DHF epidemics invaded the island at regular intervals during the next two decades.

Epidemics were reported in 1962, 1963, 1964, and 1966 (630 reported cases and 24 deaths), all caused by dengue virus types 3 and 4. During these four epidemics, 897 patients were hospitalized. Singapore's biggest DHF outbreak occurred in 1973 when 1,187 people were reportedly infected. Another epidemic struck in 1978.

DHF, caused by a virus carried by the *Aedes aegypti* mosquito, is primarily a disease affecting children, particularly those between ages four and nine. The joint pains characteristic of "classic" dengue fever are absent in DHF, which is distinguished by symptoms of hemorrhagia and, quite frequently, of shock (drop in blood pressure, collapse, and semicoma). Asian children seem particularly susceptible to DHF.

The Singapore Government promptly instituted measures to reduce the incidence of DHF, by destroying the breeding places of the *Aedes aegypti*, 95 percent of which were man-made. Residents who allowed mosquitoes to breed on their property were either fined or imprisoned. Slums, the primary breeding quarters of the mosquitoes, were cleared and an educational campaign was launched by the Ministry of Environment.

Many Southeast Asian countries were similarly afflicted during the 1960s, among them Malaysia, Indonesia, Vietnam, the Philippines, Thailand (see THAI DENGUE HEMORRHAGIC FEVER EPIDEMICS), and the city of Calcutta in India.

Further reading: Howe, ed., *A World Geography of Human Diseases;* Service, ed., *Demography and Vector-Borne Diseases;* World Health Organization, *Dengue Haemorrhagic Fever.*

Singapore Poliomyelitis Epidemic of 1958–59

Epidemic of poliomyelitis (infantile paralysis) in the tiny island nation of Singapore, situated off the southern end of the Malay Peninsula.

Previously endemic on the island, poliomyelitis had erupted to cause small outbreaks in 1946, 1948 and 1950–51. In these outbreaks, the infection had singled out children under two years of age. The epidemic of 1958–59 represented a shift in that it affected mainly older children, above eight years of age. The epidemic began in August 1958 when there was a significant increase in the reported polio cases. When it ended in mid-March 1959, a total of 415 cases had been reported. Of these, 314 occurred in the Chinese community, 46 among the Malays, 43 in the Indian-Pakistani-Sri Lankan community, and the rest among the city's European and Eurasian residents. The outbreak was discovered to be caused by the type 1 polio virus.

Eleven weeks after the notification of the first case, Singapore's Health Ministry decided to use the attenuated type 2 polio vaccine. Some 198,965 children three months to 10 years of age were vaccinated with the type 2 vaccine. As the epidemic progressed, six members of this group suffered from paralytic polio (weakness/paralysis of one or more muscles) caused by the type 1 polio virus. During this period, 179 paralytic polio cases were detected among 300,000 non-vaccinated children in the same age group.

Further reading: Hale et al., "Large-scale Use of Sabin Type 2 Attenuated Poliovirus Vaccine in Singapore during a Type 1 Polio Epidemic"; World Health Organization, *Poliomyelitis.*

Solomon Islands Poliomyelitis Epidemic of 1951

Most explosive of many poliomyelitis outbreaks on the Solomon Islands, infecting untold thousands of people and maiming hundreds of them. An acute viral illness, poliomyelitis had attacked the Solomon Islands, a volcanic archipelago in the Western Pacific Ocean, several times, most notably in 1925, 1929,

1932–33, 1947–48, 1958, and 1959, but the 1951 epidemic was the most extensive and severest of them all.

The first polio case was reported from the Central Hospital in the capital of Honiara (on Guadalcanal Island) in early March 1951. Thereafter, patients began streaming in; the hospital recorded 11 deaths in the first two weeks and treated 95 paralytic cases during the epidemic. The infection spread rapidly along the Guadalcanal coast and was especially severe in the Marau Sound area. Only the high-altitude villages in the interior escaped.

From Honiara, polio traveled to the Solomon island of Malaita at the end of March (the first cases were in Takwa) and spread quickly across the entire island, peaking within a week. The last case there occurred in Fauabu late in September. It is not known exactly how many were affected on Malaita. Auki Hospital reported 59 cases and five deaths, 645 cases were reported from the surrounding areas, and the Rohinari Catholic Mission had 28 paralytic cases, 17 of them fatal. From the northern part of the island where quarantine was more rigidly enforced, 172 cases and 27 deaths occurred. South Malaita was also infected, but since the villagers refused to divulge any information about the extent of the outbreak in their community, no information is available. The confirmed figure of 961 cases and 110 deaths on Malaita apparently represented only a quarter of the cases that actually occurred on that island.

The epidemic spread to the Western Solomons in March 1951 (11 cases and two deaths at Gizo Hospital) and all over the district and subsequently subsided after it reached the Shortland Islands late in July. Seventy-two paralytic cases and four deaths occurred in Vella Lavella (an island) and Roviana (a lagoon). The islands of Simbo, Ranongga, and Choiseul were also badly infected. Choiseul was invaded in mid-May and, despite a quarantine, the epidemic spread everywhere; there were more than 100 confirmed cases, 40 of them permanently paralyzed, and 20 or more deaths.

The Eastern Solomons escaped infection until later in the epidemic. Less than 100 cases and 10 deaths were reported from the island of Makira or San Cristobal, and nearby Ugi had many paralytic cases and four deaths and Santa Ana had more than 30 paralytic cases. The Russell Islands and Santa Isabel Island recorded very few cases and no fatalities.

According to the official statistics, there were 1,280 paralytic polio cases and 156 deaths (mainly due to bulbar palsy and respiratory failure) during the epidemic, which undoubtedly was far more intense than these figures indicate and exposed the limitations of the medical services and facilities on the Solomon Islands. The mission stations tried to help but were ill-equipped to deal with an outbreak of this magnitude and complexity. Most of the residents, therefore, had nowhere to turn for medical assistance and relied on traditional remedies such as applying heat or countering with another irritant, which were ineffective and relatively harmless. Two other practices—drinking lots of water (which led to urine retention) and exercising during the most painful phase of the infection—were decidedly harmful. For those left paralyzed, the government and the churches encouraged water exercises. Nevertheless, the epidemic left the islanders confused and devastated. When polio struck again in epidemic form during 1958, they lined up to receive the newly developed Salk polio vaccine. That outbreak fortunately was relatively minor.

Further reading: Cross, "The Solomon Islands Tragedy: A Tale of Epidemic Poliomyelitis."

Somalian Malaria Epidemic of 1961

Outbreak of malaria occurring mainly among nomadic Somalis (who make up the majority of Somalia's population) and killing untold thousands of them. (The number of infections and deaths were not registered in the country during the 1961 epidemic, which was especially fatal for infants and children under five years old.)

In 1961, following a long period of drought, abnormally heavy and prolonged rains and flooding occurred over much of northeast Africa during the year's first rainy season (April to June). The Haud region (a semidesert area with some grassy plains in southeast Ethiopia and southwest Somalia) had many areas of open water formed by the rains, which provided breeding grounds for *Anopheles gambiae* mosquitoes (through whose bites the disease is transmitted from person to person). The Somali nomads, who wander for most of the year with their livestock in search of water and pastures, were at risk of contracting malaria during the wet seasons in Somalia (April–June, September–November), when the 1961 epidemic mainly raged. A number of Somalis also suffered from the infection during the non-malarious dry seasons and had no immunity to fight the debilitating disease during the sudden changes in weather.

In the Haud, where there is an absence of perennial streams and underground sources to exploit to improve water supplies, rainwater was conserved in large tanks holding 20,000 to 100,000 gallons of water. These tanks were located along either side of the Ethiopian-Somalian border, then under dispute. In 1961, the nomads remained longer in the Haud because there was available water and grazing for their cattle, camels, and other animals. Malaria-carrying mosquitoes, abundantly breeding in the tanks, infected large numbers of nomads. At the time it was possible to treat the water in the tanks with briquettes impregnated with chemicals to prevent mosquito breeding; the treatment would not foul the water for drinking by either humans or animals. But this method proved ineffective because although the tanks on the Somali side were treated, those on the Ethiopian side (less than 100 yards across the border) were not, and mosquito-breeding was allowed to continue there without interruption. And the longer periods the nomads spent in the Haud added to the political problems between Somalia and Ethiopia and also exercised an important concern about public health in the former country.

Further reading: Colbourne, *Malaria in Africa*; Prothero, *Migrants and Malaria*.

Somalian Smallpox Epidemic of 1936

Outbreak of the variola (smallpox) virus in what is now Somalia, killing 471 persons out of 1,142 reported infected during its six-weeks duration in 1936.

During the Italo-Ethiopian War of 1935–36, numerous unvaccinated Ethiopian troops carried the highly contagious virus (which may be airborne or spread by direct contact) into Italian Somaliland, where nomads contracted the disease and carried it to others. Some inhabitants at the seaport of Berbera in British Somaliland became infected, as well as some people in Mogadiscio (Mogadishu), the seaport capital of Italian Somaliland, and in smaller seaports, such as Obbia and Eil, on the eastern Somali coast bordering the Indian Ocean. In this largely desert region, with its arid climate, the smallpox, filterable virus is capable of surviving very well, and consequently the infection was able to escalate. All Somali age groups were affected, except adults who had built up an immunity from previous infection. During the epidemic, Somalis practiced strict isolation of patients and burned their houses and clothing to prevent the spread of smallpox. Many survivors were blinded and nearly all were disfigured in some way by the epidemic, which occurred about when Italy merged Italian Somaliland, Eritrea, and the newly conquered Ethiopia into the colonial federation of Italian East Africa (May 9, 1936).

Further reading: Cahill, *Health on the Horn of Africa*; Hopkins, *Princes and Peasants: Smallpox in History*.

South African Dengue Epidemic of 1926–27

See DURBAN DENGUE EPIDEMIC OF 1926–27.

South African Diphtheria Epidemics of 1938–43

Series of severe outbreaks of diphtheria (an infectious disease of childhood) that infected a total of 18,969 persons (at least 1,000 of whom died) in the Union of South Africa. For many decades South Africans, black and white, had suffered greatly from the ravages of diphtheria, caused by the bacillus *Corynebacterium diphtheriae*, which primarily infects the throat and secretes a strong toxin that strikes the nervous and circulatory systems and the heart.

In 1938 South Africa's reported case-incidence of diphtheria greatly increased to 2,673, almost double the number usually recorded yearly. Because about 50 percent of the country's native black and Asiatic populations lived barely at "subsistence level," these people were not always able to provide their children with adequate health care; consequently, the mortality rate was higher among these children than among white Europeans. In 1939 there were 3,480 diphtheria cases, and 3,050 cases in 1940.

Diphtheria patients are infective to others as long as the virulent bacilli are present in their throat secretions; close contact spreads the disease. Many South African children contracted it in schools, sometimes through articles (pencils, crockery, and cutlery) contaminated with discharges from infected persons. In addition, cows carrying diphtheria bacilli in their udders helped spread the disease in their raw milk.

South African physicians could diagnose susceptibility to diphtheria by means of the Schick test, before preventive measures of inoculation with modified diphtheria toxoid were initiated. A certain proportion of the children were immune to the disease, having recovered from an attack or acquired immunity through inapparent infection. The Schick test was performed on many throughout the country, but epidemics continued to occur for the next three years: 3,032 cases were reported in 1941, 3,317 in 1942, and 3,417 in 1943. More than 500 deaths (mainly children) occurred during these three years, and many children became permanently disabled by the disease. Since then, mass immunization for diphtheria in South Africa has been carried out among all infants in their first year.

Further reading: Cluver, *Public Health in South Africa*; Simmons et al., *Global Epidemiology*.

South African Malaria Epidemics of 1929–35

Outbreaks of malaria on South African sugar estates in the eastern province of Natal that killed a reported 2,751 persons in the first episode (1929–30) and more than 10,000 in 1932 in the heart of Zululand (a part of Natal).

In the 1850s sugar plantations began to be established in the British colony of Natal, whose plains had been used mainly for livestock grazing. Later, in 1897, the Zulu kingdom was annexed to Natal after the British had invaded and taken control of it. Sugar became an important crop for the economy of the Union of South Africa (granted dominion status by Britain in 1910), and by 1929 landowners had established some 650 sugar estates, employing about a million-and-a-half black African workers.

After the first malaria outbreak in Natal, which apparently originated among susceptible emigrant laborers recruited from other African areas and India, South Africa's senior assistant health officer, Dr. G. A. Park Ross, organized dispensaries of free quinine, an antimalarial salt drug. There were less severe outbreaks in the following summers (1930 and 1931), but many people had little faith in the drug and preferred the herbalist cures of tribal witch doctors. Though quinine was a remedy for malaria, Ross realized it would not control the epidemic in Natal and, in the summer of 1931, decided to attack the infectious malaria-carrying mosquitoes by spraying the insecticide pyrethrum on workers' barracks and other places on the sugar estates. Not all the plantation owners were receptive to spraying until many thousands of workers died in the 1932 epidemic.

At first most South Africans were reluctant to spray water bodies, natural breeding environments of the *Anopheles gambiae* and *Anopheles funestus* mosquitoes, the chief vectors of the malaria parasite that had invaded Natal. They thought it would "spoil" their water supply and their cattle in some way. Instead, the breeding sites in the barracks were sprayed, while the mosquito-breeding places along Natal's large area of river beds were not. Later, native village huts were also sprayed, and the epidemic waned. Still later, numerous water pools were targeted, and a successful eradication of malaria resulted.

Further reading: Harrison, *Mosquitoes, Malaria and Man;* Scott, *A History of Tropical Medicine.*

South African Meningitis Epidemics of 1967–72

Various localized outbreaks of cerebrospinal meningitis (CSM) in South Africa, infecting a total of nearly 10,000 persons. Since 1919, when the country recorded its first CSM outbreak of 21 cases, the disease occurred sporadically, with as many as 2,168 cases in a severe outbreak in 1954.

Incidence of CSM then decreased for about a dozen years until 1967, when many infections were reported in South African urban centers such as Cape Town (Capetown) and Johannesburg, as well as in the Transvaal's rich gold-producing region (the extensive Witwatersrand, or the Rand). Poorly ventilated and crowded mining compounds, such as the Rand mines, were conducive to the spread of the infectious meningococcus *Neisseria meningitidis* and certain other bacteria. Often spread to and from

persons by droplet infection through sneezing and coughing, CSM's usual source of infection in the South African epidemics was asymptomatic carriers, who had no serious symptoms (fever, headache, vomiting, and stiff neck), yet harbored the bacteria in their throats and noses.

In 1967 there were a reported 1,994 CSM cases in South Africa; the infections rose to 2,135 cases in 1968 and then declined to 1,934 and 1,490 cases in 1969 and 1970 respectively. Many children under five years old were attacked and treated with sulfonamide drugs and antibiotics, along with sick older children and adults. Depending on the location, about seven percent to 12 percent of the patients died between 1967 and 1970; some recovering patients were in danger of becoming deaf or mentally deficient. During the epidemics and afterward in South Africa, certain strains of CSM became resistant to sulfonamide drugs and penicillin, thus indicating the adaptability of the meningococcal organism. After the 1972 outbreak, when 2,080 persons were infected, the disease subsided once again, thanks to increasingly effective and fast-acting medications.

Further reading: Cluver, *Public Health in South Africa;* Hartwig and Patterson, *Cerebrospinal Meningitis in West Africa and Sudan in the Twentieth Century.*

South African Plagues of 1935 and 1936

Epidemics of mainly pneumonic plague that killed 349 persons out of 543 infected in the *veldt* regions (grasslands) of South Africa.

Following serious outbreaks of plague in the coastal areas of South Africa between 1900 and 1905, the plague bacillus (*Yersinia* or *Pasteurella pestis*) had died out among domestic rodents (reservoirs of plague) in the towns and cities, but it had smoldered among wild rodents in the *veldts* in southwestern Transvaal, northwestern Orange Free State, the Cape midlands, and the Uitenhagen district near Port Elizabeth. After 1912, sporadic local outbreaks of plague had occurred with annual epizootics among the wild gerbil populations in the above-mentioned regions of South Africa.

After a great number of wild rodents in the *veldt* regions died of plague in the summer of 1935, multimammate mice or rats picked up the plague-infected fleas (one way of transmitting the disease) from gerbil burrows in sandy areas and carried them into native huts, where persons were seriously infected; there were a reported 290 cases of the disease in 1935. A small number of these cases were bubonic plague, with victims having splitting headaches, bouts of diarrhea, and vomiting; they also ran high fevers and had painful golfball-size buboes (swellings) in their groin or armpits. These bubonic patients often developed pneumonic plague, became highly contagious, and thus spread the disease to numerous others (pneumonic plague is the most serious and highly infectious form); victims usually perished within two to four days after the initial infections. There were also cases of septicemic plague, in which the human blood stream is invaded and poisoned by the virulent bacillus; it may include pharyngeal and tonsillar infections, too.

By the end of 1935, human fatalities totaled 184. The mortality rate was highest among the Asiatic population of South Africa (76 percent); lower among the native Bantu people (59 percent); and lowest among the white European population (30 percent).

The plague disease again broke out in these same regions of South Africa in 1936, displaying similar characteristics of the 1935 epidemic. There were 165 human deaths out of 253 reported cases. Preventive measures were instituted: isolation of patients with plague; sanitary programs; rodent suppression by poisoning and trapping. Thus, the potential for epizootic plague was fairly checked. In 1937 only 52 plague cases were recorded, along with 17 deaths. But plague continued to be a serious health problem in South Africa until 1949, when public education, rodent control, and vaccination of persons helped prevent outbreaks.

Further reading: Cluver, *Public Health in South Africa;* Pollitzer, *Plague.*

South African Pneumonia Epidemics of the Early 1900s
Severe annual outbreaks of pneumonia in the Johannesburg area of South Africa during the early years of the twentieth century, killing more than 40,000 black African miners working the rich gold fields of the Witwatersrand, commonly called the Rand (an enormous rock ridge).

Since 1893 blacks from the tropical areas of Africa had been recruited each year to work in the South African gold mines for periods of six to nine months. Many blacks barely survived long, difficult journeys from their native villages to arrive at the vast mine compounds. Suffering from malnutrition and the change in temperature from tropical heat to the cool, high Rand, they were often assigned to live in unsanitary barracks, where they contracted pneumonia as easily as in the mines. This disease of bacterial (or viral) origin attacks the lungs, bringing fever, chest pain, usually dyspnea and leucocytosis, and coughing.

In 1900 more than 111,500 native Africans were working in the gold mines of the Crown Mines Company in Johannesburg. During the five-year period of 1900–1904, about 45,000 miners caught pneumonia and some 6,500 of them died. Public attention was

drawn to the disease situation in the mines; church and social groups denounced the exploitation of the miners, who also caused a labor strike in the Rand mines. The South African mineowners, however, continued to recruit cheap native labor.

By 1910 more than one out of three miners was perishing from pneumonia; this resulted in South Africa's British government announcing that the recruitment of laborers would have to end unless better health protection was assured the miners. In 1913, the Bureau of Native Affairs prohibited further importation of mine workers from tropical areas north of 22° S. latitude. Afterward the mineowners, realizing the financial consequences, became very interested in the control and eradication of pneumonia in their workers. Owners attempted to select blacks less susceptible to the disease and gave protective inoculations from time to time, but pneumonia remained a dangerous health problem for South African miners until 1933, when sulfonamide drugs were first introduced and dramatically reduced the disease's mortality rate by 1939.

Further reading: Chase, *Magic Shots;* Cluver, *Public Health in South Africa.*

South African Pneumonia Epidemics of 1926–40
Serious outbreaks of pneumonia that claimed the lives of 4,495 miners out of 41,394 infected in the Union (now Republic) of South Africa.

In its various forms, pneumonia was prevalent throughout South Africa, particularly affecting infant mortality in the poor classes of Europeans and the non-Europeans. It was a severe health problem for the Bantu natives employed in the gold mines of the Witwatersrand (or the Rand), an enormous ridge of auriferous rock in the southern Transvaal (a province). Before 1926, the incidence of pneumonia was about 80 per 1,000 miners, and there were about 12 deaths per 1,000 workers in the Central-Mining Rand Mines Group. High mortality in the mines in the early 1900s made it difficult to recruit natives, who often refused to work.

In South Africa, pneumonia's infectious agent was principally *Streptococcus pneumoniae* (pneumococci). Pneumonia's inflammation of the lungs was caused by changes in temperature, the presence of other infections (which lowered the resistance of the respiratory system to pneumococci), malnutrition, and bad housing; other factors for predisposing pneumonia infection were alcoholism, trauma, and influenza. In 1926 some 50 to 60 percent of the Bantu workers lived at subsistence level and were unable to buy food to meet minimum dietary requirements. Working conditions in the mines was very strenuous, adding to the susceptibility of Rand Mines' workers,

15,430 of whom contracted pneumonia from 1926 to 1930; there were 1,829 reported deaths during those five years, the worst year being 1928, with 3,637 infections and 475 deaths. From 1931 to 1935 there were 13,304 infected workers and 1,672 fatalities from pneumonia. During four of those five years, the use of vaccines helped reduce morbidity and mortality rates, but in 1935 the incidence of the disease escalated to 3,382 cases, with the death of 410 miners that year.

The following year special attention began to be paid to the acclimatization of the Rand miners; in the winter months when the miners came up from the warm, humid depths of the gold mines into the cold, dry air above ground, they were supplied with warm coverings and hot meals before they went home. The incidence of pneumonia began to decline slowly; from 1936 to 1940 there were 12,600 cases and 994 fatalties. With the use of sulfonamide drugs to treat patients, mortality fell to 56 deaths in 1939 and 69 in 1940.

Further reading: Cluver, *Public Health in South Africa;* Simmons et al., *Global Epidemiology.*

South African Smallpox Epidemics   See CAPE COLONY AND CAPE TOWN SMALLPOX EPIDEMICS OF 1713, 1755, 1882–85.

South African Tuberculosis Epidemics of 1906–14
Serious outbreaks of tuberculosis (TB) that killed more than 5,000 persons in South Africa. Since the late nineteenth century, the South African seaports of Cape Town, East London, Port Elizabeth, and Durban had recorded increases in TB, a chronic communicable mycobacterial infection of the lungs, bones, and other body organs. In some places, there were more than 15 deaths per thousand residents annually; overcrowded housing, lack of sanitation, and inadequate diets helped spread the infection.

The largest number of TB cases occurred in Johannesburg, the center of South Africa's important gold-mining industry, where 1,129 persons perished from the disease between 1906 and 1909. TB claimed 810 victims in Johannesburg from 1909 to 1911 and an additional 1,217 victims from 1911 to 1914. Overall death rates in the mining centers (the Rand, Kimberley, and Johannesburg mines) climbed to more than 100 fatalities per thousand persons in 1908. However, numerous cases were misdiagnosed as pneumonia, and since mine owners often sent home sick black African laborers, the actual mortality figures for TB probably were inaccurate.

Some authorities claimed TB arrived with infected European miners, who spread the disease by coughing and expectorating infectious tubercle bacilli while working closely with black recruits in narrow, poorly ventilated stopes (excavations) for long hours. But the mine operators and managers objected to this claim and argued that TB was common in rural regions of South Africa and the recruits brought the disease with them; TB surveys conducted between 1910 and 1912 disputed this argument. The disease remained a serious health problem in South Africa until the development of streptomycin and other effective anti-TB drugs during the early 1950s.

Further reading: Cluver, *Public Health in South Africa;* Packard, *White Plague, Black Labor.*

South African Typhus Epidemics of 1934 and 1935
Outbreaks of louse-borne typhus fever in the Union of South Africa, killing about 13 percent of the reported 12,782 persons infected by *rickettsia prowazeki,* carried by body lice.

In 1934 South Africa suffered a prolonged drought and subsequent crop failure that impaired the nutrition and health of the native population; these conditions, along with native unhygienic ways, helped the occurrence of typhus. The province of the former Orange Free State reported 3,636 typhus cases, followed by the Cape province with 1,905 cases, the Transvaal with 208, and Natal with 207. In these four provinces in 1934, only 45 Europeans contracted the disease, which struck the natives living in the reserves (Transkei and Ciskei) much more critically. There were no cases reported in Swaziland and Bechuanaland, where louse-borne typhus had never been known to have occurred.

Another outbreak hit the four abovementioned provinces in 1935, resulting in a higher mortality rate than the year before. Of the 6,826 typhus-infected persons, there were 998 deaths, five of which were Europeans (97 had contracted the disease in 1935). At times, doctors had difficulty differentiating typhus from measles and typhoid fever in Bantu patients, whose dark skin sometimes hid the characteristic dark red rash.

Further reading: Cluver, *Public Health in South Africa;* Gear, "South African Typhus."

South Pacific Islands Dysentery Epidemics of 1843
Outbreaks of dysentery that affected several islands in French Polynesia and some of the Cook Islands in the South Pacific.

Tahiti, in the Windward Island group of the Society Islands, was struck hard early in 1843. Eyewitness accounts convey the severity of the dysentery outbreak. Apparently, the disease affected children and adults of all social classes and was particularly devastating along Tahiti's southern coast. Mortality was extremely high during the first six months of the year.

Dysentery also invaded Huahine and some of the other Society Islands of the Leeward group in 1843. At least 50 Huahine residents died during the outbreak by October 1843. Raiatéa and Tahaa, in the same island group, also suffered an epidemic of dysentery during 1843. Twenty people died, most of them children. Borabora (a Leeward island) was similarly invaded by the disease in that year. While mortality statistics are not available, many people died; some were hastened to their end by the practices of native healers. Mortality in these islands during the epidemic was estimated at a maximum of three percent.

Aitutaki and Mangaia, two of the smaller Cook Islands, were attacked by dysentery in 1843. About a hundred people died during the outbreak in Aitutaki. A crewmember of a whaling vessel is credited with introducing the disease into Rarotonga, largest of the Cook Islands, in July 1843. There, dysentery claimed 130 of the 443 persons who died on the island during the year.

Further reading: McArthur, *Island Populations of the Pacific.*

South Pacific Islands Influenza Epidemic of 1918–19

Part of the Spanish Influenza Epidemic of 1917–19 (q.v.), which wreaked havoc across much of the world and which attacked most countries in two separate waves of varying intensity. Among the island populations of the South Seas (South Pacific Ocean), previously unexposed to such infections, the epidemic had a devastating effect.

The infection is believed to have been introduced into the South Pacific islands by a ship from Auckland, New Zealand (see NEW ZEALAND INFLUENZA EPIDEMIC OF 1918–19; AUSTRALIAN INFLUENZA EPIDEMIC OF 1918–19). The steamer *Talune* left Auckland late in October 1918 and arrived at Suva in the Fiji Islands on November 4, 1918, with some influenza-infected patients on board. Within a few days, the infection spread inland and, in a relatively short period, across most of Fiji. In some areas, the mortality rate was as high as ten percent. The death toll was registered at 8,145 persons in a population of 163,972.

From Fiji the *Talune* set sail northeastward for Samoa with Fijian workers on board. It arrived in the Western Samoan islands of Upolu and Savaii on November 7, 1918, unleashing a devastating epidemic upon a highly susceptible population. By December 31, 1918, almost 8,000 people (mainly native islanders) had died of influenza in three Samoan island groups, a mortality rate of nearly 20 percent.

The *Talune* departed Samoa southward for Tonga, arriving there on November 12, 1918. A few days after it had left on its return journey to Suva, influenza broke out and spread across the Tonga Islands, affecting almost all the natives. About 1,800 Tongans died; the mortality rate there was eight percent, considerably lower than in Samoa. The Australian government dispatched a Medical Relief Expedition headed by Surgeon Grey to Samoa and Tonga. The epidemic led to the establishment of the Department of Health in Tonga.

The western Pacific island of Guam lost 858 people to the epidemic within two months (in 1898 Guam was ceded by Spain and became a U.S. possession administered by the Department of the Navy).

Tahiti, in the Society Islands (French Polynesia), was also devastated, losing one seventh of its 4,500 inhabitants between November 25 and December 10, 1918. Among the natives, the morbidity was nearly two thirds. The death toll was so high that proper burials were not possible. Instead, the streets in Tahiti were full of trucks transporting the dead to mass cremation sites.

The rest of the Society Islands suffered considerable damage too. Makatea Island reported 80 deaths in a population of less than 800. Uturoa, a town on Raiatea Island, lost 70 of its 500 residents. Of the 15,300 people living in French settlements in Oceania, 1,498 died during this epidemic.

New Caledonia (annexed by the French in 1853) was not infected until July 1921, when a ship bearing the influenza infection arrived from Sydney, Australia. The epidemic was much milder here than elsewhere in the region, but the attack rate among native islanders was very high.

Overall, there were upwards of 50,000 human deaths in the sparsely populated and relatively isolated South Sea islands during this influenza epidemic.

Further reading: Jordan, *Epidemic Influenza: A Survey.*

South-West African Typhoid Epidemic of 1904–07

Outburst of typhoid fever that killed 439 German troops engaged in fighting the Herero and Nama native people in South-West Africa (Namibia). In early 1904 the Herero nation (comprised of Bantu natives) revolted against the German occupying forces, which were soon reinforced by 14,000 additional German troops.

Poor sanitation and hygiene in the German military camps led to the first outbreak of typhoid at Onjatu (midway between Windhoek and Waterberg) in April 1904. Exposed to cold and rainy weather and extreme hardships, 25 officers and 509 soldiers (the first to be infected) most likely contracted the disease from contaminated water, and ten days later 60 more men became infected, with symptoms of severe abdominal pain, diarrhea, intense headache, and high fever. The entire German division was then moved to Otji-haenena, where the sick received more adequate medical treatment and the healthy were quarantined.

Typhoid remained a serious problem for the duration of the war against the Hereros, who were joined by the Nama nation (Hottentots of Khoi-Khoi origin) in October 1904. It is not known why the German soldiers were not initially inoculated with an effective vaccine against typhoid (available since 1897) before they were sent to Africa. Of the 1,491 German troops who died during the war, only 802 of them perished from battle wounds; many of the rest succumbed to typhoid.

Further reading: Hallett, *Africa Since 1875;* Prinzing, *Epidemics Resulting from Wars.*

Southwest Pacific Dengue Epidemics of the 1970s

Dengue epidemics that occurred in various island groups of the southwest Pacific (see FIJI ISLANDS DENGUE EPIDEMICS OF 1971–73 AND 1975).

The region's first epidemic of the decade began almost simultaneously in Fiji and Tahiti around March 1971. Toward the end of May, the number of reported cases in Tahiti began to increase. The epidemic peaked in late June–early July and subsided by September. Tahiti's rural and urban areas were affected, as were the islands of Moorea, Huahine, Raiatea, Tahaa, Bora Bora, and Maupiti. Many dengue cases were not diagnosed or reported, so precise numbers are not available, but it is estimated that 50 percent of Tahiti's population was attacked during the epidemic. Exceptionally severe hemorrhagic symptoms—mainly gastrointestinal—were observed in a large number of cases, particularly in adults. The severity of this outbreak was attributed to a highly virulent strain of the dengue type 2 virus.

In September 1971, the type 2 virus arrived in New Caledonia where it caused a major outbreak that reportedly affected 25,000 people. Some people suffered from the hemorrhagic form of the disease and there was at least one recorded death.

During March–August 1972, Niue Island suffered a major epidemic of dengue, with 90 percent of its 4,600 residents being struck by it. While all age groups were equally affected, young children experienced a more severe form (shock and hemorrhages) of the disease. Twelve deaths were reported, mainly among children. The virus was apparently introduced on the island in February 1972 by Europeans arriving from Fiji or Samoa. The outbreak began in the south, then spread to Alofi (commercial and administrative hub of Niue) and, subsequently, to the north and east. The Health Department reported treating 790 dengue cases. However, since many

people with mild symptoms did not even seek treatment, these figures are not accurate. The *Aëdes cooki* mosquito was incriminated as the main vector of the dengue type 2 virus, which caused this outbreak. An intensive mosquito control campaign, including mass education and spraying, did not noticeably affect the course of the epidemic. In addition, another outbreak of dengue caused by the type 2 virus occurred on American Samoa during 1972.

The region-wide dengue epidemics of 1974–75, caused by the type 1 virus, were more explosive. The first outbreaks were reported from the Marshall Islands early in 1974, from Nauru in mid-1974, and from the Gilbert and Ellice Islands (Kiribati and Tuvalu respectively) in late 1974; Fiji and the island of New Hebrides became infected in January 1975, New Caledonia and Tonga in March 1975, and French Polynesia and Western and American Samoa by mid-1975.

The dengue type 2 virus caused a minor outbreak in Tonga during March–April 1974. By all accounts, it was a mild and brief epidemic with a low attack rate. In 1975, however, Tonga experienced an explosive epidemic caused by the type 1 virus. Though the earliest cases were identified in March, dengue had been prevalent for weeks before that. The epidemic rapidly intensified and, barely six weeks after the notification of the first case, almost 1,000 cases were reported from Tongatabu alone. Twelve deaths were recorded, but the actual figure may have been higher. It also spread to the Haabai and Vavau group of islands, with the Vavau group recording more than 1,400 cases by the end of April. In August, outbreaks occurred on some islands of the Niuatobu-tabu group. Overall, a lower incidence was found in children under five years and adults over 45 years of age. Hemorrhagic symptoms were frequently observed in many cases. The infection, in a majority of cases, was primary. The *Aëdes aegypti* and *Aëdes tabu* mosquitoes were the main vectors involved.

In New Caledonia, where dengue was prevalent on Noumea Island in March 1975 and on Ouvea Island in July of that year, the epidemic did not take root until March 1976. When it ended in October 1978, more than 3,000 clinical cases had been observed. The Wallis and Futuna Islands (dependencies of New Caledonia) reported 20 cases and 400 cases of dengue respectively.

In 1979, another series of dengue outbreaks occurred in this region, the causative agent being the dengue type 4 virus. It all started in Tahiti early in 1979 and spread rapidly to other island groups. Noumea, where the earliest cases occurred in March 1979, did not suffer an outbreak until 1980, when 587 confirmed cases were reported. Minor outbreaks also occurred in Wallis (October 1979) and Futuna (January 1980).

Further reading: Mackenzie, ed., *Viral Diseases in South-East Asia and the Western Pacific.*

Southwest Pacific Malaria Epidemics of 1942–45

Malaria outbreaks that caused serious problems for Allied troops fighting in the southwest Pacific military campaigns of World War II.

For the Australian troops, the suffering began early in January 1942 as they walked across the jungles of the island of New Britain in the South Pacific. Their base at Rabaul had just been captured by the Japanese, and the soldiers were trying to escape capture themselves by moving away from the area. Armed with adequate doses of quinine, they set out on the long trek. Before long, malaria was striking them. The unit's supplies of quinine were exhausted by the end of the first month. Within the next four to five weeks, at least 50 soldiers died of malignant tertian malaria. Many of the survivors who fled via New Guinea to Australia apparently suffered from malignant and benign tertian malaria infections. The benign tertian infection was discovered to be quite different from that which had plagued the troops during the Middle East campaign. Whereas relapses were common in both cases, in the Middle East they usually occurred some six to nine months after the initial attack of fever, thus giving the patient time to gather strength and the prescribed medicine time to take effect. In the southwest Pacific, relapses were prompt and frequent, and many patients were often too ill for combat duty.

Throughout the military campaigns in the region, malaria was a far bigger threat than enemy action. For instance, at Milne Bay, Buna-Gona, and the Markham and Ramu River valleys in New Guinea and at Guadalcanal, mortality from malaria was considerably higher (sometimes 30 to 1) than death by enemy fire. The military, deprived of valuable manpower at a critical juncture, authorized the establishment of a research group in Queensland, Australia, to study the stock of anti-malarial drugs for value and efficacy, with special attention to Atabrine (quinacrine). The study found that Atabrine, administered regularly in the right dosage, was effective against malaria. Subsequently, Atabrine therapy was made compulsory in the South Pacific (and elsewhere in the military campaign), and the results were remarkable. From a case fatality rate of 740 per 1,000 soldiers in New Guinea in December 1943, it declined to 26 per 1,000 by November 1944. At the end of the war, as soon as Atabrine was discontinued, relapses of benign tertian malaria occurred frequently, even though the medicine had been taken for many years.

The American troops suffered severely as well. For instance, during the Bataan campaign in the Philippine Islands, nearly 85 percent of the besieged soldiers were struck by malaria and had no access to relief supplies. Early in 1942, the Americans occupied the New Hebrides Islands, where troops landing in advance on the island of Efate (Vaté) to build an airfield were promptly attacked by malaria. Within two months, nearly two thirds of the soldiers were struck. Anti-malarial drugs and other preventive supplies such as screens (around tents) were inadequate. Also, the spraying of insecticide was performed by untrained personnel and was not well-coordinated.

The Americans arrived at Guadalcanal in the Solomon Islands in August 1942. Within a month, malaria incidence had increased twelve-fold and, by October, it exploded into a major epidemic that lasted for over eight months. Reportedly, over 100,000 American army, navy, and marine personnel suffered from malaria, some of them twice. Sometimes, entire units had to be evacuated because almost everyone had malaria. For instance, nearly 80 percent of the command of the U.S. 1st Marine Division was in hospital with malaria, thus paralyzing the unit for months. Initially, *Plasmodium falciparum* (malaria parasite) infections were more common but, during the second phase, *Plasmodium vivax* (malaria parasite) infections were observed in over 95 percent of all cases.

Once again, wartime exigencies precluded the implementation of any massive anti-malarial efforts. The situation was apparently even worse in the Japanese camp and may have been an important contributing factor in America's eventual victory.

Preventive medical efforts began rather slowly. In July 1942, a malariologist was despatched to Efate; supplies and additional manpower arrived much later. Help arrived on the New Hebrides island of Espíritu Santo in September and on Guadalcanal in November. This eventually became the nucleus of a large (5,000 man strong) and effective anti-malaria force, consisting of skilled technicians and specialists drawn from all branches of the American military, as well as some from New Zealand's units. Wherever possible, natives were employed to handle the manual labor. However, anti-malaria work was relegated to second place once the fighting began and often delayed indefinitely for weeks or months.

Malaria education was an important element in the anti-malaria strategy, with special emphasis on individual preventive measures. In the area headquarters at New Caledonia, special training centers were established to train and equip personnel to deal with malaria in the field. Spraying with larvicide (mainly diesel oil until the advent of DDT) was one of the earliest control activities to be undertaken. During the remainder of the military campaign in the region, the malaria control program became a well-coordinated and highly effective one. The science of malariology advanced far more rapidly during the latter phase of World War II than during any other period in history.

Further reading: Warshaw, *Malaria: The Biography of a Killer*; Spink, *Infectious Diseases*.

Southwest Pacific Ross River Fever Epidemics of 1979–80

Ross River fever or epidemic polyarthritis that erupted across many island groups in the southwest Pacific; considered the first outbreaks of the disease outside Australia. Isolated cases had apparently occurred earlier in Papua New Guinea, the Solomon Islands, the Moluccas or Spice Islands, and Vietnam.

The first reports were from the Fiji Islands, where cases of polyarthritis with rash were observed in many people living around Nadi in western Viti Levu, Fiji's main island, in April 1979. On April 26, the matter was brought to the attention of the Fijian health authorities. The disease spread rapidly across Viti Levu, even penetrating the inland town of Namosi, but Suva, the capital of Fiji, recorded only scattered cases. In May, the Fiji islands of Vanua Levu and Taveuni were infected, some areas suffering a higher rate of infection than others. Twenty percent of the patients suffered from an itchy rash mainly on their extremities. The highest infection rate (23 percent) was reported from Nawaka. An estimated 30,000 people were affected by the disease throughout the island country.

Laboratory analysis identified the Ross River virus, an alphavirus of the *Togaviridae* family, as the infectious, causative agent. The virus is transmitted by mosquitoes; among the known mosquito vectors in the southwest Pacific are the *Aedes vigilax*, the *Culex annulirostris*, and the *Aedes polynesiensis*. The Fijian epidemic may have been caused either by a recent introduction of the virus into the country (possibly from Australia or Papua New Guinea, where it was endemic) or by an upset in the hitherto balanced host-virus relationship.

In the early stages, Ross River fever is difficult to diagnose because of the vagueness of the symptoms—fatigue, anorexia, myalgia, headache, and low-grade fever. Its most characteristic feature—arthralgia—usually develops two or three days after onset. The arthralgia usually involves more than one joint and ranges from a mere stiffness of the joints to unbearable neuralgic pain and sometimes persists long after the patient has recovered from all other symptoms.

In August 1979, the Ross River virus caused outbreaks in American Samoa. Subsequently, it was reported from the Wallis and Futuna Islands, New Caledonia, Tonga, and the Cook Islands. The virus was isolated from patients in Futuna (where the *Aedes polynesiensis* mosquito was the vector) in November 1979, and later in the year, from Wallis (two cases) and New Caledonia (31 cases). In the latter outbreak, the *Aedes aegypti* mosquito was determined as the vector in the urban areas.

Early in 1980, the virus invaded Rarotonga, the most populous of the Cook Islands. The first cases occurred late in January but were apparently not diagnosed until more cases occurred during the next month. Most of Rarotonga's cases began in March 1980; very few cases were observed after that. Other islands in the group were also affected; by the end of July 1980, Aitutaki, Mangaia, Mauke, Manihiki, Penrhyn, and Rakahanga had reported cases of polyarthritis. Studies of this outbreak revealed the disease's incubation period to be as short as three days, and the *Aedes polynesiensis* mosquito to be the mostly likely vector. Currently, the only protection against the disease is controlling the mosquito population and taking steps against getting bitten oneself.

Further reading: Mackenzie, ed., *Viral Diseases in South-East Asia and the Western Pacific*; Warren and Mahmoud, eds., *Tropical and Geographical Medicine*.

Southwest Pacific Typhus Epidemics of 1942–45

Several outbreaks of scrub typhus (*febris tsutsugamushi*, Japanese river fever, mite-borne typhus) occurring among American and Australian troops.

The disease was first noticed during the late summer and fall of 1942 around the Port Moresby and Milne Bay areas in New Guinea. It intensified as the troops traveled to the north coast of Papua (New Guinea's eastern territory) in November-December and continued to infect them during the spring and summer of 1943 as the units moved toward Finschafen. Fighting in the forefront, the Australian troops suffered far more from scrub typhus than their American counterparts did. Even the troops on adjacent Pacific islands were affected to varying degrees. Cases were reported among the military on the islands of Espíritu Santo, New Georgia, and Bougainville. A small but intense outbreak occurred on Goodenough Island (Rarotonga) where, during the period November 1, 1943–January 15, 1944, 75 cases and 19 deaths were reported from a hospital on Malauna Bay. Soldiers landing at Cape Gloucester on New Britain Island (off the east coast of New Guinea) were also infected.

Overall, during the initial phase (1942–43) of the operations, 957 cases of scrub typhus and 53 deaths were reported from American Army bases, a case fatality rate of 5.9 percent. This varied dramatically; for instance, at Finschafen, it rose to 35.3 percent.

During late 1943–early 1944, there was an outbreak of scrub typhus on Batanta Island. By far the most serious outbreaks in the region occurred between June and August 1944, immediately following the landings at Owi-Biak and Sansapor (in west Irian Jaya). In the outbreak at Owi-Biak, almost one fourth to one third of the active personnel of three battalions of ground forces and two air force squadrons were hospitalized with scrub typhus. Some units could not be mobilized until their sick members had been replaced. A total of 1,469 cases of scrub typhus and seven deaths (0.5 percent mortality) were recorded at Owi-Biak by December 1944. It is estimated that this cost the army 90,000 lost man-days.

The epidemic at Sansapor led to the hospitalization of 931 patients over a 53-day period and a case fatality rate of 3.4 percent. In the first 20 days after the outbreak began, 308 members of one regiment were admitted to the hospital and ten deaths were reported. An estimated 60,000 man-days were lost in this outbreak.

During 1944–45, scattered outbreaks occurred in six islands of the Philippines (Leyte, Samar, Mindoro, Luzon, Negros, and Mindanao). American forces in these islands reported 222 cases of scrub typhus and ten deaths.

According to one account, 5,663 cases of scrub typhus and 234 deaths were reported by the United States Army between January 1943 and August 1945, during its military operations in the southwest Pacific. Overall, 18,000 cases apparently occurred among Allied troops during World War II in this area and in the China-Burma-India region. Early in the Allied campaign, it became obvious that proper clearing and preparation of campsites was the first and most important step toward reducing the incidence of scrub typhus. This was done preferably before or immediately after a military unit had moved into an area. Troops engaged in combat or patrol duties had their uniforms and blankets sprayed with disinfectant, which protected them from mites for a week or so.

The disease begins rather suddenly and is characterized by a high fever usually lasting two weeks, chills, headache, and a skin rash, which appears on or around the fifth day. Mortality occurs when complications such as secondary pneumonia, cardiac failure, or encephalitis set in, usually in untreated or inadequately treated patients. The disease is caused when the infectious agent, *Rickettsia tsutsugamushi*, a microbe found naturally in field mice or rats, is transmitted to man through the bite of the harvest mite, *Trombicula akamushi*. It has been reported from the river valleys of China and Japan, as well as from Korea, Taiwan, Burma, and India.

Further reading: Moulton, ed., *The Rickettsial Diseases of Man*; Horsfall and Tamm, eds., *Viral and Rickettsial Infections of Man*; Davey and Wilson, *The Control of Disease in the Tropics*.

Spanish Cholera Epidemic of 1833–34 First of four deadly epidemics of cholera that affected nearly all of Spain's provinces in 1834, 1854, 1865, and 1885, coinciding with other outbreaks of major proportions in most regions of Europe and elsewhere around the world. All of these outbreaks were part of global pandemics that originated in India (see ASIATIC CHOLERA PANDEMIC OF 1826–37).

Cholera was introduced into Spain in January 1833 by some passengers on Portuguese ships unloading at the northwestern port city of Vigo. Despite forced quarantines and guards posted along the Portuguese frontier, cholera spread to many towns throughout Galicia (region in northwest Spain). In August cholera made its way from the Algarve in southern Portugal into the southern Spanish province of Andalusia, attacking first Huelva and Ayamonte, where troops guarded houses with cholera victims, and subsequently the other main cities of the region, Cádiz, Málaga, and Seville. With the onset of winter cholera briefly ceased, but arose again in January with increased virulence, appearing first in Granada. Throughout the spring it appeared in most other Andalusian cities, subsequently moving along the Mediterranean coast toward Barcelona and north through Toledo, Madrid, Segovia, Valladolid, and Burgos. Although most human deaths occurred in the late summer and fall of 1834, cases continued to be reported until the end of 1835.

A typical cholera outbreak lasted from 12 to 16 weeks, usually with a peak period of two to four weeks during which perhaps half of the total deaths occurred. Madrid suffered the majority of its fatalities in the second half of July. As reported in the *Boletín de Medicina*, cholera's progress was "so rapid, that many people passed from health to death in a few hours, some instantly and as if hit by lightning, and most in the space of twenty-four to forty-eight hours." The rapid demise of cholera's victims and its terrible ravaging of the body, which shrivels from dehydration, suffers acute diarrhea, and turns blue (cholera was called "the blue plague" in Spain), made cholera the most feared disease—although not the deadliest in absolute numbers—since bubonic plague. An estimated 5,000 people died in Madrid out of a population of less than 200,000. Throughout Spain, cholera caused approximately 300,000 deaths in 1833–34.

Spain followed the same anti-cholera measures other European countries practiced, including military cordons placed around infected cities, quarantines of many weeks' duration for both people and goods, expulsion of beggars and vagrants, and checking of health certificates. In August 1834 most of these measures were suspended under pressure from doctors, who maintained they were useless, and from cities whose economies were seriously damaged by the resultant cessation of inter-city commerce. Public and personal hygiene was then advocated as the best means of preventing cholera; sanitary commissions ordered the cleaning of streets, markets, factories, and private dwellings. Unfortunately it was not suspected that cholera bacteria live in water, although efforts were made to clean sewers and prevent use of polluted wells. Many medical reports declared that indigent people and others who led dissolute lives were far more likely to contract cholera than those with wholesome and regular habits. Poor neighborhoods experienced the majority of cholera cases due to overcrowding and lesser access to clean drinking water.

Further reading: Peset-Reig, *Muerte en España (política y sociedad entre la peste y el cólera)*; Fernández, *Epidemias y sociedad en Madrid*; Rodríguez Ocăna, *El cólera de 1834 en Granada*.

Spanish Cholera Epidemic of 1854–55   Second of four major cholera epidemics to afflict Spain in the nineteenth century (see SPANISH CHOLERA EPIDEMIC OF 1833–34). The disease entered Spain through the Atlantic port city of Vigo in early November 1853 (it had also entered through this point in 1833), purportedly by the agency of three infected sailors aboard the warship *Isabel la Católica*. It spread rapidly through the surrounding area, became extinguished in the winter of 1854, and then appeared in Vigo once again in early May.

In July 1854 a ship from Marseilles carried cholera to Barcelona, and by August it had become epidemic in most places along Spain's Mediterranean coast as far south as Cádiz and Huelva. Most of Andalusia (a region in southern Spain) became infected near the end of September, and in October cholera appeared in Castile, Navarre, and Aragon; these central and northern areas suffered the highest mortality rate. In 1855 cholera was less deadly than the year before in the northern provinces, with the exception of Aragon, but retained its virulence in the southern half of the peninsula. Although its force had finally diminished by the end of 1855, cases continued to be reported throughout 1856, especially in Seville, where cholera claimed 3,000 to 4,000 victims. More than 236,000 people died of cholera during these

years, the vast majority in 1854 and 1855. An estimated 830,000 cases occurred, rendering a case-mortality rate of 28 percent.

Madrid's worst period was the summer and fall of 1855, especially October, when 50 people died of cholera every day; approximately 4,200 cholera deaths occurred there in 1855—two percent of its population. The case-mortality rate was more than 50 percent. Other localities lost as much as ten percent of their population to cholera.

Anti-cholera measures such as military cordons surrounding infected cities, roadblocks for checking health documentation and stringent quarantine regulations, which had been imposed vigorously in the first months of the epidemic of 1834 and then abandoned, were not used in 1854–55. Municipal health boards stressed public and private hygiene as the best protection against cholera. The commission of public health in Córdoba advised practicing "the rules of sanitary maintenance, the observation of which can avoid, check, or modify the influence of the deadly germs spread by the atmosphere and which only await local or individual predisposition to become active." This is a reference to the idea that miasmatic air causes disease; although the theory was erroneous, the emphasis on cleanliness was salutary.

Calming the body with powerful sedatives and stimulating it through rubbing and use of drugs remained the standard method of treatment for cholera until the last decade of the century. Tea mixed with mustard or gum arabic, opium in drinks or enemas, diaphoretics, camphorated liniments, and alkaline baths were among the most frequently used treatments.

A minor epidemic of cholera occurred in Spain in 1859–60; out of an estimated 17,200 cases, approximately 6,830 people died.

Further reading: Peset Reig, *Muerte en España (política y sociedad entre la peste y el cólera)*; Fernandez, *Epidemias y sociedad en Madrid*; Arjona Castro, *La población de Córdoba en el siglo XIX*.

Spanish Cholera Epidemic of 1865   Third cholera epidemic in a series of four that broke out in Spain in the nineteenth century. Less devastating than the first two, it claimed approximately 120,000 victims compared with about 300,000 in 1833–34 and more than 236,000 in 1854–55 (see SPANISH CHOLERA EPIDEMIC OF 1854–55).

The first cases were reported from the city of Valencia in early July 1865, where cholera was introduced by an infected passenger on a ship from Marseilles. During August it spread north along the Mediterranean coast to Barcelona and south to Murcia. By the end of September it reached three quarters of Spain's provinces. Madrid lost most of its 2,900 victims in the second week of October. Eastern Spain suffered the highest mortality, particularly the province of Valencia.

Medical treatments, controversy over how cholera spreads, and anti-cholera regulations imposed by local and federal health boards remained much the same throughout the century. See also ASIATIC CHOLERA PANDEMIC OF 1846–63; ASIATIC CHOLERA PANDEMIC OF 1865–75.

Further reading: Peset Reig, *Muerte en España (política y sociedad entre la peste y el cólera)*; Fernández, *Epidemias y sociedad en Madrid*.

Spanish Cholera Epidemic of 1884–85

Last and least destructive of the great cholera epidemics experienced by Spain in the nineteenth century. A boat from the Algerian city of Oran carried infected passengers to Alicante on Spain's Mediterranean coast in August 1884, whence it spread throughout the immediate area, reappearing with intensified virulence in the summer of 1885. Municipal health commissions monitored cleaning and ventilation of public places and private houses, which was the basic preventive measure used in epidemics of every type throughout the nineteenth century. As in the Spanish Cholera Epidemic of 1865 (q.v.), Spain's eastern provinces suffered most, especially Valencia and Saragossa; the Andalusian city of Granada was also violently affected. Madrid suffered comparatively few fatalities (1,366). Total deaths numbered approximately 120,200, with a case-mortality rate of about 28 percent.

The mystery of cholera was solved when Robert Koch, German pioneer bacteriologist, discovered the cholera bacillus in 1883. In 1884 the Valencian physician Jaime Ferrán developed a cholera vaccine, which was largely ignored despite a massive vaccination campaign.

Cholera appeared in Spain for the last time in 1890. Four thousand people died, mostly in and around Valencia, although cases appeared in provinces as far west as Seville and Badajoz. See also ASIATIC CHOLERA PANDEMIC OF 1881–96; HAMBURG CHOLERA EPIDEMIC OF 1892.

Further reading: Peset Reig, *Muerte en España (política y sociedad entre la peste y el cólera)*; Arjona Castro, *La población de Córdoba en el siglo XIX*.

Spanish Diphtheria Epidemics of 1583–1618

Series of epidemics of "angina maligna" or diphtheritic angina that struck various parts of Spain for 35 years. The disease (named diphtheria in 1826) was popularly called by the name of "garrotillo" in Spain ("garrote" is a Spanish mode of execution by strangulation).

Spanish physicians knew little about the disease at the time. Infected children (the disease's chief victims) first had a sore throat with a low fever; then they had difficulty breathing (a grayish membrane forms in the throat to block the trachea [wind-pipe] and causes death through strangulation). Three centuries later, in 1883, German pathologist Edwin Klebs first described the diphtheria bacillus (*Corynebacterium diphtheriae*), which secretes a powerful toxin or bacterial poison that affects the human nervous and circulatory systems and heart, and may have fatal effects if there is no prompt medical treatment. In addition, the disease is contagious from a day before the first symptoms appear to at least two weeks afterward. In 1890 German bacteriologist Emil von Behring developed immunization against diphtheria by the use of an antitoxin (a word he introduced, meaning an antibody capable of counteracting a specific toxin or infective agent).

"Angina maligna" first appeared among the inhabitants of the city of Seville in southwest Spain in 1583. The frightening illness invaded most of the region (Andalusia) during the following decade. In 1596 the city of Granada (southern Spain) was struck by it; the region of Estramadura (west-central Spain) was hit in 1600 and the region of New Castile (central Spain) in 1603. Most of Spain was affected by "garrotillo" from 1610 to 1618; the year 1613 had great morbidity (incidence of disease) and mortality (frequency of death), gaining the name "anno de los garrotillos." The disease subsided but remained endemic throughout the country and reappeared repeatedly in various places throughout the seventeenth century. The city of Saragossa and other parts of Aragón (a region in northeast Spain) suffered through a diphtheria outbreak in 1630. The city of Antequera in southern Spain was also hard hit that year. In 1645 and 1646 the people of Alaejos (a town in Valladolid province) were terrorized by disease, which again spread over many parts of Spain in 1666. The Iberian Peninsula (Spain and Portugal) continued to fear the malady into the next century; especially severe outbreaks occurred in Palencia (a northern Spanish province) in 1715, in Lisbon and other cities and towns in Portugal in 1749, in New Castile and Galicia (regions in northwest Spain) in 1750–62, and in the city of Valencia on the Spanish Mediterranean coast in 1764–71.

Further reading: Burnet and White, *Natural History of Infectious Disease*; Hirsch, *Handbook on Geographical and Historical Pathology*.

Spanish Influenza Epidemic of 1917–19   Virulent pandemic that killed more people than did all the armies in World War I. The final death toll worldwide was estimated at more than 20,000,000 lives, and at least 200,000,000 (possibly as high as 500,000,000) persons became ill with the "grippe," as first the French and then others called this mysterious influenza. Though it ranks with the Plague of Justinian and the Black Death (qq.v.) as one of the most disastrous outbreaks of disease in history, it caused far less panic and dislocation than other epidemics of the past. Perhaps the sensibilities of people were too dulled by World War I and battle casualties and deaths.

Exactly when and where the Spanish Influenza began remains uncertain; however, it was so-called because Spain was the first serious point of attack (some 8,000,000 Spaniards fell ill in 1917–18). It struck military bases throughout Europe, putting tens of thousands of British, French, German, and other soldiers out of action. The British called it "Flanders grippe," and the Germans named it "Blitz Katarrh." In Paris and in French seaports like Brest, death rates from the sickness began to mount ominously in 1918, and at the same time acute respiratory infections suddenly began to be noticed at military installations in the United States (Fort Riley, Kansas, was the first to be hit by the disease, in March 1918). By October, some U.S. Army camps were reporting a death every hour, and Britain then was counting 2,000 deaths per week, with London at about 300 deaths per week. Country after country felt the ravages of the disease.

While manifesting the ordinary symptoms of influenza (headache, severe cold, fever, chills, aching bones and muscles), the Spanish form also generated complications such as severe pneumonia (with purplish lips and ears and a pallid face), purulent bronchitis, mastoid abscess, and heart problems. Called by some the "three-day fever," it developed quietly at first with a cold in the head and later with a high temperature, thus being diagnosed by some as pneumonia. But physicians did not know how to treat it to prevent death in many victims. There were suggestions that carrying asafetida (gum-resin with a garlic-like odor), camphor, cucumbers, or potatoes helped ward off the disease. To prevent its spread, U.S. public health officials recommended that persons avoid crowds, that schools and businesses be less congested, that people smother coughs and sneezes in handkerchiefs, and that buildings and homes be well ventilated. Vaccines were used with some effect, but the U.S. medical community was unable to check the spread of the disease, which swept across the country in 1918.

At least one American in four fell sick to the flu. In various cities, such as Boston, Philadelphia, and New York, public meetings were temporarily banned, and churches, theaters, and saloons shut their doors. The death toll mounted, morgues grew crowded with corpses, coffins became scarce, and some mass burials occurred. Emergency hospitals were set up in town halls, schools, and churches. Many industries and stores went on half-day schedules. And health authorities established quarantine regulations for varying periods. The influenza occurred frequently in children from age five to 14; however, persons sick between 20 and 40 years of age were most likely to die from it (about 500,000 Americans died). U.S. government and health officials were criticized for failing to cope with the emergency; yet there was insufficient scientific knowledge at the time about the exact nature of the influenza in order to uncover its vulnerable spot or cause. Consequently medical quackery prospered, with various "sure cure" remedies offered for sale across America and around the world. People's anxiety only grew.

After the armistice was signed (November 11, 1918), ending the war, the frightening disease seemed to subside, and within a year it was no longer a menace. It later vanished completely. In the 1930s scientists, using the new electron microscope, pinpointed the very tiny cottonball-shaped virus that had caused the influenza, which had reached every country of the world. Among those most affected and devastated were China (where coolies were said to have brought it to France), India (where some 12,500,000 died), Persia (Iran), South Africa, Britain, France, Spain, Germany, Mexico, Canada, the United States, and Australia. Virologists now know that radical genetic mutation, called antigenic shift, accounts for the appearance of new viral subtypes capable of engendering influenza pandemics. New viral types originate in ducks, chickens, pigs, and other animals, in which reservoirs of influenza viruses change genetically and then are passed into the environment, and to human beings. The strain that caused the 1918 epidemic, H1N1 (the first designated strain of the main type of influenza virus, called Type A), was found inside pigs (hence the label "swine flu"). Virologists always fear that the H1N1 strain may resurface, perhaps in as virulent a form as in 1918. Many pandemics originate in Asia, notably China, where enormous numbers of ducks, pigs, and other virus-producing animals live in close proximity to human beings. See also CHINESE INFLUENZA EPIDEMIC OF 1918; CANADIAN INFLUENZA EPIDEMIC OF 1918–19; INDIAN INFLUENZA EPIDEMIC OF

1918–19; BRITISH INFLUENZA EPIDEMIC OF 1918–19; PER-
SIAN INFLUENZA EPIDEMIC OF 1918.

Further reading: Collier, *The Plague of the Spanish Lady:
The Influenza Pandemic of 1918–19;* Crosby, *Epidemic and
Peace, 1918;* Beveridge, *Influenza: The Last Great Plague;*
Smith, *Plague on Us.*

Spanish Plague of 1596–1602

One of the most
destructive epidemics of bubonic plague to occur in
Spain in the 1500s and 1600s. Unlike many other
plague epidemics, which began in Spain's Mediterranean ports, especially Barcelona, in this instance
plague was introduced into northern Spain through
the Atlantic port city of Santander, where the ship
Rodamundo supposedly unloaded plague-bearing
cloth it had picked up in the French port of Dunkirk.
Very likely the ship was carrying infected rats and the
rat-fleas that transmit the plague bacteria to human
beings. The disease spread rapidly west and south
through the regions of Asturias, Galicia, and Old
Castile, then eastward through Vizcaya (Biscay) and
Logroño, until it penetrated, over a six-year period,
the entire expanse of Spain.

The actions taken in the face of plague by the small
city of Segovia, which lost some 12,000 inhabitants
to plague in a six-month period, were typical of
all Spanish cities and towns: creation of provisional
hospitals, often in hermitages; the guarding of town
gates to protect the city from infected travelers; rapid
burial of plague victims to avoid contamination by
their corpses (an erroneous belief that persisted
throughout the plague centuries); burning the bedclothes of the sick.

Historians note that this crushing epidemic of
1596–1602 coincided with a decline in national morale
caused by Spain's military defeats in Europe, political
ineffectiveness within its own borders, and the collapse of its economy. Many Spaniards considered
these epidemic years, which claimed an estimated
500,000 to 600,000 lives (six to eight percent of the
population), an additional punishment God was in-
flicting upon their already burdened nation.

Further reading: Bennassar, *Recherches sur les grandes
épidémies dans le norde de l'Espagne à la fin du XVI siècle;*
Carreras Panchón, *La peste y los médicos en la España del
renacimiento;* Ayuntamiento de Barcelona, *Datos históricos
sobre las epidemias de peste ocurridas en Barcelona.*

Spanish Plagues of the 1400s

Plague epidemics
of varying intensity and widespread incidence that
occurred throughout Spain. The devastating Black
Death (q.v.) of the mid-fourteenth century was only
the beginning of hundreds of years of physical illness, psychological distress, and economic and social
disruption that bubonic plague would continue to
bring to Europe.

Spain hosted plague continuously through the second half of the fifteenth century, although the first
large-scale epidemic of the period occurred in Seville
as early as 1400–1402, during which Seville's arch-
bishop fled the city (only to die from plague in April
1401), a common practice for those who could afford
to do so. Despite the measures a town would routinely take when faced with plague—for example,
the burning of a plague victim's belongings, fumigation of houses, and strictly enforced quarantines—
flight would remain the most highly recommended
method for preserving one's life. Seville suffered
another major epidemic in 1410.

The city of Barcelona was invaded by plague in
1408 and again in 1410, when it created a Council of
One Hundred to oversee anti-plague regulations, one
of the first such councils established in Europe. An
important Mediterranean port into which plague-
bearing rats could be easily introduced aboard ships
from other plague-ridden cities, Barcelona continued
to suffer from plague throughout the century, most
notably in 1429, 1439, 1448, 1457, 1465–66, 1468,
1475, 1483, and 1489–90. Seville, a river port with a
busy trade and known for its gross lack of public
sanitation (at a time when no locality was free of
dirty wells, drains, streets, and houses), was again
struck by plague in 1485, which spread through the
entire Guadalquivir region the following year.
Spain's northern region of Aragón, particularly the
city of Zaragoza (Saragossa), experienced damaging
epidemics in 1486, 1490, and 1495. Valencia, a region
lying on the Mediterranean coast, suffered especially
high mortality from plague in 1450 and 1465–66.
Andalusia, in the south, was overrun with a deadly
epidemic (which may have been typhus fever rather
than plague) in 1489–90, and experienced continuous
outbreaks of plague over much of its area during the
last decade of the century, as did the central region
of Castile.

In addition to the cities, provinces, and regions
mentioned, many other Spanish localities suffered
from plague at one time or another during the fifteenth century, including the cities of Valladolid,
Salamanca, Burgos, and Murcia. Madrid, which was
not yet the seat of the Spanish royal court, would
not suffer badly from plague until 1507. Palma de
Majorca was one of the first Spanish cities to draw
up a comprehensive set of plague regulations (*Ordi-
naciones del Morbo,* 1459), which included enforcement of quarantines and the requirement of
certificates of health from ships entering its port.

Further reading: Carrera Panchon, *La peste y los médicos
en la España del renacimiento;* Ayuntamiento de Barcelona,

Datos históricos sobre las epidemias de peste ocurridas en Barcelona; Ballesteros Rodríguez, *La peste en Córdoba.*

Spanish Plagues of the 1500s

Period during which dozens of epidemics of bubonic plague occurred throughout Spain, blighting the country with illness such as had not been experienced since the Black Death (q.v.) of 1350. Beginning in 1501 with a severe outbreak in Barcelona, nearly every decade thereafter was marked by the unrelenting presence of the plague. Two years later Santander, Oviedo, Pravia and other towns on Spain's Atlantic coast were badly afflicted. One of the worst epidemics of the century, whose miseries were accompanied by severe drought and food shortage, started in 1505; by 1507, about 100,000 people had died in Andalusia (southern Spain) alone, and many major cities, including Barcelona, Madrid, Valladolid, Ávila, and Zaragoza (Saragossa), suffered extremely high mortality as well. In 1510, plague drove away a high proportion of the inhabitants of Seville, many of whom died upon a premature return to the city.

A devastating epidemic again spread through Spain from 1518 to 1521. Civil unrest erupted in several places during these years (as it usually did during serious epidemics of any kind), caused both by the flight of municipal councils, which left a town ungoverned and its ordinary citizens resentful, and by economic hardship, which the cutting off of commerce, demanded by anti-plague regulations, always created. Outbreaks of plague, or even threats of one, always accentuated the division between rich and poor. Wealthy citizens, whose lives were not as drastically affected by a temporary cessation of commercial activity, were able to flee a town easily, whereas those without resources were usually trapped within an infected community. In Andalusia this plague was combined with a terrible subsistence crisis on a scale comparable to that of 1505. The city of Seville was once again the host to a very deadly epidemic in 1524. From 1527 to 1530 another great epidemic swept central and northern Spain.

A few localized, sometimes quite lethal, epidemics occurred in various parts of Spain until 1557–58, when plague broke out simultaneously in Barcelona, Valencia and Murcia. In 1564 Zaragoza was visited with a ten-month epidemic that killed about 10,000 people. Juan Tomás Porcell stands out as one of the most dedicated Spanish physicians of the period, attending hundreds of patients during this plague and credited with performing the first autopsies in an effort to understand the disease. Seville experienced plague again in 1564–68 and 1581–82; the cause of the latter outbreak was attributed to soldiers and slaves who disembarked in the city's port. The northeast region of Cataluña (Catalonia) suffered from plague from 1583 through 1591, the worst outbreak occurring in Barcelona in 1590, when more than 10,000 people died in just four months.

The gradual decline of Spain as a world power and its domestic disintegration during the last two decades of the sixteenth century was aggravated by the persistent presence of bubonic plague, a continuing scourge that harassed an already demoralized people. The century ended with the Spanish Plague of 1596–1602 (q.v.), which over a period of seven years covered most of Spain and caused at least half a million human deaths.

Further reading: Carrera Panchón, *La peste y los médicos en la España del renacimiento;* Ayuntamiento de Barcelona, *Datos históricos sobre las epidemias de peste ocurridas en Barcelona;* Ballesteros Rodríguez, *La peste en Córdoba.*

Spanish Plagues of 1637, 1646–52, and 1678–82

Three serious epidemics of plague (mainly bubonic) in Spain that caused extraordinarily high human mortality in the southern and northeastern provinces. After recovering from the calamitous Spanish Plague of 1596–1602 (q.v.), Spain was relatively free from plague until 1637, when the port city of Málaga and its surrounding area in Andalusia lost an estimated 20,000 people to the disease in less than four months. The cause of a particular outbreak of plague was always sought. Usually imported goods or recently arrived soldiers or foreign travelers were identified as the culpable agents; in the case of Málaga in 1637, the infection allegedly was imported in a shipment of wheat. So urgent was the situation that Spain's King Philip IV sent financial aid, and veterinarians were recruited to help the city's physicians. The following year plague appeared throughout the regions of Andalusia, Murcia, Valencia, and Aragon.

Andalusia was struck once again in 1646. For three years plague haunted the entire region, causing perhaps as many as 200,000 deaths, especially in Málaga and Seville (where the disease was traced to a shipment of silk). Thirty thousand people died in Valencia in 1647. During the next few years plague spread north along the Mediterranean coast until it reached Barcelona, where it caused great devastation in 1651, killing at least a third of the city's 45,000 inhabitants. In 1652 it moved through Aragon, where Zaragoza (Saragossa), the region's main city, lost a quarter of its population of 28,000. The Spanish islands of Majorca and Ibiza, in the western Mediterranean, which often escaped the pestilences of the mainland, were invaded by plague in 1652. Nearly 500,000 people lost their lives over the course of this terrible epidemic.

The last great epidemic of bubonic plague to occur in Spain started in 1678, when sailors from the Algerian city of Orán—who became sick and thus were thought to be the agents of the disease—disembarked at Málaga at the end of May. Plague swept through the southern regions of Andalusia and Murcia until it finally diminished in 1682.

It is estimated that more than one million Spaniards died from plague in the seventeenth century. During this time a great number of learned medical tracts were published containing information and advice abut the cause, spread, prevention, and treatment of the disease. Most of this material, which had remained fundamentally unchanged since the fourteenth century, was both etiologically and epidemiologically mistaken, and medically almost useless, although some treatments, such as the application of warm herbal preparations, could increase a patient's comfort. Spanish municipal authorities employed many of the same anti-plague measures as city councils everywhere in Europe, among them searching ships before allowing them to unload their cargoes, guarding town gates and requiring "certificates of health" from outsiders who wished to enter, imposing quarantines, ceasing commercial activity with other cities, cleansing or burning a plague victim's clothing, "purifying" houses with vinegar, and burning herbs and resins in city streets, all of which were designed to keep infected persons from spreading the "contagion" and to disperse what was considered corrupted, disease-causing air. These measures, so strictly and universally enforced, did little to impede bubonic plague, whose vector is a flea that transmits the plague bacterium to human beings from infected rats.

The Catholic Church was an important presence during times of plague, its monasteries operating as hospitals, its monks serving as sick-attendants. Religious processions were organized to beg protection from plague, to implore God's mercy if plague arrived, or to give thanks once an epidemic had ceased. Visitations of plague were generally believed to be scourges of an angry deity. ("It would be fitting to mention the pitiful travails this wretched and unfortunate city [Barcelona] suffers thanks to the sins of its citizens.") The movements of planets and other astronomical phenomena such as comets were also considered factors that caused plague and other diseases to appear.

Further reading: Ayuntamiento de Barcelona, *Datos históricos sobre las epidemias de peste ocurridas en Barcelona*; Ballesteros Rodríguez, *La peste en Córdoba*; González, *La peste Aragonese de 1648 a 1654*.

Spanish Plagues of 1905–06 and 1923

Epidemics of mainly bubonic plague—localized outbreaks—remembered for the uniqueness of their occurrence.

The Iberian Peninsula had been virtually free of plague after 1682, the final year of Spain's last large-scale epidemic. What was feared by contemporaries to be plague in Seville in 1709 was in fact typhus fever; and aside from an alleged outbreak in Catalonia in 1793, which was also probably a different disease, no outbreaks were recorded during the eighteenth and nineteenth centuries in either mainland Spain or Portugal. (Plague broke out on the Spanish island of Majorca in 1819 and 1820.)

After more than 200 years' absence the disease suddenly reappeared in 1899 in the Portuguese coastal city of Oporto, believed to have been imported by a ship from Bombay, India, where plague had been epidemic during the preceding few years. Although this outbreak was fleeting and caused few deaths, it spread considerable alarm, as evidenced by the many medical commissions sent to Oporto from around the world. Notably, a Valencian physician called Jaime Ferrán, who was a member of the commission from Spain, had developed some years previously a vaccination against cholera, the disease that had replaced bubonic plague as the scourge of nineteenth-century Europe (smallpox having been the great killer the century before).

Plague appeared twice more in the early twentieth century: in Barcelona from June 1905 to April 1906, during which time 23 people died, and once again in Málaga in 1923, when the rare and deadly septicemia type of plague struck the city and caused several fatalities. This latter outbreak, Spain's last, was quickly extinguished; finally armed with knowledge of the true source of plague, the infected rat (a discovery made only in the previous decade), epidemiologists and public health officials could at last successfully control this ubiquitous disease. (Although it had ceased to be a serious threat to Europe, it was still widespread in other parts of the world, particularly India.)

Further reading: Ayuntamiento de Barcelona, *Datos históricos sobre las epidemias de peste ocurridas en Barcelona*; Ballesteros Rodríguez, *La peste en Córdoba*.

Spanish Typhus Epidemic of 1489

See GRANADA TYPHUS EPIDEMIC OF 1489.

Spanish Yellow Fever Epidemics of 1803–05

Outbreaks of yellow fever that caused thousands of human deaths in three consecutive summer seasons throughout Spain's southern province of Andalusia and along Spain's Mediterranean coast in Murcia, Valencia, and Catalonia.

Abnormally prolonged high temperatures during the summer and fall of 1803 created an environment in which *Aëdes aegypti* mosquitoes, the vectors of yellow fever, could thrive. Because yellow fever is not native to Europe, it was presumed that the infection—which was not known at that time to be carried by mosquitoes—was imported from tropic or subtropic areas, particularly the Americas, with which Spain conducted an active transatlantic trade.

In 1803 the Andalusian coastal city of Málaga was ravaged by the disease, which killed nearly 7,000 people (13 percent of the population) from August to December, and in 1804, in an even worse visitation, 36 percent of the population died. The military commander of Andalusia ordered that every person leaving Málaga or its environs be quarantined and, if sick, isolated in a house separated from the town; further, the furniture and other belongings of a sick individual were to be "perfumed" with burned sulfur. Infected or not, persons without an official pass that stated their origin were subjected to quarantine. These measures were adopted reluctantly by Málaga's municipal authorities, who knew that news of yellow fever would seriously disrupt the city's commerce.

In the last months of 1804 yellow fever appeared in Córdoba, where strict preventive measures had been enforced since 1801, including posting soldiers at the city gates, cutting communication with infected places, placing a "sanitary cordon" around the city and sending travelers to isolation stations for observation or quarantine. City authorities also ordered a general cleansing of streets and houses in the belief, common until well into the nineteenth century, that ventilation and fumigation would dissipate what were thought to be poisonous disease-causing miasmas.

Other Andalusian cities that were similarly attacked by yellow fever in these years included Cádiz (see CÁDIZ YELLOW FEVER EPIDEMIC OF 1800), Seville, Granada, Écija, and Gibraltar. The cities of Alicante and Valencia on the northern Mediterranean coast were also severely affected.

In addition to more homely remedies such as garlic, quinine was widely used as a treatment against yellow fever; effective against intermittent fever, with which yellow fever was confused, it was useless against the latter disease.

Bad harvests, a seriously faltering economy, and war with England added to the miseries of southern Spain during these epidemic years.

Further reading: Peset Reig, *Muerte en España (política y sociedad entre la peste y el cólera)*; Arjona Castro, *La población de Córdoba en el siglo XIX*.

Sri Lankan (Ceylonese) Dysentery Epidemic of 1942
Severe epidemic of dysentery that affected the pear-shaped, Indian Ocean island of Sri Lanka (called Ceylon until 1978).

Dysentery, an acute waterborne infection of the intestines, can be either amoebic (amebic) or bacillary in form. Both types are spread through contaminated water and food, a process often aided by insects such as the housefly. Amoebic dysentery is caused by the *Endamoeba histolytica* while bacillary dysentery is caused by one of the four *Shigella* bacilli (*S. dysenteriae, S. flexneri, S. sonnei* and *S. boydii*).

The disease was rampant in Sri Lanka during 1938 and 1941, killing more than 2,000 people each of those two years. In 1942 it apparently caused another outbreak during which 6,052 patients were treated at government hospitals. Of these, 2,799 were found to be suffering from bacillary dysentery and 1,833 from amoebic dysentery, while in 1,420 patients the type of dysentery was not identified. Also in the same year, 59,180 dysentery patients received treatment at dispensaries and at outpatient facilities of government hospitals. The disease claimed 2,275 human lives in 1942 (a mortality rate of 38 per 100,000).

Mortality rates often vary widely during an outbreak of dysentery, depending on the type of bacillus involved. In Sri Lanka, the chief culprit behind the bacillary dysentery was discovered to be the *Shigella flexneri* bacillus. Other enteric infections were also widespread that year in the country; over 6,000 cases (1,675 of them were children under two years) of diarrhea and enteritis were treated in 1942.

Further reading: McGrew, *Encyclopedia of Medical History*; Simmons et al., eds., *Global Epidemiology*.

Sri Lankan (Ceylonese) Malaria Epidemic of 1934–35
Catastrophic malaria epidemic that extended over 5,800 square miles and claimed 254,968 victims during a 15-month period from September 1934 to December 1935. Already endemic on the island of Sri Lanka (Ceylon), malaria quickly flared into an epidemic triggered by immense hardships such as the failure of the 1934 monsoon to occur, the resultant drought of 1935, and the extreme poverty and malnutrition already experienced by much of the rural population.

The failure of the monsoon in 1934 reduced the rivers in the south to a series of pools—fertile breeding grounds for the larvae of the mosquito *anopheles culcifacies* that for a long time had been confined to the dry zone in the north. Later in the year, the explosion of the mosquito population coincided with large numbers of people being admitted into hospitals with high fever. The outbreak appeared rather suddenly in October 1934 around a river basin to the north of Colombo, Sri Lanka's capital. A month later, hospitals in the wet zone (southwestern part of the island) were reporting ten times the normal incidence of fever cases. By mid-December, the epidemic had engulfed 500,000 people, ten percent of the island's population. *Plasmodium vivax*, which spreads faster but is not as lethal, was the malaria parasite responsible for the first wave of infections.

The epidemic intensified and peaked in April 1935, with one and a half million cases reported by the end of April. Children under ten years of age were hardest hit. Nineteen of the country's 20 districts were severely affected; only Jaffna escaped infection. During this last phase, *Plasmodium falciparum*, the most lethal of the malaria parasites, was most active. The epidemic slowly waned in intensity and disappeared with the advent of normal rains in November and December 1935.

The state council, pressurized by public demand, instituted extensive relief measures. A malaria surveillance service was established, its function being to gather information on carriers and vectors and to watch for a resurgence of the disease. Internationally, the epidemic was the focus of specialized research in malariology and was thus studied in great detail. Scientists learned from it that the alternating of drought and floods produced conditions ideal for an epidemic. Sri Lanka was invaded by another epidemic in 1968 that was not as damaging as this one.

Further reading: Harrison, *Mosquitoes, Malaria and Man;* Ludowyk, *The Modern History of Ceylon.*

Sri Lankan (Ceylonese) Malaria Epidemic of 1968–69

Epidemic that struck the island of Sri Lanka (Ceylon) rather suddenly, infecting more than 500,000 people with malaria.

Though not as severe as the Sri Lankan Malaria Epidemic of 1934–35 (q.v.), it took the authorities by surprise because it marked the resurgence of a disease (malaria) they had made intensive efforts to eradicate. Over two decades of an expensive spraying and surveillance campaign had thus come to nought. Ironically, the malaria parasites had reestablished themselves in the very areas where eradication efforts had been the strongest.

Once more, the Sri Lankan authorities resorted to spraying DDT (dichloro-diphenyl-trichloroethane) using spray guns. In 1972, malaria cases declined to 150,000. However, in 1975, malaria incidence soared to 400,000 cases.

Further reading: Harrison, *Mosquitoes, Malaria and Man.*

Stockholm Poliomyelitis Epidemic of 1887

Forty-four cases of polio studied by the Swedish pediatrician Karl Medin, the first researcher to recognize the epidemic nature of the disease. Although endemic poliomyelitis had for centuries sporadically afflicted infants and young children, it did not become epidemic until the mid to late 1800s. During those years advances in public health and sanitation were gradually suppressing the polio virus, which can be spread by fecal contamination of food and water. As a result, many people did not develop the immunity that comes with childhood exposure. Once the virus was introduced into such a population group, it could take epidemic form, even striking adolescents and young adults.

Since the 1830s doctors throughout Europe had reported small groups of simultaneous cases. As the century went on, the number of victims in each outbreak began to increase, until a new peak was reached with the 1887 epidemic in Stockholm. Medin himself had seen only one or two cases annually in the previous 15 years of his clinical practice, although he knew of an 1881 epidemic of 13 cases in northern Sweden.

Because he had a large patient group to study, Medin could describe the clinical features of poliomyelitis more precisely and more completely than anyone had done before. He observed that the first symptoms were minor, generalized ones, such as a slight fever that could even disappear entirely before coming back again. Damage to the central nervous system occurred only later and even then only in some of the sufferers.

When Medin presented his findings at the Tenth International Medical Congress in Berlin in 1890, physicians from around the world took note. To recognize Medin's ground-breaking work, many medical scientists for a time termed poliomyelitis "Heine-Medin disease," pairing the Swedish doctor with Jacob von Heine, a German orthopedist whose 1840 report described polio's effects on the spinal cord. Yet the announcement of the 1887 outbreak had an unfortunate consequence. By linking Sweden with polio, Medin's work gave his country an ill-deserved reputation as the breeding ground of the disease—a reputation strengthened with the Swedish Poliomyelitis Epidemics of 1905 and 1911 (qq.v.). Polio may have been especially severe in Sweden because the country is located far to the north and because its population was widely scattered, but other countries, including the United States and several in western Europe, also suffered epidemics of polio in the last decades of the nineteenth century.

Further reading: Paul, *A History of Poliomyelitis;* Marks and Beatty, *Epidemics;* Bollet, *Plagues and Poxes.*

Strasbourg Dancing Mania (St. Vitus's Dance)

Bizarre affliction apparently confined mostly to inhabitants of the city of Strasbourg, France, manifesting itself in a maniacal or possessed state of uncontrolled dancing. Contemporary accounts differ widely as to the supposed cause of the phenomenon, which suddenly appeared in 1518 and affected several hundreds of people, men and women of all ages, who would form groups of up to 100 and dance literally until they dropped to the ground from exhaustion; some reportedly danced themselves to death. In an effort to contain the disruption the dancers produced, the town prohibited public gatherings, and set aside special places for the victims to dance with attendants to watch over them. One chronicler says the dancers were cured at a Mass given them at the nearby monastery of St. Vitus of the Rock. It is unknown whether the malady was physical or psychic in origin.

Similar types of delirium, variously called St. John's Dance, St. Guy's Dance, and Tarantism, appeared in Europe from the fourteenth through seventeenth centuries (see DANCING MANIA).

Further reading: Nohl, *The Black Death: A Chronicle of the Plague*; Rosen, *Locura y sociedad: sociología histórica de le enfermedad mental*.

Sudanese Leishmaniasis Epidemic of 1988–93

One of the largest recorded epidemics of visceral leishmaniasis (also called kala-azar and "dumdum fever"), killing as many as 40,000 persons in the African country of Sudan.

Transmitted through the bite of infective sandflies, the chronic systemic disease was thought to be typhoid fever when the first cases began to appear in southern Sudan's Upper Nile province early in 1988. But by mid-year Dutch medical authorities had determined that the infections were visceral leishmaniasis, which initially struck nomadic cattle herders who were bitten by diseased sandflies carrying the protozoan parasite *Leishmania donovani*. The insects lived in the river regions or in wet organic debris. Thousands of inhabitants in and around Bentiu became infected, as well as thousands of people in the capital of Khartoum, about 500 miles to the north in the central part of the country. Many Sudanese refugees from the south had fled to Khartoum for security because of on-going civil war.

Before 1988 leishmaniasis normally affected only a limited number of people in southern Sudan. With famine, displacement of populations, and disruption of health services because of war, conditions were advantageous for an epidemic. Malnourished persons can develop severe forms of the disease, which brings fever, inflammation of the spleen and liver, swelling of the lymph nodes, and sometimes anemia. Prompt diagnosis of the disease and early treatment of patients (such as daily injections of pentavalent antimonials for 30 days) had helped control outbreaks in the past, but the war was an obstacle,

preventing the sick from reaching special clinics or medical facilities set up in western Upper Nile province and Khartoum, where about 13,000 and 2,500 patients were treated, respectively, by mid-1989. These clinical cases represented only a small fraction of the many reported in the large area between Bentiu and Khartoum. There was insufficient medication to treat all the sick at the newly established clinic run by Sudanese physicians and public health employees at Bentiu. An estimated 600,000 to 700,000 people in Sudan became infected with leishmaniasis, for which there is no available vaccine. In some villages in the south, the disease killed 30 percent to 40 percent of the inhabitants.

Further reading: Ackerknecht, *History and Geography of the Most Important Diseases*; World Health Organization, "Leishmaniasis Epidemic in Southern Sudan," *Weekly Epidemiological Record*.

Sudanese Relapsing Fever Epidemic of 1926–28

Unexpected, severe outbreak of louse-borne relapsing fever in Sudan's western province of Darfur, where the systemic spirochetal disease raged for 18 months between 1926 and 1928. The epidemic, which probably killed at least 200,000 persons in Darfur, was successfully contained within the province by the efforts of a small team of medical officials and assistants.

Between 1908 and 1925, only five human deaths out of 200 cases of relapsing fever were recorded in Sudan, then a British colony. The next year, in September, the towns of Nyala and Kebkebia in Darfur reported much fever, along with the district of Zalingei. The senior medical officer of Darfur, G. K. Maurice, and his staff of seven were not certain at first which vector, the louse or the tick, was responsible for the disease, so dual methods of elimination were first employed.

Maurice ordered the burning of all infected living quarters in villages in order to get rid of ticks, which are carried by rodents and other animals. However, when lice were found to be the culprits, the burning ceased, and all efforts were concentrated on systematically delousing the inhabitants of the infected areas. Clothing was repeatedly boiled. To rid their heads of lice, men had their hair shaved off, and women applied a mixture of fat and kerosene to their heads. The sick were isolated in temporary shelters and treated with the drug Novarsenobillon. To prevent the disease from spreading to other provinces, sick travelers were detained and deloused at newly established border stations. Darfur's native Fur people, after whom the province was named, suffered from recurring high fever with pain and nausea but strongly resisted medical treatment; many concealed their sick, hid their clothing, and refused to be isolated. Nearly a quarter of the Fur people perished in the epidemic, which was under control by the beginning of 1928.

The actual number of human deaths from the epidemic varied in different reports. The Sudan Medical Service's Annual Report for 1926 recorded 10,000 deaths in Zalingei, an area with a population of 40,000. Another official report in 1933 listed 20,000 deaths attributed to relapsing fever in the 1926–28 epidemic. However, a British official in the Sudan Medical Service, C. E. G. Beveridge, recorded and published that at least 200,000 persons died from the epidemic in Darfur; this figure seems most probable because the province's estimated population had dropped from 750,000 in 1926 to 500,000 in 1929.

Relapsing fever continued to be a health problem in Sudan, whose Blue Nile province, the home of rich cottonfields, had 386 reported cases and 46 deaths in 1930. There were more than 22,600 cases in all the provinces of Sudan between 1935 and 1942; afterward the disease declined considerably in the country.

Further reading: Hartwig and Patterson, *Disease in African History*; Scott, *A History of Tropical Medicine*.

Sudanese Yellow Fever Epidemic of 1940 Severe yellow fever epidemic in the Nuba Mountains of Sudan, killing more than 1,500 people out of some 15,000 who were infected in 1940.

During the annual rainy months in the Nuba Mountains, yellow fever broke out in the southern areas of Moro, Tira, Limon, Heiban, and Tira Okhdar. Those stricken with the virus suffered high fevers, acute headaches, agonizing pain, and jaundice; some vomited large amounts of blood and sometimes died quickly. Medical authorities were unable to determine which species of mosquito was transmitting the virus and feared that the localized epidemic in the southern Nuba Mountains could easily spread (due to an increased number of infested mosquitoes) to adjacent areas and to the eastern frontier of Sudan (then known as Anglo-Egyptian Sudan), where allied soldiers were stationed at the start of World War II. Consequently, authorities instituted the first preventive measures against a rural epidemic of yellow fever in Central or East Africa. The entire Nuba Mountains area was isolated under a quarantine measure; railway, river, and air traffic to and from the region was stopped. To the north, the city of El Obeid (more than 100 miles from the epidemic area) established precautions and cordons because some hospital patients were jaundiced (later they were determined to have hepatitis); house-to-house inspections for yellow fever were made there as well. El Obeid was a major terminus of the Sudan

Railway, and its population was known to be entirely non-immune to yellow fever.

In early December 1940, as the epidemic was abating after the virus-carrying mosquitoes had disappeared following the rainy season, vaccine for the disease arrived in Sudan, and massive inoculation of inhabitants took place in and around the epidemic area. Afterward a survey of immunity indicated that an estimated 40,000 cases of yellow fever might have occurred in Sudan in 1940; also, a study determined that the disease may or may not be transmitted by the mosquito *Aëdes aegypti* (its usual vector in Africa). Since the epidemic in the Nuba Mountains area, there have been only rare and minor outbreaks of the disease in Sudan.

Further reading: Kirk, "Some Observations on the Study and Control of Yellow Fever in Africa"; Horsfall and Rivers, eds., *Viral and Rickettsial Infections of Man*.

Swedish Epidemics of the Early 1740s Outbreaks of typhus, dysentery, and relapsing fever that attacked all of Sweden, although they were especially lethal in southwest counties. The stage had been set for the epidemics with the winter of 1739–40, when temperatures were below average, according to the observations of the Swedish scientist Anders Celsius, and the country's interior lakes thawed much later in the spring than usual. Winters remained abnormally cold for the next few years in all western Europe as well as in Sweden.

As people spent more time indoors during the harsh winters, they made it easier for a louse-borne infection such as typhus to spread. By cutting short the growing season, the cold weather also led to unusually low harvests; as draft animals starved, died of exposure, or were slaughtered as food, it became harder to plow and sow the fields for the next year's crop. With little grain left to harvest and little work to do in the countryside, peasants either joined the ranks of the army (Sweden had declared war on Russia in July 1741) or migrated to the city to find work or food. As beggars, soldiers, and displaced peasants traveled the country, they carried diseases with them.

Doctors throughout Sweden had been sending regular medical reports to Stockholm since 1736, when a central bureau had been established to collect statistics on births and deaths and to monitor outbreaks of disease. (The detailed records allow us to track the epidemics of the early 1740s.) According to the reports, typhus first arrived in southwest Sweden in February 1742, brought by beggars from Norway, where it had been epidemic since the previous autumn. The outbreak was intensified as Swedish Finns crossed the border to claim inheritances from relatives who had died. The typhus they carried back with them to Sweden was as fatal as the plague, according to one doctor, who noted that it often caused a hemorrhage just before killing its victims.

Somewhat less lethal was "hot fever" (perhaps relapsing fever), which began to strike southwest Sweden in the spring of 1742, peaked that autumn, and continued into the following year. Dysentery had appeared earlier, in 1741, and went on to infect all areas of the country; it did not dissipate until 1743, perhaps because warm, dry summers allowed the bacteria responsible for the disease to proliferate.

The epidemics were particularly severe in southwest Sweden. In Varmland county the death rate in 1742 was 121.6 per 1,000 people—that is, about 12 percent of the population died in just one year. Although other parts of Sweden were not affected to the same degree, they did suffer from the epidemics, mostly because of military activities. As troops gathered and traveled to scenes of battle (none of which were on Swedish soil), as military ships put in at Swedish ports, and as soldiers returned home from the fighting, they carried typhus and dysentery to the people in those areas. The end of the Russo-Swedish War of 1741–43 coincided with a return to normal climatic conditions and harvest yields, and the epidemics rapidly abated. In 1744 only one small area in central Sweden experienced a population deficit (an excess of deaths over births).

Further reading: Post, *Food Shortages, Climatic Variability, and Epidemic Disease in Preindustrial Europe;* Utterstrom, "Some Population Problems in Pre-Industrial Sweden."

Swedish Poliomyelitis Epidemic of 1905 Outbreak of 1,031 cases of poliomyelitis (infantile paralysis), mostly in the rural areas of Sweden, that occurred in the summer and autumn of 1905. During those months, the Swedish doctor Ivar Wickman traveled the countryside, collecting reports of cases and following possible lines of transmission. His painstaking investigations were a milestone in polio epidemiology: He proved not only that the disease was highly contagious, but also that it could be spread by people who suffered only mild symptoms and escaped lasting paralysis.

Until the late nineteenth century polio seems to have been an endemic but sporadic disease. In the last few decades of the 1800s, however, physicians had begun to observe clusters of polio cases, with several dozen victims in each. Credit for recognizing that polio could take on epidemic form in immune populations is given to Karl Oskar Medin, Wickman's teacher, who analyzed the Stockholm Poliomyelitis Epidemic of 1887 (q.v.). Despite Medin's contribu-

tions, researchers were still not certain whether the disease was actually contagious and if so, how it could be transmitted from person to person. Once polio cases were reported in 1905, Wickman saw an opportunity to answer those questions.

While the epidemic bypassed the larger cities, it struck with a vengeance in the countryside of Sweden, afflicting five or six out of every 1,000 inhabitants. Because most rural communities were remote and self-sufficient, it was fairly easy for Wickman to re-create the dates and means of contact between them; the disease, he found, tended to travel along the major roads and railways. Once it reached a village, it could be spread mainly through school contacts. Wickman identified at least four local outbreaks in which the school was the primary infection site—which is not surprising, since polio is mostly a disease of the young. The highest incidence of severe cases (those that led to paralysis) occurred among children three to six years in age, with infants up to age three forming the next most susceptible group. Even among children between the ages of six and 15, the attack rate was still high, with more than 30 patients per 100,000 individuals.

Wickman concentrated not on such paralytic cases, however, but on the so-called abortive ones, in which people came down only with the fever that marks the first stage of the disease. Claiming that polio does not always attack the central nervous system to cause permanent weakness or paralysis, Wickman included the abortive cases in his total count and found that they equaled or surpassed the number of paralytic cases. Wickman's focus on patients with only mild manifestations of polio enabled him to make two findings essential to understanding polio. Patients with abortive cases were just as capable as the paralytic ones of transmitting the disease, and the time between contact with an afflicted person and the appearance of minor symptoms averaged only three to four days.

Although Wickman later proved to be right, for more than 50 years researchers persisted in thinking that the incubation period was at least twice as long—lasting until the major symptoms of stiffness and paralysis became evident. One reason Wickman's findings were not widely recognized was that research on polio changed direction only a year after he published his monograph on the 1905 epidemic. In 1908 scientists in Vienna, Austria, isolated the polio virus, and from then on attention shifted to laboratory work on the pathology of the disease and away from epidemiological field studies like Wickman's. In the course of such lab experiments, however, investigators studying the Swedish Poliomyelitis Epidemic of 1911 (q.v.) confirmed Wickman's hypothesis when they found the virus present even in people who were only mildly afflicted.

Nevertheless, Wickman's work on abortive cases was largely overlooked for several decades, as researchers concentrated on using animal models to study the virus's effects on the central nervous system. While Wickman watched his ideas on polio being supplanted, he still hoped to be named to Medin's professorship in pediatrics by the Stockholm Faculty of Medicine. When he was passed over for the position, despite his brilliance and his extensive training, the disappointment proved too much for him. Wickman took his own life in 1914, at the age of 42.

Further reading: Paul, *A History of Poliomyelitis;* Olin, "The Epidemiological Pattern of Poliomyelitis in Sweden from 1905 to 1950."

Swedish Poliomyelitis Epidemic of 1911   Largest epidemic of poliomyelitis known until that time, with 3,840 officially reported cases. Besides furthering the inaccurate view that polio originated in Scandinavia, the 1911 epidemic had a beneficial result. By studying several dozen of its victims, Swedish researchers clarified some aspects of the clinical epidemiology of the disease.

In the three or four years preceding the 1911 outbreak, investigators in Europe and the United States discovered the virus responsible for polio, isolating it in autopsies of human patients and experimentally infected monkeys. During the summer of 1911, when the Swedish epidemic was in full force, three researchers at the State Bacteriological Institute in Stockholm decided to build on these experiments. Carl Kling, Alfred Pettersson, and Wilhelm Wernstedt performed autopsies on 14 fatal cases and took samples from 11 acutely ill patients. In both groups the scientists found the virus present, not only in the pharynx and trachea, but also in the wall of the small intestine. The findings suggested that after the virus entered the body through the mouth or nose, it was eliminated through the intestinal tract—a claim that later proved to be correct.

The Swedish scientists also studied six families whose members exhibited slight symptoms or none at all; some of them, however, reported having close contact with victims of paralytic poliomyelitis. These subjects were considered carriers once they were found to have the polio virus in their throats and intenstines. After studying the Swedish Poliomyelitis Epidemic of 1905 (q.v.), Ivan Wickman had speculated that "abortive" cases—those that did not develop paralysis—could be responsible for spreading the disease; the research done by Kling and his colleagues provided proof of Wickman's theory.

The 1911 team extended Wickman's studies in another way. After noticing that the areas hardest hit by the 1905 epidemic had no polio cases in 1911, Wernstedt concluded that their inhabitants must have acquired immunity during the earlier epidemic. That is why, he claimed, most polio cases occurred in infants and young children; older children and adults were resistant because they had previously been exposed. His theories, along with the other results of the Swedish team, were presented in 1912 at the Fifteenth International Congress on Hygiene and Demography in Washington, D.C. It was not until the late 1930s that their findings were widely accepted.

Further reading: Paul, *A History of Poliomyelitis;* Marks and Beatty, *Epidemics.*

Swiss Plague of 1610–11   See BASEL PLAGUE OF 1610–11.

Sydney Influenza Epidemics of 1890–91   Two severe influenza epidemics that were part of the Asiatic Influenza Pandemic of 1889–90 (q.v.); other places in Australia were hit, too.

The first epidemic began when the disease reached the cities of Sydney and Melbourne and the island of Tasmania in March 1890. Adelaide and Queensland province were infected in April and Perth in May 1890. New Zealand was also affected around this time. From Sydney, the epidemic spread to the surrounding rural areas, where it continued to smoulder through the year. In the city of Sydney, the outbreak subsided around May 1890.

In September 1891, during the third wave of the pandemic, epidemic influenza erupted once more in the rural areas outside of Sydney and spread to the city early in September. When it waned early in December, it had already infected about 120,000 to 130,000 people in the province of New South Wales and had killed 234 (the first death being recorded on September 30). Most of the cases occurred in the five-week period beginning in mid-October. Nearly 44 percent of the cases treated in Sydney's institutions occurred in the last two weeks. No doubt many cases were not even reported to the authorities.

The onset of the disease was generally sudden, with a patient first complaining of being run-down, having a headache, chills, fever, and pain behind the eyeballs. Shortly thereafter, his or her temperature would increase and a dry cough and muscle pains develop. While the fever subsided after three to five days, the cough and run-down feeling often lingered for days. In older patients, secondary complications such as pneumonia and bronchitis would often develop at this stage. In fact, during this epidemic the majority of deaths (68 percent) resulted from complications following the disease.

Nearly a quarter of Sydney's population caught the "flu" infection in 1891; total morbidity was thus very high. In some parts of the city, morbidity was higher than in other sections. Mortality during this epidemic was relatively low: 0.6 per 1,000 cases. Children below four years of age and adults above the age of 60 suffered 54 percent of the total casualties.

Aware of the highly communicable nature of the disease, Sydney's board of health launched a public education campaign urging citizens to avoid crowds and public gatherings, to observe rules of simple hygiene, and to allow no visitors if there was a sickness in the family. Sick children were to be kept home from school. Since few families in the city escaped the infection, there was a major disruption in everyday life in the city; a sense of despair flooded the people of Sydney.

Further reading: Curson, *Times of Crisis: Epidemics in Sydney, 1788–1900;* Patterson, *Pandemic Influenza, 1700–1900.*

Sydney Measles Epidemics of the 1800s
Measles epidemics of varying intensity that struck the city of Sydney, Australia, several times during the nineteenth century.

Sydney's first contact with measles came in 1829, when a ship that had passengers suffering from measles arrived at the harbor. But the disease does not seem to have affected those onshore, at least not to any recorded degree. The city's first epidemic has been traced to the arrival of the ship *David Scott* on October 25, 1834. The infectious passengers on board no doubt sparked an outbreak that lasted into 1835 and spread, in January, to Hobart in Tasmania and, in March, to New Zealand's South Island by means of a native returning home from Sydney on board the *Children.* It was particularly devastating in its impact upon the highly susceptible native Maori population of New Zealand.

The first severe outbreak of measles in Sydney began in March 1854, courtesy of the *Beejapore,* which arrived from Liverpool, England, with measles and scarlet fever on board. Of its 1,023 passengers, 124 (106 of them children) died during the long sea voyage, and the ship was placed in quarantine for 54 days. Over the next seven years, at least 20 ships were quarantined at Sydney.

During March and April 1854, there was a noticeable rise in mortality in the city. From the burial registers at one city cemetery, 285 deaths (67 percent of children under five years of age) reportedly occurred during those two months alone. The Sydney

Dispensary's records show that 57 patients were treated for the disease in 1854.

Measles invaded Sydney again in 1860, when it was responsible for nearly ten percent of the city's total deaths for that year. Of the 272 people who died of measles, 83 percent were less than five years old. Mortality statistics, even where available, do not convey the whole picture. Those who were lucky enough to recover from measles often fell prey, because of their general debility, to infections like diarrhea, dysentery, and broncho-pneumonia. Clearly, by the mid-1850s, measles had established itself as the most dreaded childhood infection in Sydney.

No one, however, was prepared for the worst epidemic of measles ever to strike Sydney. It began early in February 1867, when the three-year-old daughter of a shopkeeper died of measles. A few weeks later, it became clear that an epidemic was in progress. The weekly human death toll shot from about 14 to 20 in mid-February to more than 60 by late March and early April. The epidemic peaked between late March and the first week of May, when 370 children (representing more than 50 percent of all deaths) died of the disease. Forty deaths were recorded during the first week of May, only 20 a week in June and less than ten a week in July. It is estimated that 13,000 children (nearly 70 percent of the city's under-five population) were struck by measles in 1867; 748 persons died over a five-month period (a fifth of all deaths for that year). Almost 50 percent of the deaths in the one to five year age-group in 1867 were caused by measles.

This epidemic was particularly severe in the city of Sydney, where 70 percent of all measles deaths were reported. Among the city wards that suffered acutely were those in Brisbane, Randwick, Botany, and Phillip. Given the fact that the majority of deaths occurred in children one to five years old, it is clear that the infection was acquired in the home or in the immediate neighborhood. The crowded living conditions in most city apartments must have aided the rapid spread of the disease. Eighty-one percent of the deaths occurred among Sydney's working class residents.

Almost 50 percent of the deaths resulted from complications following the actual attack. Measles exacerbated the protein-deficient stage of many young patients. The main complications were gastrointestinal and broncho-pneumonial.

Though it was one of the most disastrous childhood epidemics of the century and had a considerable impact on the family structure of Sydney's working classes, the public response to the crisis was negligible.

Further reading: Curson, *Times of Crisis: Epidemics in Sydney, 1788–1900*, Marks and Beatty, *Epidemics*.

Sydney Plague of 1900   Australia's first major outbreak of bubonic plague, part of a plague pandemic that hit southern China in the 1890s (see HONG KONG PLAGUE OF 1894) and spread to many countries (see INDIAN PLAGUE OF 1896–97).

During its course, the pandemic infected many ports around the world—Hong Kong, Singapore, Bombay, Calcutta, Port Louis, Honolulu, Manila, and Nouméa, to name a few. Between October 1899 and January 1900, some 13 ships from plague-infested ports reportedly called in at Sydney's Darling Harbor and Central Wharves (Sydney is Australia's chief port). The infection has been attributed to these sources because Sydney's first case was observed on January 19 when a dockworker fell ill.

The epidemic raged from late February to mid-August 1900, during which time 303 cases and 103 deaths were reported in the city of Sydney. Forty percent of the cases and half of the deaths occurred at the height of the epidemic between late April and early May. Just as the outbreak seemed to be subsiding in early May, another one began a week later and lasted until the end of June. The worst of the epidemic ended then, even though isolated cases were reported until mid-August.

Geographically, the epidemic remained concentrated in Sydney's harbor and main business areas. Seventy percent of the cases and fatalities were reported from here. No doubt, the crowded, unhygienic and insanitary living and working conditions in the vicinity of the harbor fostered a flourishing rat population, which facilitated transmission of the disease. Hardest hit were young and working-class males in the 15 to 45 year age-group, whose jobs involved direct contact with the harbor area or with the goods and people transiting through there. Apparently, 60 percent of all cases and deaths were from this age-group. Statistics show that only one woman was affected for every four males struck by the disease. Upper- and middle-class males generally escaped infection. Fifty children were infected too; twelve of them died.

By early April, the epidemic extended over all of Sydney except one ward; it also spread to North Sydney and Waverley and to many suburbs south and west of the city. It was most widespread in early May, when many of the eastern suburbs were also infected.

The mass hysteria and panic that accompanied the outbreak far outweighed its relatively marginal demographic impact. Nevertheless, once the epidemic began to spread, local and federal authorities quickly went into action. The localized nature of the outbreak made it easier for containment strategies to be implemented.

A very strict isolation and quarantine policy was launched that involved not only plague patients but also anyone who had come into contact with them. They were forced to leave their homes at little or no notice and transported to the Woolloomooloo quarantine depot from where they boarded launches for the Quarantine Station at North Head. Over 1,800 people were officially sequestered (generally for about seven weeks each) in this manner, with 460 removals coming in two weeks in late April. Naturally, people often resisted these evictions, leading to confrontations with the police.

Late in March, the government also began an intensive cleansing and fumigation campaign in and around Sydney's dock area. Infected streets were barricaded while the operations were carried out. Inside the dwellings, residents were allowed to do their own fumigating and scouring, but usually this arduous task was done by an army (nearly 3,000 men) of specially trained people. When the job was completed, a placard testifying to it was displayed on the house. Four thousand dwellings were cleaned in this manner.

An important step was the extermination of rats. Sydney's city council and the federal government employed separate so-called rat-squads, which rid the city of more than 100,000 rats. In addition, citizens were offered a small fee for every rat they brought in to the central depot.

The vaccination campaign began rather slowly. At first, only plague patients, their contacts, and the medical staff were vaccinated. After May, all public employees were also included. Once the vaccines became more freely available, members of the general public who lived and/or worked in the infected area were given preference. Citizens banded together to form vigilance committees in various areas.

The mass hysteria attending this epidemic was in fact fanned by newspapers' sensational reporting, which alleged that the city's Chinese community had introduced plague into Sydney and then tried to hide its own members suffering from it. Newspapers also described in lurid detail the burial methods followed for plague victims. Medical statements notwithstanding, many people still believed that the disease was spread by personal contact and thus avoided the quarantined areas. Australia's other territories and states and New Zealand took strict precautions against goods and passengers arriving from New South Wales (where Sydney is the state capital), which caused financial suffering to many in the shipping business. The epidemic caused a tremendous dislocation in Sydney's social and economic life. However, by highlighting the filthy living and working conditions in the city, the epidemic also prompted eventual reform of the city's health and sanitation facilities.

Further reading: Curson, *Times of Crisis: Epidemics in Sydney, 1788–1900*; Shaw, ed., *Australian Encyclopedia.*

Sydney Smallpox Epidemic of 1881–82

Relatively small outbreak of smallpox in Sydney that, nevertheless, created much panic and public hysteria and disrupted normal life in the city (see SYDNEY PLAGUE OF 1900). The epidemic, however, had important consequences for the public health reform movement in Australia.

The epidemic began with the notification of Sydney's first case of smallpox on May 25, 1881. The patient was the infant son of a Chinese merchant, who had apparently caught the infection from his nurse. Just as he recovered, fresh outbreaks were reported from other areas of the inner city. By late June, the epidemic began to spread more rapidly, peaking initially from late July to late September and again between early October and early December. When the epidemic officially ended (February 19, 1882), 163 cases and 41 deaths were reported. The total number of cases may have been closer to 250 since many cases were not recorded for fear of evictions and quarantine, and many others were incorrectly diagnosed.

The residential areas in and around the city center suffered the brunt of the outbreak, with 66 percent of all cases and 68 percent of all deaths being reported from five localities. The crowded and insanitary living and working conditions in these areas no doubt aided the transmission of the virus. Children under ten years of age suffered the most in terms of morbidity (34 percent) and mortality (41 percent). Mortality was also higher (61 percent) among men than women. Case fatality rates were highest in the 40 to 50 year age-group, where a third of those who were affected died.

The city of Sydney was caught unawares and unprepared to cope with this disaster. No guidelines had been established for dealing with public health problems and infectious diseases. Hence, the official reaction was sometimes muddled and vague, often contradictory. A concurrent outbreak of chicken pox often confused doctors into making the wrong diagnosis. There were rumors of doctors neglecting quarantined patients. Stories such as these were fodder to a populace terror-stricken by images of the disease, of vaccination, and of the terrible conditions at Sydney's Quarantine Station. There was a loud clamor from the public for compulsory vaccination, notification of infectious diseases, and the creation of a central public health authority.

The government-appointed Board of Health took charge of the epidemic in mid-July 1881. In mid-September, an official committee was established to study the issue of compulsory vaccination but it did not reach any resolution. Meanwhile, the number of cases continued to rise and the government's response to the crisis came in for severe criticism. In mid-December when the epidemic was almost over, legislation requiring compulsory registration of all smallpox cases was enacted.

One of the government's first policies was the quarantining of all patients and their immediate contacts—initially at home (under medical supervision, supposedly) and subsequently at the Quarantine Station at North Head. The patient's house was barricaded and guarded, screens attached to the windows, a yellow flag displayed on the property, and neighbors notified by circular. All human contacts were vaccinated, if willing. Sequestering at the Quarantine Station was apparently not made compulsory, except for Chinese residents, who were forcibly evicted, until almost the end of the epidemic. Nine hundred people (163 cases; the rest were contacts) were officially quarantined. Seven hundred were detained on board ships in Sydney harbor. A permanent new isolation hospital (Coast Hospital) was declared open in December 1881.

The Ambulance and Disinfecting Corps was established by the Board of Health late in July and charged with cleaning, fumigating, and scavenging all infected homes and their surroundings. Large areas of Sydney were cleaned in this manner; Chinese-owned residences and businesses received strong-arm measures. The city council urged residents to properly dispose of their household wastes and to buy disinfectants and fumigants at special depots.

People's tempers ran so high that even the issue of compulsory vaccination was hotly debated. Government officers and staff and inmates of institutions were routinely vaccinated while those in high-risk areas were urged to undergo the procedure. The Chinese were forced into it. More than 61,000 people were vaccinated in 1881 alone.

Though only three cases occurred among Sydney's Chinese residents, the epidemic exacerbated anti-Chinese feelings, forcing the government to declare all Chinese ports infected and to quarantine all ships arriving from China. Chinese goods and services were boycotted, Chinese property vandalized, and the Chinese themselves harassed on the streets. This culminated in the passage of the Chinese Restrictions Bill by the provincial parliament late in August (limiting Chinese immigration and quarantining any ship with Chinese passengers on board). Ships from New Zealand refused to enter the Sydney docks and even neighboring Victoria insisted on a thorough inspection of ships from New South Wales, before allowing them entry.

Further reading: Curson, *Times of Crisis: Epidemics in Sydney, 1788–1900;* MacLeod and Lewis, eds., *Disease, Medicine, and Empire.*

Syphilis Epidemic in Naples See FRENCH ARMY SYPHILIS EPIDEMIC OF 1494–45.

Syrian Cholera Epidemic of 1822–23 Epidemic brought into Syria by caravans traveling from the Persian Gulf region (see PERSIAN CHOLERA EPIDEMICS OF 1821–22). It was part of the Asiatic Cholera Pandemic of 1817–23 (q.v.), originating in India (see INDIAN CHOLERA EPIDEMIC OF 1817–18), which caused havoc over much of Asia (see THAI CHOLERA EPIDEMIC OF 1820; INDONESIAN CHOLERA EPIDEMIC OF 1821; CHINESE CHOLERA EPIDEMIC OF 1820–22; JAPANESE CHOLERA EPIDEMIC OF 1822).

Cholera first broke out in Aleppo (northwest Syria) in early November 1822—almost within days of the caravans' arrival in the town, as the French consul there pointed out. He and some 200 of his friends isolated themselves in his country house until the epidemic passed by, thus escaping infection.

In 1823 cholera reappeared, this time at Alexandretta (Iskenderun), revisited many places it had passed through in 1822, and also erupted in several ports on the Caspian Sea. In June 1823, it infected the cities of Laodicea and Antioch and then moved along Syria's Mediterranean frontiers. By late 1823, cholera had disappeared entirely from the region.

Strict measures were introduced by the pasha (Turkish governor) to prevent the epidemic from spilling over into Egypt.

Further reading: Pollitzer, *Cholera;* Macnamara, *A History of Asiatic Cholera.*

Syrian Cholera Epidemic of 1947–48 Isolated outbreak of cholera that began in Syria a year after the nation gained full independence.

The origin of this relatively minor outbreak is uncertain. Cholera was first reported from two adjacent villages in Hauran province along the Dera-Damascus highway on December 19–20, 1947. Simultaneously, cholera broke out in three villages in the Al Ghouta plain on the outskirts of Damascus (Syria's capital). Officially, 45 cases and 18 human deaths were reported from these five villages; actually, at least 77 cases were believed to have occurred.

Hauran and Damascus provinces were promptly cordoned off. No one was allowed to enter or leave these areas unless he or she produced a certificate of immunization against cholera. With the assistance of the World Health Organization and generous financial contributions from companies and charitable foundations, nearly 1,500,000 Syrians living in the affected areas and in the Syrian city of Aleppo were administered the cholera vaccine. No new cases were reported after the initial outbreak, and the epidemic was officially declared ended on January 17, 1948.

Further reading: Pollitzer, *Cholera;* Simmons et al., *Global Epidemiology.*

Syrian Plague of A.D. 638–39 (Plague of Amwās) Severe epidemic of plague that virtually decimated the Syrian army. The infectious disease apparently struck in two waves in A.D. 638 and 639. The villages of Muharram and Safar were infected in the first wave. The second wave came down particularly hard on the Syrian Army fighting in Amwās (Amawās), much to the relief of its Byzantine opposition. Nearly 25,000 Arab soldiers reportedly died of the plague. The disease then spread very rapidly through most of Syria, which had only recently been devastated by famine, before it spread to Iraq and Egypt.

Alarmed, the caliph urgently recalled his military commander, Abu 'Ubaydah, from Amwās to Medina, seeking to prevent his death in the epidemic. Mindful of the Prophet Muhammad's teachings forbidding Muslims from entering or leaving plague-infected areas, the commander refused the caliph's request and stayed with his troops in Syria. The caliph himself then journeyed to Syria and met the commander and other leaders at Sargh. They disagreed on future strategy regarding the epidemic, so the caliph finally accepted the advice of the leaders of the Prophet's tribe to quit the infested area and commanded Abu 'Ubaydah to move his troops into a safe area.

Pious Muslims believed plague to be an act of mercy and martyrdom for the faithful and a punishment for non-believers. Further, because of the disease's divine origin it was not considered contagious. These beliefs caused much controversy in the face of recurring plague epidemics, when the infectiousness of the disease became obvious and caused people to flee in panic.

This visitation on Syria occurred, some said, because its inhabitants drank wine, a practice forbidden by Islam. The caliph promptly punished the offenders. Abu 'Ubaydah meanwhile moved his army to Hauran, but himself succumbed to the disease at al-Jabiyah.

Further reading: Dols, *The Black Death in the Middle East.*

T

Tahitian Poliomyelitis Epidemic of 1951 Epidemic that gripped Tahiti and some of the nearby Tuamotu Islands.

Tahiti was just recovering from a devastating measles outbreak, when the infectious poliovirus struck in March 1951. Like the measles virus, it spread rapidly (most likely by direct contact) throughout Tahiti and the nearer Tuamotu Islands. The five-week period from March 18 to April 21 was particularly intense. By the end of May 1951, 128 cases of paralytic poliomyelitis were reported, 109 of them on Tahiti (see VIETNAMESE POLIOMYELITIS EPIDEMICS OF 1958–60). There were eight fatalities. It is important to remember that only the most severe (paralytic) polio cases were included in these statistics. Many milder and non-paralytic cases were often unreported and perhaps even undiagnosed in these South Pacific islands.

Tahiti's paralytic rate (360 per 100,000) was significantly high. Most of the cases occurred in the 11 to 19 year age-group. The disease's attack rate among infants and children below age five was relatively low in comparison to polio outbreaks in other tropical countries. See also NICOBAR ISLANDS POLIOMYELITIS EPIDEMIC OF 1947.

Further reading: McArthur, *Island Populations of the Pacific;* World Health Organization, *Poliomyelitis.*

Tahitian Smallpox Epidemic of 1841 French Polynesia's first recorded contact with smallpox, its impact on Tahiti mitigated by widespread vaccination in these French-controlled islands of the South Pacific.

Smallpox was brought into Tahiti early in June 1841 by an American ship en route from Valparaiso, Chile, to Hawaii; there had already been six deaths from smallpox on board, including five Hawaiians and the captain's brother. However, because the American consul had requested some supplies from Tahiti and a local doctor had concluded that there was no illness on the ship, it was allowed to anchor in Matavai Bay, Tahiti. Quarantine procedures were not adhered to and eventually were abandoned during the two weeks it was anchored here, where the doctor and three passengers debarked. Almost immediately after the ship had left Papeete (Tahiti's capital), one of the passengers died and the infection spread to many of the natives.

Soon afterward, an American warship arrived with vaccine material, which was distributed across Tahiti and nearby islands. Its timely arrival, together with travel restrictions imposed on the natives, helped contain the spread of the disease and avert a major disaster. Everywhere, the unvaccinated were the first to be struck. In Matavai, where many had been vaccinated, only six people died; five children recovered from the infection. Northeastern Tahiti lost 20 people and Darling's Station about ten people. The district of Faaa suffered the most: more than 100 people died during the outbreak, sometimes as many as five a day. Sixty deaths were recorded in Papeete during the two- or three-week period before October 2, 1841; most of them had refused to be vaccinated. The outbreak appeared to be concentrated in northwestern Tahiti and claimed some 200 lives. The overall mortality rate could not have exceeded 2.5 percent except in certain key areas, where it may have been as high as ten percent.

Smallpox also spread to the nearby island of Moorea soon after it erupted in Tahiti. A Moorean chief visiting Tahiti for medical treatment apparently brought the virus back to the island. While he survived, 13 family members and a priest who had accompanied him to Moorea died. Fifty-four cases occurred in eastern Moorea (29 of them fatal), and 13 people died along the northern coast.

The the northwest, Huahine and the rest of the Leeward Islands in French Polynesia were not attacked; the island of Bora Bora's harbor was declared closed to all shipping until the epidemic in Tahiti had ended.

Further reading: McArthur, *Island Populations of the Pacific.*

Tahitian Venereal Disease Epidemic of 1768–69

Widespread occurrence of venereal disease on the South Pacific island of Tahiti following its introduction there by a visiting European expedition in 1768.

Exactly which expedition was responsible for introducing venereal disease on the island remains a matter of controversy. Tahiti was apparently free from any such diseases when a British expedition under Captain Samuel Wallis landed there in the *Dolphin* in 1767. He was followed nine months later, in 1768, by a French expedition led by Louis Antoine de Bougainville; this group had been traveling from one Pacific island to another and hence is more likely to have acquired and transmitted these infections. Bougainville's men suffered from venereal disease soon after their arrival in Tahiti and were widely regarded as having brought it into the island. Naturally, Bougainville denied this and instead accused Wallis of having done it. According to another report, the infection arrived on two Spanish ships about ten months after the *Dolphin*'s visit. However, it is possible that the Spanish expedition was mistaken and was actually a French one.

Upon landing in Tahiti in 1769, Captain James Cook of England found that venereal disease was rampant among the natives and that they did not seem unduly worried about it. Gonorrhea was probably the main disease involved in this outbreak, but syphilis was also present. On his next visit to Tahiti in 1773, Cook recorded that venereal disease was not as common among the natives as in 1769; the Tahitians now feared it and called it *Apa no Pretane* (British disease) because they thought that Bougainville was British. The Tahitians also claimed to have found a cure for gonorrhea. Syphilis they apparently could not treat.

Cook initially thought that perhaps his crew had been guilty of bringing the disease into Tahiti. However, he later remembered that everyone on board the *Endeavour* had been examined by the ship's surgeon about a month before arriving in Tahiti and pronounced infection-free. By July 1769, more than 40 of his crewmembers had been infected with gonorrhea and syphilis. Following a three-month stay, the *Endeavour* set sail for New Zealand, arriving there in October 1769 after a ten-week voyage. Gonorrhea, which can remain actively infectious for long periods, was undoubtedly one of the venereal infections introduced by Cook's crew into New Zealand.

Further reading: McArthur, *Island Populations of the Pacific*; Gluckman, *Medical History of New Zealand Prior to 1860*.

Taiwanese Cholera Epidemic of 1962

Brief but explosive outbreak of cholera, part of the Asiatic Cholera Pandemic of 1961–75 (q.v.) that invaded Taiwan (Republic of China) during the summer of 1962. This island country had been cholera-free since an outbreak in 1946 (3,809 cases and 2,210 deaths), with not a single case reported during the intervening period.

The *el tor* cholera first struck Taiwan in July 1962; the earliest cholera cases were observed on July 17, and the *Vibrio el tor* bacterium was identified as the causative agent soon thereafter. During the second week, the infection spread very rapidly. The number of new cases slackened somewhat in the third and fourth weeks, but the epidemic did not start subsiding until the fifth week and was officially declared over on September 19, 1962.

During this eight-week period, 1,548 people suspected of harboring the *Vibrio el tor* or having the disease were admitted to Taiwan's provincial hospitals. Of these, 383 were confirmed as cholera patients and 380 as symptomless carriers. There were 24 deaths, a 6.2 percent fatality rate. Generally, there were more cases and more fatalities among the nonvaccinated than among the vaccinated. As a group, males with outdoor occupations suffered the maximum number of cases (99) while housewives had the highest incidence among women. Also, a higher incidence was noted among adults, especially those above 50 years of age, than among children.

The government responded promptly to this crisis by setting up a three-tiered administrative system charged with taking immediate steps to control the epidemic. The entire country was divided into "emergency" zones (where cholera had already occurred or adjacent areas) and "alert" zones (the rest of the country). Inoculation against cholera was made compulsory for everyone except pregnant women, sick people, and children below one year of age. All confirmed and suspected patients were isolated, and every infected household was quarantined and financially compensated for the loss in income. Water supplies in each area were inspected, and vendors in the markets were banned from selling uncovered food (especially fruit) and drink during the outbreak. Sewage and drainage systems were updated and a public health education campaign launched throughout Taiwan. Undoubtedly, these intensive measures helped control the spread of the epidemic.

Further reading: Yen, "A Recent Study of Cholera with Reference to an Outbreak in Taiwan in 1962"; Barua and Burrows, eds., *Cholera*.

Taiwanese Encephalitis Epidemics of 1958–61

Several outbreaks of Japanese B Encephalitis (JBE) that occurred in 1958–61 on the island of Taiwan (formerly Formosa) in the China Sea.

JBE was known in Taiwan as "summer encephalitis," an illness with high mortality that primarily affected young children. Since July 1955, physicians had been urged to report cases of encephalitis but notification was not mandatory, so there may have been considerable underreporting. The first recognized outbreak of JBE in Taiwan was in 1958, a year when there were severe outbreaks in Korea and Japan (see JAPANESE ENCEPHALITIS EPIDEMICS OF THE 1920S AND 1930S; INDIAN ENCEPHALITIS EPIDEMIC OF 1977–78).

During March–April 1958, the incidence of JBE in Taiwan began to rise gradually until it peaked in mid-July, when most of the cases occurred. According to one account, 140 cases occurred in July alone. Another account put the tally for the entire epidemic at 142 cases and 50 deaths. The epidemic was at its most intense on the Pescadore Islands.

JBE struck Taiwan again during the summer of 1960, a year when 287 cases and 87 deaths (case-fatality rate was 30.3 percent) were reported. The overall attack rate was 2.91 percent per 100,000 people. Children between three and 15 years old suffered most of the cases (230) and deaths (61), but case-fatality rates were the highest in those immediately below and above this age-group. The port of I-lan in northeast Taiwan bore the brunt of the 1960 outbreak and also suffered in 1961.

Taiwan's largest outbreak of JBE occurred in 1961, when 704 cases (overall attack rate was 7.15 per 100,000 people) and 146 deaths (case-fatality rate was 20.7 percent) were reported. Most of the cases (655) were in children below age 15. Case-fatality rates were highest in children under three years of age (37.1 percent) and declined progressively with age. Stray cases of JBE occurred in May and June, but the epidemic did not intensify until July–August. It peaked between July 11 and August 10, 1961, when 490 people came down with the disease. Although the epidemic subsided as rapidly as it had begun, a few cases lingered through early November. The outbreak mainly affected the northern and central regions, being particularly severe in the cities of Taipei (111 cases) and Hsinchu (102 cases, 24 per 100,000). Men suffered a higher attack rate (8.3 per 100,000 people) than women (6.0 per 100,000 people).

JBE is an illness that begins rather suddenly with high fever, vomiting, convulsions, headache, listlessness, and stiffness of the extremities. It is caused by an arbovirus that is transmitted by *Culex tritaeniorhynchus* and *Culex fuscocephalus*, two species of mosquitoes.

Further reading: Grayston, "Encephalitis on Taiwan"; Green et al., "The Epidemiology of Japanese Encephalitis Virus on Taiwan in 1961."

Taiwanese Rubella Epidemics of 1957–58 and 1968–69

Two large rubella (German measles) epidemics that affected the island of Taiwan (formerly Formosa).

The epidemic of 1957–58 began during the 1957 summer break (July–August) in and around Taipei, the country's commercial capital. When schools reopened in September, the incidence of rubella increased, and by October, it was clear that an epidemic was in progress. The infection apparently arrived in northern Taiwan from Japan and spread rapidly from north to south all over the country and even to the outlying Pescadores, a group of islands between Taiwan and mainland China.

Between mid-November 1957, when the epidemic peaked in the northern cities of Taipei and Keelung (Kirun) and mid-March 1958, when it peaked in Taitung, most of the main island had been affected. Rubella reached the Pescadores late in March and peaked soon thereafter. Everywhere, school-going children born since the previous rubella epidemic of 1944 (i.e., in the 7 to 13 year age group) suffered the highest attack rates (30 percent). Nearly 50 percent of the 10- to 12-year-olds in Taipei came down with the clinical symptoms of rubella; the figures were only slightly lower for the other cities. Preschoolers with siblings in this age-group suffered an attack rate between 7 percent and 23 percent. Attack rates were markedly lower in the teenage and young adult population.

The epidemic of 1968–69 began in Taipei in January 1968. Once again, schoolchildren born since the previous epidemic (i.e., those under 11 years of age) were the most susceptible. Nearly half of that population came down with the disease in Taipei, 24 percent in Taichung, and 21 percent in Kaoshiung. The epidemic was at its peak in Taipei in April and was over by the end of May before schools closed for the summer. Attack rates in the central and southern regions of Taiwan, where the epidemic peaked in May and early June, were considerably lower. Kaoshiung suffered two mild waves of rubella—in May 1968 and in 1969. Taken together, they were far weaker than the outbreak that hit Taipei in 1968. Rubella invaded the Pescadores in 1969 but did not reach epidemic proportions.

Further reading: Evans, ed., *Viral Infections of Humans*; Grayston et al., "The Epidemiology of Rubella on Taiwan."

Tanganyikan Influenza Epidemic of 1957

Serious six-month-long epidemic of Asian influenza in Tanganyika (Tanzania). By the end of the epidemic in December, there were a total of 93,725 reported cases in Tanganyika, where it is believed the influenza was under-reported. Almost every country worldwide, except for a few isolated islands and remote regions (such as Africa's interior), experienced this new Asian-strain virus mutation of influenza in 1957–58.

First reported in China in late February 1957, the A-strain virus spread along the eastern fringe of Asia to many areas in Europe, the Middle East, Africa, and the United States. In late June 1957 the virus reached the Tanganyikan port city of Dar es Salaam on board a steamship and was soon infecting Morogoro (a town inland, west of Dar es Salaam) and the seaport of Tanga. From the coastal seaports, the virus was transmitted along railways and roads to almost all parts of Tanganyika that summer. The inhabitants of the neighboring, populous towns of Dodoma and Manyoni were severely infected in September. However, because of the use of antibiotics, the mortality rate in Tanganyika was not nearly as high in 1957 as it had been in the worldwide Spanish Influenza Epidemic of 1917–19 (q.v.); there were no deaths among the 8,468 persons infected in Dar es Salaam, and for Tanganyika as a whole, most of the 158 fatalities occurred among the elderly.

Further reading: Clyde, *History of the Medical Services of Tanganyika*; Dunn, "Pandemic Influenza in 1957."

Tanganyikan Meningitis Epidemic of 1942 Outbreak of cerebrospinal meningitis (CSM) that killed a reported 6,960 persons out of 11,687 infected in the British territorial mandate of Tanganyika (Tanzania) in East Africa. It was the worst outbreak of this acute bacterial disease in East Africa since World War I.

From 1921 to 1933 CSM appeared in serious, isolated outbreaks confined to Tanganyika's northwestern area. At that time it was endemic (and still is) in the country's Masasi area in the south (the Southern Province). In 1933 the CSM infection began to increase when migrant workers from the Belgian territory of Rwanda-Urundi (Rwanda and Burundi) carried the disease with them when they crossed Tanganyika's northwest border to find work on the estates and in the diamond fields in the northern and eastern areas. By 1939 cases of CSM were found throughout Tanganyika and increased during the next three years.

In 1942 the disease severely infected the northwestern Tanganyikan towns of Kigoma and Kasulu, through which the African laborers from Rwanda-Urundi passed, and for the first time ever, it spread to the north-central area (the Lake Province), where more than 5,843 persons became infected with CSM, and 1,719 of them eventually died. The spread of CSM was not halted despite quarantine restrictions and the use of prophylactic and sulfa-pyridine drugs in Tanganyika.

During the dry months (September and October of 1942), the CSM epidemic was particularly serious because the human mucous membrane is weakened as a barrier to infection, which is commonly transferred by sneezing and coughing patients; the disease attacks the meninges (the three membranes—dura mater, pia mater, and arachnoid—enveloping the spinal chord and brain). It takes only a small number of infected people to spread CSM; many people can harbor the pathogen (disease-producing bacterium) in their noses and throats, without displaying symptoms of CSM, and spread the infection to others. Also, the pathogen can be easily stored in contaminated bedclothes and floor dust, which can be inhaled. After contracting the disease, patients soon experience fever, violent headaches, dizziness, vomiting, a rash, and a stiff neck; delirium and coma often appear. Most patients remain sick for one to three weeks, and in acute cases, death can occur within a day or two.

In Tanganyika, although professional health authorities worked hard to control the epidemic, the mortality for CSM was the highest rate ever to occur there: almost 57 percent. The next year about 8,800 CSM cases occurred in the country, and from then until 1971, annual outbreaks were reported with less severity (curative drugs helped control the disease after 1950).

Further reading: Clyde, *History of the Medical Services of Tanganyika*; Hartwig and Patterson, *Cerebrospinal Meningitis in West Africa and Sudan in the Twentieth Century*.

Tanganyikan Plague of 1951–53 Outbreak of mainly bubonic plague that killed over 250 persons out of about 1,600 infected in various towns and villages in northeast and central Tanganyika (Tanzania), East Africa. The disease had long been endemic in this United Nations trust territory under British administration, occurring irregularly but at times acutely in certain areas.

In November 1951 in the South Pare Mountains in northeastern Tanganyika, plague took the lives of 16 people in Suji within three weeks. The epidemic worsened in the region and lasted until January 1952, during which time there were 135 human deaths out of the 665 persons infected. Compared to earlier outbreaks of plague there, the mortality rate (proportion of deaths to those infected) was considerably lower due to efficient medical treatment, which provided massive doses of the antibiotic streptomycin to patients; in addition, there were effective restrictions on the movement of people and extensive cleansing of houses and the destruction of rat fleas with insecticide. Also important that year (1951) was the inoculation of about 45,000 Africans with plague vaccine, which at first was resisted by the Masai (Massai) people, who finally submitted to vaccination after being convinced it was the only way to prevent plague from spreading to their cattle.

Apparently a plague patient from the Mbulu area, on the western Masai Steppe, carried a diseased rat flea in his luggage to the hospital at Singida, some 90 miles to the south; a ward servant at the Singida hospital contracted plague. At the time heavy rainfall forced many rats to seek shelter in houses and helped spread the infection to the natives (plague is a zoono-sis—a disease communicable from animals to human beings under natural conditions). The epidemic in the Singida area continued throughout 1952, striking a reported 357 people. Streptomycin and the surgical removal of buboes (inflamed swellings of lymph glands in the groin or armpit) kept human fatalities to 48, most of these dying from pneumonic plague. The Singida and Mbulu plague foci were linked by the nomadic, warlike M'angati people, whose unsanitary camps were infested with the multimannate mouse or rat, a common plague-tolerant African rodent. Plague in Tanganyika is mainly sylvatic (occurring in wild animals) and did not spread to the common house rat in the towns, except in the village of Ilongero near Singida, where wild rodents carried their fleas into the grain stores; the fleas and the house rats (when they died) transmitted plague to the people.

From Singida, plague spread south to the towns of Manyoni and Itigi and the surrounding area, infecting 302 natives and killing 48 of them by March 1952. After the epidemic subsided in 1953, the number of plague cases decreased considerably, and the disease was not a serious problem in Tanganyika during the following decade, when it was granted (1961) independent status in the British Commonwealth.

Further reading: Clyde, *History of the Medical Services of Tanganyika*; Gregg, *Plague: An Ancient Disease in the Twentieth Century*.

Tarantism   See DANCING MANIA.

Thai Beriberi Epidemics of 1890–1910   Outbreaks of beriberi occurring at various institutions in Thailand. Data gleaned from hospitals, police, and army and navy officials revealed 22,670 cases of beriberi and 1,063 deaths during 1901–10 alone. Little is known about the incidence of beriberi among much of the civilian population.

Thailand's first recorded outbreak occurred in 1890 at the central jail in Bangkok, one of the first institu-

tions to be supplied with white, steam-milled rice. At the time few people, even among medical practitioners, knew about the disease. The epidemic subsided soon after the authorities substituted hand-milled rice for the steam-milled variety. Beriberi is caused by the lack of thiamine or vitamin B_1, a nutrient that is often lost in the process of steam-milling.

In August 1900, the first case of beriberi was admitted to the police hospital. In the years following, beriberi admissions became fairly commonplace. The rise in the incidence of beriberi coincided with the local availability of white, steam-milled rice, which had, until then, mainly been exported to Europe.

Another epidemic raged in Bangkok's insane asylum when white rice replaced hand-milled rice in 1900. Over the following nine years, beriberi gained in intensity in the asylum and led to 783 deaths. Then, in February 1908, hand-milled rice was reintroduced; since then, no new cases were recorded.

Further outbreaks were also reported from several jails near Bangkok and from a reform school at Koh Si Chang in 1908. In all these cases, the simple substitution of hand-milled rice for the steam-milled kind brought the outbreak under control.

Another major outbreak occurred at a police school in Bangkok in early 1909, when 353 of 400 new police recruits developed beriberi. All had been eating white rice. Late in April another group of 400 recruits were admitted to the school and given hand-milled rice. No new cases of beriberi were reported after that.

Beriberi incidence was the highest along the riverbanks in the province of Bangkok, where white rice was easily available. In 1910, there was a small outbreak among the custom guards positioned at various places along the main rivers; it ended when under-milled rice was introduced instead of white rice. See also PHILIPPINE BERIBERI EPIDEMICS OF 1901–02 AND 1909; SINGAPORE BERIBERI EPIDEMICS OF 1942–45.

Further reading: Williams, *Toward the Conquest of Beriberi*.

Thai Cholera Epidemic of 1820   Epidemic that arrived in Thailand (then known as Siam) from India (see INDIAN CHOLERA EPIDEMIC OF 1817–18), a wave of the Asiatic Cholera Pandemic of 1817–23 (q.v.).

The cholera epidemic entered Saiburi, a town in southern Thailand, in March 1820 from Penang (Malaysia) and moved west via Songkhla to the mouth of the Chaophraya River. Heavy fatalities were reported from the town of Samut Prakan, leading to a mass exodus of people (carrying the disease with them) to Bangkok and other places. Bangkok was invaded in late May. Here, the death toll was very high—30,000 people, approximately one fifth of the city's population, died within a short time. Corpses lay scattered in cemeteries and on monastery grounds, and those that could not be cremated were left floating in rivers and in canals. Many panic-stricken citizens fled their homes and monasteries, leaving the markets and streets deserted. People stopped drinking the contaminated river water and subsisted on a meager diet.

Rama II, the Thai king, ordered all his subjects to suspend their regular duties and to devote themselves to the chanting of sacred verses and to the giving of alms to Buddhist monks. He also ordered the release of all captive animals and persons, except Burmese prisoners. The government held a religious ceremony accompanied by gunfire to ward off the evil forces.

Medically, local authorities were ill-equipped to handle a disaster of this magnitude. The experience eventually led to the introduction of Western medicine in Thailand. The epidemic, which severely affected the coastal towns, began to subside in April 1821. Moving north from Bangkok, it later invaded Vietnam.

Further reading: Owen, ed., *Death and Disease in Southeast Asia*.

Thai Dengue Hemorrhagic Fever Epidemics Several epidemics of dengue hemorrhagic fever (DHF), more deadly than "classic" dengue, occurring in Thailand from the late 1950s to the mid-1980s.

DHF, an urban disease that initially strikes port cities, first burst on the scene in Southeast Asia during the 1950s, and was identified as a new disease in the Philippines in 1953. Thailand's first DHF epidemic struck the capital city of Bangkok rather suddenly, or so it seemed, in 1958. It was a very severe epidemic with high attack and death rates; 2,418 cases were reported in Bangkok. The causative agent was later discovered to be the dengue virus type 1.

Epidemic activity initially seemed to follow a biennial cycle but, a decade later, became more irregular. In Bangkok, DHF incidence mounted again in 1960, with 1,742 reported cases. The epidemic of 1962 was better documented. For the first time, all the 72 provinces in Thailand were asked to send in annual DHF reports. Of the 870,000 children under 15 years of age in the Bangkok-Thonburi area, a staggering 150,000 to 200,000 were affected by minor illnesses caused by the dengue or chikungunya viruses. Hospital records show that 4,187 DHF patients were hospitalized during this period; one third of them experienced the shock syndrome. Another 4,000 city residents were treated privately, either in clinics or

at home. Over 6,000 DHF cases were recorded elsewhere in the country—chiefly from areas close to the main railway lines, where population density and adequate breeding grounds created a thriving atmosphere for the DHF vector, the mosquito *Aëdes aegypti* (see SINGAPORE DENGUE HEMORRHAGIC FEVER EPIDEMICS). (The dengue virus is transmitted not person-to-person but via the mosquito's bite.)

In 1964, there were 5,358 cases reported in Bangkok-Thonburi and 9,020 in the Thai provinces. Over the next few years, DHF cases declined in Bangkok but showed a marked rise in the provinces. It became endemo-epidemic, the infectious disease with the most deaths per year in Thailand. There is no immunization against DHF.

In 1970, Thailand's Ministry of Health assumed record-keeping of DHF cases for the entire country. For the 1975–78 period, it recorded 71,312 hospitalized cases of DHF and 1,676 deaths. Other years of high DHF incidence were 1972, 1975, 1977, 1980, and 1984–85.

DHF, a disease that particularly affects children under age 14 and attacks the circulatory system and precipitates bleeding from the nose, mouth, and other areas, has been observed in many countries in Southeast Asia, the Western Pacific, and, in the last decade, the South Pacific. DHF can be caused by dengue serotypes 1, 2, 3, and 4 and is characterized by the presence of hemorrhagia and, frequently, shock. Some medical experts now believe that DHF is the human body's reaction to invasion by more than one serotype.

Further reading: McGlashan and Blunden, eds., *Geographical Aspects of Health*; World Health Organization, *Dengue Haemorrhagic Fever*.

Thasian Mumps Epidemic First recorded outbreak of mumps, described by the Greek physician Hippocrates, who was probably present on the Greek island of Thasos in the Aegean Sea when the epidemic occurred in the late fifth century B.C. (perhaps around 410). Although the previous autumn and winter had been unusually mild, spring that year was marked by northerly winds. A number of people then came down with dry coughs that left them hoarse and with swellings beside one or both ears. These swellings, neither inflamed nor painful, disappeared in every case without a sign, and all sufferers recovered.

Few women caught the disease, presumably because they (like most Greek women in ancient times) remained inside the home for much of the day. The majority of sufferers were instead young men, usually those who frequented the gymnasium or the wrestling school—gathering places in which a contagious disease could spread quickly. Transmission was undoubtedly easier since most victims did not have fevers that confined them to bed. Most of the men eventually developed inflammations in one or both testicles, sometimes accompanied by pain and fever; this characteristic orchitis enables modern scholars to identify the disease as mumps.

Although Hippocrates's description is our first written account of mumps, the disease was almost certainly present earlier in the classical world. The mildness of the Thasian epidemic, and its primary focus on adolescents, suggest that by the late fifth century B.C. mumps had been around long enough to become a less virulent childhood disease.

Further reading: Hippocrates, *Epidemics*; Grmek, *Diseases in the Ancient Greek World*; Patrick, "Disease in Antiquity: Ancient Greece and Rome."

Third Plague Pandemic   See PLAGUE PANDEMIC, THIRD.

Thirty Years' War Epidemics

Pestilences that raged among combatants and civilians alike in Germany and surrounding lands from 1618 to 1648. Although the leading killers were typhus fever, bubonic plague, and dysentery, other infectious diseases such as scurvy broke out as well. The struggle for hegemony in Europe and the ideological conflicts between Roman Catholics and Protestants that marked the war were played out mainly in Germany. The constant movement of troops across the country led to repeated outbreaks of disease; a number of local epidemics, however, were unrelated to military action.

Information about these numerous epidemics comes mainly from local chronicles, such as parish registers and tax records, that are often exaggerated and incomplete. Many give so little description of symptoms that often one cannot determine whether a person died from an infectious disease or from the extensive famine during the war. The flight of thousands of refugees from country to city during the war also makes epidemiological analysis difficult.

What the chronicles do show us is that disease was not a condition exclusive to wartime; pestilences attacked many parts of Germany for a decade or two prior to 1618. In that year Protestants in Bohemia rebelled against growing Catholic power in the region. When a Catholic Habsburg, Ferdinand II, was chosen Holy Roman emperor in 1619, they set up a German Protestant prince in his place. A decisive Catholic win at White Mountain near Prague in late 1620 suppressed the revolt and inaugurated both a decade of victories for the imperial Habsburg forces and a series of epidemics. As the Protestant troops dispersed after the battle, they spread disease throughout the Palatinate and Alsace in southwest Germany.

From the start, however, the war was not merely a Catholic-Protestant conflict or even solely a German one. A Catholic country that nonetheless wanted to contain growing Habsburg power, France first intervened in 1624 and intermittently over the next decade supported attacks by Germany's enemies. In addition, Christian IV, the Protestant king of Denmark, invaded Germany in 1625. As the Danish and the imperial armies fought in Saxony and Thuringia in central Germany during 1625 and 1626, and later in the northern part of the country, the diseases that followed in their wake infected many cities and towns. The chronicles, though often imprecise about symptoms, include repeated accounts of "head disease," Hungarian disease, and red or black spots like flea bites that must refer to typhus.

Although a defeated King Christian returned to Denmark in 1629, another Scandinavian ruler invaded Germany in the following year. Gustavus Adolphus or Gustavus II, the Protestant king of Sweden, took advantage of the power struggle between Ferdinand, who was trying to centralize his power as emperor, and many German princes, who were resisting the imperial consolidation. The emperor had to confront the Swedish troops unaided, because his Italian allies could not recruit soldiers. After the just-ended Mantuan War (a three-year-long offshoot of the Thirty Years' War in which France and the Habsburgs fought over the inheritance of some imperial lands in Italy), the northern half of the Italian peninsula was in the throes of a plague epidemic.

For two years after Gustavus's invasion, his army conquered the imperial forces again and again, but the Swedes experienced a setback in 1632 with the unsuccessful siege of Nuremberg in southern Germany. As both the Swedes and the imperialists camped before the city, food and supplies soon ran out and thousands of soldiers in each army succumbed to typhus and scurvy. Without engaging each other in battle, both armies left in September, spreading the diseases to surrounding areas. The final defeat of the Swedes, however, did not come until two years later, when they were beaten at Nördlingen in Bavaria by Ferdinand and his troops from Spain and Italy. As they pursued the defeated Swedes, the imperial soldiers carried disease through Württemberg in southwest Germany. During the next few years, human deaths from epidemics reached high rates, especially along the Rhine River, where fighting was now concentrated.

Bubonic plague made its first recorded appearance of the war in 1630, but after 1634 it seems to have become especially prominent. The chronicles of the German city of Dresden for 1634–35, for example, mention "swellings" that were undoubtedly buboes. Unlike typhus, bubonic plague is not carried by armies, but the crowding of refugees into cities aided the spread of the disease. One city sought by uprooted peasants was Munich in Bavaria, which closed all but two gates and sequestered newcomers outside the walls. The measures were of little avail; in late 1634 an epidemic, perhaps of bubonic plague, is said to have killed about 15,000 residents. The pestilence broke out again the following year and did not abate until 1637.

Nor were smaller towns in Bavaria immune. In 1634 Oberammergau was struck by a plague that killed about 85 people, one fifth of its inhabitants. The survivors claimed that if the epidemic would cease, they would perform the drama of Christ's sufferings and death once every ten years—a vow their descendants have kept to this day. A famine so severe that people resorted to eating the bodies of criminals taken down from the gallows exacerbated many other epidemics throughout Germany in the mid-1630s.

The Peace of Prague of 1635, which reconciled the Holy Roman emperor and the German princes, may have promised relief to the suffering Germans, but the war went on. France and Sweden remained adversaries of the Habsburgs, and fighting continued in Germany, especially in the north, until 1648. Little of the military action was systematic or centralized, and the endless marches of small armies continued to bring disease. Although severe outbreaks were almost nonexistent in the last decade of the war, typhus had become practically endemic in Germany.

Disease did not spare other countries. The Netherlands, France, Italy, and England endured outbreaks throughout the war, as fighting spilled over the German borders and as soldiers returned home. Even neutral Switzerland suffered from its proximity to Germany; a severe epidemic, of unknown type, ravaged the country in 1635. Disease spread through Austria and Hungary as well, particularly after 1644.

Many features of the Thirty Years' War facilitated disease transmission, including the ongoing troop movements, the influx of fresh soldiers from foreign countries, the constantly shifting areas of battle, the displacement of the German population, and the overcrowding of refugees into cities. In the war the line between the military and the civilian spheres was blurred as it had never been before. The baggage trains of armies, for example, often attacked villages along their route to get supplies, as did small groups of demobilized foreign soldiers. Forced to fend for

themselves on their way home, they used their weapons to extort food from the villagers, many of whom fought back in armed struggles. At other times, sick soldiers were cared for in private homes. With such extensive contact between soldier and peasant, the usual army diseases such as typhus and dysentery could easily cross over into a weakened civilian population.

Using local chronicles, previous generations of historians had claimed that one third or one half of the German population died during the war. The observed population losses, however, seem due as much to internal displacement, as refugees moved away from the fighting and then returned home once peace was restored, as to death from sickness and combat. The mortality rate was perhaps closer to 15 percent to 20 percent, but no one can say with certainty what portion died of infectious disease.

Further reading: Langer, *The Thirty Years' War*; Parker, *The Thirty Years' War*; Prinzing, *Epidemics Resulting from Wars*.

Tiverton Typhus Epidemic of 1644

Devastating epidemic of lice-borne typhus fever that erupted among the inhabitants of Tiverton, a town in the west of England, in the summer of 1644 during the English Civil Wars. The fever was probably brought into Tiverton when the Earl of Essex garrisoned his Parliamentary troops there from July 5 to July 18, as the epidemic began shortly thereafter, in August. Tiverton's parish records show the worst mortality in October, with 105 human deaths, which was 8 to 10 times the monthly average. Although no medical description of this disease exists, the arrival of Essex's undoubtedly lice-ridden troops points almost certainly to typhus fever. The cause of many deaths was recorded in burial registers as "the sweating sickness," indicating profuse sweating as a symptom. This evidently recalled to the minds of the townspeople the famous "English sweats" of a century before (see ENGLISH SWEATING SICKNESS EPIDEMICS).

On September 21, 1644, about 200 troops of the opposing Royalist army occupied Tiverton and remained there till October 1645. It is not known how many men among the Parliamentary or Royalist forces involved in the occupation of Tiverton were infected by typhus fever (see OXFORD TYPHUS EPIDEMIC OF 1643; READING TYPHUS EPIDEMIC OF 1643).

Further reading: Creighton, *A History of Epidemics in Britain*; Zinsser, *Rats, Lice and History*.

Tongan and Samoan Measles Epidemics of 1893

Two seemingly unrelated outbreaks of measles that began first in the Tonga Islands in the South Pacific and then in the Samoa Islands to the north.

The Tongan epidemic, which started on the island of Tongatapu, was attributed to an importation from New Zealand. It is not clear how far the infection spread, although one account implies that it spread throughout the island. Remembering the lethal measles epidemic of 1875 in the Fiji Islands, many people took what little precaution they could against the after-effects of the disease. An estimated 1,000 people, representing five percent of the population, died during this epidemic. The survivors, many in a state of panic and far too discombobulated to attend to daily chores, also faced a possible threat from famine.

Later, during the same year (1893), measles attacked the islands of Samoa. The virulence or malignity of this first visitation of measles on Samoa has often been disputed. In one contemporary account, it was described as being widespread (the attack rate was very high), with mortality ranging from zero to ten percent in some areas. An editorial in a local Samoan newspaper commented in September 1893 on the mildness of the epidemic. In October, it was reported that measles had claimed only 25 human lives along the northern section of Upolu (one of the main Samoan islands). The epidemic subsided in February 1894. According to the newspaper editor, it caused at least 300 human deaths, some of them from dysentery, however.

The Methodist mission on Savaii (Samoa's largest island) gave a different account of this same epidemic, reporting high mortality despite many precautions. Fearful of meeting the same fate that befell many islanders in Tonga and earlier in Fiji, the natives were apparently more conscientious in following the advice of doctors and missionaries. Another Methodist missionary reported that 1,600 Samoans died of measles and/or related complications. It is not possible to verify this since there was no civil registration of deaths then. Mortality may have also varied substantially from place to place.

Measles was not the only outbreak Samoans had to contend with in 1893. The epidemic had been preceded by a short but brutal civil war whose repercussions continued through 1894 as well. Both these outbreaks caused people to neglect their plantations. Soon many of the islands were gripped by famine-like conditions. See also FIJI ISLANDS MEASLES EPIDEMICS OF 1875, 1903, AND 1911.

Further reading: McArthur, *Island Populations of the Pacific*.

Torgau Typhus and Dysentery Epidemic of 1813

Catastrophic outbreak of louse-borne typhus fever and dysentery that killed more than 30,000 people in the garrison town of Torgau in eastern Germany (northeast of Leipzig) during one of the most destructive sieges of the Napoleonic Wars.

Over the course of the summer of 1813 thousands of sick and convalescing French soldiers poured into the 5,000-inhabitant town on the Elbe River; for example, 4,000 arrived from Dresden on July 18. By September, people were forced to leave their homes to make room for the sick, who now numbered about 6,000; one third of those who contracted typhus fever died. After the Battle of Dennewitz on September 6, about 10,000 more men arrived, along with 5,000 horses. Six weeks later the Prussian Army besieged Torgau. The situation became critical, hundreds of people dying every day: "Then the pestilence began to spread at an alarming rate among the inhabitants and among the Frenchmen quartered in the homes of citizens, so that the entire city of Torgau came to resemble a large, overcrowded lazaret." The number of men suffering from dysentery and typhus fever increased to about 12,000; 8,000 patients died in November alone.

An Austrian physician described the appalling conditions of the hospitals, floors ankle-deep in excrement, men drinking the urine of others to quench their thirst, dead bodies lying next to live men shivering in unheated rooms: "The French lazarets in the city represented scenes of horror such as repel human nature, and such as one must actually witness in order to appreciate fully their dreadfulness." Heaps of corpses were thrown into the Elbe River. Streets and houses were piled with refuse, dead horses filled the ditches, a sickening smell permeated the air. Over a 12-month period, an estimated 30,000 soldiers died in Torgau, mostly from dysentery and typhus fever. Nearly 700 town inhabitants died, the majority from typhus. Typhus also circulated among the Prussian troops surrounding the town, killing 300 soldiers in three months. The epidemic gradually abated through the early part of 1814.

Further reading: Dohm, *Die Typhusepidemie in der Festung Torgau, 1813–1814*; Prinzing, *Epidemics Resulting from Wars*.

Tours Diphtheria Epidemic of 1818–20

Outbreak studied by the French physician Pierre-Fidèle Bretonneau, the first researcher to define diphtheria as a clinical entity. Prior to his investigations, cases of diphtheria were often diagnosed as croup (the term used for any obstruction of breathing), malignant angina, or scorbutic gangrene. In performing dozens of autopsies on people said to have died from one of these diseases, Bretonneau found in them the same type of false membrane, a sign that only one pathological process, not several, was at work. Furthermore, he claimed, the disease it caused was contagious, although most doctors of the time believed that croup at least was not. By tracing diphtheria among family members, Bretonneau proved that it could be spread from person to person.

Early in 1818, soon after soldiers of the Vendée Legion arrived in Tours in west-central France, many of them became sick with what was called scorbutic gangrene. Ulcers formed on their gums, then spread to the mucous membranes of their lips and cheeks. Within a short time doctors began to see civilian cases of what they termed malignant angina, a highly fatal throat disease; its symptoms, however, were found in only one tenth of the infected soldiers. As the patients—from 120 to 400 at any given time—filled the hospital, its chief physician, Bretonneau, had the opportunity to observe numerous cases firsthand. Before the epidemic stopped in 1820, he studied in detail 130 military and 20 civilian cases, performing autopsies on 60 of them.

In the next few years Bretonneau was able to investigate other similar outbreaks: one in 1824–25 at La Ferrière, where 21 people out of a population of 250 were afflicted, 18 of them fatally; and the other, much more severe, at nearby Chenusson, in 1825–26. These later epidemics confirmed the theory he had developed during the 1818 epidemic: malignant angina, scorbutic gangrene, and "true" croup were just manifestations of the same disease, for which he coined the name diphtheritis (he or one of his pupils later changed it to diphtheria). It was characterized by a false membrane covering the mouth, pharynx, and air passages, a symptom found in other diseases; nonetheless, diphtheria could be distinguished from these illnesses by its epidemic nature.

Bretonneau communicated his ideas in an 1821 address to the Academy of Medicine in Paris, and five years later in a treatise that has become a classic medical study. His research on diphtheria was only one of his contributions to medicine. In 1825 he became the first to perform a successful tracheotomy; he wrote an important work on typhoid fever; and he formulated the influential doctrine of specificity—the concept that each disease has its own cause and specific clinical symptoms. Although his theories about diphtheria were widely accepted in France, physicians in Britain and the rest of Europe were more skeptical. One reason may have been their unfamiliarity with diphtheria; until the European Diphtheria Epidemic of the Late 1850s (q.v.), the disease had scarcely been seen outside of Norway, Denmark, and France.

Further reading: Andrews et al., *Diphtheria*; Major, *Classic Descriptions of Disease.*

Tripoli Cholera Epidemic of 1911

Outbreak of cholera in Tripoli in Libya from mid-October to mid-December 1911, infecting at least 10,000 persons and killing about 3,000 of them.

From a source in Mecca, in what is now Saudi Arabia, cholera spread to the Alexandria-Cairo area in Egypt, from where it moved south up the Nile Valley and west into Tripoli. During the course of the epidemic, the disease was confined to Tripoli, Libya's capital and largest port and city, and was spread mainly by contaminated dates, infected by flies; cholera, caused by the *Vibrio comma* bacterium, is usually ingested in contaminated water but can also be spread by flies carrying the bacteria from excrement to food.

In Tripoli, the first persons contracting the acute intestinal infection were the native beggars on the streets, who quickly spread the disease to the rest of the city's population (mainly Arabs, Berbers, and blacks). It soon spread among hundreds of Italian soldiers stationed in Tripoli after Italy annexed Libya on November 5, 1911. At first, many thought that cholera had been conveyed to Libya with the Italian soldiers; however, this idea was discounted because the disease did not break out in the Libyan seaports of Benghazi (Bengasi), Derna, Homs, and Tobruk, where thousands of other Italian soldiers had disembarked. To prevent the spread of cholera to Italy, sick soldiers were not allowed to return home until they had fully recovered from it.

Further reading: Stock, *African Environment Special Report 3: Cholera in Africa*; Prinzing, *Epidemics Resulting from Wars.*

Tunisian Cholera Epidemic of 1849–50

Major outbreak of cholera in Tunisia in North Africa, killing about 56,000 persons out of some 118,500 stricken with the acute intestinal disease over ten months (see ASIATIC CHOLERA PANDEMIC OF 1846–63). The French had apparently carried cholera into Algeria, where it was carried by land and sea into neighboring Tunisia.

In early January 1848 Tunisia's Muslim ruler, Ahmed Bey, closed his country's seaports to all ships from known cholera-infected countries, such as Egypt and Turkey; other vessels coming from uninfected regions were to be quarantined for inspection for 24 days. In mid-October 1849 a Tunisian ship, arriving from Algeria, entered the port of Tabarca without permission; to ward off contagion, the ship's cargo was disinfected with vinegar (at the time, the bacterial cause of cholera was not known). However, infected crew members carried the disease into Tabarca. In a short time an epidemic erupted in the Tunisian-Algerian border area that advanced eastward to the capital city of Tunis in mid-December, where the disease killed untold thousands of Muslims, Jews, and others before the epidemic abated in midsummer of 1850.

A battalion of Tunisian troops, quarantined in Tunis, was allowed to return home and unwittingly carried the infection to the Sahel region (it is spread by contaminated water and food). There, many members of the Mahdiya tribe were stricken. The contagion spread to Gabes on the coast, as well as to the Djerid region, where some 8,000 persons died within a few days. Meanwhile Ahmed Bey fled from the disease in Tunis from Muhammadiya to Porto Farina on the coast, where it followed him. Muslim and European medical treatment continued to concentrate mainly on bloodletting, one of the worst treatments for a disease that causes death by dehydration from vomiting and diarrhea.

In Tunis, about 7,600 persons perished from cholera during the epidemic; the Muslim community suffered the worst, 3,900 deaths; the Jewish sector nearly as badly, 3,400 deaths; and the much less populated Catholic sector, only 300 deaths (although it had the highest mortality rate of those who contracted cholera: 300 out of 475).

Further reading: Ackerknecht, *History and Geography of the Most Important Diseases;* Gallagher, *Medicine and Power in Tunisia, 1780–1900.*

Tunisian Plague of 1818–20

Major epidemic of plague that killed possibly a quarter of the people in Tunisia (then a Muslim kingdom under a Turkish bey, or governor), including some 30,000 inhabitants of the city of Tunis.

Traders or travelers by land or by sea from Algiers were thought to have brought the plague disease into the port of Tunis in 1818. Mahmud Bey, the ruler of Tunis, knew the horrors of plague because of an earlier outbreak in Tunisia in 1784–85; when a physician diagnosed the disease spreading through Tunis in 1818, Mahmud ordered the physician to be beaten and thrown into jail, for he wanted to hear or learn nothing about it. Nonetheless, the three forms of plague broke out: bubonic (with painful buboes [swellings] of lymph nodes), septicemic, and pneumonic (the most serious and highly infectious form).

Although Jews were frequently blamed for disasters, they were not so accused in 1818 in Tunis; when a Jewish citizen was burned at the stake, his death seemed to increase the severity of the plague epidemic, and many citizens looked on it as a God-sent sign of disapproval of Jews' executions (which were stopped). Mahmud Bey's quarantine regulations were disobeyed by some Muslims, who preferred religious invocations as a defense against the plague and sometimes tried to convert plague-stricken Jews to Islam (with the saying "there is no flight from destiny"). Many Muslims who took precautions were spared and believed their lives had been saved as an "act of God." Undoubtedly the bey's sanitary cordons to restrict traffic and trade helped.

In July 1820 the disease subsided considerably in Tunis and Tunisia. The mortality rate had been high; between 30 percent and 50 percent of the victims of simple bubonic plague had perished, and nearly all those who contracted pneumonic and septicemic plague had died. In the city of Tunis, estimated mortality ranged from about 30,000 to as high as 50,000 (in a total population of about 120,000). The Tunisian kingdom possibly suffered a fatality rate of 25 percent, and much of its land was left uncultivated, causing more hardship and increasing dependency on European countries for food and assistance.

Further reading: Gallagher, *Epidemics in the Regency of Tunis, 1780–1880;* Shattuck, *Diseases of the Tropics.*

Tunis Typhus Epidemic of 1868

Serious outbreak of louse-borne typhus fever that killed at least 5,000 inhabitants of Tunisia's capital city of Tunis. Dirty, crowded conditions and food shortages in Tunisia in 1867 favored epidemic typhus, characterized by high fever, severe pains, blood in the stool and urine, and a red rash.

Along with famine in the winter of 1867–68, unusually cold weather struck the city of Tunis, where sometimes the corpses of animals and people were left unburied in the streets. Human body lice, which carry the rickettsial infection, thrived in these conditions, and many typhus cases began to be reported after mid-February 1868. When the Tunisian government appeared indifferent to the typhus problem, a European sanitary council initiated steps to control it, enacting public health rules such as disposal of all human and animal cadavers from the streets, isolation of typhus patients, and disinfection of prisons and army barracks.

The epidemic was most severe in the overcrowded Muslim, Jewish, and Catholic sections of Tunis, where typhus was not subject then to quarantine procedures (as cholera was). The diffusion of the epidemic was not closely documented by French and local officials, and there is speculation some 50,000 persons may have died from it in Tunis and the provinces outside the city.

Further reading: Gallagher, *Medicine and Power in Tunisia, 1780–1900;* Gelfand, *The Sick African.*

Turkish Influenza Epidemic of 1957–58

Offshoot of the Asian Influenza Pandemic of 1957 (q.v.), leading to a severe outbreak of influenza in Turkey during 1957–58 (see INDIAN INFLUENZA EPIDEMIC OF 1957–58; JAPANESE INFLUENZA EPIDEMIC OF 1957–58).

Influenza arrived in Turkey at the end of June 1957, on a course through Pakistan, Iran, and Syria.

In July, it fanned out across the country and became epidemic. Over the next few months, incidence or morbidity soared, with 53,565 cases recorded in August and 106,970 cases in September, and peaked in October, when 128,277 cases were reported. During November, the incidence dropped to 50,580 cases and, in December, to 17,587 cases. Thereafter, the epidemic began to subside, with 10,088 cases recorded in January and 2,188 cases in February. Actual incidence of the disease during the outbreak is believed to have been much higher. In Turkey, influenza was not considered a notifiable disease, and many cases, especially in the rural areas, no doubt escaped detection and treatment.

Many and varied complications were noted in the wake of this epidemic. Predominant among them were eye hemorrhages and psychiatric and neurological complaints.

Further reading: Payzin et al., "Neurological and Psychiatric Complications of Asiatic Flue."

U

Ugandan AIDS Epidemic   See AFRICAN AIDS EPIDEMIC.

Ugandan Plagues of 1926–31   Series of devastating epidemics of bubonic, pneumonic, and septicemic plague (the three clinical forms of the disease) in Uganda in east-central Africa.

Following a plague outbreak in the Far East in 1893, this highly infectious disease entered North Africa in 1896, spread to both West and South Africa by 1899, and reached British East Africa by 1902. In some areas, it disappeared after one or two localized outbreaks; in other regions, the disease remained endemic for about 20 years until more severe, widespread outbreaks began to occur, such as in Uganda.

Between June and August 1926, bubonic plague broke out in the native kingdom of Buganda in southeastern Uganda and in the nearby eastern province; out of the 1,844 cases reported, 1,574 were fatal. In 1927 a second outbreak in these same areas took the lives of 1,863 persons (out of 2,171 infected). Most of the infected had contracted the disease from plague-carrying fleas, which had moved from dead rats or other rodents (their hosts) to infest man (another host). Bitten by the fleas, the Ugandans became ill with splitting headaches, bouts of diarrhea and vomiting, and high fevers (as high as 107° F); they also were in agony when golf-ball-size buboes (swellings) appeared in their groin or armpits. In 1929 the number of Ugandans who contracted the disease soared to 5,960 (more than double the total cases reported in 1926–28); total fatalities were 5,118 that year (almost half the human deaths [2,518] occurred in the country's Mengo district).

Uganda's eastern province experienced almost annual plague outbreaks; workers on the cotton plantations there came down with the disease, which had reached epizootic proportions (temporary prevalence among many animals in a wide area) by 1930. Western areas of Uganda reported no outbreaks of plague, but the north-central district of Lango was hit in 1931.

Uganda's mortality rate reached nearly 90 percent (14,899 persons contracted plague, 13,124 of them died, between 1926 and 1931); many of the cases had been pneumonic and speticemic plague, along with the bubonic form. A form of pneumonia set in when the lungs of bubonic-infected patients were attacked; pneumonic patients (who easily passed the disease from person to person) frequently coughed up blood and usually died within two to four days after their initial infection. Patients with septicemic plague (in which the human bloodstream is invaded by the virulent bacillus carried by the diseased flea) sometimes died hours after contracting it, before buboes had time to form; recovery was rare in these cases, with or without treatment.

In 1932 only 60 plague cases (with 40 deaths) occurred in Uganda, where medical help, drugs, and vaccinations were offered and effective. The following year there were 858 cases (with 833 deaths). Localized outbreaks of plague continued until the 1980s, when the disease seemed to have disappeared.

Further reading: Marks and Beatty, *Epidemics;* Scott, *A History of Tropical Medicine.*

Ugandan Sleeping Sickness Epidemic of 1940–43
First recorded epidemic of African sleeping sickness (African trypanosomiasis) in Uganda, killing about 250 persons of the 2,500 infected, mainly in the Busoga region.

When the disease's first victim (a schoolboy) died in late December 1940, he was thought to have contracted the Gambian strain of the disease *(Trypanosoma gambiense)*, which more than 30 years earlier had killed at least 100,000 people in Uganda and Tanganyika (see UGANDAN-TANGANYIKAN SLEEPING SICKNESS EPIDEMIC OF 1900–1909); some 11,000 had died in the Busoga region in southeastern Uganda in that earlier epidemic. While visiting Busoga's Lake Victoria area between the towns of Iganga and Jinja in November 1940, the schoolboy was painfully bitten by a disease-carrying tsetse fly. Within three weeks the boy (then in Uganda's capital of Kampala) had a high fever and intense headache, followed by anemia, swelling limbs, heart problems, tremors, and rapid wasting; he died before the sleeping phase of the disease. At the same time, two immigrant laborers at a Kakira sugar estate on the western edge of the Busoga forest became ill and later died in Jinja's hospital with symptoms similar to the schoolboy's. A local Soga (native Bantu-speaking person on the north shore of Lake Victoria) also fatally contracted the disease in December 1940. All the victims were found to be infected with the Rhodesian strain *(Trypanosoma rhodesiense)*, generally a more virulent form of sleeping sickness and, at that time, believed to be confined to the semi-arid savannah and woodland of eastern Africa south of the equator.

Uganda (then a British protectorate) had taken elaborate precautions to prevent the transport of disease across its borders after the devastating sleeping sickness epidemic in 1900–1909. Nonetheless, authorities believed that the two immigrant workers (on the sugar estate at Kakira) had entered Uganda with sleeping sickness (they came from what is now Rwanda and Burundi, to the south). Ugandan authorities ordered native Luo fishermen to return home—to the eastern shores of Lake Victoria in Kenya (where the Gambian sleeping sickness was active). Evacuation of inhabitants of Uganda's Lake Victoria area between Jinja and Kakira was carried out, but the disease spread eastward to the leper colony of Buluba (at the head of Thurston Bay) and then farther east to Kityerera, where it infected forestry workers. By this time (June 1941), 80 persons had contracted the disease. Soon additional cases were diagnosed at Kityerera, Ikulwe (deeper in the Busoga forest area), and Kyemeire (farther east, 12 miles from Lake Victoria); by January 1942 the disease had moved into Kenya.

During the peak of the Ugandan epidemic in 1942, a temporary "sleeping sickness camp" was built at Bugiri (in the eastern end of the Busoga "fly belt"), where numerous people were sick and many new cases were brought. Because of the rapid removal of infected persons to the camp, the infection rate declined considerably by the end of 1943. The end of abnormally heavy rainfall also contributed to the tsetse fly receding and thus the abatement of the disease, which has remained endemic in Uganda since 1944.

Further reading: Ford, *The Role of Trypanosomiasis in African Ecology;* Ormerod, "The Epidemic Spread of Rhodesian Sleeping Sickness, 1908–1960."

Ugandan-Tanganyikan Sleeping Sickness Epidemic of 1900–1909

Major epidemic of African sleeping sickness (African trypanosomiasis) in territories around Lake Victoria, killing at least 100,000 people in what became Uganda and Tanganyika in east-central Africa.

In the last quarter of the nineteenth century, new trading routes opened in Africa's equatorial belt, notably the Congo River basin. The increasing number of riverboats helped spread infectious disease as traders and travelers moved about. An estimated half a million persons perished from sleeping sickness in the Congo region between 1895 and 1905; by 1900 this killer disease had reached the shores and islands of Lake Victoria.

British physicians Albert and Jack Cook, brothers working then in Uganda, were the first to diagnose sleeping sickness in patients' blood—a major breakthrough in analysis of this disease that brings physical wasting and growing somnolence, leading to death. After two years of research by the British government and thousands of deaths, the Gambian form of sleeping sickness was isolated and its vector identified as the tsetse fly (later, in 1910, a second and more acute form of the disease was identified as the Rhodesian strain).

In Uganda, the hardest hit region was Busoga, a prosperous banana-growing area on Lake Victoria's north shore; more than 11,000 people there died of the sickness by 1909. In the Buvuma islands on the lake, about 43,000 were reportedly killed by the disease between 1900 and 1905.

German East Africa (Tanganyika, now Tanzania) also suffered, but less severely, reporting sleeping-sickness deaths on the German-held islands of Kome, Bumbire, Maisome, and Ukerewe on Lake Victoria. In 1905 ten percent of the lake port of Mwanza (2,000 people) died from the disease, which was then well established in the hinterlands around Lake Victoria.

At the time there was no known cure, and many Africans were just abandoned when they became sick. There were too few hospitals in British and German East Africa to treat the growing number of sick. British and German authorities sought a cure and a solution to rid the regions of the tsetse fly. Robert Koch, a leading German bacteriologist, arrived (1906) at Tanga on Tanganyika's seacoast and found a cure with atoxyl, a derivative of arsenic. The drug had some remedial effect, but heavy doses caused blindness in over 20 patients.

When the epidemic continued to rage along Lake Victoria's shores and the tsetse fly could not be exterminated, British Commissioner Sir Hesketh Bell arranged for the native people to evacuate their homes in the disease zones. More than 25,000 inhabitants of the Sese and Buvuma islands alone were moved to the mainland. The evacuation, along with stricter border patrols by both British and German officials, led to a sharp decline in sleeping-sickness cases reported; the epidemic waned before the end of 1909.

Further reading: Clyde, *History of the Medical Services of Tanganyika*; McKelvey Jr., *Man Against Tsetse*.

Upper Voltaic Meningitis Epidemic of 1939 Severe outbreak of cerebrospinal meningitis (CSM) that killed 3,118 out of 6,783 infected persons in Upper Volta (Burkina Faso) in West Africa in 1939. This acute bacterial disease had broken out sporadically in the southern and central regions of Upper Volta since 1907, and had occurred in other areas in the so-called "CSM belt" (stretching from northern Uganda in East Africa to Senegal in the westernmost part of the continent). In 1939 Upper Volta (then a French colony) suffered the most fatalities recorded in an outbreak of CSM that swept across Africa.

CSM attacks the meninges (the three membranes enveloping the spinal cord and brain), and its pathogen (disease-producing micro-organism) is commonly transmitted by sneezing and coughing of sick patients, who suffer from fever, intense headache, stiff neck, nausea, photophobia, eye muscle paralysis, and petechial rash. CSM epidemics occur during months when cold weather forces people to stay inside and dry air weakens the effectiveness of mucous membranes as a barrier to infection. The dark, crowded, poorly ventilated houses in the densely populated areas of Upper Volta facilitated the rapid spread of CSM among the inhabitants.

In January 1939, at the beginning of the cold, dry season, the town of Kiembara first reported an outbreak of CSM (a traveler from Niger had evidently brought the infectious bacteria there). Then the nearby town of Tougan reported 19 cases between January and April 1939, months when the disease spread south to Tenkodogo (where 2,552 people were infected) and to nearby Fada N'Gourma (where 2,310 people became infected). Upper Volta's capital, Ouagadougou (with a population of about 537,000 people), reported 987 CSM cases, and the town of Kaya to the north had 857 cases. Very few persons were infected in other places that recorded the disease, including Bobo-Dioulasso (a city of 297,000 people), Gaoua, Dori, and Koudougou. Little could be done for the sick during the epidemic, which ended with the spring rains in April 1939. Authorities isolated the sick, put restrictions on travel and public gatherings, and banned funerals, but the infection was not able to be curtailed by administrative measures. CSM remained seasonally epidemic throughout Upper Volta after 1939, and it spread from the country into neighboring southern French Sudan (Mali) and what is now northeast Ghana and northern Togo.

In the 1940s effective sulfa drugs became available to help lower the fatality rate in Upper Volta; by 1962 the rate had dropped to ten percent. Afterward, incidence of CSM reported in the country declined considerably, especially from 1972 to 1977, with no fatalities during the early 1980s.

Further reading: Hartwig and Patterson, *Disease in African History*; Hartwig and Patterson, *Cerebrospinal Meningitis in West Africa and Sudan in the Twentieth Century*.

U.S. AIDS Epidemic Outbreak of AIDS (acquired immunodeficiency syndrome) that began in the United States in 1981 and killed more than 240,000 Americans by late 1994. The disease will claim still more victims: Experts estimate that as of late 1989 about one million Americans were infected with the virus that causes AIDS, which is today (1994) one of the main causes of death in Americans aged 20 to 40. Although many of them do not realize it yet, the virus has already set in motion a progressive deterioration of their immune system that, as far as scientists can determine, inevitably leads to death.

Despite its lethality, AIDS is not a highly contagious disease. The virus is transmitted not through casual contact, but only through the exchange of body fluids, especially blood and semen. As a result, although AIDS cases have been reported in all 50 U.S. states, the disease is not widespread in the population at large. Before 1993 the epidemic had hit hardest in large cities (such as New York City and San Francisco) and among gay (homosexual) males (many of whom are white and middle-class) and among injecting-drug users and their sex partners and children (who are predominantly poor minorities). Because AIDS is concentrated in groups whose behavior many Americans condemn, the epidemic has sparked controversy and highlighted deep political, religious, and ideological differences in U.S. society. Yet it has also improved the way medical researchers and public health officials deal with infectious disease, and increased our understanding of the human immune system.

AIDS made its first official appearance in the United States in June 1981, when the Centers for Disease Control (CDC) reported on five gay men from Los Angeles who had a rare infection, *Pneumocystis carinii pneumonia*. Before long other doctors published accounts of gay male patients with uncommon illnesses, such as the cancerous skin lesions of Kaposi's sarcoma. Soon after, similar disorders were observed in hemophiliacs, and the condition was given the name "acquired immune deficiency syndrome" in 1982.

Much about AIDS remains unknown, including its origin (it appears to have arisen in Africa at least several decades ago), but the pace of scientific discovery once the disease was identified has been remarkable. In 1983 the mutant agent proclaimed to cause AIDS—the human immunodeficiency virus (HIV)—was isolated by French scientists led by Dr. Luc Montagnier of the Pasteur Institute in Paris and its structure and functioning determined in the following years. In 1985 a test became available to screen blood donations for the antibodies to HIV; in March 1987 the U.S. Food and Drug Administration (FDA) approved zidovudine (also known as AZT), the first antiviral drug against HIV. Since then, the FDA has sanctioned scores of other therapies for people with AIDS, while vaccine trials are under way.

HIV attacks the cells that coordinate virtually all phases of the immune response. Shortly after it invades the body, HIV may trigger a brief, febrile illness that resembles influenza or mononucleosis, but it then remains latent, in some cases for at least ten years, causing only minor symptoms such as persistent swollen lymph nodes, night sweats, fatigue, and diarrhea. Eventually, something kicks the virus into high gear. It reproduces rapidly, cripples the immune system, and leaves the person vulnerable to opportunistic infections that can affect every organ system of the body. Caused by organisms that are usually harmless in humans, these illnesses signal the start of AIDS, the final stage of HIV infection. (In 1992 scientists reported people suffering from an AIDS-like illness but having no HIV infection in their bodies.)

Although the course of the disease is different in each person, the ultimate prognosis is the same. The life expectancy of someone diagnosed with AIDS now averages two years, with nearly 100 percent of patients dead within five years. The overwhelming number of victims are young adults; in 1991 nearly three quarters of the people who died from AIDS were between 25 and 44 years old.

To take into account the increasing awareness of the many clinical manifestations of HIV infection, the CDC has expanded its definition of HIV/AIDS several times since publishing the first one in 1982. Even with the updated criteria, the CDC estimates that its figures (which include all 50 states, the District of Columbia, and U.S. territories) indicate only about 70 percent to 90 percent of HIV-related deaths. Even so, by 1992, there was one such reported death every 12 minutes.

The long latency period of HIV evidently allowed the virus to spread unchecked for years before anyone knew what it was. It first made inroads among homosexual and bisexual men, especially those in large cities, where the opportunities existed for sex with numerous partners (often anal intercourse,

which can tear skin). Although the number of new cases among them leveled off by the early 1990s, gay males continue to be heavily represented among AIDS patients. Of the 47,095 official cases counted in 1992, 50.8 percent were homosexual men. Once the disease was identified, the gay community quickly formed volunteer organizations to care for people with AIDS and to disseminate information about prevention and treatment.

Many gays, along with others alarmed by the toll of the epidemic, turned to political activism. They resisted public health measures, such as mandatory reporting of those infected, that they thought would further stigmatize homosexuals. They also called for more funding for the disease and its victims, quicker access to promising treatments, and a role in supervising clinical trials. Their persistence paid off: since late 1989, for instance, a "parallel track" policy has allowed AIDS patients not enrolled in drug trials to be treated with experimental therapies while testing continues, while in late 1990 the government announced that all AIDS drug trials receiving federal funds must include patient advocates on their supervising committees. These innovations will likely be carried over to the drug development process for other diseases.

Unfortunately, the attention AIDS activists were fighting for sometimes came in the form of hysteria and blame. In the late 1980s children with AIDS (many of them hemophiliacs, who had acquired the virus from transfusions before the screening test was marketed) were prevented from attending school, and they and their families were ostracized. After the CDC reported in 1990 on five patients in Florida who may have contracted AIDS from their dentist, congresspeople and worried citizens called for mandatory testing of all health care practitioners. In fact, the risk of transmission remains much higher from patient to provider than the other way around.

The groups that the infection is targeting right now are not white, middle-class Americans, but rather inner-city minorities and users of injectable drugs (IDUs) and their sex partners. As the shift from gay males to drug users began in the late 1980s, some public health officials set up controversial needle-exchange programs, the first one of which began in Tacoma, Washington, in August 1988. Intended to prevent the sharing of drug equipment, which often contains residues of blood after use, the programs allow drug users to exchange used needles and syringes for clean ones at no charge.

Through drug users the disease is gaining access to the heterosexual population: In 1992, 56.8 percent of new AIDS cases among heterosexuals were the result of sex with an IDU, and many of these newly diagnosed patients were women. As women pick up the virus, they are capable of spreading it to non-drug using partners or to their own children. Although only about two percent of total AIDS patients are under 13 years of age, the number of pediatric cases will continue to grow; about one third to one half of all babies born to HIV-infected mothers acquire the virus.

Some experts fear that among IDUs and poor minorities, the infection may become endemic by the end of the 1990s. Overall, however, the rate of increase in AIDS has been slowing down, and the CDC estimates that the number of new cases may level off at about 60,000 to 70,000 per year by 1995. HIV-related deaths will remain high, however, since there are so many infected people. Research continues on ways to slow the progression to AIDS and fight off opportunistic infections. As HIV-infected people stay alive longer, however, the government, insurance companies, and health care providers will keep arguing over the costs of caring for them (which can now run to tens of thousands of dollars per person).

The close connection of AIDS with marginalized social groups and with behavior of which many Americans do not approve guarantees that controversies will continue throughout the 1990s. Needle-exchange programs, mandatory testing, sex education and the promotion of condoms, confidentiality of patient information, and other topics will be debated for years to come. See also AFRICAN AIDS EPIDEMIC.

Further reading: Centers for Disease Control, *Morbidity and Mortality Weekly Report*; National Research Council, *The Social Impact of AIDS in the United States*; Stine, *Acquired Immune Deficiency Syndrome*.

Usambara Malaria Epidemic of 1941–42

Unusual epidemic of malaria that claimed the lives of 240 of the 1,500 persons infected in five native villages along the western Usambara Mountains in northeast Tanzania.

In December 1941 visiting workers from sisal estates on Tanzania's lower plains unwittingly introduced malaria parasites to the mountain village of Ngulwi. At an altitude of 4,500 feet, Ngulwi is too high in the Usambaras for the Anopheles mosquitoes (malaria's vectors) to live long enough to breed. However, unusually warm rains created an environment on the mountains' west side for the mosquitoes to breed. Malaria subsequently struck Ngulwi and the nearby village of Ubiri (near Lushoto) and then Vuga and Bungu, leaving villagers, who had never built up an immunity to the disease, with recurring high fevers. By February 1942 the epidemic had extended as far as Bumbuli, the fifth village struck.

Many of those who survived the illness suffered kidney, liver, or blood complications. Along Tanzania's coast and on its plains, malaria is endemic (peculiar to a locality), enabling inhabitants there to acquire much immunity after recovering from it. But in the Usambaras, where malaria seldom occurs, the morbidity is always acute.

Further reading: Clyde, *Malaria in Tanzania*; Colbourne, *Malaria in Africa*.

U.S.-British-Chinese Armies' Typhus Epidemics of 1943–45

Outbreaks of scrub typhus (*febris tsutsugamushi*, Japanese river fever, mite-borne typhus) among United States, British, and Chinese troops in Burma and India during World War II (see SOUTHWEST PACIFIC TYPHUS EPIDEMICS OF 1942–45).

Scrub typhus fever initially broke out in 1943 among British soldiers training in the jungles of Ceylon (Sri Lanka) and later intensified as troops positioned themselves along the Burmese-Indian border. The next year it struck American and Chinese army units based near Ledo in Assam (northeastern corner of India). Initially called "CBI Fever" (Chinese-Burmese-Indian Fever), the disease was discovered to be quite widespread, extending from Fort Hertz (Putao) in northernmost Burma through Assam to Imphal and south to Cox's Bazar (in southernmost Bangladesh). It was a serious health hazard for most of the military units in the region. From November 1, 1943, to September 1, 1945, 1,098 cases of scrub typhus were reported among the American (695 cases, 58 deaths) and Chinese (403 cases, 40 deaths) troops. The average case fatality rate was 8.9 percent, but this varied from site to site.

In December 1944, the United States Typhus Commission (see JAPANESE-KOREAN TYPHUS EPIDEMIC OF 1945–46) established a field office in Ledo to study individual case records from the American Army hospitals and learn more about the incidence and distribution of the disease and about where it was acquired. These studies revealed that most of the outbreaks here and in the 1942–45 southwest Pacific region were caused by the *Rickettsia tsutsugamushi* or *Rickettsia orientalis*, transmitted to man by the mite *Trombicula akamushi* or *Trombicula deliensis*. The general pattern was similar to that of the southwest Pacific epidemics. The outbreaks in Burma and India ended rather abruptly when the troops were transferred out of the region.

Scrub typhus proved to be a formidable threat to the Allied troops fighting against Japan in this region and in the southwest Pacific during the Second World War. In fact, it was far more serious in its consequences than the louse-borne typhus epidemics that plagued Allied operations in Europe and the

Middle East (see IRANIAN [PERSIAN] TYPHUS EPIDEMIC OF 1942–44).

Further reading: Moulton, ed., *The Rickettsial Diseases of Man.*

U.S. and Caribbean Dengue Epidemic of 1826–28

Serious outbreak of dengue fever that struck parts of the southern United States and the Caribbean from 1826 to 1828.

Dengue is an infectious tropical and subtropical disease, known also as breakbone fever because of its characteristic and severe pain in bones, joints, and muscles. It is caused by the same viruses responsible for hemorrhagic fever (a more critical form of dengue), transmitted not person-to-person, but by the bite of particular mosquitoes (*Aëdes aegypti, Aëdes albopictus,* and *Aëdes scutellaris*) found in regions where the disease is endemic. The onset of the disease is sudden, with symptoms of high fever, nausea, intense headache (particularly behind the eyes), vomiting, unbearable pain in bones and joints, and pink rashes over parts of the body. A victim normally recovers fully after a week, but may experience prolonged fatigue and sometimes depression. There are no known effective drugs against dengue; treatment is usually cool sponging to lower the fever and pain relieving drugs.

In the autumn of 1826 officials in Savannah, Georgia, first reported an outbreak of dengue, which subsequently erupted in other parts of the American South (notably at Pensacola, Florida, in May 1828 and at Charleston, South Carolina, and New Orleans, Louisiana, in June 1828); Savannah was again struck by epidemic dengue in August 1828. The acute febrile disease also invaded the Virgin Islands in the West Indies, infecting many inhabitants in St. Thomas and St. Croix between September 1827 and March 1828. From these two islands, dengue apparently moved westward and southward. Jamaica reported an epidemic in December 1827 and Cuba had one in March 1828; the smaller islands of St. Barthelemy, St. Kitts (St. Christopher), Antigua, Guadeloupe, Martinique, Barbados, and Tobago also recorded many illnesses from dengue at various times between November 1827 and May 1828. Persons on the Dutch island of Curaçao off the Venezuelan coast also fell gravely ill (November 1827), and in New Granada (Colombia) there were numerous cases in Cartagena, a Caribbean seaport, and in Bogotá. In the latter months of 1828, the epidemic reached the Mexican seaport of Veracruz on the Gulf of Mexico and the British island colony of Bermuda in the North Atlantic. Both places had much sickness; Bermuda again suffered a dengue epidemic in 1837.

The 1826–28 dengue epidemic did not extend into the northern U.S. although Philadelphia reported a few isolated cases among crewmembers of a ship arriving there from Havana, Cuba, in 1828. Soon afterward the epidemic subsided.

Further reading: Marks and Beatty, *Epidemics;* Hirsch, *Handbook on Geographical and Historical Pathology;* Nash, *Evolution and Disease.*

U.S. Cholera Epidemic of 1832

Worldwide pandemic from Europe that invaded New York first; the disease was known more for its social effects than for the number of people killed. The poor were the hardest hit, which eventually led to public health innovations and social reform. The epidemic also precipitated a bitter clash between the "haves" and "have nots." The rich feared the mob, and the poor viewed the cholera as a means of oppression, perhaps even deliberately let loose to wipe out society's lowest tier. Cholera had been linked to immoral or dissolute behavior long before it reached North America. In the United States, all excesses were uniformly condemned as unhealthy and equated to sin. The same vices that predisposed a person to poverty could also predispose him to contracting cholera. The respectable associated material well-being with their regularity and, by implication, virtuousness. According to some, cholera was punishment from God to remind Man of his mortality and promote virtue by destroying the immoral and dissolute.

Cholera *asiatica* (Asiatic cholera) is caused by the bacteria *cholera vibrio* or *vibrio comma,* which enters the human intestine and works quickly to kill on the same day. In the nineteenth century, one half of all cholera victims died. The bacteria is excreted and commonly transmitted by polluted water, by flies that carry the contamination from fecal matter to food, unwashed hands, and uncooked fruits and vegetables. Symptoms approximate those of acute arsenic poisoning. Characteristics of the disease include diarrhea, acute cramps, and chronic vomiting. Dehydration and cyanosis result, exemplified by a blue, shrunken face, cold and darkened extremities with skin of the feet and hands puckered. In the first half of the nineteenth century, cholera's true cause was unknown and there was no effective treatment.

From New York, cholera spread along the eastern coast and moved westward to the Pacific by 1834. Large towns established hospitals and raised money. Boston collected $50,000 at the very suggestion of a cholera epidemic. As it turned out, Boston and Charleston (only at first) evaded the epidemic. Because most towns lacked permanent boards of health, they were created. Volunteer organizations helped collect funds and control the disease. Not until August and September did cholera sweep through the South. Some areas, lightly touched in 1832, were more severely hit in 1833 after the disease remained dormant over the winter. Then cholera broke out in the West and South, as virulent as ever. Cholera reentered the United States from Cuba in 1833, moving into New Orleans and Charleston and then northward toward Canada. Steamboats, railroads, and canals all perpetuated the spread of the disease. New Orleans was the hardest hit, with 5,000 dead of cholera, and another 5,000 dead of yellow fever.

By June 14, cholera invaded the United States in New York state. By July, every New York City inhabitant who was able had fled. New York City streets were cleaned and covered with lime. There was no noise or crime. Almshouse inmates were released on their own recognizance. Penitentiary criminals were taken to Blackwell's Island. The board of health issued terribly inaccurate daily cholera reports (because physicians failed to report cases despite the threat of a heavy penalty). Nonetheless, the reports riveted the city's attention. Five cholera hospitals were established.

When 45 New York City dwellers died on July 10, newspapers stated that the special medical council indicated that the disease had killed only people overindulging in drink or drugs or otherwise taking risks and published a list of rules for minimizing the risk of getting cholera. As business came to a halt, even hard-working poor people had no means of support. Various associations donated food, funds, and clothing. When the disease peaked around July 20, more than 100 people per day were dying. Carts going through the streets collected bodies. Smoke from preventatives like tar and pitch filled the air. The poor resented the intrusion of outside authority into their lives, violently discouraging efforts to remove their sick and dead. Mobs attacked officials and doctors. The red light district was by far the hardest hit.

After July 20, the number of cases subsided. Once the dense population of people in crowded, filthy circumstances had transferred to a new location or died, cholera faded out. New York City returned to normal by the end of August. All but one of the hospitals closed. The expatriates returned. Businesses resumed their normal pace. However, many still died of cholera. Many families without fathers faced the coming severe winter, and the needy lined the streets. By Christmas, the disease ended. After the epidemic, all the reforms evaporated. The streets were no longer kept hygienically clean. Boards of health either disappeared or settled back into their previous apathy.

Cholera always started with the poor even if it spread to other classes. It was socially inexcusable to contract cholera. New York buried 95 percent of the dead in pauper's graves. Richmond, Virginia, buried 90 percent in the poorhouse cemetery. Cholera ravaged mainly the poor because they were packed in close, often squalid, housing circumstances and could not flee to the country, as did those who had means. Confined to the city, the poor had to depend on very polluted city wells and river water. Many helping the poor were shocked by their living conditions. By mid-nineteenth century, cholera had provoked much more social reform than indignation against sinners and the poor.

Further reading: Ackerknecht, *History and Geography of the Most Important Diseases*; McGrew, *Encyclopedia of Medical History*; Rosenberg, *The Cholera Years*.

U.S. Cholera Epidemic of 1849

Pandemic from Europe that penetrated first at New York and then at New Orleans; it was quickly carried nationwide by immigrants, California-bound gold seekers, and the transportation system—the railroad, steamboat, and stagecoach. Although exact figures were unavailable, mortality approximated less than 10 percent of the country's population. From every European port, families and adventurers with gold fever made their way to America. In the U.S. epidemic, cholera killed more immigrants than any other grouping. Cities with the highest death tolls—New Orleans, Cincinnati, St. Louis, and New York—held the most immigrants. In battling cholera, cities, towns, and settlements fared according to the quality of their water supply and sanitation. Unwilling to pay, most towns either had a volunteer health board or none, and could not afford cholera hospitals. To the majority, both cholera and poverty were moral rather than social problems. As in 1832, cholera was thought to scourge the poor and sinful.

Cholera *asiatica*, caused by the bacteria *cholera vibrio* or *vibrio comma*, entered the human intestine and worked quickly to kill, often on the same day. In the nineteenth century, one-half of all cholera victims died. The bacteria was excreted and commonly transmitted by polluted water, flies that carried the contamination from fecal matter to food, unwashed hands and uncooked fruits and vegetables. Symptoms approximated those of acute arsenic poisoning. Disease characteristics included diarrhea, acute cramps, and chronic vomiting. Dehydration and cyanosis resulted, indicated by a blue face, as well as cold and darkened extremities with shrunken skin of the feet and hands. Until 1849, cholera had been causally linked to filth and immorality. By means of the microscope, biologists were breaking new ground that would reveal the bacterial source.

In the South, German ships brought cholera to New Orleans in December 1848. Once cholera deaths had been reported, business stopped because people fled and traders refused to enter the city. In New Orleans alone, the pestilence killed at least 4,000 people. Mild winter weather permitted the disease to spread up the Mississippi, Tennessee, and Arkansas rivers by riverboat, but cold temperatures limited any immediate outbreak to the Deep South. Cholera killed an estimated 10,000 slaves, which led to higher slave prices and wiped out 10 percent of the population in the Rio Grande Valley.

On December 1, 1848, the steamship *New York* from Le Havre brought cholera to New York City. Despite a quarantine and passenger hospital, cholera soon appeared in the city's immigrant domiciles. However, winter prevented a general outbreak. By summer, cholera spread to New York from the west, also. As in 1832, New York was still the dirtiest American city. Between the middle of May to the middle of August, cholera had killed at least 5,000 New Yorkers out of a population of 500,000, many of whom had fled by July. Five hospitals were established over the summer. The board of health had failed to get politically-awarded street cleaning contracts enforced, and corpse removal was slow. Before August, business was at a standstill. Working people, not equipped for an indefinite length of unemployment, suffered. The epidemic peaked in New York City around the beginning of August, with 100 dying daily. Although ships were quarantined, no control measures had been placed on trains. Suddenly, the disease subsided. Within two weeks, business resumed a healthy pace.

From New York City, cholera spread in the East. Health boards in Boston, Philadelphia, and Baltimore prepared for the epidemic. As in 1832, many medical reports appeared in journals and newspapers. Dire descriptions of death were counterbalanced by reassurance that temperance, prudence, and proper habits preserved people. Water supplies, garbage disposal, and sanitation were usually inadequate anywhere. Boston spent nearly $30,000 mounting a successful campaign against cholera. Fatalities numbered only 160 of 262 hospitalized. Although Philadelphia lost only 700 in a population of 408,000, cholera killed 858 of Buffalo's 21,000 residents.

By spring, cholera spread throughout the Mississippi Valley and westward. In Cincinnati, an estimated 6,000 people in a population of 110,000 died of cholera. St. Louis lost at least 10 percent of its population. No town was too isolated or too small. In Washington, Indiana, cholera killed around 60 of the 200 residents who had not left. Western towns were hardest hit because of poor sanitation, inadequate water supplies, and large transient populations crowded into small living quarters. Graves of gold seekers lined the trails to California. Indian villages were often decimated. Although San Francisco did not suffer heavily, Sacramento lost 1,000 out of a population of 8,090 (4,000 had already fled).

Although the epidemic began to abate by the end of 1849, it recurred sporadically until 1854 because immigrants kept it alive. In 1850, cholera spread through the waterways between New Orleans and St. Louis, where 1,448 died that year. Other cities also suffered. After 1854, cholera abruptly disappeared. See also U.S. CHOLERA EPIDEMIC OF 1832; U.S. CHOLERA EPIDEMIC OF 1866.

Further reading: Ackerknecht, *History and Geography of the Most Important Diseases*; Chambers, *The Conquest of Cholera*; Rosenberg, *The Cholera Years*.

U.S. Cholera Epidemic of 1866 Pandemic that killed less than five percent of the U.S. population due to effective public health measures. In October 1865, the English steamer *Atalanta*, which had stopped in Le Havre, France, brought immigrants with cholera to New York. The ship was quarantined until passengers had been transferred to a hospital ship. Carried by soldiers, immigrants, and the railroad, the disease spread quickly. The medical community joined moralists in decrying the lack of decent housing for immigrants, who were crowded into slums. In scientific thought, statistics and observation were superceding abstract reasoning. Microorganisms as the cause of disease were coming to be accepted, as in the work of Louis Pasteur. While cholera in 1832 America had been a moral dilemma, it had evolved into a social problem by 1866. Nevertheless, people still believed cholera to be contagious, and attacked cholera hospitals as they had during the 1832 and 1849 epidemics.

Cholera *asiatica* was caused by the bacteria *cholera vibrio* or *vibrio comma*, which entered the human intestine and worked quickly to kill on the same day. In the nineteenth century, one-half of all cholera victims died. The excreted bacteria was commonly transmitted by polluted water, flies that carried the contamination from fecal matter to food, unwashed hands, and uncooked fruits and vegetables. Symptoms approximated those of acute arsenic poisoning. Characteristics of the disease included diarrhea, acute cramps, and chronic vomiting. Dehydration and cyanosis resulted, as indicated by a blue face, as well as cold and darkened extremities, with shrunken skin of the feet and hands. In 1854, Dr. John Snow, proved that vomit and excretion of cholera victims carried in water supplies was the common cause of epidemics. By 1855, Snow's principles were practiced in New York state's quarantine hospital.

New York City proved that disease—not just cholera—could be stopped. While winter delayed the disease's spread, the city prepared. Public health reformers managed to get a reform bill for the city passed by the state legislature in the winter of 1866. The legislation sought to establish a board of health made up of medical men trained in public health, rather than political appointees. New York streets were caked with ice, snow and filth. As in 1832 and 1849, pigs remained the only normal means of street cleaning. Although the board managed to get much filth removed from the streets, their efforts were slowed by court orders.

The disease was prevalent throughout the country before it made inroads at its point of initiation. Cholera arrived in New York in April 1866. Around May 1, cholera killed its first three victims at three geographically separate sites, which caused concern. To prevent spread of the disease, victims' belongings were burned, and lime and disinfectants were strewn throughout the evacuated buildings. Cholera did not recur at those locations. Although more than 20 new cases occurred in June, there was no general outbreak, due to the preventive measures taken. Although New York City reported 1,200 deaths and Brooklyn reported 800 to 900 deaths, the count was probably at least 50 percent too low. The board had succeeded. Between March and November, over 31,000 stop orders, 4,000 yard cleaning orders, and 770 cistern cleanup orders had been given out. New York City's Board of Health had taught a powerful lesson by preventing an epidemic in America's largest, most crowded, and (previously) dirtiest city. Although the disease spread from New York, the eastern cities never had a big outbreak; only 834 died in Philadelphia.

Other U.S. cities, in turn, demanded such a board, but none had the power of New York City's. Cincinnati's board controlled the public domain well, but could not force the private sector to clean up. Both Chicago and Cincinnati were hard hit by cholera. Chicago had no board of health, and Cincinnati waited until the death rate reached 90 before setting up a hospital. Twelve hundred died in Cincinnati. St. Louis lost 3,500. In 1867, Illinois set up a Chicago Board of Health with powers approximating those of New York City's board.

In New Orleans, a riot instigated by newly freed blacks and quelled by infected soldiers led to 1,350 cholera deaths. Disease spread by boat from New Orleans into the Deep South; 510 died in Vicksburg between August and September. A steamship carrying army recruits from New York to Texas brought cholera there. Many soldiers died as a result. San Antonio lost 500 people, although most of the usual inhabitants had fled.

The disease persisted until the end of 1867, especially in the West. From New Orleans, it spread along the Gulf Coast and the Mississippi River. Only isolated cases developed between St. Louis and New York. For 12 cities and three army posts, deaths ranged between 10,000 and 12,000. Estimates of losses for the whole country were four or five times greater than the numbers given, according to one source. See also U.S. CHOLERA EPIDEMIC OF 1832; U.S. CHOLERA EPIDEMIC OF 1849.

Further reading: Ackerknecht, *History and Geography of the Most Important Diseases*; Chambers, *The Conquest of Cholera*; Rosenberg, *The Cholera Years*.

U.S. Cholera Epidemic of 1873

Pandemic that primarily ravaged the South and Midwest, first taking root in New Orleans and the Delta area before spreading northward to Dakota territory, Pittsburgh, and Minnesota. The disease entered New Orleans on ships either from Europe or Rio de Janeiro, infected by Mediterrean trade. Now besieged by cholera in addition to poverty and carpetbaggers, the Southern states so desperately needed commerce that news of the disease's spread was hushed up, especially in trade centers along the major waterways, where the infection spread fastest. The pestilence hit small towns and the countryside much harder than it did large cities, which by this date had instituted public health reforms. As a result, the epidemic of 1873 was far less lethal and widespread than the 1832, 1849, and 1866 epidemics.

Cholera *asiatica* was caused by the bacteria *cholera vibrio* or *vibrio comma*, which entered the human intestine and worked quickly to kill, often on the same day. The excreted bacteria was commonly transmitted by polluted water, flies that carried the contamination from fecal matter to food, and unwashed hands. Symptoms, approximating those of acute arsenic poisoning, included diarrhea, acute cramps, and chronic vomiting. Dehydration and cyanosis resulted, as indicated by a blue face, as well as cold, dark extremities, with shrunken skin of the feet and hands. The cure was antibiotics to kill the bacteria and water pumped into the system intravenously to counteract dehydration.

The pestilence killed 259 people in New Orleans before July 1873. Cholera spread first through the parishes of southern Louisiana and then up the Mississippi River. In Mississippi, the disease haunted plantations and boat landings, especially because steamboats tossed untreated sewage overboard. Cholera spread into Arkansas by both railroad and boat. Characterized by squalor, absence of a sanitation system, and stagnant ponds, Memphis, Tennessee, lost 275 of the 1,000 inhabitants infected. In Nashville, with its own waste disposal problems, cholera was thought to have killed over 1,000. The epidemic peaked on June 20, when 72 died. Visitors attending an industrial exposition broadcast cholera throughout the state and into other states. As a result, Murfreesboro, Chattanooga, Knoxville, Shelbyville, and Gallatin all sustained heavy losses. Infection was carried from Nashville to Huntsville and Birmingham, Alabama.

Cholera penetrated the Ohio Valley by rail and boat. Kentucky was the hardest hit. North of the Ohio River, only the southernmost regions of adjacent states suffered losses from the disease. Infection spread along the Ohio River in the wake of the steamboat *John Kilgore*, which carried cholera sickness and death. In some areas, mortality was high. Louisville, Kentucky, having succeeded as a transportation center, concealed its cholera outbreak. From May 11 to October, cholera raged in St. Louis, Missouri, which suffered 700 deaths. From St. Louis, disease spread via the railroad and along the Missouri and Mississippi rivers. See also U.S. CHOLERA EPIDEMIC OF 1832; U.S. CHOLERA EPIDEMIC OF 1849; U.S. CHOLERA EPIDEMIC OF 1866.

Further reading: Ackerknecht, *History and Geography of the Most Important Diseases;* Chambers, *The Conquest of Cholera.*

U.S. Civil War Epidemics Outbreaks of various diseases that hit Union and Confederate troops during the U.S. Civil War (April 12, 1861–June 30, 1865) and ultimately spurred a public health revolution in the United States. Infectious diseases played a major role during this war, killing thrice as many soldiers (71 died per thousand) as succumbed to battle wounds.

In the Union Army, the reported mortality rate was 32 per thousand per year in the regular army, 55 per thousand in the white volunteers, and 133 per thousand in the black troops. Both sides estimated that each soldier suffered six rounds of sickness during the war. Throughout the summer of 1861, approximately 30 percent of all troops were sick. Outbreaks of viral diseases were widespread (given the movement of soldiers and civilians) in the crowded military camps, but even more debilitating were the recurrent fevers and enteric disorders caused by poor food and unhygienic living conditions. The U.S. Army Medical Corps lacked both the numbers (corpsmen) and the training to cope with an expanding army and the rapidly worsening health conditions. But in June 1861, the U.S. Sanitary Commission was established, an act that was to have a lasting impact on public health in the country.

The diseases of dysentery and diarrhea (in acute and chronic forms) were probably the most devastating of all. Together, they affected 1,739,135 soldiers and killed 44,558 over four years, an average annual attack rate of 711 per thousand people. Many already weakened Union and Confederate troops living near primitive, uncovered latrines and eating improperly cooked food readily fell prey to a variety of enteric ailments. The attack rate for these during the Civil War was 29 times higher than during World War I, and the death rate was 258 times higher.

Typhoid fever, then a killer disease, was also rampant, especially among new recruits; 79,462 cases of typhoid and 29,336 deaths (37 percent mortality) were reported in the Union Army. Some regiments were dubbed "typhoid" regiments because of the high incidence of the disease. With one attack conferring immunity, typhoid incidence declined as the pool of susceptible soldiers shrank. Nevertheless, case mortality increased from 17 percent in 1861 to 56 percent in 1865. Typho-malarial fevers were recorded but classified separately.

Infectious hepatitis (in epidemic and scattered form) affected about 72,000 soldiers in the Union Army. While it debilitated thousands of them, it was generally mild and did not cause many fatalities. During the Peninsular Campaign of 1862, some 3,400 Union soldiers were infected.

Malaria, the second most common camp disease, occurred in virtually every department (territory) but was more intense in the South. Regional and seasonal in its distribution, it killed many but left thousands more weakened and prone to further attacks and relapses. Among the Union troops, there were 1,315,955 cases and 10,063 deaths reported. In July 1861, the U.S. Sanitary Commission recommended that every Union soldier in a malarious region be given a daily dose of quinine sulphate (dissolved in whiskey). This prophylactic use of a drug was a milestone in the evolution of preventive medicine within the nation's military. But another disease of warm climates, the much dreaded yellow fever, did not become a serious threat, except in South Carolina in 1862 and in a few other areas.

Fresh meat and vegetables intended for the soldiers often did not reach them. Thus scurvy (caused by lack of vitamin C) was a constant presence, particularly among units living on field rations. However, few physicians had seen it in their regular practice, so it sometimes went undiagnosed. Considerably more dangerous and widespread was incipient scurvy (scorbutic diathesis).

Although vaccination had altered the epidemiology of smallpox, the poor quality of the vaccine led to growing resistance against the procedure. That and the social disruptions of war were reflected in an increased incidence of smallpox. Most of the hastily recruited soldiers and volunteers had not been vaccinated (though vaccination was an army requirement) and the vaccine was in short supply, so smallpox was rampant (albeit in scattered fashion) on both sides. The Union Army reported 6,716 cases of smallpox and 2,341 deaths among its 61,132 black soldiers, and 12,236 cases and 4,717 deaths among its 431,237 white troops. Severe outbreaks occurred in Washington, D.C., during 1861–62, mainly among 40,000 recently freed blacks living there in temporary housing and among the new recruits. By 1863, all the city's neighborhoods, including the White House, had been infected; President Abraham Lincoln apparently delivered the Gettysburg Address while suffering from the initial symptoms of smallpox. Smallpox also erupted in the Confederate and Union prison camps; for instance, more than 2,000 cases and 618 deaths occurred between February 1862 and June 1865 among Confederate prisoners at Camp Douglas, Illinois. In the South, poor vaccine quality sometimes made vaccination almost as dangerous as smallpox itself; some 5,000 Confederate troops were invalided by the disease during the Battle of Chancellorsville in early May 1863.

Wave upon wave of measles also invaded the army camps, and few new recruits (especially from the rural areas) escaped infection. Early in the war, there was gross undercounting of measles cases; a reported 67,763 cases and 4,246 deaths occurred among white Union troops. Outbreaks of measles were common in 1861–62, and many of the deaths resulted from pulmonary complications such as pneumonia. Further, diseases such as mumps, typhus, dengue, meningitis, venereal disease, diphtheria, scarlet fever, and a variety of respiratory ailments were also prevalent among some troops during the Civil War.

The Sanitary Commission helped change the way medicine was practiced in the United States. Far exceeding its original mandate as an advisory body, it reformed the Medical Bureau, prepared monographs on the treatment of important military diseases, gave respectability to the nursing profession, and stressed the importance of compiling national vital statistics and of volunteerism in the health field.

It also sponsored "Sanitary Fairs," which not only raised funds for the medical care of soldiers but also increased public awareness of health issues.

Further reading: Adams, *Doctors in Blue: The Medical History of the Union Army in the Civil War;* Steiner, *Disease in the Civil War.*

U.S. Dengue Epidemics of 1850–51 and 1878–80

Two extensive epidemics of dengue fever (breakbone fever) that occurred in the southern United States. Thousands of people, bitten by certain mosquitoes carrying the dengue virus, suffered high fever (up to 106° F), severe headaches, agonizing pain in their back and limbs, and pale pink rashes (petechiae) on their feet and legs. The fatality rate was very low, as is usual with dengue, a fever of warm climates that typically lasts for six or seven days. A victim may be left in a state of fatigue and depression for some weeks after the disease has run its course. Children usually have a milder fever than adults. No known drugs are effective against dengue, which can be controlled by eliminating the breeding places of the *Aëdes* mosquitoes' larvae.

The first epidemic erupted in Charleston, South Carolina, in July 1850 and then appeared in Savannah and Augusta, Georgia, and New Orleans, Louisiana, in August. By autumn the disease was prevalent in Mobile, Alabama, and moved down the coast of the Gulf of Mexico to Galveston, Texas, which was hard-hit in October 1850. It continued south to Matagorda and then to Brownsville on the Texas-Mexico border before gradually subsiding thereafter.

At that time, 1851, the dengue epidemic was present in Havana, Cuba, and in Lima, Peru, and its port, Callao. During the next decade the nonfatal but very unpleasant disease attacked many inhabitants in various Caribbean islands (notably Martinique) and struck Mobile, Alabama, again in 1854. New Orleans suffered from dengue again in 1873, when about 40,000 residents became ill. This Southern city, along with Charleston, Augusta, Savannah, and other smaller cities, endured another severe dengue epidemic five years later (1878–80), and the residents of Galveston and Austin, Texas, were afflicted by still another dengue outbreak in 1885–86. See also U.S. AND CARIBBEAN DENGUE EPIDEMIC OF 1826–28.

Further reading: Marks and Beatty, *Epidemics;* Ehrenkranz et al., "Pandemic Dengue in Caribbean Countries and the Southern United States."

U.S. Influenza Epidemic of 1889–90   See ASIATIC INFLUENZA PANDEMIC OF 1889–90; EUROPEAN INFLUENZA PANDEMIC OF 1889–90.

U.S. Influenza Epidemic of 1918–19   See SPANISH INFLUENZA EPIDEMIC OF 1917–19.

U.S. Influenza Epidemic of 1957–58   Offshoot of the Asian Influenza Pandemic of 1957–58 (q.v.) that spread across the continental United States (see INDIAN INFLUENZA EPIDEMIC OF 1957–58; JAPANESE INFLUENZA EPIDEMIC OF 1957–58; TURKISH INFLUENZA EPIDEMIC OF 1957–58).

The H2N2 virus, a subtype of the Asian A2 influenza virus and closely related to that which caused the Asiatic Influenza Pandemic of 1889–90 (q.v.), first arrived in the United States in June 1957: at Newport, Rhode Island, where naval exercises were being held offshore (June 2), and shortly thereafter at various military bases in California (June 11–20). These outbreaks were characterized by mild cases and high attack rates but did not involve the civilian communities nearby. During the summer, small localized outbreaks were reported from far-flung areas of the country, such as California, Virginia, Iowa, and Pennsylvania; most of these occurred among groups of summer campers living and traveling in crowded conditions and also among migrant workers. They were closely monitored by the local health authorities, who feared that a major epidemic might erupt at anytime.

The U.S. government released an additional $800,000 to deal with the imminent epidemic, and the Influenza Surveillance Unit was established in July 1957 as an arm of the United States Public Health Service; its job was to collect and disseminate information about the disease and especially to measure general epidemiological trends. Facilities were provided so that laboratory and epidemiological studies could be conducted. Emergency health services were organized and vaccine production accelerated to meet the anticipated demand. However, the government did not provide funding for a nationwide vaccination campaign, and out of the 30 million vaccine doses tested for release when the epidemic peaked, only seven million were given to the public, and that was on a purely voluntary basis.

During August 1957, the pace began to quicken, with intense outbreaks reported from agricultural communities across Louisiana and Mississippi; they began among schoolchildren and spread very rapidly throughout a locality. Early in September, the epidemic erupted along the densely populated East Coast; New York City was one of the earliest of the big cities to be attacked. Almost simultaneously, the flu virus caused serious eruptions in communities across New Mexico, Utah, and Arizona. School openings played a crucial role in the diffusion of the epidemic, which continued to move from the West, East, and Gulf coasts toward the central and northern sections of the country during October. North and South Dakota were among the last areas to be involved.

In general, the epidemic peaked over most areas in mid-October. Forty-five million cases of influenza were estimated to have occurred during October–November 1957 alone. The epidemic subsided with the onset of winter, but incidence (mainly intense outbreaks affecting older people in scattered localities) increased briefly during late February and early March 1958. Mortality reports indicate that most of the deaths occurred in two distinct flu waves; the first wave peaked early in November 1957, and the second wave peaked during the week of March 1, 1958, even though the morbidity levels then were far lower than late in 1957. Secondary bacterial pneumonia caused many of the deaths during this second phase. Overall, the epidemic was apparently responsible for 70,000 deaths across the country—a greater proportion of them among the very young and among the elderly and the infirm, as opposed to the adult (middle-aged and young) population. Officials estimated that children in the five-to-fifteen age group suffered attack rates as high as 60 percent, but their mortality rates were low. See also U.S. INFLUENZA EPIDEMIC OF 1968–69.

Further reading: Trotter Jr. et al., "Asian Influenza in the United States, 1957–58"; Pyle, *The Diffusion of Influenza*.

U.S. Influenza Epidemic of 1968–69   Epidemic marking the arrival of the Hong Kong Influenza Pandemic of 1968 (q.v.) in the United States. The so-called "Hong Kong flu" was first identified and subsequently drew much international attention when it broke out in Hong Kong in July 1968, apparently immediately following a similar outbreak in southeastern China. During August, outbreaks were reported from many countries in southeast Asia, including Vietnam, where U.S. forces were deeply engaged in the Vietnam War (1956–75). Consequently the viral disease arrived in the United States before it reached Europe (see BRITISH INFLUENZA EPIDEMIC OF 1968–70) or other parts of the world (see RUSSIAN INFLUENZA EPIDEMIC OF 1968–69).

The Hong Kong flu virus was first isolated in the United States on September 2, 1968, from a patient who had just returned from Vietnam. During the same week, it was also identified during a flu outbreak at a military school in San Diego, California. Alaska and Hawaii also reported cases among military personnel that week. On September 6, the U.S. surgeon general alerted the health authorities in all 50 states about the possibility of an epidemic spread of influenza and invited their cooperation in monitoring the disease. Those at risk were urged to get immunized with a new vaccine being manufactured at the time.

During September, scattered cases occurred among civilians in 16 U.S. states; many cases were in the eastern section of the country, mainly in people recently returned from Vietnam. Civilian outbreaks were first reported from Puerto Rico and Alaska during late September and early October. In the continental United States, the first civilian outbreak occurred in Needles, California, in the third week of October. Nearly 35 percent to 40 percent of that town's citizens were struck with an influenza-like disease. Over the next few weeks (October 19 to November 9), influenza attacked four other western states and Hawaii. The disease continued to spread eastward. The first outbreaks on the East Coast occurred in Pennsylvania and New Jersey in the week ending November 16. By November 23, the disease had invaded 21 widely scattered states and, by December 28, all 50 states had been infected. The southeast and south-central regions were the last to be involved in the epidemic. However, according to Pyle (see below) the disease may have spread simultaneously from several urban centers.

The 1968–69 epidemic was widespread and led to school and college closings in 23 states; the week before Christmas was the peak flu period in many (37) states. In fact, 29 states and the District of Columbia reported maximum flu activity between December 15 and January 4, 1969. Mortality due to pneumonia-influenza peaked during the week ending January 11, 1969; there were 1,688 deaths reported that week alone. Generally, mortality curves trailed morbidity curves by three to four weeks. Overall, some 33,000 influenza-related deaths occurred nationwide during the epidemic.

The Hong Kong viral strain (H3N2) was estimated to have infected 30,000,000 Americans during the last quarter of 1968. Attack rates ranged from 15 percent to 50 percent. The main course of the disease lasted three to seven days, with some symptoms (coughing and listlessness) lingering for weeks; pneumococcal pneumonia was the main bacterial complication. Studies indicated that all age-groups were affected; the highest attack rates were in children below five years of age and in adults 45 to 64 years of age. The newly manufactured flu vaccine was not released for use until mid-November, three weeks after the Needles outbreak. At the height of the epidemic, ten million doses of the vaccine had been distributed and only six million Americans had been immunized. This policy came in for considerable public criticism following the epidemic.

The epidemic gradually declined during January 1969; the H3N2 virus, a subtype of the influenza A virus, did not cause a second wave. However, outbreaks of influenza B were reported from 20 states from late January to the end of March, particularly among elementary schoolchildren. Eight neighboring midwestern states recorded the maximum influenza B activity.

Further reading: Pyle, *The Diffusion of Influenza;* Sharrar, "National Influenza Experience in the USA, 1968–69."

U.S. Poliomyelitis Epidemic of 1916

First widespread outbreak of poliomyelitis (infantile paralysis, or Heine-Medin disease) in the United States, affecting 26 states (especially those in the northeast). There were about 27,000 reported cases and about 7,000 human deaths from polio during the epidemic. The New York City area was particularly hard-hit, with some 9,000 cases (97 percent of them being in children under 16 years old) and 2,448 deaths; this was a rate of 28.5 cases per 100,000 people. (Between 1909 and 1915, the largest yearly rate in the United States had been 7.9 polio cases per 100,000.) The epidemic, which frightened the public and the medical community, began in midsummer and abated in late October with the arrival of cool, autumn weather.

At first a victim of polio may seem as if he or she has a summer cold or a flush from playing outside on a hot day. A headache and low fever may appear the next day. Later, unexpectedly, paralysis may occur; the limbs cannot move, or worse, the lungs stop knowing how to breathe (the poliovirus destroys certain nerve cells so that muscles involved in breathing are paralyzed). By 1905 physicians knew that poliomyelitis did not always paralyze, but this continued to be the disease's main sign for diagnosis.

At the onset of the 1916 epidemic, polio was popularly thought to be caused by a bizarre variety of possible sources, such as moldy flour, gooseberries, poisonous caterpillars, sewage odors, and infected milk bottles. The viral derivation of polio had, however, been established by 1909, and scientists optimistically expected to discover easily how the disease spread and how to treat it. But they were disappointed; no vaccine against polio emerged until 1955 when a vaccine containing three types of dead poliovirus was developed by Dr. Jonas Salk and his colleagues.

Some scientists at New York City's Rockefeller Institute for Medical Research (founded in 1901, now Rockefeller University) had discovered a poliovirus in the aural and nasal body areas and had surmised that the disease was transmitted by close contact (by sneezes or kissing); yet the intestinal virus's pattern of affecting only one person in a family seemed to contradict this logic. Also, polio affected adults as well as children and thus was not very accurately called infantile paralysis. The disease attacked every social group, not just the lower classes. Epidemiologists had often insisted on linking the disease to filth and poverty, although evidence supported a random type of spread of polio.

The 1916 epidemic was distinguished by the high degree of isolation and quarantine that was enforced; since health officials did not know how polio was spread, they used strictures appropriate for fighting and controlling other infectious diseases. Along with quarantine, strictures included posting of signs at the homes of polio victims, screening of windows, disinfecting bed clothing, nurses changing their clothes immediately after attending patients, and preventing animal pets from entering sick persons' rooms. A new restriction, announced on July 14, 1916, which limited all travel into and out of the epidemic area in New York City caused an angry outcry. Only identification cards (health certificates) permitted children 16 years old and under to leave New York City from July 18 to October 3, provided there was or had been no polio in their homes. The city's commissioner of health, Dr. Haven Emerson, zealously enforced these disease control measures, and the city's mayor, John P. Mitchel, put to use the sizable aid offered by the U.S. Public Health Service, which included sanitary engineers, epidemiologists, clinicians, and an entomologist.

During the summer of 1916 New Yorkers who could left the city and stayed away until October. In the nearby Westchester suburbs, New Rochelle suffered the worst outbreak of the disease, which some people blamed on a large number of immigrants. Hudson Park's beach banned swimming by nonresidents, local vaudeville theaters could not entertain children under 16, and Sunday school was eliminated there. Physicians held daily meetings with parents to talk about childcare. Sutton Manor, a wealthy suburb, voluntarily isolated itself from interacting with the rest of the New York City area; health department officials posted quarantine signs in English, Italian, and Yiddish. A hospital strictly for infectious disease was erected in less than two weeks, due to overtime cooperation among the workers. But by then (September) the worst of the epidemic was over; most of the stricken had either recovered or could not be helped anymore.

A federal public health team then amassed extensive, significant statistical data about the epidemic; behavior characteristics of polio were mapped out, such as its routes of spread, victims' ages in rural and city settings, and racial differences and effects. The team's summary report, which did not appear until 1918, showed that quarantine had not worked, animals had not played a part in spreading the disease to people, and marked age differences existed

between urban and rural polio victims. The report also stated that polio was transmitted between people by unknown means, that most cases were not recognizable by classic symptoms (like paralysis), and that abortive cases might be the key to understanding the spread of the disease. Finally, the report declared that two to three cases of polio per thousand people can sufficiently immunize a population so that an epidemic declines. See NEW YORK POLIOMYELITIS EPIDEMIC OF 1907; U.S. POLIOMYELITIS EPIDEMIC OF 1942–53.

Further reading: Paul, *A History of Poliomyelitis;* Smith, *Patenting the Sun: Polio and the Salk Vaccine.*

U.S. Poliomyelitis Epidemic of 1931   Poliomyelitis outbreak nearly rivaling the U.S. Poliomyelitis Epidemic of 1916 (q.v.) and occurring when the disease was no longer considered a "new" scourge in the United States. The 1931 polio epidemic killed 4,138 people (12.2 percent of the reported cases) and was centered, like most outbreaks up to that time, in the northeast; New York City had almost 4,500 cases and New Haven had 149. The epidemic began in July, peaked in August, and ended in October with the onset of colder weather—a pattern typical for poliomyelitis, also called infantile paralysis.

Because prevention, cure, and proper treatment of polio were unknown then, physicians and health officers felt helpless and could provide only a few, often erroneous, guidelines, such as staying away from crowds and isolation in quarantine if the disease struck a family. Also recommended were checklists of commonsense personal and household hygiene habits. New York City's Department of Health received the following strange array of suggestions for treatment: camphor hung around the neck, eating salt, spinal injections of saliva, nose sprays, and blood injected into muscles. In 1931 oral-nasal secretions were blamed for the spread of polio, which doctors now know is transmitted by direct contact with pharyngeal secretions or feces of infected people through close association.

In its first stage, polio could seem like a cold or flu, with symptoms of fever, headache, nausea, sore throat, vomiting, and body aches. Then muscle weakness, convulsions, neck and spine stiffness, and finally (in stage two) paralysis clearly identify the illness as poliomyelitis. In 1931 the slightest muscle weakness was cause to encase limbs in casts, which were often suspended by pulleys above patients' beds. For those with paralyzed lungs, there were "iron lung" respirators to make breathing possible.

As a result of the 1931 epidemic, the Yale Poliomyelitis Commission (also known as the Yale Poliomyelitis Study Unit) was formed in June 1931 under the direction of Dr. James Trask; its purpose was to study clinical virology and to attempt to isolate the poliovirus from extremely ill patients, especially abortive cases (which still had to be proven to be poliomyelitis, despite past research). At the time it was still widely believed that the variety of minor illnesses accompanying an epidemic had nothing to do with poliomyelitis.

The Yale commission declared that isolation of the virus was an impractical method for trying to control the disease because there were too many cases that lacked the classic characteristics of poliomyelitis. The commission set about to probe abortive, minor cases to prove their infectiousness. It eventually established a precedent that would be followed thereafter: with the outbreak of a disease, a research team or teams would be invited to the disease area to study it. For 40 years, the Yale commission would be called to consult on epidemics all over the United States. See also U.S. POLIOMYELITIS EPIDEMIC OF 1942–53.

Further reading: Landon, *Poliomyelitis: A Handbook for Physicians and Medical Students*; Paul, *A History of Poliomyelitis*.

U.S. Poliomyelitis Epidemic of 1942–53

One of the worst outbreaks of a disease dreaded because of the paralysis that came to symbolize it; peaked in 1952 at about 60,000 cases.

Poliomyelitis, or polio, affected affluent, hygienic, advanced civilizations, and it hit virulently in the United States. Less sanitary civilizations had little problem with polio because of a general immunity gained through early exposure. But once public health reform had improved sanitation by the end of the nineteenth century, poliomyelitis changed from a mild endemic condition to a seemingly new and virulent pestilence. From lack of exposure, people became more vulnerable to infection. When the disease was introduced at wide intervals, the impact was epidemic.

Because of poor sanitation, polio had existed as a worldwide, endemic children's disease. In past centuries when childhood mortality was typical, polio was thought to be the last children's plague. Exposure to the disease produced immunity; most cases were unnoticeable. Due to lack of exposure resulting from good sanitation, the disease became more lethal and attacked older age groups. By 1940, poliomyelitis was more fitting a name than infantile paralysis, because the number of afflicted younger children had decreased while the number of individuals age 10 and up had increased. There were outbreaks among the U.S. military during World War II, and the incidence of infection among the especially vulnerable American troops was ten times higher in

Africa than in the United States, for example. Wherever troops traveled abroad, poliomyelitis was endemic.

The National Foundation for Infantile Paralysis (NFIP) spearheaded a massive effort against polio, inspired by the leadership of President Franklin D. Roosevelt, himself a symbol of victory over the disease, and his one-time law partner Basil O'Connor. The organization not only was the most important in the fight against polio, but also served as a role model for all fund-raising foundations and coordinated research efforts to come. The NFIP's emphasis on promotion and propaganda techniques caused the evolution to present attitudes where any important research should get public funding. The NFIP was the first "democratic" organization of its kind, relying as it did on small contributions from anyone (as during the March of Dimes campaign) and on common people instead of socialites in its organization.

The period from 1941 through 1955 was the NFIP's years of glory. President Roosevelt, paralyzed by polio from the age of 39, was the power and personality propelling the search for a polio antidote. Between 1938 and 1962, the NFIP raised $630 million. Despite, or perhaps because of hardship, people, especially women, helped the foundation thrive during World War II. The NFIP's mission was threefold: the care of any polio victims lacking the means adequate for treatment; research and training in polio for medical people; and information for the public, about both NFIP and the disease, through promotional activities.

Scientists and physicians came to understand that polio was most commonly a gastrointestinal infection that could be transmitted by healthy people, especially children with low reservoirs of immunity. An acute viral illness, polio's severity can range from inapparent infection to nonparalytic and paralytic complications. It is caused by the picornavirus (It., *piccolo*, small) containing ribonucleic acid (RNA). There were three forms of polio: types 1, 2, and 3. The virus, ingested or inhaled by mouth, can settle in the tonsils, pharnyx, or ileum. Later passing to the gut, the virus can eventually be retrieved from feces. In 90 percent to 95 percent of the cases, the virus never passes beyond the lymph nodes, so the infection has either no symptoms or only flu-like symptoms. It is sometimes thought that polio passes from human excretion through hands not thoroughly washed.

If poliovirus enters the human bloodstream and subsequently the central nervous system, paralysis results, although the severity varies with the quantity of the virus, its point of attack, and the damage incurred. Although thought of as symptomatic of polio, paralysis occurs infrequently. Victims of acute polio can be returned to normal breathing by using the "iron lung," developed during the 1920s, other types of respirators, or a "rocking bed" that helps victims breathe by causing the abdominal contents to push up against the lungs.

Up to the 1940s, paralyzed limbs were put in splints or braces to prevent muscle contractions, and to allow the victim the freedom to walk. Sister Elizabeth Kenny, an Australian nurse, influenced an about-face in therapeutic treatment of polio, although controversy surrounded her as she became embroiled in politics. She took on the medical community in the United States when she advocated physical therapy to treat the disease's symptoms and reawaken healthy muscle and nerve response, and rejected splints and casts, which could result in permanent nerve and muscle atrophy.

There was no cure or antidote once the infection had begun. Vaccinations could only control the disease. Only high immunity levels could prevent polio's spread. Dr. Jonas Salk developed a dead virus vaccine that was widely tested in 1953–54. The following year the U.S. Public Health Service approved the use of the Salk vaccine, which has to be injected. Although the vaccine was "safe," it was thought to be only 50 percent effective. Also, three shots and a booster were necessary to administer it. In 1957, Dr. Albert B. Sabin developed an oral vaccine with a live, attenuated virus that was much more effective. By 1961, the average number of polio cases in the United States had diminished to 570. Successful vaccination in the Western Hemisphere has resulted in an absence of "wild" cases since August 1991. A few cases have occurred each year in reaction to vaccination.

Further reading: McGrew, *Encyclopedia of Medical History;* Paul, *A History of Poliomyelitis.*

U.S. Rubella Epidemic of 1964   Largest rubella epidemic ever recorded in the United States, infecting about 12,500,000 people, ending some 30,000 pregnancies in miscarriage, abortion, or stillbirth, and leaving about 20,000 rubella victims congenitally handicapped. Because of its size, the epidemic dramatically illustrated as never before the effect of rubella on the unborn. The cost of the 1964–65 epidemic was put at between $1 billion and $2 billion. That number might triple if it included the cost of educating the victims of the epidemic. During the epidemic, it was discovered that rubella could lead to any number of infant defects—blindness and deafness were most common—and that a child could be born with rubella itself.

Also known as German measles and now distinguished from rubeola, rubella was first written up by Germans Sennert, Horst, and Pechlin in the seven-

teenth century. Rubella emerged in the eighteenth century as a disease with similarities to scarlet fever and measles. In the 1930s, the cause of the disease was established to be a virus. Rubella remained an unimportant disease until it was linked to birth defects. In 1941, Sir Norman McAlister Gregg, an Australian ophthalmologist, first correlated rubella in pregnant women with congenital deformities, especially related to the eyes and heart.

A mild, viral epidemic disease, rubella is characterized by swollen lymph nodes in the neck and behind the ears, moderate fever, and rash, all of which can be so mild as to escape recognition. Other common symptoms include arthritis and arthralgia. Rarely, complications like encephalomyelitis and purpura can result. Rubella is spread by direct contact with an infected person. Incubation runs from 10 to 20 days. Treatment consists of bed rest, lots of fluids, and light meals.

Depending upon the stage of differentiation of the organs in the human fetus, rubella can cause damage to one or many organs, including the brain, which can later retard the physical and emotional development of the child. The younger the fetus, the more total damage is possible. Brain dysfunction can lead to a multitude of handicaps, including psychiatric disorders and behavioral problems. Other defects can include deafness, heart problems, cataracts, glaucoma, retarded growth, enlarged spleen and/or liver, and encephalitis, to name but a few. Congenital rubella is the primary cause of deafness among older children and teenagers involved in hearing-impaired educational programs. If rubella has caused central nervous system damage along with other defects, the effect on the victim and his or her family can be catastrophic.

During the 1964–65 rubella outbreak, more than half of about 20,000 babies afflicted with congenital handicaps were deaf. In 1964, the number of children born deaf rose 30 percent over those of the previous year, which suggests that the number of children made deaf by rubella was in fact higher than 50 percent in the 1964–65 epidemic. In one study, half of those who had had congenital rubella suffered eye defects. In the same study, there was a 95 percent correlation between heart and eye problems.

The rubella virus was isolated in 1962, which led to development of vaccines. Since the invention of a rubella vaccine in 1969, the rate of cases has drastically declined. Introduction of vaccines will supposedly reduce deafness in future generations by 20 percent. Vaccinations made of live rubella can also damage the fetus, and are therefore to be avoided by women two months before impregnation and anytime during pregnancy. Because of widespread immunization of children, rubella infection has shifted to older (post-puberty) age groups. Development of a rubella vaccine and liberal abortion laws have curtailed the lasting effects of rubella.

Further reading: Chess et al., *Psychiatric Disorders of Children with Congenital Rubella*; Gruenberg et al., *Vaccinating Against Brain Syndromes: The Campaign Against Measles and Rubella*.

U.S. Smallpox Epidemic of 1901–03

Series of intense smallpox outbreaks that occurred principally in Boston, New York, and Philadelphia, as well as in New Jersey and Ohio. America's second-to-last significant epidemic of *variola major* (the severe form of smallpox), it raged even as *variola minor* (the milder form of the disease that often escaped detection) was rampant throughout the midwestern sections of the country.

In New York City, the epidemic began in November 1900 when the disease was introduced there by a traveling theater troupe. During November and December, about 100 smallpox cases were reported in the city; in 1901 the incidence rapidly increased. That year, the city's health board requested, and was granted, $30,000 to build additional facilities to tend the sick on North Brother Island. In August 1901, Dr. A. N. Bell alleged in *The Sanitarian* that the city's health department had let the epidemic get out of control. Apparently, by then, Manhattan alone had reported more than 900 cases, and 1,521 cases and 221 deaths had occurred in Brooklyn since the outbreak began. Gradually, the health department awakened to its responsibility and began a mass vaccination program. There were 398 smallpox deaths recorded by year's end.

The fatal *variola major* remained rampant in the city, where an additional five vaccination centers opened for business by March 1902, and 155 vaccinators were on the job immunizing nearly 10,000 people daily at times. And thus, more than 810,000 people were immunized over a six-month period—twice more than in any previous year. This was an important factor in controlling the epidemic, since 40 percent of the cases occurred in the city's newly arrived immigrant population. Patients checking into the municipal hospitals were required to be vaccinated. There were 1,516 smallpox cases and 309 deaths in the city during 1902. The city's private hospitals preferred not to admit patients with contagious diseases, and conditions at the municipal hospitals established specially for this purpose were so primitive and disgusting that many poor families tried to hide their sick rather than have them treated at such facilities. Some of the patients reportedly likened the facilities to the "Black Hole of Calcutta."

(The "Hole" was a notoriously small, suffocating lockup in Calcutta, India, where most of the Europeans confined overnight died from heat, thirst, or lack of air on June 20–21, 1756).

Philadelphia reported 1,342 cases and 231 deaths, and Cleveland had 1,034 cases and 182 deaths during 1902. That year, 1,024 cases and 190 deaths were reported in Boston; the last big outbreak of *variola major* in that city, it prompted a detailed pathological study of some of the victims. The study is considered a landmark for its time; doctors experimented with erythrotherapy or red light treatment during this outbreak.

A total of 5,332 smallpox cases and 980 deaths (18.4 percent case-fatality rate) were reported in the United States in 1901, 10,334 cases and 1,841 deaths (17.8 percent case-fatality rate) in 1902, and 6,113 cases and 752 deaths (12.3 percent case-fatality rate) in 1903. Thereafter the incidence of smallpox steadily declined until the 1920s, when it briefly surged again.

Further reading: Fenner et al., *Smallpox and Its Eradication*; Duffy, *A History of Public Health in New York City, 1866–1966*.

U.S. Yellow Fever Epidemics of 1878–79

Devastating outbreaks of yellow fever occurring mainly in cities and towns in the Mississippi and Ohio river valleys and infecting more than 100,000 persons (of whom at least 20,000 died). Caused by a virus, yellow fever is a communicable disease transmitted from person to person by the bite of infective *Aëdes aegypti* mosquitoes (this was not known in 1878–79).

In early July 1878 the deadly viral infection entered the port city of New Orleans, Louisiana, probably aboard ships from Havana, Cuba. More than 20,000 inhabitants of New Orleans became infected during the next four months; when the epidemic ended there in October, as mosquito activity dropped off with the cooler weather, more than 4,000 people had perished from the fever. About a third of New Orleans' approximately 150,000 inhabitants usually left the city every year during the hot summer months; thus, the epidemic's morbidity rate was 20 percent, and its mortality rate was also 20 percent among those stricken remaining in the city.

After the first fatalities were reported in New Orleans, officials at Mobile, Alabama, established a rigid quarantine against ships from the Louisiana port. Yellow fever then moved northward up the Mississippi River with fever-ridden crewmembers aboard the *John D. Porter*, a new towboat hauling a string of barges for Pittsburgh. The disease entered Vicksburg, Mississippi, when the boat's engineer and fireman were taken ashore to be buried. Farther up the river, the towboat was barred from docking at Memphis, which nonetheless became infected somehow that summer and saw more than 5,000 persons perish from yellow fever. Some 25,000 inhabitants of Memphis fled during the epidemic, during which corpses were found in abandoned buildings and public parks.

Meanwhile, the virus traveled with the crew of the towboat to Cairo, Illinois, at the confluence of the Mississippi and Ohio rivers. The substitute engineer (recruited at Vicksburg) died, and one of the doctors at Cairo fell victim to the disease while treating patients. The towboat continued up the Ohio River to Louisville and Cincinnati, where four crewmembers eventually succumbed after docking there. Some of the crew refused to continue the voyage and later debarked at Gallipolis, Ohio, where 31 villagers fatally contracted the virus. By the time the boat arrived at Pittsburgh, 23 members of its crew had died of yellow fever, which had spread to scores of cities and towns in the southern Gulf states and the Midwest. It reached St. Louis and traveled along the Tennessee River to Chattanooga in 1878.

Special attention was directed at the small town of Grenada in north-central Mississippi in August 1878. The town's telegrapher sent daily dispatches about the yellow fever epidemic there; about 2,000 out of Grenada's 2,200 white residents fled by August 17, and about 170 of the remaining 200 whites contracted the disease, most of them fatally (there was no account of the infection among the black population). On August 29, the dispatcher reported 22 deaths in 24 hours, and two days later he died of the fever at his telegraph key.

Local officials enforced quarantines during the epidemics, sometimes enforcing them at the point of a shotgun. State health boards in the Mississippi Valley planned joint actions in the event of another siege of yellow fever, which again broke out severely in Memphis in July 1879 and caused another mass evacuation. Notification of the pestilential danger was sent to all the states up the Mississippi River. However, there were objections from cotton brokers and other businessmen to the quarantines and evacuations, as well as to the lack of support for the refugees camped outside Memphis. New Orleans was also infected that summer (1879) but suffered less severely (like Memphis) than the previous year; afterward, sanitary programs were more strictly established in both of these cities.

Further reading: Duffy, *The Sanitarians*; Williams, *The United States Public Health Service, 1798–1950*; Smith, *Plague on Us.*

V

Venezuelan Smallpox Epidemic of 1580 Severe outbreak of smallpox that struck the Caracas and other Indians in northern Venezuela (then an adjunct of New Granada). It greatly weakened Indian resistance to the Spanish colonizing of the region.

Spaniards first explored northern Venezuela in the early 1500s, fruitlessly searching for the mythical kingdom of El Dorado (a city or realm of fabulous wealth). They then confined themselves to slave hunting in the area and transported Indian slave labor to work on the Spanish plantations in Cuba and Haiti. These slave raids left the Venezuelan Indians extremely hostile to any future Spanish expeditions. By the mid-1500s, Spain began to consider Venezuela an important agricultural resource; the Spanish had control of the Venezuelan coast from the town of Coro (founded in 1527) in the west to the island of Margarita and the seaport of Cumaná (founded in 1523) in the east. They then pushed inland and founded the town of Valencia on Lake Tacarigua, but soon encountered hostile Indians; a succession of Spanish settlements in the Caracas Valley failed to survive repeated Indian attacks.

In 1567 the Spanish government sponsored an expedition led by Diego de Losada, a Spanish explorer, to secure the fertile Caracas Valley and other inland valleys of Venezuela. Losada established the town of Caracas (1567), and a decade of fighting between the Spaniards and Indians ensued before smallpox, an acute infectious disease, began attacking the latter. Brought to Venezuela by the Spanish, smallpox further decimated the Caracas, Carib, and other Indians, who had concentrated their forces against the enemy and grown weak and suffered malnutrition after many years of war. In the Caracas Valley, it is estimated that the native population fell from about 30,000 Indians to about 10,000 or 12,000 because of the 1580 smallpox epidemic, which ended much of the Indian resistance. Caracas became a major base for further Spanish expansion into Venezuela.

Further reading: Lombardi, *Venezuela*; Ramenofsky, *Vectors of Death*.

Venezuelan Yellow Fever Epidemic of 1929 Outbreak of jungle yellow fever infecting about a thousand persons in the Cuyuni River valley area of eastern Venezuela. In the forest areas, many male workers contracted the viral disease through the bite of several species of mosquitoes, including the *Aëdes aegypti*. At first their symptoms were so mild that physicians misdiagnosed the cases; as the seriousness of the infections increased, pathological changes and serological tests confirmed that yellow fever was the culprit.

In the small inland towns of El Callao, Curi, El Palmar, and Guasipati in eastern Venezuela, inhabitants first succumbed to jungle yellow fever in the summer of 1929. The overall fatality rate was at least five percent at the close of the epidemic a few months later. Some "fever fighters" in Venezuela remained baffled by the unexplained outbreak in this region, for usually yellow fever had broken out in coastal regions, in mainly urban areas where the reservoir of infection is man and *Aëdes aegypti* mosquitoes (man has no essential role in the transmission of jungle yellow fever). Later researchers discovered that the Cuyuni valley region was a silent, endemic focus for yellow fever, and that monkeys, susceptible to the disease, and some forest-dwelling mosquitoes there could carry the disease. Eventually large numbers of Venezuelans became immune to jungle yellow fever, which was fatal to only 122 persons in the country from 1951 to 1975.

Further reading: Scott, *A History of Tropical Medicine*; Strode, ed., *Yellow Fever*.

Venice Plague of 1477–78 See ITALIAN PLAGUES OF 1477–79.

Venice Plague of 1575–77 Virulent epidemic of mainly bubonic plague that killed about 50,000 inhabitants of Venice, Italy, during the Renaissance.

By the sixteenth century, the city of Venice had experienced numerous plague outbreaks (an estimated 100,000 Venetians died during the Black Death [q.v.] in the mid-fourteenth century) and had acquired probably more knowledge than any other European city in dealing with the plague disease. By 1575 Venice, one of the four major states of northern Italy (along with Milan, Genoa, and Florence), had developed a public health organization far in advance of the rest of Europe. Though the Venetian health officials were anxious to fight the epidemic in 1575, the plague pathogen (microorganism) and vectors (rodents and fleas) had not been identified yet. Officials did not know that plague-infected fleas can survive from six weeks up to a year and can easily lodge in clothing, straw mattresses, furs, carpets, and rags. Though the Venetians had long suspected that cotton, wool, and other goods harbored the infection, they were unaware that grain was the main vehicle for the transport of plague from one place to another. In Venice and other pre-industrial European cities, people (both rich and poor) often lived in unsanitary conditions where rats and fleas flourished, and dogs and cats in Venice were frequently slaughtered en masse in the belief that the coats of these animals harbored plague-carrying germs (this actually made life easier for the rats, natural reservoirs of plague).

An estimated 50 percent of Venice's population of some 180,000 people contracted the disease during the epidemic; they developed painful lumps and boils (called buboes) mainly in the groin, armpit, and neck, along with high fevers, severe headaches, giddiness, and congested eyes. Doctors administered various ineffective treatments, such as phlebotomy (bloodletting), emetics (agents that induce vomiting), theriacas (antidotes to poison), and ointments. Many people opposed these treatments and the ordinances (with severe penalties for breaking them) that required that plague cases be promptly reported, that the sick be immediately isolated, and that clothes and bedding of those who died from plague be burned. Innkeepers ignored the controls; gravediggers trafficked in the clothes of the dead; carriers forged or exchanged health passes; and rich merchants continually obstructed health inspectors, quarantines, and any limitations on trade. The mortality was 28 percent at the close of the epidemic in 1577. Very few of the deaths evidently resulted from the pneumonic and septicemic forms of plague (transmitted from person to person by coughing, via droplets).

Earlier, in gratitude for their deliverance from a plague outbreak in 1535, the Venetians had erected a magnificent church, Santa Maria della Salute, on the Grand Canal. In the church's sacristy hangs a famous painting (*St. Mark Triumphant*) by the Venetian painter Titian, a supposed victim of plague who actually died of old age in 1576; the painting shows two patron saints of plague, Saint Sebastian (being pierced by arrows) and Saint Roch (pointing to his plague boil).

Further reading: Cipolla, *Fighting the Plague in Seventeenth Century Italy;* Hirst, *The Conquest of Plague.*

Venice Plague of 1630–31   See ITALIAN PLAGUES OF 1629–31.

Vermont Poliomyelitis Epidemic of 1894   World's first relatively large outbreak of poliomyelitis (infantile paralysis or Heine-Medin disease), with a total of 132 cases fully documented by Dr. Charles S. Caverly, president of the Vermont State Board of Health. The epidemic occurred in Rutland County, Vermont.

The year before (1893) 26 cases of polio were reported in the Boston, Massachusetts, area, which had averaged only three to six cases a year between 1889 and 1892. At the time, two physicians, John J. Putnam and E. W. Taylor, wrote and published a paper entitled "Is Acute Poliomyelitis Unusually Prevalent This Season?" concerning the upsurge in cases. The outbreak in Vermont was thought perhaps to be a continuation of the 1893 Boston outbreak, interrupted by the cold of winter.

In mid-June 1894 the Vermont towns of Rutland and Wallingford hosted this acute viral illness of the central nervous system, which is highly contagious and frequently epidemic in the summer months among children. The disease brings on fever, headache, gastrointestinal problems, malaise, and sometimes paralysis. By July it had spread to other Vermont towns. Young children were the first victims, but as time went on, the average age of those infected moved upward, and older children were attacked in later polio outbreaks.

The Vermont epidemic was the first to receive the full examination and documentation of a health officer (Dr. Caverly), who diligently tracked down polio patients and made observations. The epidemic killed 13.5 percent of the 132 persons afflicted with the poliovirus; 56 persons recovered completely from the disease, while 30 people became permanently paralyzed. The mortality rate was high because many victims were older children and adults (the older a patient is, the more severe the effect of the disease). Caverly observed that six of the 132 cases exhibited polio symptoms but no paralysis. The abortive cases had not gone unnoticed; only many years later were such cases recognized as a major part of a polio epidemic. In addition, Caverly made certain that medical facilities were provided for the rehabilitation of polio survivors. See also U.S. POLIOMYELITIS EPIDEMIC OF 1916.

Further reading: Paul, *A History of Poliomyelitis;* Smith, *Patenting the Sun: Polio and the Salk Vaccine;* Marks and Beatty, *Epidemics.*

Vienna Plague of 1349   Severe epidemic of bubonic plague that broke out in Vienna, Austria, lasting from four to six months. It was a part of the Black Death (q.v.) sweeping Europe then. No clear medical descriptions of the plague are available from Viennese sources, but several unofficial eyewitness accounts of the illness are available. It began in April 1349 and, according to the descriptions, appeared in two phases. The first phase lasted for about two months, and the victims had high fever, pains in the chest, and foul breath. Those who coughed out blood during this phase usually died. In the second phase, which lasted for approximately three to five months, the victims developed large and painful boils all over their bodies, extreme thirst, and high fever. Death occurred between the fourth and seventh days of the illness in the second phase, and in both phases the victims had black spots all over their bodies. In addition, their tongues and throats often turned black, thus giving the name of Black Death to the illness.

Mortality reports from Vienna at the time of this plague are vague, but there are some reports that there were many deaths. There are also reports of mass graves with up to 40,000 human corpses in just one of them. These are most likely overestimates, but it is clear that the illness was devastating and killed possibly ten percent of the population living in Vienna.

Physicians and astrologers of the time believed that the illness was caused by cosmic forces. Many people believed that epidemics were caused by natural catastrophes such as flooding, earthquakes, climatic changes, and famines. This particular plague fell into such a paradigm because Vienna and the country around it had suffered from a sequence of natural phenomena and disasters. There had been an outbreak of locusts, an eclipse of the sun, unusually warm weather in December of 1340, storms, fires, an extremely rainy summer the year before the plague hit, and a severe earthquake in the southern Alps. In Vienna specifically, there are reports that in 1349 the sun and moon lost color and 12 rainstorms devastated vineyards and cornfields.

The disease was reported to have been extremely contagious and was spread from person to person. It was believed at the time that the disease could be communicated through the skin or just by looking at a patient. Gravediggers seem to have caught the disease in great numbers, and yet many people who nursed the sick were able to escape catching it. Poor people were more affected than the wealthy, and

Jews seemed particularly susceptible, possibly because of their crowded and restricted living quarters in the city. During the epidemic, many people seemed to remain in the city. They often went to church and prayed for their lives. Legacies to churches and monasteries increased, and money and property were given to the church in return for promises to hold masses in memory of the deceased. Consequently, many churches were enlarged during this time, and several new ones were built.

There are no official, detailed accounts of the day-to-day behavior of the Viennese citizens during the plague epidemic. As a result, no comparisons can be made with people's behavior in other countries during epidemics—such as the heartless behavior of the Florentines as described by Boccacio (see PLAGUE OF FLORENCE [BLACK VOMIT]). At the time of this epidemic, Vienna suffered from poor general hygiene. Garbage was thrown in the streets, and open-air markets were held in most parts of the city. The spread of the epidemic was most likely caused by the germs from rot in the streets, as well as carried by the rats who roamed there. Public bath houses, brothels, and the extensive merchant travel in the region may also have been significant factors in the spread of the plague epidemic, which came to an end in Vienna in September of 1349. Recovery was short, as plague struck a decade later and lasted for an entire year.

Further reading: McNeill, *Plagues and Peoples;* Velimirovic and Velimirovic, "Plague in Vienna."

Vienna Sleeping Sickness Epidemic   See ENCEPHALITIS LETHARGICA (VON ECONOMO'S DISEASE) EPIDEMIC OF 1915–26.

Vietnamese Dengue Epidemics of the 1950s, 1960s, and 1970s   Several recorded outbreaks of dengue hemorrhagic fever (DHF) in Vietnam.

The first epidemic, apparently severe and extensive, was reported from Hanoi in North Vietnam during the rainy season of 1958. The actual number of cases that occurred is not known, but experts believe them to be in the hundreds. One study of 68 patients hospitalized during the outbreak revealed that the clinical aspects (collapse, gastrointestinal hemorrhage, and so on) were identical to those seen in patients suffering from DHF in other southeast Asian countries. The mortality rate for the 68 cases in the above study was seven percent.

South Vietnam's first recorded outbreak of hemorrhagic fever occurred between April and July 1960. The town of Cai-Be in Dinh Tuong province, southwest of Saigon, was the focus of this outbreak. Since most of the cases were not hospitalized, the true extent of the epidemic remains a matter of conjecture. Fifty children died during the outbreak. The Saigon-based representative of the World Health Organization observed that the disease clinically resembled Philippine hemorrhagic fever. At the same time as the Cai-Be outbreak, DHF also infected village children in An Giang province (40 to 80 miles north along the Mekong River from Cai-Be). Mortality among these children was reportedly high.

Another severe outbreak of hemorrhagic fever occurred during 1963 in the delta region of the Mekong River in South Vietnam. The Delta outbreak, as it came to be known, apparently began in May 1963, when the local authorities received word of a disease with high mortality affecting young children in the area. Identified as hemorrhagic fever in August, the disease spread to small villages along the Mekong River, just south of the Cambodian border. From May to October 1963, 331 cases and 116 deaths were reported. Subsequently, cases were also observed in Saigon, where the disease first made its appearance in 1960. Of the 331 cases, 104 had hemorrhagic signs and 64 of these ended fatally. The dengue type 2 virus was isolated during the Delta outbreak. The next epidemic, a large one, occurred in 1969, when 2,813 cases and 87 deaths occurred in the southern part of the country.

There was a major outbreak in Vietnam in 1973, when a staggering 14,320 cases and 986 deaths were said to have occurred. The following year, incidence dropped to 4,261 cases and 438 deaths. During the early 1970s, DHF incidence also increased dramatically in Thailand.

In most of the southeast Asian countries, DHF outbreaks had begun in large urban areas. In South Vietnam, however, the rural communities were the first to be infected. Undoubtedly, trade and the constant movement of goods and people along the Mekong River, the country's main artery, dictated the course of the epidemics.

Further reading: Halstead, "Mosquito-borne Haemorrhagic Fevers of South and South-East Asia"; Halstead et al., "Dengue Haemorrhagic Fever in South Vietnam: Report of the 1963 Outbreak."

Vietnamese Plagues of the Early 1900s   Epidemics of bubonic and pneumonic plague that invaded Vietnam during the third pandemic (see HONG KONG PLAGUE OF 1894; INDIAN PLAGUE OF 1896–97; SYDNEY PLAGUE OF 1900). The disease was first observed in the country in 1898, the earliest recorded case occurring in Annam in the port city of Nha Trang. In 1901, the northern region of Tonkin was affected. Little is known about the extent and severity of these early outbreaks.

Later, in 1906, plague was observed in Cochin China or southern Vietnam. The outbreak was centered around Saigon's main market and was found to be caused by rat-infested cargo shipments arriving from Canton and Hong Kong, both plague-ridden then. The earliest confirmed cases were among the Indians of Saigon and most of the cases were concentrated in the Saigon-Cholon area.

An outbreak of pneumonic plague struck the nearby Mekong River Delta in 1911. Official reports indicate that 1,018 cases and 886 deaths occurred in the towns of Gia Dinh, Chau Doc, Thu Dau Mot, and Soc Trang. In the Saigon-Cholon zone, 233 people died. On the delta, another small but severe epidemic of pneumonic plague was reported from the town of Vinh Long in 1915. Most of the 24 deaths (including three medical workers) occurred barely two days after the initial symptoms had been noted. The incubation period was three to four days for the plague.

Pneumonic plague erupted again in 1925. Reportedly, this outbreak was extremely serious and its mortality rate very high. This time, it infected the boat-dwellers along the Gia Long canal in Chau Doc province. In these cases, a postmortem helped confirm the cause of death. Chau Doc province was infected again in 1941, when one person was found to have transmitted the disease to six families during his brief incubation period. Everyone so infected died less than 48 hours after the primary symptoms had set in.

Vietnam's most devastating plague outbreaks occurred in the mid-1960s during the American military presence in the country.

Further reading: Trong et al., "A Mixed Pneumonic Bubonic Plague Outbreak in Vietnam"; Gregg, *Plague: An Ancient Disease in the Twentieth Century*.

Vietnamese Plagues of the 1960s   Series of plague outbreaks, some extensive, that devastated Vietnam, accounting for 90 percent of the world's reported plague incidence at the time.

Plague had invaded Vietnam during the Third Plague Pandemic (q.v.) at the turn of the century (see VIETNAMESE PLAGUES OF THE EARLY 1900S), but the virulent disease's severity then was nothing compared to that of the outbreaks in the 1960s. In 1961, plague broke out over the southern island province of Long Khanh; three more provinces, all of them along the South China Sea, came under attack in 1962. The next year, plague invaded twice as many Vietnamese provinces, most of them adjacent to the previously infected areas. Two additional provinces were affected in 1964.

In 1965, as the American military campaign in Vietnam intensified during the Vietnam War (1956–

75), so did the plague outbreaks, which soon covered 24 of 44 provinces, from the province of Quang Tri in the north to well beyond Saigon (Ho Chi Minh City) in the south. The distribution of plague cases changed slightly from year to year, but the overall area under attack remained the same. In South Vietnam, from just 15 cases annually in 1956–60, the incidence soared to over 4,000 cases annually in 1965–70 (more than 25,000 cases reportedly occurred during this period); undoubtedly, the actual figures were far more than this. Widespread bombing and aerial spraying of Vietnam's thickly forested and arable areas forced plague-bearing rodents and human beings into crowded refugee camps around urban areas, thus stimulating the rapid spread of infection. Bandicoots (large rats) were found to be the carriers of the infected rat flea, *Xenopsylla cheopis*, in these areas, and more than half of them were apparently diseased also.

In 1965, plague outbreaks occurred in widely scattered areas in Vietnam. A mixed bubonic-pneumonic outbreak (43 cases and 16 deaths in six hamlets over two months) was reported from the disputed An Khe district in Binh Dinh (An Nhon) province in August 1965. In Long Khanh province, pneumonic plague infected six people in one family within a very short time. The city of Da Nang recorded 270 cases between September 1965 and June 1966. From there the infection spread to Hue, where a massive vaccination effort was launched, and DDT was sprayed in and around infected homes. Slightly more than 400 cases occurred.

Cam Ranh city reported a plague epidemic in January–February 1966; there were 44 cases, 80 percent of them fatal. Another epidemic in February 1967 infected 58 people; the affected area in Cam Ranh was cordoned off and dusted with insecticide. Military personnel in the vicinity were given booster shots, and many civilians vaccinated for the first time. Also in 1967, plague erupted for the first time in the central highlands of Kontum province, home of the Montagnard tribes. This outbreak consisted of two distinct phases; a majority of the cases and all the deaths were among women and children since the men were on duty in the Civilian Defense Group. None had been vaccinated before the outbreak began.

The withdrawal of the American forces from Vietnam began in 1970, and by 1972 plague incidence had dropped to around 2,500 cases a year. It is estimated that between 100,000 and 250,000 plague cases occurred in Vietnam during 1964–74, and 90 percent of them were distributed over 13 provinces. Most of these occurred in sparsely populated areas;

otherwise the incidence would have been much higher. In 1974, a third of the country's cases were from Quang Nam province. Vietnam's limited medical facilities were already severely strained by the difficult circumstances. While fatality rates were high among untreated cases, they were five percent or lower among patients lucky to get treatment. Most American personnel were vaccinated; not so the Vietnamese. The war spurred the development of a longer-lasting freeze-dried vaccine, and the Americans established a facility in Saigon to study the disease.

Further reading: Gregg, *Plague: An Ancient Disease in the Twentieth Century*; Trong et al., "A Mixed Pneumonic Bubonic Plague Outbreak in Vietnam."

Vietnamese Poliomyelitis Epidemics of 1958–60
Outbreaks of poliomyelitis (infantile paralysis) that struck numerous areas (urban and rural) in Vietnam.

For three years, from 1958 to 1960, Vietnam was invaded by epidemic poliomyelitis every year. The outbreaks were widespread and quite severe and children were among the primary victims. The three types of poliovirus were isolated during these epidemics. In 1959, the incidence was quite high: 52.16 polio cases for every 100,000 people. By 1960, this rate had declined to 0.45 per 100,000.

Poliomyelitis is an acute but common viral infection characterized by a sore throat, headache, vomiting, and sometimes a stiffening of the neck and back. Early in the illness, lower neuron paralysis may develop. Abortive poliomyelitis, as this form of the disease is sometimes called, begins after a two- to five-day incubation period. Over 96 percent of all polio infections fall into this category. However, in about three percent to four percent of polio cases, the central nervous system becomes infected, resulting in paralysis.

The government of the former Soviet Union sent vast quantities of the live Sabin-Shumakov polio vaccine, which was found to be effective against the three types of poliovirus. Subsequently, Hanoi's Institute of Hygiene and Epidemiology began manufacture of the triple oral vaccine with the technical assistance of the Soviet Academy of Medical Sciences. Vietnam became one of the first countries to achieve polio-free status almost entirely through its own efforts.

Further reading: McMichael, ed., *Health in the Third World: Studies from Vietnam*; Paul, *A History of Poliomyelitis.*

von Economo's Disease See ENCEPHALITIS LETHARGICA (VON ECONOMO'S DISEASE) EPIDEMIC OF 1915–26.

W

Walcheren Island Malaria Epidemic of 1809 See EUROPEAN MALARIA EPIDEMICS OF 1805–12 AND 1823–27.

West African Cholera Epidemics of 1970–71 Outbreaks of cholera spreading down the West African coast from Guinea to Cameroon and claiming at least 1,400 human lives out of more than 28,000 infected people.

The cholera disease was brought back from Russia with some returning Guinean students who had vacationed there in the summer of 1970; an outbreak was occurring on the Russian coast of the Black Sea. In August 1970 cholera broke out in Conakry, Guinea, among Fanti fishermen; the Fanti (an African black nation in Ghana) fished along the West African coast. Evidently the Fanti peddling of cholera-contaminated fish helped spread the disease among the inhabitants of Conakry. Since the Fanti were blamed for spreading the disease, Ghanians were expelled from Guinea. Other fishing groups besides the Fanti were also responsible for introducing cholera into coastal areas of other countries.

The Fanti fishermen moving from Guinea to neighboring Sierra Leone carried the disease with them; an outbreak was reported in the fishing village of Bailoh from September 19 to 25, 1970, and Freetown, Sierra Leone's capital, had a few cases. Sierra Leone's eastern provinces eventually reported 292 cholera cases in 1970 and 211 cases in 1971; the disease disappeared from the country after an outbreak in December 1971.

Liberia, south of Sierra Leone, suffered more seriously after cholera first appeared in Monrovia (Liberia's capital) in early October 1970; all Liberian counties except Lofa reported outbreaks. Monrovian authorities reported an average of 100 cholera cases a month. After infecting Liberia, the disease next appeared in the Ivory Coast village of Bingerville, close to the capital of Abidjan, where it afflicted 447 persons (killing 25 of them). In several of the nearby Ivory Coast villages between October and December 1970, about 1,500 people became sick with diarrhea, vomiting, abdominal cramps, and dehydration (cholera's symptoms); 120 victims perished.

A Togolese citizen with cholera brought the disease into Ghana while on an airplane flight from Guinea on September 1, 1970. Two months later serious outbreaks occurred in various coastal places, including Ghana's capital city of Accra; there were 73 deaths among the 2,886 people infected during November and December 1970. In 1971 human fatalities increased to 609, with 12,623 persons having contracted the disease (which never reached the upper Ghanian regions). The Fanti fishermen of Ghana were largely responsible, it is now believed, for carrying cholera into their country and neighboring Togo, where the epidemic peaked with 158 cases reported in January 1971.

From Togo, it traveled to Dahomey (Benin), where the first cholera case occurred in the fishing village of Agoné Kané on December 7, 1970; it then spread to Porto-Novo in late December. The epidemic raged in Dahomey until April 1971, causing 260 human deaths out of 1,812 afflicted. Nigeria was the next country to be hit, and its capital, Lagos, became the center from which other parts of the country became infected. Ijow native fishermen and local gin dealers who traveled from Lagos to the marketplaces at Bomadi and Ojobo helped spread cholera to the western Niger River delta, where 758 persons were infected (39 died) between January and March 1971. In addition, 75 people died out of about 135 cases in six remote Nigerian villages before medical aid arrived, and more than 1,600 cases occurred in coastal areas from February to June 1971.

Cameroon was struck when the first cholera case was reported in a fishing village near Douala on the Atlantic coast in mid-1971; a subsequent four-week-long epidemic occurred in Douala and its vicinity, with 55 deaths out of 333 cases. The transmission of cholera was once again attributed to the movement of fishermen along the coast. Equatorial Guinea and the Central African Republic, south and east of Cameroon respectively, were also infected to a lesser degree. With the help of the World Health Organization (called in by Guinean officials at the onset of the initial epidemic in 1970), immunization programs were set up to curtail the mortality rates in the infected regions.

Further reading: Cartwright, *Disease and History;* Stock, *African Environment Special Report 3: Cholera in Africa.*

West Indian Dengue Epidemic of 1826–28   See U.S. AND CARIBBEAN DENGUE EPIDEMIC OF 1826–28.

X

Xerxes's Army Epidemic See PLAGUE OF XERXES.

Xinjiang (Sinkiang) Hepatitis Epidemic of 1986–88 Extensive epidemic of Hepatitis E that occurred in the southern section of western China's Xinjiang (Sinkiang) Uighur Autonomous Region (see SHANGHAI HEPATITIS EPIDEMIC OF 1988).

The epidemic, caused by contaminated drinking water, attacked 23 counties and towns in two phases over a 20-month period from September 1986 to April 1988. During this time, 119,280 cases were reported—an attack rate of three percent. However, members of the Uighur, or Uigur, tribe suffered a higher attack rate (7.1 percent) than people of other nationalities in the region. This has been attributed to their habit of drinking water straight (without boiling) from pools and canals that were often heavily contaminated by fecal matter. Members of the Han and Hui nationalities, who usually drink boiled or well water, did not suffer as much.

More than 77 percent of the patients were in the 15 to 49 year age group, which suffered an attack rate of 5.1 percent. The attack rate for children under 14 years old was 0.9 percent and for adults over 50 years, 0.2 percent. The attack rate was slightly higher in men, no doubt because of greater exposure to contaminated water. A study conducted during this outbreak found that those in close contact with Hepatitis E patients ran a greater risk of contracting the disease than those without any contact.

In China, epidemics of Hepatitis E usually occur during or just after the rainy season (mostly in the summer months). The incubation period ranges between 15 and 75 days, the average being 36 days. Its onset is generally abrupt, with many patients developing fever. In most cases, the hepatitis jaundice disappears within a week, but it takes about six weeks for the patient to recover completely. The mortality rate can be high in pregnant women in their last trimester.

During this 1986–88 epidemic, the government launched an extensive campaign aimed at arresting the spread of the disease by educating the people about the need for improved personal hygiene and better water, food, and sanitation facilities. Thereby, it did succeed in reducing Hepatitis E infection rates in the country.

Further reading: Wen et al., eds., *Viral Hepatitis in China: Problems and Control Strategies;* Szmuness et al., eds., *Viral Hepatitis: 1981 International Symposium.*

Y

Yellow Plague of A.D. **664**   First major epidemic recorded in English history, coinciding with a total eclipse of the sun. After remarking on the eclipse, an event always full of portent for medieval people, the Venerable Bede (author of *The Ecclesiastical History of the English Nation*) wrote: "In the same year of our Lord's incarnation, 664, a sudden pestilence also depopulated the southern coasts of Britain, and afterwards extending into the province of the Northumbrians, ravaged the country far and near, and destroyed a great multitude of men . . ." The Old English word for epidemic disease, "on-flyge" or "the on-flying," captured the essence of the fast-traveling destruction of the many diseases to which medieval populations were so frequently subject.

The term "yellow plague" was not used by contemporaries to describe this pestilence, but was employed by later writers, who apparently assumed that the Irish Yellow Plague ("buidhe conaill") of the 540s was the same disease as the pestilence of 664. It remains a matter of debate among medical historians as to whether the great epidemic of 664 was in fact a recurrence of the first Yellow Plague in Ireland, itself unidentified. Bede unfortunately did not describe symptoms in his history, so the precise nature of the pestilence, like most medieval epidemics, is open to question. Smallpox seems a likely possibility. Those who have argued for bubonic plague have not demonstrated a large population of plague-infected house-rats, necessary for the presence and spreading of bubonic plague; claims for pneumonic plague have also been unconvincing (see PLAGUE OF ENGLAND, GREAT).

The Yellow Plague held on tenaciously for 20 or 25 years, causing, as contemporary records indicate, widespread mortality with attendant social disruption and abandonment of religious faith.

Further reading: Marks and Beatty, *Epidemics*; Creighton, *A History of Epidemics in Britain*; Shrewsbury, *A History of Bubonic Plague in the British Isles*; Winslow, *The Conquest of Epidemic Disease*.

Yukon Indian Influenza Epidemic of 1900   Unexpected outburst of influenza among the Kutchin and other Indian tribes inhabiting the Yukon River area. The native Indians called influenza the "white man's disease" because it evidently arrived with ailing whites—explorers, missionaries, and settlers in the region.

In June 1900 the disease suddenly struck the Aleut Indians in western Alaska; its contagious, infectious virus then attacked the Eskimos to the east and at the same time (early August 1900) spread to the Kutchin and other bands living in the present-day Yukon Territory. Many Indians became severely ill, with headaches, fevers, and respiratory inflammation. One Kutchin tribe on the Yukon River had 71 members out of 335 perish. The infection soon attacked other Indian camps along the river with even more intensity, and several missionary priests in the area tried to assist the sick Indians in late September. But with frost and cold arriving in the Yukon by this time, the disease situation worsened, with desolation and death in every Indian camp along the river. There was at least one corpse in every Indian hut in the camps, where sometimes entire families were wiped out by influenza. Without knowledge of prevention and any modern medicines, the missionaries were unable to help the natives. A woodcutter who accompanied the priests to the camps wanted to burn 16 Indian corpses too putrid to handle; the Indian survivors, however, refused to allow him to build cremation bonfires. Untold hundreds of Indians died from influenza during the epidemic, which spread south into British Columbia by December 1900.

Further reading: Mathews, *The Yukon*.

Z

Zairian Ebola Epidemic of 1976 Outbreak of ebola, an unusual new African hemorrhagic fever disease, that killed at least 218 persons between mid-August and September 22, 1976, in a part of northern Zaire (formerly the Congo). The infectious agent, discovered to be a togavirus, was later called "ebola," after the Ebola River, which flowed in the vicinity of the Zairian epidemic. This acute hemorrhagic virus, confined largely to the tropics, was proven to be one of the deadliest known to modern medicine. To date there is no treatment for ebola, and the reservoir host for the ebola organism is still unknown.

In the small village of Yambuku in Zaire's northern rain forest, more than 200 inhabitants died from a mysterious, painful bleeding infection in August–September 1976. On September 23 a Belgian nun who had been nursing patients at the Roman Catholic missionary hospital contracted the infection herself. Two physicians from Kinshasa (Zaire's capital) were then called in to deal with this baffling disease, but they quickly retreated to Kinshasa, bringing the seriously ill nun with them. At Kinshasa's Ngaliema Hospital, the nun was isolated, continued to suffer from severe head pain, vomiting, 103° F temperature, and dehydration, for which intravenous fluids and blood transfusions could not compensate. Massive doses of antibiotics had no effect on her ailment. Seven days after becoming infected, the nun bled from her gums and died the next day, bleeding from other orifices. During the next weeks in Yambuku, three other nuns, a priest, and several other members of the missionary hospital died from the same illness.

Blood samples from a victim of the disease in Maridi in southernmost Sudan (near Zaire's northeastern border) were then sent to the U.S. Centers for Disease Control in Atlanta, Georgia. The "ebola" virus was discovered, and shortly afterward a member of the Centers for Disease Control (part of the newly formed International Medical Commission) arrived in Kinshasa to study the ebola infection, which had killed another nun and a native nurse there (the former had accompanied the first stricken nun to the capital city in September). The main concern of the commission became the prevention of the spread of the disease in Kinshasa, where hospital staff and others who came into contact with the three victims there were quarantined. Ebola did not spread, and no link was found between the cases in Zaire and Sudan.

In the following months, the epidemic's first cases in Yambuku were traced to contaminated hypodermic injections, but no effort was made to isolate numerous other patients contracting the virus, who returned to their homes and spread the disease by person-to-person contact, presumably. In 1977 a young native girl living in Tandala, Zaire (about 200 miles from Yambuku), died from ebola; she had never been in contact with anyone from the 1976 epidemic.

Further reading: Astor, *The Disease Detectives;* Smith Jr. and Wyngaarden, eds., *Cecil Textbook of Medicine;* Garrett, *The Coming Plague.*

Zairian Plague of 1992 Outburst of plague in northeastern Zaire (formerly the Congo) from January to August 1992, killing 78 persons out of 191 who were infected. This highly contagious, bacterial disease is endemic in Zaire and other parts of Africa.

In January 1992 the first cases of plague (the bubonic form) were reported in the Ituri forest region of northeast Zaire. All the patients recovered following antibiotic treatments. In February and March several more persons contracted bubonic plague in the same area (the health zone of Logo in the Ituri forest) and survived the infection, which is carried to humans from rodents (usually by infective fleas). Other health zones in northeastern Zaire—Rimba and Nyarembe and Rethy—successively reported more cases of plague in the following months. In the health zone of Nyarembe, most of the cases were pneumonic and septicemic in form; in the former, the lungs are attacked, and in the latter, the bloodstream. (Plague pneumonia in a person can easily be transmitted to another person through coughing.)

During the eight-month-long epidemic, the four above-mentioned health zones were affected by bubonic, pneumonic, and septicemic plague and had difficulty treating sick inhabitants. There was no telephone service in the Ituri forest area; local roads were in poor shape; and armed conflict among groups was taking place there. For the most part, the plague was concentrated in Logo, where more than 60 percent of the infections and fatalities occurred. The epidemic's 41 percent fatality rate overall was the highest in recent years in Zaire.

Further reading: McGrew, *Encyclopedia of Medical History*; World Health Organization, "Epidemic of Plague," *Weekly Epidemiological Records*, 42.

Zambian Plague of 1917–18   See NORTHERN RHODESIAN PLAGUE OF 1917–18.

Zambian Smallpox Epidemic of 1955   Serious epidemic of smallpox in the central African country of Zambia (then called Northern Rhodesia), killing 501 persons out of 3,538 who were infected.

In early January 1955 small outbreaks of smallpox were first reported in the mineral-rich Copperbelt (a mining region in north-central Zambia). By April the disease had moved from the mining towns into the rest of the country; many victims were either blinded or disfigured as the variola virus (the infectious agent) spread among the natives, either by close contact with the diseased through respiratory discharges or by airborne means. The epidemic worsened during the dry season (May to October) when the greater mobility and social activities of the rural people helped increase its spread; the dry season, with its low amount of humid air, increased the survival of the deadly virus. People of all ages were affected, except adults who had acquired immunity from contracting smallpox in previous outbreaks in 1927–30 and 1945.

Most of the large mining towns in the Copperbelt were badly infected by smallpox; a total of 2,772 cases were reported there; in just one week in mid-June 1955, there were 42 cases (out of which 37 were fatal) in the mining town of Mufulira. Though officials put into use highly stable freeze-dried vaccines (which were developed in the early 1950s), the fatality rate in the Copperbelt was 16.85 percent. Mortality was 14.16 percent for the entire country.

Zambia experienced another smallpox outbreak in 1963–64, when the British were granting it self-government and then full independence as a republic. Smallpox was eliminated in Zambia after the World Health Organization's global eradication campaign (1964).

Further reading: Hopkins, *Princes & Peasants Smallpox in History*; Kimble, *Tropical Africa*.

Zanzibar Cholera Epidemic of 1869   Devastating epidemic of cholera that killed an estimated 70,000 persons in one year (1869) on the island of Zanzibar (now part of Tanzania) off the coast of East Africa in the Indian Ocean. It was part of the Asiatic Cholera Pandemic of 1865–75 (q.v.).

Cholera, an acute intestinal disease, apparently made its way into Zanzibar from the northern Somali seaport of Berbera, which had been infected via a ship most likely from Bombay, India, in November 1864. The disease moved westward from Somaliland into Abyssinia (Ethiopia) in 1865; from there it spread southward and eventually reached the Masai people's country in Kenya and Tanganyika (Tanzania) in 1869. The nomadic Masais helped spread cholera during their raids on other tribal groups, notably those around Laikipia, Kenya. Traders evidently carried cholera with them to Zanzibar in 1869. At the time environmental sanitation was nearly nonexistent in most of Africa, despite knowledge that cholera-epidemic control could be achieved by stopping the distribution of polluted water. (In 1849 British physician John Snow had published his discovery that the disease might enter the human system in contaminated water.)

In Zanzibar, cholera-diseased human corpses were cast into stagnant harbor waters as well as into ponds and wells. The people did not know that the infection was carried by a bacterium (*Vibrio comma*) and was transmitted through ingestion of water or food contaminated by human feces or vomit. Flies may also carry the bacteria from excrement to food. The inhabitants of Zanzibar suffered diarrhea and colicky abdominal pain followed by nausea and vomiting (cholera's symptoms); many had painful deaths often on the same day as infection. Authorities estimate that at least 100,000 people were infected by cholera on Zanzibar, and about 70,000 of them perished. Numerous ships from other countries docked at the island's chief seaport (called Zanzibar) and filled their vessel tanks with water taken from contaminated wells and ponds. The result was that the ships reintroduced cholera along the East African coast as they traveled from Cabo Delgado (Cape Delgado, Mozambique) to Cape Horn, South Africa, in 1870.

Further reading: Ackerknecht, *History and Geography of the Most Important Diseases*; Stock, *African Environment Special Report 3: Cholera in Africa*.

Timetable of Plague and Pestilence

Date	Disease	Locality
11th cent. B.C.	Plague? Dysentery?	Ashdod (Israel)
480 B.C.	Dysentery?	Asia Minor, Greece
451 B.C.	Tuberculosis? Anthrax?	Rome
430–429 B.C.	Plague? Smallpox? Typhus?	Athens (Greece)
c. 410 B.C.	Mumps	Thasos (Greece)
c. 400 B.C.	Diphtheria? Influenza? Whooping Cough?	Perinthus (Turkey)
396 B.C.	Smallpox? Plague?	Carthage (Tunisia)
c. 250–243 B.C.	"Hunpox" (Smallpox?)	China
212 B.C.	Influenza?	Syracuse (Sicily)
A.D. 1st cent.	Plague	Libya, Egypt, Syria
A.D. 165–80	Smallpox? Measles?	Roman Empire
A.D. 251–66?	Smallpox? Measles?	Roman Empire
A.D. 6th cent.	Plague	Frankish kingdom (France)
A.D. 542	Plague	Byzantine Empire, Europe
A.D. 569–71	Smallpox	Saudi Arabia
A.D. 580	Smallpox	Frankish kingdom (France)
A.D. 585–87	Smallpox?	Japan
A.D. 638–39	Plague	Syria, Iraq, Egypt
A.D. 664	Plague? Smallpox?	Britain
A.D. 680	Plague	Rome, northern Italy
A.D. 8th–9th cent.	Smallpox	Japan
A.D. 735–37	Smallpox	Japan
c. A.D. 746–48	Plague	Constantinople (Turkey), Greece
A.D. 10th cent.	Smallpox	Japan
A.D. 994–95	Smallpox?	Japan
A.D. 998–1025	Measles	Japan
1081–83	Malaria, Typhoid, Dysentery	Rome—Henry IV's army
1083	Typhus	Cava (Italy)
1098	Typhoid, Scurvy, Malaria?	Antioch (Turkey)—Crusaders
1148	Typhoid, Scurvy	Adalia (Turkey)—Crusaders
1167	Malaria? Typhus?	Rome—Frederick Barbarossa's army
1189	Typhoid, Scurvy	Acre (Israel)
1218–19	Scurvy	Damietta (Egypt)—Crusaders
1250	Scurvy, Typhoid	Al Mansurah (Egypt)—Crusaders
1347–80s	Plague	Europe, Britain, Middle East
1374	Dancing Mania	Germany, France
1400s	Plague, Dysentery, Typhus	Britain, Spain, Portugal
1400s	Plague? Typhus? Smallpox?	Ireland
1402–04	Plague	Iceland
1417	Plague	Florence
1425	Dysentery	Florence
1430	Plague	Florence
1450–1520	Plague, Measles, Smallpox, Syphilis	France
1462–65	Plague	Germany
1466	Plague	Paris
1477–79	Plague	Italy
1485	Sweating Sickness	England
1489	Typhus	Granada (Spain)
1494–95	Syphilis	Naples—French army
1494–95	Plague	Iceland

Date	Disease	Locality
1499–1500	Plague	London
1500s	Plague	Spain, Portugal
1500s	Plague	Germany, Austria, Switzerland
1500s–1600s	Tarantism	Taranto, southern Italy
1507	Smallpox	Hispaniola
1507–08	Sweating Sickness	England
1512	Syphilis	Japan
1516–17	Sweating Sickness	England
1518	Dancing Mania Smallpox	Strasbourg (France) Hispaniola
1519–25	Plague? Typhus? Smallpox? Influenza?	Ireland
1520–1600	Plague	France
1520–21	Smallpox	Mexico
1522	Typhus	Cambridge (England)
1525–27	Smallpox	Peru
1528	Typhus	Naples—French army
1529	Sweating Sickness	England, Germany, northern Europe
1530	Plague	Edinburgh (Scotland)
1535–36	Plague? Typhus? Smallpox? Relapsing Fever?	Ireland
1542	Typhus	Hungary—Joachim's army
1551	Sweating Sickness	England
1552	Typhus, Dysentery	Metz (France)—Charles V's army
1555–62	Smallpox	Brazil
1563	Plague	London
1564	Plague	Lyon (France)
1566	Typhus	Hungary—Maximilian II's army
1574–76	Plague	Ireland
1575–77	Plague	Venice
1576	Typhus Diphtheria	Mexico Paris
1577	Typhus	Oxford (England)
1578	Whooping Cough Plague	Paris London
1580	Influenza Smallpox	Italy Venezuela
1585	Smallpox Plague	Peru Edinburgh (Scotland)
1586	Typhus	Exeter (England)
1591	Smallpox	Philippines
1592–96	Measles	Western New York
1593	Plague	London
1596–1602	Plague	Spain
1597	Plague	Edinburgh (Scotland)
1600–1608	Plague	Scotland
1602	Plague	Prussia
1603	Plague	London
1604–05	Plague	Ireland
1610–11	Plague	Basel (Switzerland)
c. 1617–19	Smallpox	Massachusetts
1618	Diphtheria	Italy

Timetable of Plague and Pestilence (*continued*)

Date	Disease	Locality
1618–48	Typhus, Plague, Scurvy, Dysentery	Germany, central Europe
1625	Plague	London
1625–40	Plague	France
1628–29	Plague	Lyon (France)
1629–31	Plague	Italy
1630–33	Plague	Florence
c. 1633	Smallpox	Massachusetts
1634–40	Measles? Influenza?	Quebec, eastern Canada
1634	Smallpox	Connecticut
1636	Plague	London
1637	Plague	Spain
1643	Typhus	Oxford (England)
	Typhus	Reading (England)
1644	Typhus	Tiverton (England)
1644–48	Plague	Scotland
1646–52	Plague	Spain
1647	Yellow Fever	Barbados
1648–49	Smallpox	Massachusetts
1650–51	Plague	Ireland
1655	Yellow Fever	Jamaica
1656–57	Plague	Italy
1660	Smallpox	Brazil
1661–65	Typhus	London
1662	Smallpox	Central New York
1663–68	Plague	Germany, Austria, Switzerland
1665	Plague	London
1665–66	Smallpox	Brazil
1666	Smallpox	Boston
1667–68	Smallpox	London
1668	Yellow Fever	New York
1674	Smallpox	London
1675–76	Plague	Malta
1675–83	Plague	Germany, Austria, Switzerland
1677–78	Smallpox	Boston
1678–82	Plague	Spain
	Malaria	Britain, Europe
1679	Plague	Vienna
1681	Smallpox	London
1684	Rubella	Japan
1685–86	Typhus	London
1689	Typhus, Dysentery	Londonderry, Dundalk (Ireland)
1690–91	Measles	Japan
1699	Yellow Fever	Charleston (South Carolina)
1702	Yellow Fever	New York
1702–03	Smallpox	Boston
1703–04	Typhus	Augsburg (Germany)
1706	Yellow Fever	Charleston (South Carolina)
1707–09	Smallpox	Iceland
1708–09	Measles	Japan
	Influenza	Europe
1708–10	Typhus	Ireland
1709	Plague	Danzig (Prussia)

Date	Disease	Locality
1709–20	Typhus	London
1710	Yellow Fever	Quebec
1712	Influenza	Europe
1713	Smallpox	Cape Colony (South Africa)
1718	Sweating Sickness	Picardy (France)
1718–20	Typhus	Ireland
1718–22	Influenza	Europe
1720–22	Plague	Marseilles
1721	Smallpox	London
1721–22	Smallpox	Boston
1722	Ergotism	Russia
1726–29	Typhus	London
1727–28	Plague	Astrakhan (Russia)
1728	Yellow Fever	Charleston (South Carolina)
1728–30	Typhus	Ireland
1729–30	Influenza	Europe
1730–31	Measles	Japan
1732	Yellow Fever	Charleston (South Carolina)
1732–33	Influenza	Europe, Britain
1733–34	Smallpox	Greenland
1734	Typhus	Germany
1735–40	Diphtheria, Scarlet Fever	New England
1736–39	Influenza, Dysentery, Smallpox	Scandinavia
1738–39	Plague	Russia
1738–42	Dysentery	France
1740	Influenza	France
	Yellow Fever	Guayaquil (Ecuador)
1740–41	Typhus, Dysentery	Ireland
1740–42	Typhus, Typhoid	France
1741–42	Typhus	London
1741–43	Typhus, Typhoid, Dysentery	Germany
1740s	Typhus, Relapsing Fever, Dysentery	Sweden
1742–43	Influenza	Europe, Britain
1743	Yellow Fever	Guayaquil (Ecuador), New York
1745	Yellow Fever	New York
1747–48	Diphtheria	Cremona (Italy)
1748–50	Malaria	Europe
1750	Typhus	London
1751–53	Smallpox	England
1753	Measles	Japan
1755	Smallpox	Canada, Cape Colony (South Africa)
1757–63	Typhus, Dysentery	Germany
1762	Influenza	Europe, Britain
	Yellow Fever	Philadelphia
1763–64	Smallpox	Boston
1764	Typhus	Naples (Italy)
1767	Influenza	Britain
1768–69	Venereal Disease	Tahiti (South Pacific)
1769–70	Smallpox	India, Bengal
1770–72	Malaria	Europe
1772–73	Plague	Persia
1775–76	Influenza	Britain

Timetable of Plague and Pestilence (*continued*)

Date	Disease	Locality
1776	Smallpox	Quebec, Colombia
	Measles	Japan, Hawaii
1778	Yellow Fever	St. Louis (Senegal)—British army
1779	Dysentery	France
	Smallpox	Mexico City
1779–83	Malaria	Europe
1780–82	Smallpox	Canada
1781–82	Influenza	Europe, Asia
1781–83	Cholera	India
1782	Influenza	Britain
1783–84	Plague	Dalmatia (Croatia)
1788–89	Influenza	Europe, Britain
	Smallpox	Australia
1789	Influenza	New England
1790s	Dysentery? Influenza?	New Zealand, Fiji Islands
1792	Dysentery	France—Prussian army
1792–99	Yellow Fever	Charleston (South Carolina)
1793	Yellow Fever	Philadelphia
1793–95	Scarlet Fever	New England
1794	Yellow Fever	New Haven (Connecticut)
1794–98	Yellow Fever	Haiti, U.S. Atlantic coast
1795	Yellow Fever	New York
1796	Smallpox	Britain
1796–1800	Typhus	Italy
1797	Smallpox	Mexico, Guatemala
1798	Yellow Fever	New York, Philadelphia, Baltimore
1798–1801	Plague	Near East—Napoleon's army
1800	Yellow Fever	Cádiz (Spain)
	Plague	Persia
1802	Yellow Fever	Haiti
	Smallpox	Northeast Nebraska
1803	Influenza	Britain
	Measles	Japan
1803–05	Yellow Fever	Spain
1804	Yellow Fever	Livorno, Lucca (Italy)
1804–28	Yellow Fever	Gibraltar (Spain)
1805–07	Typhus	Austria, Prussia
1805–12	Malaria	Europe
1807	Typhus	Danzig (Prussia)
1810	Yellow Fever	Cádiz (Spain)
1812–13	Typhus, Dysentery	Russia—Napoleon's army
1812–14	Typhus	Prussia
1813	Typhus, Dysentery	Torgau (Germany)
	Typhus	Danzig (Prussia), Mexico City
	Plague	Malta
1813–14	Typhus	Mainz, Germany, France
1814	Smallpox	Italy
1815	Yellow Fever	Mauritius
	Meningitis	Albenga (Italy)
1815–85	Yellow Fever	Sierra Leone (West Africa)
1816–18	Typhus	Italy
1816–19	Smallpox, Typhus	Britain

Date	Disease	Locality
1817–18	Smallpox	Madagascar
	Cholera	India
1817–19	Typhus, Dysentery	Ireland
1817–23	Cholera	Asia, Africa
1818–20	Plague	Tunisia
1818–21	Diphtheria	Tours (France)
1820–21	Cholera	Philippines
1820–22	Cholera	China
1820–40	Influenza, Whooping Cough	New Zealand
1821	Yellow Fever	Barcelona
	Cholera	Indonesia
	Miliary Fever	France
1822	Cholera	Japan
1823	Cholera	Astrakhan (Russia)
1823–24	Measles	Japan
1823–27	Malaria	Europe
1823–31	Smallpox	Scotland
1825–26	Smallpox	England
1826–27	Cholera	India
1826–28	Dengue	United States, Caribbean
1826–37	Cholera	Asia, Europe, North America
1829–30	Cholera	Persia
1829–31	Cholera	Russia
1829–33	Malaria	Oregon
1830	Plague	Persia
	Influenza	Britain
1830–31	Influenza	Asia, Europe, North America
1831	Cholera	Mecca (Saudi Arabia)
1831–32	Cholera	Germany
1832	Cholera	Britain, United States, Canada
1832–33	Cholera	France
	Smallpox	Calcutta
1833	Influenza	Persia, Britain
	Smallpox	Mexico
1833–34	Cholera	Spain
1834	Cholera	Canada
	Measles	Sydney
1834–35	Plague	Egypt
1835	Measles	New Zealand
1836–37	Influenza	Asia, Europe, Australia, Britain, South Africa
	Measles	Japan
1836–40	Typhus	Ireland, Scotland
1837	Smallpox	North Dakota—Mandan Indians; Saskatchewan; Manitoba
	Influenza	Samoa (South Pacific)
1837–38	Smallpox	Montana, Saskatchewan, Calcutta
	Typhus	Britain
1837–40	Smallpox	Britain
1839	Influenza	Samoa
1839–45	Meningitis	Italy
1840–44	Ergotism	Finland
1841	Smallpox	Tahiti

Timetable of Plague and Pestilence (*continued*)

Date	Disease	Locality
1841–42	Miliary Fever	France
1842	Yellow Fever	Guayaquil (Ecuador)
1843	Dysentery	South Pacific Islands
1843–44	Smallpox	Calcutta
1846	Measles	Faeroe Islands
1846–47	Measles	Canada
1846–50	Typhoid Typhus, Dysentery	Java (Indonesia) Ireland
1846–63	Cholera	Asia, Europe, North and South America
1847	Typhus Yellow Fever	Canada U.S. Northwest—Cayuse Indians
1847–48	Typhus, Influenza Influenza	Britain Europe
1848–49	Cholera	Britain, France
1848–50	Cholera	Germany
1849	Cholera Yellow Fever	United States, Canada Rio de Janeiro
1849–50	Cholera Smallpox	Tunisia Calcutta
1850	Miliary Fever Yellow Fever	France Rio de Janeiro
1850–51	Dengue	United States
1850s–1959	Plague	China, India, South America, Africa
1853	Smallpox	Hawaii
1853–54	Cholera	Britain, France
1853–59	Cholera	Germany
1854	Measles Cholera	French Polynesia, New Zealand Canada, Spain
1854–56	Scurvy, Typhus, Cholera, Dysentery	Crimea (southern Ukraine)
1855–58	Diphtheria	Europe
1857	Smallpox	Calcutta
1858	Cholera	Japan
1860	Miliary Fever	France
1860–61	Cholera	India
1861–65	Dysentery, Typhoid, Typhus, Malaria, Scurvy, Measles, Smallpox	United States—Civil War armies
1862	Measles, Cholera	Japan
1862–63	Ergotism	Finland
1862–64	Yellow Fever	Bahamas, Rio de Janeiro
1862–65	Typhus	London
1863–64	Scarlet Fever	New Zealand
1864–65	Smallpox Cholera	Angola India
1865	Cholera Smallpox	Spain, Mecca (Saudi Arabia) Calcutta
1865–66	Cholera	France, Britain
1865–75	Cholera	Asia, Europe, Africa, North and South America
1866	Cholera	United States
1866–67	Cholera	Germany, Italy
1866–68	Malaria	Mauritius

Date	Disease	Locality
1867–68	Cholera	India
1868	Typhus Kala-azar	Tunis India
1868–75	Smallpox	New York, United States
1869	Smallpox Cholera	Montana—Gros Ventre Indians Zanzibar
1870s	Yellow Fever	Rio de Janeiro
1870–72	Cholera Smallpox	Central Asia Italy
1870–75	Smallpox	Europe
1871	Cholera	Germany
1871–72	Smallpox	Britain
1873	Whooping Cough Cholera Kala-azar	New Zealand United States India
1873–75	Smallpox	Calcutta
1875	Measles	Fiji Islands
1875–76	Scarlet Fever	Australia
1876	Typhus	Ethiopia
1876–77	Scarlet Fever	New Zealand
1878–79	Yellow Fever Malaria	New Orleans, Memphis, Mississippi and Ohio River valleys Punjab (India)
1880s–90s	Yellow Fever	Panama
1881–82	Scarlet Fever Smallpox	New Zealand Sydney
1881–96	Cholera	Asia, Europe, Africa, South America
1882–83	Cholera	Philippines
1882–85	Smallpox	Cape Colony (South Africa)
1882–86	Diphtheria	Cairo, Alexandria
1883	Cholera	Philippines
1884–85	Cholera	Italy, Spain
1885	Smallpox	Montreal, Calcutta
1886–98	Smallpox	Ethiopia
1887	Poliomyelitis Miliary Fever	Stockholm France
1888–89	Cholera	Philippines
1889–90	Influenza	Europe, Asia, Africa, North and South America, Australia
1890	Measles	Gilbert and Ellice Islands (Kiribati and Tuvalu)
1890–91	Influenza	Sydney
1890–1910	Beriberi	Thailand
1891–92	Cholera	India
1892	Cholera	Russia, Hamburg
1893	Measles	Tonga, Samoa
1894	Poliomyelitis Plague	Vermont Hong Kong, China
1895–1906	Sleeping Sickness	Congo
1896–97	Plague	India
1897–99	Smallpox Dengue	Kenya Caribbean, United States
1898–1913	Sleeping Sickness	Príncipe (West Africa)

Timetable of Plague and Pestilence (*continued*)

Date	Disease	Locality
1899–1900	Yellow Fever	Havana
	Plague	Hawaii
1899–1902	Typhoid	South Africa—British troops
1899–1903	Plague	Philippines, Brazil
1899–1923	Cholera	Asia, Europe
1900	Plague	Brazil, Sydney
	Cholera	India
	Influenza	Yukon, Ontong Java (South Pacific)
1900–1904	Plague	San Francisco
	Pneumonia	South Africa
1900–1909	Sleeping Sickness	Uganda, Tanganyika (Tanzania)
1901–02	Beriberi	Philippines
	Smallpox	Britain, Italy
1901–03	Smallpox	United States
1901–05	Whooping Cough	Italy
1902	Cholera	Egypt
1902–04	Cholera	Philippines
1903	Scarlet Fever	New Zealand
	Measles	Fiji Islands
1904	Smallpox	Rio de Janeiro
1904–05	Beriberi	Japan—army
1904–07	Typhoid	South-West Africa (Namibia)
	Plague	India
1905	Poliomyelitis	Sweden
	Smallpox	Brazil
1905–06	Plague	Spain, Vietnam
1906–14	Tuberculosis	South Africa
1907	Whooping Cough	New Zealand, Samoa
	Poliomyelitis	New York
1907–09	Plague	San Francisco
1908	Plague	Ecuador, Ghana
	Smallpox	Rio de Janeiro
	Malaria	Punjab (India)
1908–13	Typhoid	British Columbia
1909	Beriberi	Philippines
1910	Cholera	Russia
	Schistosomiasis	Iraq
1910–11	Plague	Manchuria
1910–14	Plague	Java (Indonesia)
1911	Poliomyelitis	Sweden
	Measles	Fiji Islands
	Cholera	Tripoli (Libya)
	Plague	Morocco
1912	Plague	Kilimanjaro (Tanzania)
1912–40	Sleeping Sickness	Chad
1914–15	Typhus	Serbia
1915–22	Typhus	Russia
1915	Plague	Vietnam
1915–16	Poliomyelitis, Measles	New Zealand
1915–22	Cholera	Russia
1915–20	Encephalitis Lethargica	Europe
1916	Poliomyelitis	United States
1917–18	Murray Valley Encephalitis	Australia
	Plague	China, Northern Rhodesia (Zambia)

Date	Disease	Locality
1917–19	Influenza	Europe, Asia, Africa, North and South America, Australia, Oceania
1918–24	Meningitis	Mongalla (southern Sudan)
1918–26	Plague	Ecuador
1919	Cholera	Manchuria
1919–31	Encephalitis	Britain
1920–21	Smallpox	Italy
	Plague	Manchuria
1921	Schistosomiasis	Iraq
1921–22	Relapsing Fever	Mali
1922	Murray Valley Encephalitis	Australia
1922–23	Smallpox	Chad
	Malaria	Russia
1923	Plague	Spain
1924	Schistosomiasis	Iraq
	Encephalitis	Japan
1924–25	Plague	Ashanti (Ghana), Madagascar, Los Angeles, Vietnam
1925–26	Influenza	Russia
	Murray Valley Encephalitis	Australia
1926	Yellow Fever	Ghana
	Miliary Fever	France
	Whooping Cough	Samoa
	Cholera	Manchuria
	Influenza	Ontong Java (South Pacific)
1926–27	Dengue	Durban (South Africa)
	Influenza	Russia
1926–28	Relapsing Fever	Sudan
1926–30	Pneumonia	South Africa
1926–31	Meningitis	Mongalla (southern Sudan)
1928	Influenza	Ontong Java (South Pacific)
	Schistosomiasis	Iraq
1928–30	Plague	Manchuria, Mongolia, Uganda
1929	Malaria	Pakistan
	Yellow Fever	Venezuela
1930s	Cholera	Afghanistan
1930–35	Smallpox	Nigeria
1931	Poliomyelitis	United States
1931–32	Plague	China
1931–35	Pneumonia	South Africa
1932–33	Encephalitis	Japan
	Plague	Java (Indonesia), Madagascar
1934	Typhus, Plague	South Africa
	Poliomyelitis	Los Angeles
1934–35	Malaria	Sri Lanka
1935	Typhus, Plague	South Africa
1935–36	Influenza	Ontong Java (South Pacific)
	Plague	Ecuador
1935–37	Encephalitis	Japan
	Plague	Madagascar
1936	Smallpox	Somalia
	Plague	South Africa
	Measles	Gilbert and Ellice Islands (Kiribati and Tuvalu)
1936–37	Whooping Cough	Samoa

Timetable of Plague and Pestilence (*continued*)

Date	Disease	Locality
1936–41	Sleeping Sickness	Ghana
1937	Poliomyelitis	New Zealand
	Encephalitis	Japan
1937–39	Meningitis	Chad
1937–42	Cholera	China
1938	Measles	New Zealand
1938–40	Malaria	Brazil
1938–41	Rubella	Australia
1938–43	Diphtheria	South Africa
1939	Meningitis	Upper Volta (Burkina Faso)
	Yellow Fever	Sudan
1940–41	Poliomyelitis	Egypt—New Zealand troops
1940–43	Sleeping Sickness	Uganda
1940–45	Typhus	Egypt
1941	Malaria	Constantine (Algeria)
1941–42	Malaria	Usambara Mtns. (Tanzania)
1941–43	Meningitis	Santiago (Chile)
1942	Dysentery	Sri Lanka
	Plague	Kenya
	Meningitis	Tanganyika (Tanzania)
1942–44	Malaria	Egypt
	Plague	Senegal
	Poliomyelitis	India, Malta
	Typhus	Persia, Algeria
	Tuberculosis	Ghana
1942–45	Malaria, Typhus	Southwest Pacific
	Beriberi	Singapore
	Typhus	Morocco
	Dengue	Japan
1942–53	Poliomyelitis	United States
1943–44	Typhus	Naples (Italy)
	Influenza	Russia
1943–45	Typhus, Sprue	India, Burma—Allied armies
	Relapsing Fever	Algeria
1944–45	Poliomyelitis, Schistosomiasis	Philippines
	Scarlet Fever	New Zealand
1944–46	Relapsing Fever	Egypt
1945–46	Typhus	Japan, Korea
	Malaria	Japan
	Relapsing Fever	Kenya, Morocco
	Cholera	China
1945–49	Meningitis	Ghana
1946	Bornholm Disease	Singapore
	Cholera	Afghanistan
1946–47	Influenza	Russia
1946–48	Smallpox	Rhodesia (Zimbabwe), Ghana
1947	Poliomyelitis	Nicobar Islands (India)
1947–48	Encephalitis, Mumps	Guam
	Cholera	Syria, Egypt
1949	Pneumonia	Peking (Beijing)
	Meningitis	Nigeria
1949–50	Leptospirosis	Israel
1950	Whooping Cough	Samoa
	Meningitis	Nigeria

Date	Disease	Locality
1950–51	Measles	French Polynesia
	Malaria	Saudi Arabia
	Hepatitis	Korea
	Diphtheria	Israel
	Influenza	Britain
1950–52	Typhoid	Italy
	Poliomyelitis	Israel
1951	Murray Valley Encephalitis	Australia
	Poliomyelitis	Tahiti, Solomon Islands
	Ergotism	France
1951–53	Plague	Tanganyika (Tanzania)
	West Nile Fever	Israel
	Hemorrhagic Fever	Korea
1952	Poliomyelitis	Bangkok, Copenhagen
1952–54	Malaria	Ghana
	Pneumonia	Peking (Beijing)
1954	Typhoid	Kenya
1955–56	Hepatitis	Delhi (India)
	Smallpox	Zambia
	Dengue	Philippines
1957	West Nile Fever	Israel
1957–58	Influenza	Asia, Europe, North America, Africa
	Kyasanur Forest Disease	India
1958	Malaria	Ethiopia
	Dengue	Vietnam, Thailand
1958–59	Poliomyelitis	Singapore
	Pneumonia	Peking (Beijing)
1958–61	Encephalitis	Taiwan
1959–64	Hemorrhagic Fever	Bolivia
1960s	Plague	Vietnam
	Dengue	Singapore
1960	Dengue	Vietnam, Thailand
1960–62	Yellow Fever	Ethiopia
1961	Malaria	Somalia
	Dengue	Philippines
1961–62	Cholera	Philippines, Indonesia
1961–75	Cholera	Asia, Africa, Europe
1963	Dengue	Vietnam, India, Caribbean
1964	Rubella	United States
	Encephalitis	Houston
	Dengue	Thailand, India, Caribbean
1964–65	Influenza	Russia
1965	Plague	New Mexico
	Yellow Fever	Senegal
	Dengue	India
1965–67	Smallpox	Indonesia
1967	Smallpox	Guinea
	Marburg Virus	Germany
1967–71	Smallpox	Brazil
1967–72	Meningitis	South Africa, Morocco
1968	Influenza	Hong Kong
1968–69	Influenza	Russia, United States, Britain, Taiwan
	Malaria	Sri Lanka
	Dengue	Caribbean, Vietnam
	Poliomyelitis	Vietnam

Timetable of Plague and Pestilence (*continued*)

Date	Disease	Locality
1969–70	Dysentery	Guatemala
	Influenza	Papua New Guinea
1969–71	Conjunctivitis	Africa, Asia
1970–72	Dengue	Burma
	Cholera	West Africa, Mali, Chad
1970–72	Smallpox	Afghanistan
1971	Cholera	India, Bangladesh
	Conjunctivitis	India, Singapore
1971–72	Poliomyelitis	Malaysia
	Dengue	Southwest Pacific
1971–73	Smallpox	Bangladesh
	Dengue	Fiji Islands
1973–74	Smallpox	India
	Dengue	Singapore
1974–75	Malaria	India
	Cholera	Kenya
	Dengue	Southwest Pacific
	Kala-azar	India
1976	Legionnaires' Disease	Philadelphia
	Ebola	Zaire
1976–78	Dengue	Southwest Pacific, Thailand
1977	Rift Valley Fever	Egypt
1977–78	Influenza	China, Russia, North and South America, Australia, Europe
	Encephalitis	India
1978	Cholera	Maldive Islands
1979–80	Kala-azar	India
	Ross River Fever	Southwest Pacific
	Dengue	China, Southwest Pacific
1980	Conjunctivitis	Singapore
1981	Kala-azar	India
1983	Plague	Ecuador
1986–88	Hepatitis	Xinjiang (China)
1986–90	Yellow Fever	Nigeria
1987–90s	AIDS	Africa, United States, Europe, Asia . . . worldwide
1988	Hepatitis	Shanghai
1988–93	Leishmaniasis (Kala-azar)	Sudan
1989–91	Cholera	Africa
1991–92	Cholera	Peru . . . Latin America
1992	Plague	Zaire
	Meningitis	Burundi
1992–93	Diphtheria	Russia
1994	Cholera	Zaire—Rwandan refugees
	Plague	India

BIBLIOGRAPHY

Ackerknecht, Erwin H. *History and Geography of the Most Important Diseases*. New York: Hafner, 1965.

———. *A Short History of Medicine*. New York: Ronald Press, 1955.

Ackerman, Evelyn Bernette. *Health Care in the Parisian Countryside, 1800–1914*. New Brunswick, N.J.: Rutgers University Press, 1990.

Ackroyd, W. R. *Conquest of Deficiency Diseases*. Geneva: World Health Organization, 1970.

Adams, George W. *Doctors in Blue: The Medical History of the Union Army in the Civil War*. New York: Collier Books, 1952.

Afzal, Mohammad. *The Population of Pakistan*. Islamabad: Pakistan Institute of Development Economics, 1974.

Akhtar, Rais, and Learmonth, A. T. A., eds. *Geographical Aspects of Health and Disease in India*. New Delhi: Concept, 1985.

Alarcon, O. J. "La Peste Bubonica: Problema de Urgente Resolucion." *Revista Ecuatoriana de Higiene y Medicina Tropical*, 15:1958.

Alexander, John T. *Bubonic Plague in Early Modern Russia: Public Health and Urban Disaster*. Baltimore: Johns Hopkins University Press, 1980.

Alivizator, Gerasimos P. *The Early Smallpox Epidemics in Europe*. Athens: University of Athens, 1950.

Altman, Robert K. "Malaria Surges in India Despite Vast Drive." *The New York Times*, October 6, 1975.

Anderson, R. M., and May, R. M., eds. *Population Biology of Infectious Diseases*. Berlin: Springer-Verlag, 1982.

Andrews, Frederick W., et al. *Diphtheria: Its Bacteriology, Pathology and Immunology*. London: His Majesty's Stationery Office, 1923.

Anna, Timothy. *The Fall of the Royal Government of Mexico City*. Lincoln: University of Nebraska Press, 1978.

Ansari, N., ed. *Epidemiology and Control of Schistosomiasis (Bilharziasis)*. Baltimore: University Park Press, 1973.

Arbuthnot, John. *An Essay Concerning the Effects of the Air on Human Bodies*. London: J. Tonson, 1733.

Arjona Castro, Antonio. *La población de Córdoba en el siglo XIX*. Córdoba, Spain: Universidad Instituto de Historia de Andalucia, 1979.

Armstrong, Edward. *The Emperor Charles V*. London: Macmillan, 1902.

Arno, Peter S., and Feiden, Karyn L. *Against the Odds: The Story of AIDS Drug Development, Politics and Profits*. New York: HarperCollins, 1992.

Arnold, David. "Cholera and Colonialism in British India." *Past and Present: A Journal of Historical Studies*, 113 (November 1986): 11.

———. "Cholera Mortality in British India, 1817–1947," in *Imperialism, Health and Medicine*. Farmingdale, N.Y.: Baywood, 1981.

———. ed. *Imperial Medicine and Indigenous Societies*. Manchester, England: Manchester University Press, 1988.

Ashburn, P. M. *The Ranks of Death: A Medical History of the Conquest of America*. New York: Coward-McCann, 1947.

Astor, Gerald. *The Disease Detectives*. New York: New American Library, 1985.

Aveling, Harry, ed. *The Development of Indonesian Society*. New York: St. Martin's Press, 1980.

Aykroyd, W. R. *The Conquest of Famine*. New York: Reader's Digest, 1975.

Ayuntamiento de Barcelona. *Datos históricos sobre las epidemias de peste ocurridas en Barcelona*, vol. 15. Barcelona: Instituto Municipal de Historia, 1965.

Bacellar, Renato Clark. *Brazil's Contribution to Tropical Medicine and Malaria: Personalities and Institutions*, tr. Anita Farquhar. Rio de Janeiro: Gráfica Olimpica Editôra, 1963.

Bailey, Norman T. J. *The Biomathematics of Malaria*. High Wycombe, England: Charles Griffin, 1982.

Baird, Henry Martyn. *The Huguenots and Henry of Navarre*. New York: Scribner, 1903.

Baldwin, Marshall W. *Alexander III and the Twelfth Century*. Glen Rock, N.J.: Newman Press, 1968.

Ballesteros Rodríguez, Juan. *La peste en Córdoba*. Córdoba, Spain: Publicaciones de la EXCMA, Disputación Provincial, 1982.

Bannister, Barbara A. *Infectious Diseases*. London: Baillière Tindall, 1983.

Bantug, Jose P. *A Short History of Medicine in the Philippines During the Spanish Regime, 1565–1898*. Manila: Colegio Medico-Farmaceutico de Filipinas, 1953.

Barclay, George W. *Colonial Development and Population in Taiwan*. Princeton, N.J.: Princeton University Press, 1954.

Barger, George. *Ergot and Ergotism*. London: Gurney and Jackson, 1931.

Barrett, Tony, and Blaikie, Piers, eds. *Aids in Africa: Its Present and Future Impact*. London: Belhaven Press, 1992.

Barua, Dhiman, and Burrows, William, eds. *Cholera*. Philadelphia: W. B. Saunders, 1974.

Bassett, Charlotte A. "Yellow Fever," in *Collier's Encyclopedia*. New York: Macmillan, 1989.

Baxby, Derrick. *Jenner's Smallpox Vaccine: The Riddle of Vaccinia Virus and Its Origin*. London: Heinemann Educational Books, 1981.

Bayne-Jones, Stanhope. *The Evolution of Preventive Medicine in the United States Army, 1607–1939*. Washington, D.C.: Office of the Surgeon General, Department of the Army, 1968.

Bedson, Sir Samuel Phillips, et al., eds. *Virus and Rickettsial Diseases of Man*. London: Edward Arnold, 1967.

Behbehani, Abbas Meshkat. *The Smallpox Story: In Words and Pictures*. Kansas City: University of Kansas Medical Center, 1988.

Bell, Walter George. *The Great Plague in London in 1665*. London: John Lane, The Bodley Head, 1924.

Benecke, G. *Society and Politics in Germany, 1500–1750*. London: Routledge and Kegan Paul, 1974.

Benenson, Abram S., ed. *Control of Communicable Diseases in Man*. Washington, D.C.: American Public Health Association, 1985.

Bennassar, Bartolomé. *Recherches sur les grandes épidémies dans le norde de l'Espagne à la fin du XVI siècle*. Paris: S.E.V.P.E.N., 1969.

Bernkopf, H., et al. "Isolation of West Nile Virus in Israel." *The Journal of Infectious Diseases*, 93 (September–October 1953): 207–18.

Berry, Virginia G. "The Second Crusade," in *A History of the Crusades*, ed. Kenneth M. Setton, vol. 1. Madison: University of Wisconsin Press, 1969.

Bett, Walter R. *The History and Conquest of Common Diseases*. Norman: University of Oklahoma Press, 1954.

Beveridge, William Ian B. *Influenza: The Last Great Plague: An Unfinished Story of Discovery*. New York: Prodist, 1977.

Bhatia, B. M. *Famines in India: A Study in Some Aspects of the Economic History of India (1860–1965)*. London: Asia Publishing House, 1963.

Billings, Malcolm. *The Cross and the Crescent: A History of the Crusades*. New York: Sterling, 1988.

Biraben, Jean-Noel. "Certain Demographic Characteristics of the Plague Epidemic in France, 1720–1722." *Daedalus*, 97 (1968): 536–45.

———. *Les hommes et la peste en France et dans les pays Européens et Méditerranéens*, vol. 1: *La peste dans l'histoire*; vol. 2: *Les hommes face à la peste*. Paris: Mouton, 1975.

Blake, John B. *Benjamin Waterhouse and the Introduction of Vaccination*. Philadelphia: University of Pennsylvania Press, 1957.

———. *Public Health in the Town of Boston, 1630–1822*. Cambridge, Mass.: Harvard University Press, 1959.

Boak, Arthur E. R. *A History of Rome to 565 A.D.*, 4th ed. New York: Macmillan, 1955.

Boase, T. S. R. *Death in the Middle Ages*. New York: McGraw-Hill, 1972.

Boccaccio, Giovanni. *The Decameron*, tr. G. H. McWilliam. Middlesex, England: Penguin, 1970.

Bollet, Alfred Jay. *Plagues and Poxes: The Rise and Fall of Epidemic Disease*. New York: Demos, 1987.

Booss, John, and Esiri, Margaret M. *Viral Encephalitis: Pathology, Diagnosis and Management*. Oxford: Blackwell Scientific Publications, 1986.

Botsford, George Willis, and Robinson, Charles A., Jr. *A Hellenic History*, 4th ed. New York: Macmillan, 1956.

Boutier, Jean; Dewerpe, Alain; and Nordman, Daniel. *Un tour de France royal: le voyage de Charles IX, 1564–1566*. Paris: Aubier, 1984.

Bove, Frank James. *The Story of Ergot*. New York: S. Karger, 1970.

Bowsky, William M., ed. *The Black Death*. Huntington, N.Y.: Robert E. Krieger, 1978.

Boyce, D. George. *Modern Ireland: The Search for Stability*. Dublin: Gill and Macmillan, 1990.

Boyd, M. F. *Malariology: A Comprehensive Survey of all Aspects of this Group of Diseases from a Global Standpoint*, 2 vols. Philadelphia: W. B. Saunders, 1949.

Bradford, William. *Of Plymouth Plantation*, notes and intro. Samuel Eliot Morison. New York: Knopf, 1952.

Bradley, W. H. "Discussion: Influenza 1951." *Proceedings of the Royal Society of Medicine*, 44 (September 1951): 789–804.

Brandi, Karl. *The Emperor Charles V*, tr. C. V. Wedgwood. London: Jonathan Cape, 1963.

Breakey, Gail F., and Voulgaropoulous, Emmanuel. *Laos Health Survey: Mekong Valley, 1968–69*. Honolulu: University Press of Hawaii, 1976.

Breman, J. G.; Alecaut, A. B.; and Lane, J. M. "Smallpox in the Republic of Guinea, West Africa. 1. History and Epidemiology." *The American Journal of Tropical Medicine and Hygiene*, 26 (July 1977): 756–64.

Brett-James, Antony. *Europe against Napoleon: The Leipzig Campaign, 1813, from Eyewitness Accounts*. London, Macmillan, 1970.

Briggs, Robin. *Early Modern France, 1560–1715*. Oxford: Oxford University Press, 1977.

Brilliant, Lawrence B. *The Management of Smallpox Eradication in India*. Ann Arbor: University of Michigan Press, 1985.

Brinkley, Capt. F. *A History of the Japanese People*. London: Encyclopaedia Britannica, 1915.

Brody, S. N. *The Disease of the Soul: Leprosy in Medieval Literature*. Ithaca, N.Y.: Cornell University Press, 1974.

Brothwell, Don, and Sandison, A. T., eds. *Diseases in Antiquity*. Springfield, Ill.: Charles C. Thomas, 1967.

Browning, Robert. *Justinian and Theodora*. London: Thames and Hudson, 1987.

Bruce-Chwatt, Leonard Jan. *Essential Malariology*. New York: Wiley Medical, 1985.

———. "The Lisbon Story." *Bulletin of the National Society of India for Malaria and other Mosquito-borne Diseases*, 7 (January 1959): 15–26.

———. "Malaria Research and Eradication in the USSR." *Bulletin of the World Health Organization*, 21 (1959): 737–72.

———. *The Rise and Fall of Malaria in Europe: A Historico-Epidemiological Study*. Oxford: Oxford University Press, 1980.

Brundage, James A. *Crusades: A Documentary Survey*. Milwaukee: Marquette University Press, 1962.

Burkholder, Mark A., and Johnson, Lyman A. *Colonial Latin America*. New York: Oxford University Press, 1990.

Burnet, F. M. *Viruses and Man*. Harmondsworth, England: Penguin, 1953.

Burnet, F. M., and Clarke, Ellen. *Influenza: A Survey of the Last Fifty Years in the Light of Modern Work on the Virus of Epidemic Influenza*. Melbourne, Australia: Macmillan, 1942.

Burnet, Sir MacFarlane, and White, David O. *Natural History of Infectious Disease*, 4th ed. Cambridge, England: Cambridge University Press, 1972.

Burrows, Edmund H. *A History of Medicine in South Africa*. Cape Town: A. A. Balkema, 1958.

Burt, Alfred LeRoy. *The Old Province of Quebec*. Minneapolis: University of Minnesota Press, 1933.

Bury, J. B. *A History of the Later Roman Empire, from Arcadius to Irene*. Chicago: Argonaut, 1967; reprint of 1889 ed.

———. *History of the Later Roman Empire, from the Death of Theodosius I to the Death of Justinian*. New York: Dover, 1958; reprint of 1923 ed.

Bury, J. B., and Meiggs, Russell. *A History of Greece*, 4th ed. New York: St. Martin's Press, 1975.

Butler, Thomas. *Plague and Other Yersinia Infections*. New York: Plenum Medical Books, 1983.

Byrne, F. J., et al., eds. *A New History of Ireland*, vol. 3. Oxford: Clarendon Press, 1976.

Cahill, Kevin M. *Health on the Horn of Africa*. London: Spottiswoode, Ballantyne, 1969.

Cambridge Ancient History, 3rd ed. London: Cambridge University Press, 1970.

Campbell, A. M. *The Black Death and Men of Learning*. New York: Columbia University Press, 1931.

Campbell, Bruce M. S., ed. *Before the Black Death: Studies in the "Crisis" of the Early Fourteenth Century*. Manchester, England: Manchester University Press, 1991.

Camus, Albert. *The Plague*, tr. Stuart French. New York: Knopf, 1969.

Canard, Jean. *Les pestes en Beaujolais, Forez, Jarez, Lyonnais du XIVème au XVIIIème siècle*. Régny: L'Abbaye de Pradines, 1979.

Carey, Mathew. *A Short Account of the Malignant Fever, Lately Prevalent in Philadelphia*. New York: Ayer, 1970; reprint of 1794 ed.

Carmichael, Ann G. *Plague and the Poor in Renaissance Florence*. Cambridge, England: Cambridge University Press, 1986.

Carreras Panchón, Antonio. *La peste y los médicos en la España del renacimiento*. Salamanca, Spain: Universidad de Salmanca, 1976.

Carroll, Vern, ed. *Pacific Atoll Populations*. Honolulu: University Press of Hawaii, 1975.

Cartwright, Frederick F. *Disease and History*. New York: Thomas Y. Crowell, 1972.

———. "Pandemics Past and Future," in *Disease in Ancient Man*, ed. Gerald D. Hart. Toronto: Clarke Irwin, 1983.

Cary, M., and Scullard, H. H. *A History of Rome Down to the Reign of Constantine*, 3rd ed. New York: Macmillan, 1979.

Cassen, R. H. *India: Population, Economy and Society*. New York: Holmes and Meier, 1978.

Castiglioni, Arturo. *A History of Medicine*, tr. E. B. Krumbhaar. New York: Jason Aronson, 1969.

Caughey, J. E., and Porteous, W. M. "An Epidemic of Poliomyelitis Occurring among Troops in the Middle East." *The Medical Journal of Australia*, 1 (1946): 5–10.

Caulaincourt, Armand de. *With Napoleon in Russia*. New York: Grosset and Dunlap, 1935.

Centers for Disease Control, U.S. *Morbidity and Mortality Weekly Report*, various issues, 1952–94.

Chambers, J. S. *The Conquest of Cholera.* New York: Macmillan, 1938.

Charbonneau, Hubert, and LaRose, André, eds. *The Great Mortalities: Methodological Studies of Demographic Crises in the Past.* Liège, Belgium: Ordina Editions, 1979.

Chase, Allen. *Magic Shots.* New York: William Morrow, 1982.

Chess, Stella; Korn, Sam; and Fernandez, Paulina. *Psychiatric Disorders of Children with Congenital Rubella.* New York: Brunner/Mazel, 1971.

Chin-Hsien, Teng. "Adenovirus Pneumonia Epidemic Among Peking Infants and Preschool Children in 1958." *Chinese Medical Journal,* 80 (April 1960): 331–39.

"Cholera in Africa: Lessons on Transmission and Control for Latin America." *The Lancet,* 338 (September 28, 1991): 791–95

"Cholera—Worldwide, 1989." *The Journal of the American Medical Association,* 264 (July 25, 1990): 441.

Christophers, Major S. R. *Malaria in the Andamans.* Calcutta: Superintendent Government Printing, 1912.

———. *Malaria in the Punjab.* Calcutta: Superintendent Government Printing, 1911.

Chronicles of the Crusades. London: George Bell and Sons, 1903.

Cipolla, Carlo M. *Faith, Reason and the Plague in Seventeenth-Century Tuscany.* Ithaca, N.Y.: Cornell University Press, 1977.

———. *Fighting the Plague in Seventeenth-Century Italy.* Madison: University of Wisconsin Press, 1981.

Clark, Andrew Hill. *The Invasion of New Zealand by People, Plants and Animals.* Westport, Conn.: Greenwood Press, 1970.

Clark, John I., et al., eds. *Population and Disaster.* Oxford: Basil Blackwell, 1989.

Cliff, Andrew D., and Haggett, Peter. *Atlas of Disease Distributions.* Oxford: Basil Blackwell, 1988.

Cloudsley-Thompson, J. L. *Insects and History.* New York: St. Martin's Press, 1976.

Cluver, E. H. *Public Health in South Africa.* Johannesburg: Central News Agency, 1944.

Clyde, David F. *History of the Medical Services of Tanganyika.* Dar es Salaam, Tanzania: Government Press, 1962.

———. *Malaria in Tanzania.* London: Oxford University Press, 1967.

Cochrane, Eric. *Florence in the Forgotten Centuries, 1527–1800: A History of Florence and the Florentines in the Age of the Grand Dukes.* Chicago: University of Chicago Press, 1973.

Colbourne, Michael. *Malaria in Africa.* London: Oxford University Press, 1966.

Coleman, William. *Yellow Fever in the North: The Methods of Early Epidemiology.* Madison: University of Wisconsin Press, 1987.

Collier, Richard. *The Plague of the Spanish Lady: The Influenza Pandemic of 1918–19.* New York: Atheneum, 1974.

Collins, Richard N., et al. "Plague Epidemic in New Mexico, 1965." *Public Health Reports,* 82 (December 1967):1077–99.

Connelly, Owen. *Blundering to Glory: Napoleon's Military Campaigns.* Wilmington, Del.: Scholarly Resources, 1987.

Cook, Noale David, and Lovell, W. George, eds. *Secret Judgments of God: Old World Disease in Colonial Spanish America.* Norman: University of Oklahoma Press, 1991.

Cook, S. F. "The Smallpox Epidemic of 1797 in Mexico." *Journal of the History of Medicine,* 7 (October 1939):937–69.

Cooper, Michael S. J., ed. *They Came to Japan: An Anthology of European Reports on Japan, 1543–1640.* Berkeley: University of California Press, 1965.

Cope, V. Zachary, ed. *History of the Second World War: Medicine and Pathology.* London: Her Majesty's Stationery Office, 1952.

Corley, T. A. B. *Democratic Despot: A Life of Napoleon III.* London: Barrie and Rockliff, 1961.

Cornell, James C., Jr. *The Great International Disaster Book.* New York: Scribner, 1976.

Corsi, Pietro, and Weindling, Paul, eds. *Information Sources in the History of Science and Medicine.* London: Butterworth Scientific, 1983.

Cossart, Yvonne E. *Virus Hepatitis and Its Control.* London: Baillière Tindall, 1977.

Covell, G., and Baily, J. D. "Malaria in Sind" and "The Study of a Regional Epidemic of Malaria in Northern Sind." *Records of the Malaria Survey of India,* 2 (June 1935).

Cowley, Geoffrey A. "The Great Disease Migration." *Newsweek,* 118 (Fall–Winter 1991):54.

Craton, Michael. *A History of the Bahamas.* London: Collins, 1962.

Crawfurd, Raymond. *Plague and Pestilence in Literature and Art.* Oxford: Clarendon Press, 1914.

Creighton, Charles. *A History of Epidemics in Britain,* 2 vols., 2nd ed. London: Frank Cass, 1965.

Croll, Neil A., and Cross, John H., eds. *Human Ecology and Infectious Diseases.* New York: Academic Press, 1983.

Crompton, D. W. T.; Nesheim, M. C.; and Pawlowshi, Z. S., eds. *Ascariasis and Its Public Health Significance.* London: Taylor and France, 1985.

Crosby, Alfred W. *America's Forgotten Pandemic: The Influenza of 1918.* Cambridge, England: Cambridge University Press, 1989.

———. *Ecological Imperialism: The Biological Expansion*

of Europe, 900–1900. New York: Cambridge University Press, 1986.

———. *Epidemic and Peace, 1918.* Westport, Conn.: Greenwood Press, 1976.

Cross, A. B. "The Solomon Islands Tragedy: A Tale of Epidemic Poliomyelitis." *Medical History,* 21 (April 1977):137–55.

Cross, Neil A., and Cross, John H., eds. *Human Ecology and Infectious Diseases.* New York: Academic Press, 1983.

Crow, John A. *The Epic of Latin America.* Garden City, N.Y.: Doubleday, 1971.

Cruls, Gastão. *Aparência do Rio de Janeiro,* 2 vols. Rio de Janeiro: Livraria José Olympio Editôra, 1965.

Currey, Bruce, and Hugo, Graeme, eds. *Famine as a Geographical Phenomenon.* Dordrecht, Netherlands: D. Reidel, 1984.

Curson, P. H. *Times of Crisis: Epidemics in Sydney, 1788–1900.* Sydney: Sydney University Press, 1985.

Daiches, David. *Edinburgh.* London: Hamish Hamilton, 1978.

Darrell, Richard W., ed. *Viral Diseases of the Eye.* Philadelphia: Lea and Febiger, 1985.

Da Silva Araújo, Carlos. *Fatos e personagens da historia da medicina e da farmacia no Brasil,* 2 vols. Rio de Janeiro: Revista Continente Editorial, 1979.

Davey, T. H., and Wilson, T. *The Control of Disease in the Tropics.* London: H. K. Lewis, 1965.

Davies, C. W., et al. "An Epidemic of Louse-Borne Relapsing Fever in Kenya." *Transactions of the Royal Society of Tropical Medicine and Hygiene,* 41 (September 1947):141–70.

Davis, Kingsley. *The Population of India and Pakistan.* Princeton, N.J.: Princeton University Press, 1951.

Davis, Natalie Zemon. *Society and Culture in Early Modern France.* Stanford, Calif.: Stanford University Press, 1975.

Daws, Gavan. *Shoal of Time: A History of the Hawaiian Islands.* Honolulu: University Press of Hawaii, 1968.

De, S. N. *Cholera: Its Pathology and Pathogenesis.* Edinburgh: Oliver and Boyd, 1961.

Debré, Robert. "Lethargic Encephalitis or von Economo's Disease," in *Clinical Virology: The Evaluation and Management of Human Viral Infections,* ed. Robert Debré and Josette Celers. Philadelphia: W. B. Saunders, 1970.

Dedijer, Vladimir, et al. *History of Yugoslavia.* New York: McGraw-Hill, 1974.

Defoe, Daniel. *A Journal of the Plague Year.* Harmondsworth, England: Penguin, 1966; originally published in 1722.

Delumeau, Jean, and Lequin, Yves. *Les malheurs des temps: histoire des fléaux et des calamités en France.* Paris: Librairie Larousse, 1987.

Desowitz, Robert S. *The Malaria Capers: More Tales of Parasites and People, Research and Reality.* New York: W. W. Norton, 1991.

de Vinsauf, Geoffrey. *The Itinerary of Richard I and Others to the Holy Land,* in *Chronicles of the Crusades.* London: George Bell and Sons, 1903.

Dickinson, W. C. *A New History of Scotland,* vol. 1. London: T. Nelson, 1961.

Dio Cassius. *Roman History,* tr. Earnest Cary. New York: Macmillan, 1954; Loeb edition.

Diodorus Siculus. *The Library of History,* tr. C. H. Oldfather. Cambridge, Mass.: Harvard University Press, 1954; Loeb edition.

Dionysius of Halicarnassus. *Roman Antiquities,* tr. Earnest Cary. Cambridge, Mass.: Harvard University Press, 1947; Loeb edition.

Disease and Society in Provincial Massachusetts: Collected Accounts, 1736–1939. New York: Arno Press, 1972.

Dixon, C. W. *Smallpox.* London: J. and A. Churchill, 1962.

Dobyns, Henry F. *Their Number Becomes Thinned: Native American Dynamics in Eastern North America.* Knoxville: University of Tennessee Press, 1983.

Dohm, Karsten. *Die Typhusepidemie in der Festung Torgau, 1813–1814.* Düsseldorf: Triltsch, 1987.

Dols, Michael W. *The Black Death in the Middle East.* Princeton, N.J.: Princeton University Press, 1977.

Donovan, J. W. "A Study in New Zealand Mortality: 6, Epidemic Diseases." *New Zealand Medical Journal,* 70 (December 1969):406.

Dowling, Harry F. *Fighting Infection: Conquests of the Twentieth Century.* Cambridge, Mass.: Harvard University Press, 1977.

Dubos, René. *Man Adapting.* New Haven, Conn.: Yale University Press, 1965.

Duffy, John. *Epidemics in Colonial America.* Baton Rouge: Louisiana State University Press, 1971.

———. *A History of Public Health in New York City, 1625–1866.* New York: Russell Sage Foundation, 1968.

———. *A History of Public Health in New York City, 1866–1966.* New York: Russell Sage Foundation, 1968.

———. *The Sanitarians: A History of American Public Health.* Urbana: University of Illinois Press, 1990.

Dunn, Frederick L. "Pandemic Influenza in 1957: Review of International Spread of New Asian Strain." *The Journal of the American Medical Association,* 166 (March 8, 1958): 1140–48.

Dyson, Tim, ed. *India's Historical Demography: Studies in Famine, Disease and Society,* Collected Papers on South Asia No. 8. Riverdale, Md.: Riverdale Company, 1989.

Ecke, D. H.; Johnson, C. W.; Miles, V. I.; Wilcomb, M. J.; and Irons, J. V. *Plague in Colorado and Texas,*

Public Health Monograph No. 6. Washington, D.C.: Government Printing Office, 1952.

Economo, Constantin von. *Encephalitis Lethargica: Its Sequelae and Treatment.* London: Oxford University Press, 1931.

Edwardes, Edward J. *A Concise History of Smallpox and Vaccination in Europe.* London: H. K. Lewis, 1902.

Ehrenkranz, N. Joel, et al. "Pandemic Dengue in Caribbean Countries and the Southern United States: Past, Present and Potential Problems." *The New England Journal of Medicine,* 285 (December 23, 1971):1160–69.

Elgood, Cyril. *A Medical History of Persia and the Eastern Caliphate.* Cambridge, England: Cambridge University Press, 1951.

Erlanger, Steven. "Diphtheria in Russia Worsens, Killing 100 in '93." *The New York Times,* August 22, 1993.

Eusebius. *The Ecclesiastical History and the Martyrs of Palestine,* tr. Hugh Jackson Lawlor and John Ernest Leonard Oulton. New York: Macmillan, 1928.

Evans, Alfred S., ed. *Viral Infections of Humans: Epidemiology and Control.* New York: Plenum Medical Books, 1989.

Evans, Alfred S., and Brachman, Philip S., eds. *Bacterial Infections of Humans: Epidemiology and Control,* 2nd ed. New York: Plenum Medical Books, 1991.

Evans, Alfred S., and Feldman, Harry A., eds. *Bacterial Infections of Humans: Epidemiology and Control.* New York: Plenum Medical Books, 1982.

Evans, Richard J. *Death in Hamburg: Society and Politics in the Cholera Years, 1830–1910.* Oxford: Clarendon Press, 1987.

Farley, John. *Bilharzia: A History of Imperial Tropical Medicine.* Cambridge, England: Cambridge University Press, 1991.

Farris, William Wayne. *Population, Disease, and Land in Early Japan, 645–900.* Cambridge, Mass.: Harvard University Press, 1985.

Farthing, M. J. G., and Keusch, G. T., eds. *Enteric Infection: Mechanisms, Manifestations and Management.* New York: Raven Press, 1988.

Fehrenbach, T. R. *Fire and Blood: A History of Mexico.* New York: Macmillan, 1973.

Felsenfeld, Oscar. "Some Observations on the Cholera (El Tor) Epidemic in 1961–62." *Bulletin of the World Health Organization,* 28 (1963):289–96.

Fenner, F., et al. *Smallpox and Its Eradication.* Geneva: World Health Organization, 1988.

Fernández, Antonio. *Epidemias y sociedad en Madrid.* Barcelona: Vicens-Vives, 1985.

Fezensac, M. de. *The Russian Campaign, 1812,* tr. Lee Kennett. Athens: University of Georgia Press, 1970.

Field, Mark G. *Soviet Socialized Medicine: An Introduction.* New York: Free Press, 1967.

Fifth International Congresses on Tropical Medicine and Malaria. Istanbul, Turkey, 1953.

Fleming, William L. "Syphilis Through the Ages." *The Medical Clinics of North America,* 48 (May 1964):587–612.

Flinn, M. W., ed. *The Sanitary Condition of the Labouring Population of Gt. Britain by Edwin Chadwick 1842.* Edinburgh, Scotland: University Press, 1965.

Ford, John. *The Role of Trypanosomiasis in African Ecology.* Oxford: Clarendon Press, 1971.

Foster, Michael, and Gaskell, J. F. *Cerebro-Spinal Fever.* Cambridge, England: Cambridge University Press, 1916.

Foster, R. F. *Modern Ireland, 1600–1972.* London: Penguin Press, 1988.

Fourth International Congresses on Tropical Medicine and Malaria, Abstracts. Washington, D.C.: Department of State, 1948.

Frank, Tenney. *A History of Rome.* New York: Henry Holt, 1923.

Franzius, Enno. *History of the Byzantine Empire.* New York: Funk and Wagnalls, 1967.

Fraser, D. W., et al. "Legionnaires' Disease: Description of an Epidemic of Pneumonia." *The New England Journal of Medicine,* 297 (December 1, 1977):1189–97.

Fraser, Walter J. *Charleston! Charleston! The History of a Southern City.* Columbia: University of South Carolina Press, 1989.

Frazer, W. M. *A History of English Public Health, 1834–1939.* London: Baillière, Tindall and Cox, 1950.

Freyre, Gilberto. *The Mansions and the Shanties,* tr. and ed. Harriet de Onís. New York: Knopf, 1963.

Frieden, Nancy M. *Russian Physicians in an Era of Reform and Revolution, 1856–1905.* Princeton, N.J.: Princeton University Press, 1981.

Fuentes, Patricia de, ed. and tr. *The Conquistadors.* New York: Orion, 1963.

Fujikawa, Yu. *Japanese Medicine.* New York: Paul B. Hoeber, 1934.

Fukumi, Hideo. "Summary Report on the Asian Influenza Epidemic in Japan, 1957." *Bulletin of the World Health Organization,* 20 (1959):187–98.

Fuller, John G. *Fever: The Hunt for a New Killer Virus.* New York: Reader's Digest Press, 1974.

Furman, Bess. *A Profile of the United States Public Health Service, 1798–1948.* Washington, D.C.: U.S. Department of Health, Education and Welfare, 1973.

Furnivall, J. S. *Netherlands India: A Study of Plural Economy.* New York: Macmillan, 1944.

Gabrieli, Francesco, ed. and tr. *Arab Historians of the Crusades*. Berkeley: University of California Press, 1969.

Gad, Finn. *History of Greenland*. Montreal: McGill-Queen's University Press, 1973.

Galdston, Iago, ed. *Man's Image in Medicine and Anthropology*. New York: International Universities Press, 1963.

Gallagher, Nancy Elizabeth. *Egypt's Other Wars: Epidemics and the Politics of Public Health*. Syracuse, N.Y.: Syracuse University Press, 1990.

———. *Epidemics in the Regency of Tunis, 1780–1880: A Study in the Special History of Medicine*. Los Angeles: University of California Press, 1978.

———. *Medicine and Power in Tunisia, 1780–1900*. New York: Cambridge University Press, 1983.

Gallagher, Richard. *Diseases that Plague Modern Man: A History of Ten Communicable Diseases*. Dobbs Ferry, N.Y.: Oceana, 1969.

Gardner, Brian. *The East India Company: A History*. New York: McCall, 1971.

Garrett, Laurie. *The Coming Plague: Newly Emerging Diseases in a World Out of Balance*. New York: Farrar, Straus and Giroux, 1994.

Garrison, Fielding H. *An Introduction to the History of Medicine*. Philadelphia: W. B. Saunders, 1929.

Gear, J. H. S. "South African Typhus." *South African Journal of Medical Sciences*, 3 (1938):134–60.

Geggus, David. *Slavery, War and Revolution: The British Occupation of St. Domingue, 1793–1798*. New York: Oxford University Press, 1982.

Gelfand, Michael. *Northern Rhodesia in the Days of the Charter*. Oxford: Basil Blackwell, 1961.

———. *The Sick African*, 2nd ed. Cape Town: Juta, 1957.

Gelfand, Michael, and Laidler, Percy Ward. *South Africa: Its Medical History, 1652–1898*. Cape Town: C. Struik, 1971.

Geoffrey de Vinsauf. *The Itinerary of Richard I and Others to the Holy Land*, in *Chronicles of the Crusades*. London: George Bell and Sons, 1903.

Gerrard, Nelson S. *The Icelandic Heritage*. Arborg, Manitoba: Sage, 1986.

Gibbon, Edward. *The History of the Decline and Fall of the Roman Empire*, ed. J. B. Bury. London: Methuen, 1911; first published, 1776–88.

Gill, Clifford A. *The Genesis of Epidemics*. London: Baillière, Tindall and Cox, 1928.

Gilman, Sander L. *Disease and Representation: Images of Illness from Madness to AIDS*. Ithaca, N.Y.: Cornell University Press, 1988.

Gjerset, Knut. *History of Iceland*. New York: Macmillan, 1924.

Gluckman, L. K. *Medical History of New Zealand Prior to 1860*. Auckland: Whitcoulls, 1976.

———. *Tangiwai: A Medical History of 19th-Century New Zealand*. Auckland: Whitcoulls, 1976.

González, Jesus Maiso. *La peste Argonese de 1648 a 1654*. Zaragoza, Spain: Universidad de Zaragoza, 1982.

Goodall, E. W. *A Short History of the Epidemic Infectious Diseases*. London: John Bale, 1934.

Gordon, Richard. *Great Medical Disasters*. New York: Stein and Day, 1983.

Gorgas, Marie D., and Hendrick, Burton J. *William Crawford Gorgas: His Life and Work*. New York: Doubleday, Page, 1924.

Gottfried, Robert S. *The Black Death*. New York: Free Press, 1983.

———. *Epidemic Disease in Fifteenth-Century England*. New Brunswick, N.J.: Rutgers University Press, 1978.

Goubert, Pierre. *The Course of French History*, tr. Maarten Utlee. New York: Franklin Watts, 1988.

Grant, Michael. *History of Rome*, rev. ed. London: Weidenfeld and Nicolson, 1978.

Grayston, J. Thomas. "Encephalitis on Taiwan." *The American Journal of Tropical Medicine and Hygiene*, 11 (January 1962):126–30.

Grayston, J. Thomas, et al. "The Epidemiology of Rubella on Taiwan." *International Journal of Epidemiology*, 1 (Autumn 1972):245–60.

Green, Irving J., et al. "The Epidemiology of Japanese Encephalitis Virus on Taiwan in 1961." *The American Journal of Tropical Medicine and Hygiene*, 12 (July 1963):668–74.

Greenwood, Major. *Epidemics and Crowd-Diseases: An Introduction to the Study of Epidemiology*. London: Williams and Norgate, 1935.

Gregg, Charles T. *Plague: An Ancient Disease in the Twentieth Century*. Albuquerque: University of New Mexico Press, 1985.

Gregorovius, Ferdinand. *History of the City of Rome in the Middle Ages*. New York: AMS Press, 1967; reprint of 1905 ed.

Gregory of Tours. *The History of the Franks*, tr. O. M. Dalton. Oxford: Clarendon Press, 1927.

Grist, Norman R., et al. *Diseases of Infection: An Illustrated Textbook*. Oxford: Oxford University Press, 1987.

Grmek, Mirko D. *Diseases in the Ancient Greek World*, tr. Mireille Muellner and Leonard Muellner. Baltimore: Johns Hopkins University Press, 1989.

Grossman, Richard. *The Other Medicines*. Garden City, N.Y.: Doubleday, 1985.

Grote, George. *A History of Greece*. New York: AMS Press, 1971; reprint of 1888 edition.

Grousset, Rene. *The Epic of the Crusades*. New York: Orion, 1970.

Gruenberg, Ernest M.; Lewis, Carol; and Goldston,

Stephen. *Vaccinating Against Brain Syndromes: The Campaign Against Measles and Rubella.* New York: Oxford University Press, 1986.

Guerard, Albert. *The Life and Death of an Ideal: France in the Classical Age.* New York: George Braziller, 1956.

Guerra, E. Sales. *Osvaldo Cruz.* Rio de Janeiro: Casa Editoria Vecchi, 1940.

Gundersheimer, Werner L., ed. *French Humanism, 1470–1600.* London: Macmillan, 1969.

Hadingham, Evan. *Lines to the Mountain Gods: Nazca and the Mysteries of Peru.* New York: Random House, 1987.

Haggard, Howard W. *Devils, Drugs, and Doctors.* Boston: Charles River Books, 1980; reprint of 1929 edition.

Hahon, Nicholas, ed. *Selected Papers on the Pathogenic Rickettsiae.* Cambridge, Mass.: Harvard University Press, 1968.

Haj, Fareed. *Disability in Antiquity.* New York: Philosophical Library, 1970.

Halasz, Zoltan. *A Short History of Hungary.* Hungary: Corvina Press, 1975.

Hale, J. H., et al. "Large-scale Use of Sabin Type 2 Attenuated Poliovirus Vaccine in Singapore during a Type 1 Polio Epidemic." *British Medical Journal,* 5137 (June 20, 1959):1041–49.

Hallett, Robin. *Africa Since 1875.* Ann Arbor: University of Michigan Press, 1974.

Halstead, Scott B. "Mosquito-borne Haemorrhagic Fevers of South and South-East Asia." *Bulletin of the World Health Organization,* 35 (1966):3–15.

Halstead, Scott B., et al. "Dengue Hemorrhagic Fever in South Vietnam: Report of the 1963 Outbreak." *The American Journal of Tropical Medicine and Hygiene,* 14 (September 1965):819–30.

Hammon, W. M., et al. "Epidemiologic Studies of Concurrent 'Virgin' Epidemics of Japanese B Encephalitis and of Mumps on Guam, 1947–48, with Subsequent Observations Including Dengue, Through 1957." *The American Journal of Tropical Medicine and Hygiene,* 7 (July 1958):441–67.

Hammond, N. G. L. *A History of Greece to 322 B.C.,* 3rd ed. Oxford: Clarendon Press, 1986.

Hampe, Karl. *Germany under the Salian and Hohenstaufen Emperors,* tr. Ralph Bennett. Oxford: Basil Blackwell, 1973.

Hanley, Susan B., and Wolf, Arthur P., eds. *Family and Population in East Asian History.* Stanford, Calif.: Stanford University Press, 1985.

Hansen, Peter. *Geschichte der Epidemien bei Menschen und Tieren im Norden.* Glückstadt, Germany: J. J. Augustin, 1925.

Hare, Ronald. "The Antiquity of Diseases Caused by Bacteria and Viruses: A Review of the Problem from a Bacteriologist's Point of View," in *Diseases in Antiquity,* ed. Don Brothwell and A. T. Sandison. Springfield, Ill.: Charles C. Thomas, 1967.

———. *Pomp and Pestilence.* London: Victor Gollancz, 1954.

Harrison, Gordon. *Mosquitoes, Malaria and Man: A History of the Hostilities Since 1880.* New York: E. P. Dutton, 1978.

Harrison's Principles of Internal Medicine, 11th ed. New York: McGraw-Hill, 1987.

Hartman, F. W., et al., eds. *Hepatitis Frontiers.* Henry Ford Hospital International Symposium. Boston: Little, Brown, 1957.

Hartwig, Gerald W., and Patterson, K. David. *Cerebrospinal Meningitis in West Africa and Sudan in the Twentieth Century.* Los Angeles: Crossroads Press, 1984.

———. *Disease in African History.* Durham, N.C.: Duke University Press, 1978.

Harvey, G. E. *History of Burma from the Earliest Times to 10 March 1924.* New York: Octagon Books, 1983.

Hastrup, Kirsten. *Nature and Policy in Iceland, 1400–1800.* Oxford: Clarendon Press, 1990.

Havens, W. Paul, Jr., ed. *Infectious Diseases,* vol. 2 of *Internal Medicine in World War II.* Washington, D.C.: Office of the Surgeon-General, Department of the Army, 1963.

———. "Viral Hepatitis." *U.S. Armed Forces Medical Journal,* 3 (July 1952):1013.

Heagerty, John J. *Four Centuries of Medical History in Canada, and a Sketch of the Medical History of Newfoundland,* 2 vols. Bristol, England: John Wright and Sons, 1928.

Health and Disease in Tribal Societies. New York: Ciba Foundation Symposium 49, 1977.

Heer, Friedrich. *The Holy Roman Empire,* tr. Janet Sondheimer. New York: Praeger, 1968.

Hehir, Sir Patrick. *Malaria in India.* London: Oxford University Press, 1927.

Heichelheim, Fritz; Yeo, Cedric; and Ward, Allen. *A History of the Roman People,* 2nd ed. Englewood Cliffs, N.J.: Prentice-Hall, 1984.

Heitland, W. E. *The Roman Republic.* Cambridge, England: Cambridge University Press, 1923.

Hemming, John. *The Conquest of the Incas.* New York: Harcourt Brace Jovanovich, 1970.

———. *Red Gold: The Conquest of the Brazilian Indians, 1500–1760.* Cambridge, Mass.: Harvard University Press, 1978.

Henig, Robin M. *A Dancing Matrix: Voyages Along the Viral Frontier.* New York: Knopf, 1993.

———. "Flu Pandemic." *The New York Times Magazine,* November 29, 1992.

Henschen, Folke. *The History and Geography of Diseases,* tr. Joan Tate. New York: Delacorte Press, 1962.

————. *The History of Diseases*, tr. Joan Tate. London: Longmans, 1966.

Heppell, Muriel, and Singleton, Frank B. *Yugoslavia*. New York: Praeger, 1961.

Herms, William B. *Malaria: Cause and Control*. New York: Macmillan, 1913.

Herodotus. *The Histories*, book 8, tr. Aubrey de Selincourt. New York: Penguin, 1972.

Herold, J. Christopher. *Bonaparte in Egypt*. New York: Harper and Row, 1962.

Hillier, S. M. and Jewell, J. A. *Health Care and Traditional Medicine in China, 1800–1982*. London: Routledge and Kegan Paul, 1983.

Hippocrates. *Epidemics*, tr. W. H. S. Jones. London: William Heinemann, 1923; Loeb edition.

————. *Hippocratic Writings*, tr. W. H. S. Jones. New York: Putnam, 1923; Loeb edition.

Hirsch, August. *Handbook on Geographical and Historical Pathology*, 3 vols, tr. from the 2nd German edition by Charles Creighton, M.D. London: New Sydenham Society, 1883 (vol. 1), 1885 (vol. 2), 1886 (vol. 3).

Hirst, L. Fabian. *The Conquest of Plague: A Study of the Evolution of Epidemiology*. Oxford: Clarendon Press, 1953.

Ho, Ping-ti. *Studies on the Population of China, 1368–1953*. Cambridge, Mass.: Harvard University Press, 1959.

Hobhouse, Henry. *Forces of Change: An Unorthodox View of History*. New York: Arcade, 1990.

Hobson, William. *World Health and History*. Bristol, England: John Wright and Sons, 1963.

Hoeprich, Paul D., ed. *Infectious Diseases: A Modern Treatise of Infectious Processes*, 3rd ed. New York: Harper and Row, 1983.

Hoff, Ebbe Curtis, ed. *Preventive Medicine in World War II*, vols. 4, 5, 6. Washington, D.C.: Office of the Surgeon-General, Department of the Army, 1958, 1960, 1963.

Hoffmann, Léon-François. *La peste a Barcelone*. Paris: Presses Universitaires de France, 1964.

Holmes, William H. *Bacillary and Rickettsial Infections: Acute and Chronic*. New York: Macmillan, 1940.

Holt, Mack P. *The Duke of Anjou and the Politique Struggle During the Wars of Religion*. Cambridge, England: Cambridge University Press, 1986.

Hookham, Hilda. *A Short History of China*. New York: New American Library, 1972.

Hopkins, Donald R. *Princes and Peasants: Smallpox in History*. Chicago: University of Chicago Press, 1983.

Hopkins, Jack W. *The Eradication of Smallpox*. Boulder, Colo.: Westview Press, 1989.

Hoppen, Theodore K. *Ireland since 1800: Conflict and Conformity*. London: Longman, 1989.

Horn, J. S. *Away with all Pests*. New York: Monthly Review Press, 1969.

Hornblower, Simon. *The Greek World, 479–323 B.C.* London: Methuen, 1983.

Horsfall, Frank L., and Rivers, Thomas M., eds. *Viral and Rickettsial Infections of Man*. Philadelphia: J. B. Lippincott, 1959.

Horsfall, Frank L., and Tamm, Igor, eds. *Viral and Rickettsial Infections of Man*. Philadelphia: J. B. Lippincott, 1965.

How, W. W., and Wells, J. *A Commentary on Herodotus*. London: Clarendon Press, 1928.

Howard, John. *Prisons and Lazarettos*, vol. 2. Montclair, N.J.: Patterson Smith, 1973; reprint of 1791 ed.

Howe, G. Melvyn, ed. *A World Geography of Human Diseases*. London: Academic Press, 1977.

Huard, Pierre, and Wong, Ming. *Chinese Medicine*, Bernard Fielding. London: Weidenfeld and Nicolson, 1968.

Hubbert, William T.; McCulloch, William F.; and Schnurrenberger, Paul R., eds. *Diseases Transmitted from Animals to Man*, 6th ed. Springfield, Ill.: Charles C. Thomas, 1975.

Huckstep, R. L. *Typhoid Fever*. Edinburgh: E. and S. Livingstone, 1962.

Hudson, Robert P. *Disease and Its Control: The Shaping of Modern Thought*. Westport, Conn.: Greenwood Press, 1983.

Hull, Thomas G. *Diseases Transmitted from Animals to Man*. Springfield, Ill.: Charles C. Thomas, 1930.

Hunter, William Wilson. *Annals of Rural Bengal*. London: Smith, Elder, 1897.

Hutchin, Elisabeth F. "Historical Summary," ch. 1 of *Poliomyelitis*, by the International Committee for the Study of Infantile Paralysis. Baltimore: Williams and Wilkins, 1932.

Hutchinson, John F. *Politics and Public Health in Revolutionary Russia, 1890–1918*. Baltimore: Johns Hopkins University Press, 1990.

Hutton, Edward. *The Cities of Lombardy*. London: Methuen, 1912.

Hyde, Gordon. *The Soviet Health Service: A Historical and Comparative Study*. London: Lawrence and Wishart, 1974.

Hyma, B., and Ramesh, A. *Cholera and Malaria Incidence in Tamil Nadu, India: Case Studies in Medical Geography*. Waterloo, Ontario: Department of Geography, University of Waterloo, 1977.

Imhof, Arthur, and Lindskog, Bengt J. "Les causes de mortalité en Suède et en Finlande entre 1749 et 1773." *Annales Economies, Sociétés, Civilisations*, 29 (July–August 1974).

Ingham, Kenneth. *A History of East Africa*. London: Cox and Wyman, 1962.

Inglis, Brian. *A History of Medicine.* Cleveland: World Publishing, 1965.

Ingram, Edward. *In Defense of British India: Great Britain in the Middle East, 1775–1842.* London: Frank Cass, 1984.

International Poliomyelitis Congress. *Poliomyelitis: Papers and Discussions Presented at the Third International Poliomyelitis Conference.* Philadelphia: J. B. Lippincott, 1955.

Isaacs, A., and Andrewes, C. H. "The Spread of Influenza." *British Medical Journal,* 4737 (October 20, 1951):921–27.

Isichei, Elizabeth. *A History of Nigeria.* New York: Longman, 1983.

Jamison, E. M., et al. *Italy, Medieval and Modern: A History.* Oxford: Clarendon Press, 1919.

Jannetta, Ann Bowman. *Epidemics and Mortality in Early Modern Japan.* Princeton, N.J.: Princeton University Press, 1987.

Jean de Joinville. *Memoirs of Saint Louis IX,* in *Chronicles of the Crusades.* London: George Bell and Sons, 1903.

Jelliffe, D. B., ed. *Diseases of Children in the Subtropics and Tropics.* London: Edwin Arnold, 1970.

Jenkins, Romilly. *Byzantium: The Imperial Centuries, A.D. 610–1071.* New York: Random House, 1966.

Jones, W. Glyn. *Denmark: A Modern History.* London: Croom Helm, 1986.

Jordan, Edwin O. *Epidemic Influenza: A Survey.* Chicago: American Medical Association, 1927.

Joseph, Stephen C. *Dragon Within the Gates: The Once and Future AIDS Epidemic.* New York: Carroll and Graf, 1992.

Kamen, Henry. "Economic and Social Consequences of the Thirty Years' War." *Past and Present: A Journal of Historical Studies,* 39 (April 1968):44–61.

Kammen, Michael G. *Colonial New York: A History.* New York: Scribner, 1975.

Keller, Hans Urs. *Die letzte grosse Epidemie von Suette Miliare.* Zurich: Juris Druck, 1970.

Kelly, Amy. *Eleanor of Aquitaine and the Four Kings.* Cambridge, Mass.: Harvard University Press, 1950.

Khairallah, Amin A. *Outline of Arabic Contributions to Medicine and the Allied Sciences.* Beirut, Lebanon: American Press, 1946.

Kilbourne, Edwin D. *Influenza.* New York: Plenum Medical Books, 1987.

———. *The Influenza Viruses and Influenza.* New York: Academic Press, 1975.

Kimble, George H. T. *Tropical Africa,* vol. 2. New York: Twentieth Century Fund, 1960.

Kiple, Kenneth F., ed. *The Cambridge World History of Human Disease.* Cambridge, England: Cambridge University Press, 1993.

Kirk, R. "Some Observations on the Study and Control of Yellow Fever in Africa, with Particular Reference to the Anglo-Egyptian Sudan." *Transactions of the Society of Tropical Medicine and Hygiene,* 37 (September 1943):125–50.

Klein, Ira. "Death in India, 1871–1921." *Journal of Asian Studies,* 32 (August 1973):639–59.

Klingberg, M. A., ed. *Rift Valley Fever,* vol. 3 of *Epidemiology and Biostatistics.* Basel, Switzerland: S. Karger, 1981.

Klingberg, M. A., et al. "Certain Aspects of the Epidemiology and Distribution of Immunity of West Nile Virus in Israel," in *Proceedings of the Sixth International Congresses on Tropical Medicine and Malaria.* Lisbon, Portugal: 1958.

Koch-Weser, Dieter, and Vanderschmidt, Hannelore, eds. *The Heterosexual Transmission of AIDS in Africa.* Cambridge, Mass.: Abt Books, 1988.

Kohn, Stanislas, and Meyendorff, Alexander F. *The Cost of the War to Russia.* New York: Howard Fertig, 1973.

Kono, Reisaku. "Apollo 11 Disease or Acute Haemorrhagic Conjunctivitis—A Pandemic of a New Enterovirus Infection of the Eyes." *The American Journal of Epidemiology,* 101 (1975):383–90.

Kosary, Dominic, and Vardy, Steven Bela. *History of the Hungarian Nation.* Astor Park, Fla.: Danubian Press, 1969.

Krautheimer, Richard. *Rome: Profile of a City, 312–1308.* Princeton, N.J.: Princeton University Press, 1980.

Kumar, Dharma, and Desai, Meghnad, eds. *The Cambridge Economic History of India,* vol. 2 (c. 1757–c. 1970). Cambridge, England: Cambridge University Press, 1983.

Kuykendall, Ralph S., and Day, A. Grove. *Hawaii: A History (From Polynesian Kingdom to American Statehood).* Englewood Cliffs, N.J.: Prentice-Hall, 1961.

Lampton, Christopher. *Predicting AIDS and Other Epidemics.* New York: Franklin Watts, 1989.

Lancaster, H. O. *Expectations of Life: A Study in the Demography, Statistics, and History of World Mortality.* New York: Springer-Verlag, 1990.

Landon, John. *Poliomyelitis: A Handbook for Physicians and Medical Students, Based on a Study of the 1931 Epidemic in New York City.* New York: Macmillan, 1934.

Langer, Herbert. *The Thirty Years' War.* Poole, England: Blandford Press, 1980.

Lapin, John H. *Whooping Cough.* Springfield, Ill.: Charles C. Thomas, 1943.

Lassen, H. C. A. "A Preliminary Report on the 1952 Epidemic of Poliomyelitis in Copenhagen." *The Lancet,* 264 (January 3, 1953):37–41.

Last, John M. *Public Health and Human Ecology.* East Norwalk, Conn.: Appleton and Lange, 1987.

Lautzas, Peter. *Die Festung Mainz im Zeitalter des Ancien Régime, der Französischen Revolution und des Empire (1736–1814)*. Wiesbaden, Germany: F. Steiner, 1973.

Learmonth, Andrew. *Disease Ecology*. Oxford: Basil Blackwell, 1988.

———. *Patterns of Disease and Hunger*, Problems in Modern Geography Series. North Pomfret, Vt.: David and Charles, 1978.

Leavy, Barbara Fass. *To Blight with Plague: Studies in a Literary Theme*. New York: New York University Press, 1992.

Lehane, B. *The Compleat Flea*. New York: Viking, 1969.

Leslie, Charles, ed. *Asian Medical Systems: A Comparative Study*. Berkeley: University of California Press, 1976.

Lewis, D. B. Wyndham. *Charles of Europe*. New York: Coward-McCann, 1931.

Lewis, R. A. *Edwin Chadwick and the Public Health Movement, 1832–1854*. London: Longmans, Green, 1952.

Lien-teh, Wu. *Plague Fighter: The Autobiography of a Modern Chinese Physician*. Cambridge, England: W. Heffer and Sons, 1959.

———. *A Treatise on Pneumonic Plague*. Geneva: League of Nations Health Organization, 1926.

Lien-teh, Wu, et al. *Plague: A Manual for Medical and Public Health Workers*. Shanghai: National Quarantine Service, 1936.

Lind, Andrew W. *Hawaii's People*. Honolulu: University of Hawaii Press, 1955.

Lindroth, Sten, ed. *Swedish Men of Science, 1650–1950*. Stockholm: Swedish Institute/Almqvist and Wiksell, 1952.

Link, Vernon B. *A History of Plague in the United States of America*, Public Health Monograph No. 26. Washington, D.C.: U.S. Government Printing Office, 1955.

Livy, *History of Rome*, tr. Frank Gardner Moore. Cambridge, Mass.: Harvard University Press, 1940; Loeb edition.

Llewellyn, Peter. *Rome in the Dark Ages*. London: Faber and Faber, 1971.

Locke, David M. *Viruses: The Smallest Enemy*. New York: Crown, 1974.

Lockwood, Charles. *Manhattan Moves Uptown: An Illustrated History*. Boston: Houghton Mifflin, 1976.

Lombardi, John V. *Venezuela: The Search for Order, the Dream of Progress*. New York: Oxford University Press, 1982.

Longmate, Norman. *King Cholera: The Biography of a Disease*. London: Hamish Hamilton, 1966.

Lord, Rexford D., et al. "Virological Studies of Avian Hosts in the Houston Epidemic of St. Louis En-

cephalitis, 1964." *The American Journal of Tropical Medicine and Hygiene*, 22 (September 1973):662–71.

Luby, James P., et al. "The Epidemiology of St. Louis Encephalitis in Houston, Texas, 1964." *The American Journal of Epidemiology*, 86 (November 1967):584–97.

Lucenet, Monique. *Lyon: malade de la peste*. Palaiseau: Sofedir, 1981.

Ludowyk, E. F. C. *The Modern History of Ceylon*. New York: Praeger, 1966.

Mackenzie, John S., ed. *Viral Diseases in South-East Asia and the Western Pacific*. Sydney, Australia: Academic Press, 1982.

MacKenzie, R. B. "Epidemiology of Machupo Virus Infection. 1. Pattern of Human Infection, San Joaquín, Bolivia, 1962–1964." *The American Journal of Tropical Medicine and Hygiene*, 14 (1965):808.

MacKenzie, R. B.; Beye, H. K.; Valverde, L.; and Garron, H. "Epidemic Hemorrhagic Fever in Bolivia." *The American Journal of Tropical Medicine and Hygiene*, 13 (1964):620.

Maclean, F. S. *Challenge for Health: A History of Public Health in New Zealand*. Wellington: Government Printers, 1964.

MacLeod, Roy, and Lewis, Milton, eds. *Disease, Medicine, and Empire*. New York: Routledge, 1988.

MacNalty, Arthur Salusbury. *Epidemic Diseases of the Central Nervous System*. London: Faber and Gwyer, 1927

———. "Epidemic Diseases of the Central Nervous System." *The Lancet*, 208 (March 1925):475–80, 532–38, 594–99.

Macnamara, C. *A History of Asiatic Cholera*. London: Macmillan, 1876.

MacPhail, Sir Andrew. *History of the Canadian Forces, 1914–19*. Ottawa: F. A. Acland, 1925.

Maehl, William Harvey. *Germany in Western Civilization*. University: University of Alabama Press, 1979.

Magner, Lois N. "Diseases of the Premodern Period in Korea," in *The Cambridge World History of Human Disease*. Cambridge, England: Cambridge University Press, 1993.

Magnusson, Sigurdur A. *Northern Sphinx: Iceland and the Icelanders from the Settlement to the Present*. Montreal: McGill-Queen's University Press, 1977.

Mahoney, Irene. *Madame Catherine*. New York: Coward, McCann and Geoghegan, 1975.

Major, Ralph H. *Classic Descriptions of Disease*, 3rd ed. Springfield, Ill.: Charles C. Thomas, 1932.

"Malta Epidemic of Poliomyelitis, The." *The Lancet*, 245 (October 30, 1943):549.

Mandrou, Robert. *Introduction to Modern France, 1500–1640*, tr. R. E. Hallmark. New York: Holmes and Meier, 1976.

Marcus Aurelius. *Meditations,* tr. and intro. Maxwell Staniforth. New York: Penguin, 1981.

Marks, Geoffrey, and Beatty, William K. *Epidemics.* New York: Scribner, 1976.

Marshall, P. J. *Bengal: The British Bridgehead.* Cambridge, England: Cambridge University Press, 1987.

Mars-Jones, Adam. *Monopolies of Loss.* London: Faber and Faber, 1992.

Martini, G. A., and Siegert, R., eds. *Marburg Virus Disease.* New York: Springer-Verlag, 1971.

Mathews, Frank P., and Mosley, Wiley Henry. "Cholera," in *Collier's Encyclopedia.* New York: Macmillan, 1989.

Mathews, Richard. *The Yukon.* New York: Holt, Rinehart and Winston, 1968.

Matossian, Mary Kilbourne. *Poisons of the Past: Molds, Epidemics, and History.* New Haven, Conn.: Yale University Press, 1989.

Mattingly, P. F. *The Biology of Mosquito-Borne Disease.* London: Allen and Unwin, 1969.

Maul, Carlos. *O Rio da bela época.* Rio de Janeiro: Livraria S. José, 1967.

Maxwell, James L. *The Diseases of China.* Shanghai: A.B.C. Press, 1929.

May, Jacques M. *The Ecology of Human Disease,* Studies in Medical Geography Series. New York: MD Publications, 1958.

———. *Studies in Disease Ecology,* Studies in Medical Geography Series. New York: Hafner, 1961.

Mayer, Hans Eberhard. *The Crusades.* Oxford: Oxford University Press, 1972.

McAlpine, Douglas. "Epidemiology of Acute Poliomyelitis in India Command." *The Lancet,* 249 (August 4, 1945):130–33.

McArthur, Norma. *Island Populations of the Pacific.* Canberra: Australian National University Press, 1968.

McCullough, David. *The Path Between the Seas: The Creation of the Panama Canal 1870–1914.* New York: Simon and Schuster, 1977.

McElwee, W. L. *The Reign of Charles V.* London: Macmillan, 1936.

McGlashan, Neil D., and Blunden, John R., eds. *Geographical Aspects of Health: Essays in Honor of Andrew Learmonth.* London: Academic Press, 1983.

McGrew, Roderick E. *Encyclopedia of Medical History.* New York: McGraw-Hill, 1985.

———. *Russia and the Cholera, 1823–1832.* Madison: University of Wisconsin Press, 1965.

McKelvey, John J., Jr. *Man Against Tsetse: Struggle for Africa.* Ithaca, N.Y.: Cornell University Press, 1973.

McKeown, Thomas. *The Modern Rise of Population.* New York: Academic Press, 1976.

———. *The Origins of Human Disease.* Oxford: Basil Blackwell, 1987.

McMichael, Joan K., ed. *Health in the Third World: Studies from Vietnam.* Nottingham, England: Bertrand Russell Peace Foundation, 1976.

McNeill, William H. *Plagues and Peoples.* Garden City, N.Y.: Anchor Press/Doubleday, 1976.

McVail, John C. *Half a Century of Smallpox and Vaccination.* Edinburgh, Scotland: Livingstone, 1919.

Medicine in Colonial Massachusetts, 1620–1820. Boston: Colonial Society of Massachusetts, 1980.

Melnick, J. L., ed. *Progress in Medical Virology.* Basil, Switzerland: S. Karger, 1984.

Menon, I. G. K. "The 1957 Pandemic of Influenza in India." *Bulletin of the World Health Organization,* 20 (1959):199–224.

Miller, D. L.; Pereira, Marguerite S.; and Clarke, M. "Epidemiology of the Hong Kong/68 Variant of Influenza A2 in Britain." *British Medical Journal,* 1 (747) (February 27, 1971):475–78.

Mociño, José Maria. *Disertación de la fiebre epidémica, que padeció Cadiz, Sevilla y la mayor parte de Andalucía desde el año 1800 y principalmente de la que sufrió Ecixa el año 1804.* Mexico: Sociedad Mexicana de Historia y Filosofía de la Medicina, 1982.

Moll, Aristides A. *Aesculapius in Latin America.* Philadelphia: W. B. Saunders, 1944.

Morgan-Witts, Max, and Gordon, Thomas. *Anatomy of an Epidemic.* Garden City, N.Y.: Doubleday, 1982.

Moss, H. St. L. B. "The History of the Byzantine Empire: An Outline," in *Byzantium: An Introduction to East Roman Civilization,* ed. by Norman H. Baynes and H. St. L. B. Moss. London: Oxford University Press, 1969.

Moulton, F. R., ed. *The Rickettsial Diseases of Man.* Washington, D.C.: American Society for the Advancement of Science, 1948.

Mukherjee, S., and Basu, S. "Cholera El Tor in India: Effect on Epidemiology of Classical Cholera." *Tropical and Geographical Medicine,* 19 (1967):138–43.

Mullen, Fitzhugh. *Plagues and Politics: The Story of the United States Public Health Service.* New York: Basic Books, 1989.

Mullet, Charles F. *The Bubonic Plague and England.* Lexington: University of Kentucky Press, 1956.

Munz, Peter. *Frederick Barbarossa: A Study in Medieval Politics.* Ithaca, N.Y.: Cornell University Press, 1969.

Myers, Jacob M., tr. and notes. *Anchor Bible: II Chronicles.* Garden City, N.Y.: Doubleday, 1965.

Nash, J. T. C. *Evolution and Disease.* New York: William Wood, 1915.

Nathan, Carl F. *Plague, Prevention and Politics in Man-*

churia, 1910–1931. Cambridge, Mass.: Harvard University Press, 1967.

National Research Council. The Social Impact of AIDS in the United States. Washington, D.C.: National Academy Press, 1993.

Navarro, Vicente, ed. Imperialism, Health and Medicine, Policy, Politics, Health and Medicine Series. Farmingdale, N.Y.: Baywood Publishing, 1981.

Neale, J. E. The Age of Catherine de Medici. New York: Harper, 1962.

Newsholme, Arthur. The Origin and Spread of Pandemic Diphtheria. London: Swan Sonnenschein, 1898.

Nicole, Christopher. The West Indies. London: Hutchinson, 1965.

Nicolson, Nigel. Napoleon 1812. New York: Harper and Row, 1985.

Nohl, Johannes. The Black Death: A Chronicle of the Plague. London: Allen and Unwin, 1926.

Norbeck, Edward, and Lock, Margaret. Health, Illness and Medical Care in Japan: Cultural and Social Dimensions. Honolulu: University of Hawaii Press, 1987.

Nordal, Johannes, and Kristinsson, Valdimir, eds. Iceland, 874–1974. Reykjavik: Central Bank of Iceland, 1975.

Oaks, Stanley C., Jr., et al., eds. Malaria: Obstacles and Opportunities. Washington, D.C.: National Academy Press, 1991.

Odo of Deuil. The Journey of Louis VII to the East, tr. and ed. Virginia G. Berry. New York: W. W. Norton, 1948.

Oldenbourg, Zoe. The Crusades. New York: Pantheon, 1966.

Olin, Gunnar. "The Epidemiological Pattern of Poliomyelitis in Sweden from 1905 to 1950," in Poliomyelitis: Papers and Discussions Presented at the Second International Poliomyelitis Congress, compiled and edited for the International Poliomyelitis Congress. Philadelphia: J. B. Lippincott, 1952.

Ormerod, W. E. "The Epidemic Spread of Rhodesian Sleeping Sickness, 1908–1960." Transactions of the Royal Society of Tropical Medicine and Hygiene, 55 (November 1961):525–38.

Osborn, June E., ed. History, Science, and Politics: Influenza in America, 1918–1976. New York: Prodist, 1977.

Ostrogorsky, George. History of the Byzantine State, tr. Joan Hussey, rev. ed. New Brunswick, N.J.: Rutgers University Press, 1969.

Owen, Norman G., ed. Death and Disease in Southeast Asia. New York: Oxford University Press, 1987.

Oxford Textbook of Medicine, 2 vols., 2nd ed. Oxford: Oxford University Press, 1987.

Pacaut, Marcel. Frederick Barbarossa, tr. A. J. Pomerans. London: Collins, 1970.

Packard, Randall M. White Plague, Black Labor. Berkeley: University of California Press, 1989.

Pan American Health Organization. Health Conditions in the Americas, 1981–1984, 2 vols. Washington, D.C.: Pan American Health Org., 1986.

———. Health Conditions in the Americas, vol. 1. Washington, D.C.: Pan American Health Org., 1990.

———. Plague in the Americas. Washington, D.C.: Pan American Health Org., 1965.

Pankhurst, Richard. Economic History of Ethiopia: 1800–1935. Addis Ababa: Haile Selassie I University, 1968.

———. An Introduction to the Medical History of Ethiopia. Trenton, N.J.: Red Sea Press, 1990.

Panum, Peter Ludwig. Observations Made During the Epidemic of Measles on the Faroe Islands in the Year 1846, tr. Ada S. Hatcher. New York: Delta Omega Society, 1940.

Parahym, Orlando da Cunha. Endemias Brasileiras. Recife, Brazil: Universidade do Recife, 1961.

Paredes Borja, Virgilo. Historia de la medicina en el Ecuador, 2 vols. Quito: Editorial Casa Dela Cultura Ecuatoriana, 1963.

Parker, Geoffrey. The Thirty Years' War. London: Routledge and Kegan Paul, 1984.

Parsons, Claire D. F., ed. Healing Practices in the South Pacific. Honolulu: University of Hawaii Press, 1985.

Partington, Wilfred. The War Against Malaria. London: Ross Institute Fund, 1923.

Parton, Roger, and Warlaw, Alastair C., eds. Pathogenesis and Immunity in Pertusis. Chichester, Scotland: John Wiley and Sons, 1988.

Patrick, Adam. "Disease in Antiquity: Ancient Greece and Rome," in Diseases in Antiquity, ed. Don Brothwell and A. T. Sandison. Springfield, Ill.: Charles C. Thomas, 1967.

Patterson, K. David. Health in Colonial Ghana: Disease, Medicine, and Socio-Economic Change 1900–1955. Waltham, Mass.: Crossroads Press, 1981.

———. Infectious Diseases in Twentieth-Century Africa: A Bibliography of their Distribution Consequences. Waltham, Mass.: African Studies Association, 1979.

———. Pandemic Influenza, 1700–1900: A Study in Historical Epidemiology. Totowa, N.J.: Rowan and Littlefield, 1986.

Paul, Benjamin D., ed. Health, Culture and Community: Case Studies of Public Reactions to Health Programs. New York: Russell Sage Foundation, 1955.

Paul, John R. A History of Poliomyelitis. New Haven, Conn.: Yale University Press, 1971.

Paul the Deacon. History of the Langobards, tr. William Dudley Foulke. Philadelphia: University of Pennsylvania Press, 1907.

Payzin, S., et al. "Neurological and Psychiatric Complications of Asiatic Flue," in Proceedings of the

Sixth International Congresses on Tropical Medicine and Malaria. Lisbon, Portugal: 1958.

Pearson, M. N. *The Portuguese in India*. Cambridge, England: Cambridge University Press, 1987.

Pelling, Margaret. *Cholera, Fever and English Medicine, 1825–1865*. Oxford: Oxford University Press, 1978.

Peset Reig, Mariano, and Peset Reig, José Luís. *Muerte en España (política y sociedad entre la peste y el cólera)*. Madrid: Seminarios y Ediciones, 1972.

Peters, Edward, ed. *The First Crusade: The Chronicle of Fulcher of Chartres and Other Source Materials*. Philadelphia: University of Pennsylvania Press, 1971.

Peters, W., and Killick-Kendrick, R., eds. *The Leishmaniases in Biology and Medicine*. London: Academic Press, 1987.

Peterson, John. *Province of Freedom: A History of Sierra Leone, 1787–1870*. Evanston, Ill.: Northwestern University Press, 1969.

Petrovich, Michael Boro. *A History of Modern Serbia, 1804–1918*, vol. 2. New York: Harcourt Brace Jovanovich, 1976.

Phelan, John Leddy. *The Hispanization of the Philippines: Spanish Aims and Filipino Responses, 1565–1700*. Madison: University of Wisconsin Press, 1959.

———. *The People and the King: The Comunero Revolution in Colombia, 1781*. Madison: University of Wisconsin Press, 1978.

Plague Reconsidered: A New Look at Its Origin and Effects in 16th and 17th Century England, A Local Population Studies Supplement. England: Hourdsprint Stafford, 1977.

Plessis, Alain. *The Rise and Fall of the Second Empire, 1852–1871*, tr. Jonathan Mandelbaum. Cambridge, England: Cambridge University Press, 1979.

Poliomyelitis: Papers and Discussions Presented at the Fourth International Poliomyelitis Conference. Philadelphia: J. B. Lippincott, 1958.

Pollitzer, R. *Cholera*. Geneva: World Health Organization, 1959.

———. *Plague*. Geneva: World Health Organization, 1954.

———. *Plague and Plague Control in the Soviet Union*. New York: Institute of Contemporary Russian Studies, Fordham University, 1966.

Pollock, John C. *A Foreign Devil in China*. Minneapolis: World Wide Publication, 1971.

Poppino, Rollie E. *Brazil, the Land and People*. New York: Oxford University Press, 1968.

Post, John D. *Food Shortages, Climatic Variability, and Epidemic Disease in Preindustrial Europe: The Mortality Peak in the Early 1740s*. Ithaca, N.Y.: Cornell University Press, 1985.

———. *The Last Great Subsistence Crisis in the Western World*. Baltimore: Johns Hopkins University Press, 1977.

Powell, J. H. *Bring Out Your Dead: The Great Plague of Yellow Fever in Philadelphia in 1793*. New York: Time-Life, 1965.

Pramanik, Major D. D. "Joy Bangla—An Epidemic of Conjunctivitis in India." *The Practitioner*, 207 (December 1971):805–06.

Prescott, Orville. *Lords of Italy: Portraits from the Middle Ages*. New York: Harper and Row, 1972.

Prescott, William Hickling. *The Rise and Decline of the Spanish Empire*, ed. Irwin R. Blacker. New York: Viking, 1963.

Preston, Richard. *The Hot Zone*. New York: Random House, 1994.

Prinzing, Friedrich. *Epidemics Resulting from Wars*. Oxford: Clarendon Press, 1916.

Pritchard, James, ed. *Ancient Near Eastern Texts Relating to the Old Testament*, 3rd ed. Princeton, N.J.: Princeton University Press, 1970.

Proceedings of the Sixth International Congresses on Tropical Medicine and Malaria. Lisbon, Portugal: 1958.

Procopius. *History of the Wars*, tr. H. B. Dewing. Cambridge, Mass.: Harvard University Press, 1961; Loeb edition.

Prothero, R. Mansell. *Migrants and Malaria*. London: Longmans, Green, 1965.

Pullan, Brian S. *Rich and Poor in Renaissance Venice: The Social Institutions of a Catholic State, to 1620*. Oxford: Basil Blackwell, 1971.

Pusey, William Allen. *The History and Epidemiology of Syphilis*. Springfield, Ill.: Charles C. Thomas, 1933.

Pushkarev, Sergei. *The Emergence of Modern Russia, 1801–1917*, tr. Robert H. McNeal and Nova Yedlin. New York: Holt, Rinehart and Winston, 1963.

Pyle, Gerald F. *The Diffusion of Influenza: Patterns and Paradigms*. Totowa, N.J.: Rowan and Littlefield, 1986.

Quennevat, Jean-Claude. *Les vrais soldats de Napoléon*. Brussels, Belgium: Sequoia-Elsevier, 1968.

Quétel, Claude. *History of Syphilis*. Baltimore: Johns Hopkins University Press, 1990.

Radetsky, Peter. *The Invisible Invaders: The Story of the Emerging Age of Viruses*. Boston: Little, Brown, 1991.

Rady, Martyn. *The Emperor Charles V*. London: Longman, 1988.

Rail, C. D. *Plague Ecotoxicology: Including Historical Aspects of the Disease in the Americas and the Eastern Hemisphere*. Springfield, Ill.: Charles C. Thomas, 1985.

Ramenofsky, Ann F. *Vectors of Death: The Archaeology of European Contact*. Albuquerque: University of New Mexico Press, 1987.

Ramsay, David. *Ramsay's History of South Carolina*, 2 vols. Newberry, S.C.: W. J. Duffie, 1858.

Ranger, Terence, and Slack, Paul, eds. *Epidemics and Ideas: Essays on the Historical Perception of Pestilence.* Cambridge, England: Cambridge University Press, 1992.

Ransford, Oliver. *"Bid the Sickness Cease": Disease in the History of Black Africa.* London: John Murray, 1983.

Raychaudhuri, Tapan, and Habib, Irfan, eds. *The Cambridge Economic History of India*, vol. 1 (c.1200–c. 1750). Cambridge, England: Cambridge University Press, 1983.

Razzell, Peter. *The Conquest of Smallpox: The Impact of Inoculation on Smallpox Mortality in Eighteenth-Century Britain.* Sussex, England: Caliban Books, 1977.

Reed, Dwayne; Maguire, Terry; and Mataika, Jona. "Type 1 Dengue with Hemorrhagic Disease in Fiji Epidemiologic Findings." *The American Journal of Tropical Medicine and Hygiene*, 26 (1977): 784–91.

Report on Progress in Manchuria, 1907–1928. Dairen, China: South Manchuria Railway, March 1929.

Reports on Public Health and Medical Subjects, No. 4. London: H. M. Stationery Office, 1920.

Rink, Henrik. *Danish Greenland: Its People and Products.* Montreal: McGill-Queen's University Press, 1974; reprint of 1877 edition.

Rivers, W. H. R., ed. *Essays on the Depopulation of Melanesia.* Cambridge, England: Cambridge University Press, 1922.

Rodríguez Ocāna, Esteban. *El cólera de 1834 en Granada: enfermedad catastófica y crisis social.* Granada, Spain: Universidad de Granada, 1983.

Roland, Charles G., ed. *Health, Disease and Medicine.* Hamilton, Ontario: Hannah Institute for the History of Medicine, 1982.

Rolleston, J. D. *The Smallpox Pandemic of 1870–74.* London: J. Bale and Danielsson, 1933.

Rosa, Francisco Ferreira da. *Rio de Janeiro: noticia historica e descritiva da capital do Brasil.* Rio de Janeiro: Official da Prefeitura, 1905.

Rosebury, Theodor. *Microbes and Morals: The Strange Story of Venereal Disease.* New York: Viking, 1971.

Rosen, George. "Acute Communicable Diseases," in *The History and Conquest of Common Diseases*, ed. Walter R. Bett. Norman: University of Oklahoma Press, 1954.

———. *Locura y sociedad: sociología histórica de la enfermedad mental.* Madrid: Alianza Editorial, 1974.

———. *Preventive Medicine in the United States, 1900–1975: Trends and Interpretations.* New York: Science History Publications, 1975.

Rosenberg, Charles E. *The Cholera Years: The United States in 1832, 1849, and 1866.* Chicago: University of Chicago Press, 1987.

Rothschild, Henry, ed. *Biocultural Aspects of Disease.* New York: Academic Press, 1981.

Ruhrah, John, and Mayer, Erwin E. *Poliomyelitis in All Its Aspects.* Philadelphia: Lea and Febiger, 1917.

Runciman, Steven. *A History of the Crusades*, 3 vols. Cambridge, England: Cambridge University Press, 1954.

———. "The First Crusade: Antioch to Ascalon," in *A History of the Crusades*, ed. Kenneth M. Setton. Madison: University of Wisconsin Press, 1969.

Russell, Paul F. *Malaria.* Oxford: Basil Blackwell, 1952.

———. *Man's Mastery of Malaria.* London: Oxford University Press, 1955.

Ryan, Frank. *The Forgotten Plague: How the Battle Against Tuberculosis Was Won and Lost.* Boston: Little, Brown, 1993.

Ryle, John. "Zero Grazing." *London Review of Books*, November 5, 1992.

Sabin, A. B. "Research on Dengue during World War II." *The American Journal of Tropical Medicine and Hygiene*, 1 (January 1952):30–50.

Salvatorelli, Luigi. *A Concise History of Italy*, tr. Bernard Miall. New York: Oxford, 1940.

Sansom, George. *A History of Japan to 1334.* Stanford, Calif.: Stanford University Press, 1958.

Santos, Francisco Agenor de Noronha. *Chorographia do Districto Federal (cidade do Rio de Janeiro).* Rio de Janeiro: Aguila, 1913.

Sasa, Manabu. *Human Filariasis: A Global Survey of Epidemiology and Control.* Tokyo: University of Tokyo Press, 1976.

Savant, Jean. *Napoleon in His Time*, tr. Katherine John. New York: Thomas Nelson, 1958.

Savitt, Todd L. *Medicine and Slavery: The Diseases and Health Care of Blacks in Antebellum Virginia.* Urbana: University of Illinois Press, 1978.

Scherman, Katharine. *The Birth of France.* New York: Random House, 1987.

Schöppler, Stabsarzt, Dr. *Die Geschichte der Pest zu Regensburg.* Munich, Germany: Otto Gmelin, 1914.

Scott, David. *Epidemic Disease in Ghana, 1901–1960.* London: Oxford University Press, 1965.

Scott, Franklin D. *Sweden: The Nation's History.* Minneapolis: University of Minnesota Press, 1977.

Scott, H. Harold. *A History of Tropical Medicine.* Baltimore: Williams and Wilkins, 1939.

Seddon, H. J., et al. "The Poliomyelitis Epidemic in Malta, 1942–3." *Quarterly Journal of Medicine*, 14 (January 1945):1–26.

Segur, Philippe-Paul de. *Napoleon's Russian Campaign*, tr. J. David Townsend. Boston: Houghton Mifflin, 1958.

Service, Michael W., ed. *Demography and Vector-Borne Diseases.* Boca Raton, Fla.: CRC Press, 1989.

Seton-Watson, Hugh. *The Russian Empire, 1801–1917.* Oxford: Clarendon Press, 1967.

Setton, Kenneth M., ed. *A History of the Crusades,* vols. 1–3, 2nd ed. Madison: University of Wisconsin Press, 1969.

Sharrar, Robert G. "National Influenza Experience in the USA, 1968–69." *Bulletin of the World Health Organization,* 41 (1969): 361–66.

Shattuck, George Cheever. *Diseases of the Tropics.* New York: Appleton-Century-Crofts, 1951.

Shaw, John, ed. *Australian Encyclopedia.* Sydney: William Collins, 1984.

Shaw, Stanford J., and Shaw, Ezel Kural. *History of the Ottoman Empire and Modern Turkey,* 2 vols. Cambridge, England: Cambridge University Press, 1977.

Shepherd, Robert, *Ireland's Fate.* London: Aurum Press, 1990.

Shortt, S. E. D., ed. *Medicine in Canadian Society.* Montreal: McGill-Queen's University Press, 1981.

Shrewsbury, J. F. D. *A History of Bubonic Plague in the British Isles.* Cambridge, England: Cambridge University Press, 1970.

———. "The Plague of the Philistines." *The Journal of Hygiene,* 47 (1949):244–52.

Shryock, Richard Harris. *Medicine and Society in America, 1660–1860.* New York: New York University Press, 1960.

Shurkin, Joel N. *The Invisible Fire: The Story of Mankind's Victory Over the Ancient Scourge of Smallpox.* New York: Putnam, 1979.

Siddiqui, Wasim A., ed. *Proceedings of the Asia and Pacific Conference on Malaria held April 21–27, 1985.* Honolulu: John A. Burns School of Medicine, University of Hawaii, 1985.

Siegfried, Andr. *Routes of Contagion.* New York: Harcourt, Brace and World, 1965.

Siegler, Hans Georg. *Danzig, Chronik eines Jahrtausends.* Düsseldorf, Germany: Droste Verlag, 1991.

Sigerist, Henry E. *Civilization and Disease.* Chicago: University of Chicago Press, 1970.

———. *Medicine and Health in the Soviet Union.* New York: Citadel Press, 1947.

———. *Socialized Medicine in the Soviet Union.* New York: W. W. Norton, 1937.

Silius Italicus. *Punica,* tr. J. D. Duff. Cambridge, Mass.: Harvard University Press, 1934; Loeb edition.

Simmons, James Stevens, et al. *Global Epidemiology: A Geography of Disease and Sanitation.* Philadelphia: J. B. Lippincott, 1954.

Simpson, D. I. H. *Marburg and Ebola Virus Infections: A Guide for Their Diagnosis, Management, and Control.* Geneva: World Health Organization, 1977.

Simpson, Howard N. *Invisible Armies.* Indianapolis: Bobbs-Merrill, 1980.

Simpson, W. J. *A Treatise on Plague.* Cambridge, England: Cambridge University Press, 1905.

Singer, Charles, and Underwood, E. Ashworth. *A Short History of Medicine.* New York: Oxford University Press, 1962.

Singleton, Fred. *A Short History of Finland.* Cambridge, England: Cambridge University Press, 1989.

Sinor, Denis. *History of Hungary.* London: Allen and Unwin, 1959.

Slack, Paul. *The Impact of Plague in Tudor and Stuart England.* London: Routledge and Kegan Paul, 1985.

Smith, Bernard. *European Vision and the South Pacific.* New Haven, Conn.: Yale University Press, 1985.

Smith, F. B. *Florence Nightingale: Reputation and Power.* London: Croom Helm, 1982.

———. *The People's Health, 1830–1910.* New York: Holmes and Meier, 1979.

Smith, Geddes. *Plague on Us.* New York: Commonwealth Fund, 1941.

Smith, Herbert H. *Brazil, the Amazons and the Coast.* New York: Scribner, 1879.

Smith, J. R. *The Speckled Monster: Smallpox in England, 1670–1970, with Particular Reference to Essex.* Chelmsford, England: Essex Record Office, 1987.

Smith, Jane S. *Patenting the Sun: Polio and the Salk Vaccine.* New York: William Morrow, 1990.

Smith, Kenneth M. *Beyond the Microscope.* Harmondsworth, England: Penguin, 1943.

Smith, Lloyd H., Jr., and Wyngaarden, James B., eds. *Cecil Textbook of Medicine.* Philadelphia: W. B. Saunders, 1988.

Smout, T. C. *A History of the Scottish People, 1560–1830.* London: Colhas, 1969.

Snow, John. *Snow on Cholera.* London: Hafner, 1965.

Solsten, Eric, and Meditz, Sandra W., eds. *Finland: A Country Study.* Washington, D.C.: Library of Congress, Federal Research Division, 1990.

Spink, Wesley W. *Infectious Diseases: Prevention and Treatment in the Nineteenth and Twentieth Centuries.* Minneapolis: University of Minnesota Press, 1978.

Squires, H. C. *The Sudan Medical Service.* London: Heinemann, 1958.

Stallybrass, C. O. "Encephalitis Lethargica: Some Observations on a Recent Outbreak." *The Lancet,* 205 (October 27, 1923):922–25.

Stamp, L. Dudley. *The Geography of Life and Death.* Ithaca, N.Y.: Cornell University Press, 1964.

Stanley, N. F., and Joske, R. A., eds. *Changing Disease Patterns and Human Behaviour.* New York: Academic Press, 1980.

Stearn, E. Wagner, and Stearn, Allen E. *The Effects of*

Smallpox on the Destiny of the Amerindians. Boston: Bruce Humphries, 1945.

Steinberg, S. H. *The Thirty Years War.* New York: W. W. Norton, 1966.

Steiner, Paul E. *Disease in the Civil War: Natural Biological Warfare in 1861–65.* Springfield, Ill.: Charles C. Thomas, 1968.

Stepan, Nancy. *Beginnings of Brazilian Science: Oswaldo Cruz, Medical Research and Policy, 1890–1920.* New York: Science History Publications, 1976.

Stine, Gerald J. *Acquired Immune Deficiency Syndrome: Biological, Medical, Social, and Legal Issues.* Englewood Cliffs, N.J.: Prentice Hall, 1993.

Stock, Robert F. *African Environment Special Report 3: Cholera in Africa.* London: International African Institute, 1976.

Stoddard, T. Lothrop. *The French Revolution in San Domingo.* New York: Negro Universities Press, 1970.

Strayer, Joseph R. "The Crusades of Louis IX," in *A History of the Crusades*, ed. Kenneth M. Setton. Madison: University of Wisconsin Press, 1969.

Strode, George K., ed. *Yellow Fever.* New York: McGraw-Hill, 1951.

Strong, Richard P., et al. *Typhus Fever with Special Reference to the Serbian Epidemic.* Cambridge, Mass.: American Red Cross at Harvard University Press, 1920.

Stuart-Harris, Charles H. "Influenza." *British Medical Journal,* 5120 (February 1959):490–91.

———. "Influenza and Its Complications." *British Medical Bulletin,* 15 (September 1959):216–20.

Stuart-Harris, Charles H., et al. *Influenza: The Viruses and the Disease,* 2nd ed. London: Edward Arnold, 1985.

Studt, Ward B.; Sorensen, Jerold G.; and Burge, Beverly. *Medicine in the Intermountain West.* Salt Lake City: Olympus, 1976.

Styler, Herman. *Plague Fighters.* Philadelphia: Chilton, 1960.

Sudhoff, Karl, and Sticker, Georg. *Zur historischen Biologie der Krankheitsreger: Materialen, Studien und Abhandlungen.* Giessen, Germany: Alfred Tröpelmann, 1910.

Sugar, Peter F., ed. *A History of Hungary.* Bloomington: Indiana University Press, 1990.

Suro, Roberto. "The Cholera Watch." *The New York Times Magazine,* March 22, 1992.

Sutherland, N. M. "Parisian Life in the Sixteenth Century," in *French Humanism, 1470–1600*, ed. Werner L. Gundersheimer. London: Macmillan, 1969.

Swedlund, Alan C., and Armelagos, George J., eds. *Disease in Populations in Transition: Anthropological and Epidemiological Perspectives.* New York: Bergin and Garvey, 1990.

Swee-Hock, Saw. *Singapore: Population in Transition.* Philadelphia: University of Pennsylvania Press, 1970.

Swerdlow, David L., et al. "Waterborne Transmission of Epidemic Cholera in Trujillo, Peru: Lessons for a Continent at Risk." *The Lancet,* 340 (July 4, 1992):28–33.

Sykes, Sir Percy. *A History of Persia,* 2 vols. London: Macmillan, 1951.

Symonds, John Addington. *Renaissance in Italy,* 2 vols. New York: Modern Library, 1935.

Szakaly, Ferenc. "The Early Ottoman Empire, Including Royal Hungary, 1526–1606," in *A History of Hungary*, ed. Peter F. Sugar. Bloomington: Indiana University Press, 1990.

Szmuness, Wolf, et al., eds. *Viral Hepatitis: 1981 International Symposium.* Philadelphia: Franklin Institute Press, 1982.

Tabrah, Ruth. *Hawaii: A Bicentennial History.* New York: W. W. Norton, 1980.

Taeuber, Irene B. *The Population of Japan.* Princeton, N.J.: Princeton University Press, 1958.

Taves, Archibald William. *The Etiology and Diagnosis of Epidemic Cerebro-Spinal Meningitis.* Providence, R.I.: Snow and Farnham, 1906.

Taylor, R. A. Russell. *Poliomyelitis and Polioencephalitis.* London: H. K. Lewis, 1955.

Taylor, Thomas E. *Running the Blockade,* 3rd ed. London: J. Murray, 1896.

Terris, Milton, ed. *Goldberger on Pellagra.* Baton Rouge: Louisiana State University Press, 1964.

Thomas, Gordon, and Morgan-Witts, Max. *Anatomy of an Epidemic.* Garden City, N.Y.: Doubleday, 1982.

Thompson, J. M. *Louis Napoleon and the Second Empire.* New York: W. W. Norton, 1955.

———. *Napoleon Bonaparte: His Rise and Fall.* New York: Oxford University Press, 1969.

Thompson, James Westfall. *Economic and Social History of the Middle Ages.* New York: Century, 1928.

———. *The Wars of Religion in France, 1559–1576.* New York: Frederick Unger, 1909.

Thompson, K. D. B. "Mortality Trends of Epidemic Meningitis in Northern Areas of Nigeria, 1961–1970." *The Journal of Tropical Medicine and Hygiene,* 76 (January 1973):8–12.

Thucydides. *History of the Peloponnesian War,* tr. Rex Warner. New York: Penguin, 1980.

Tien, H. Yuan, ed. *Population Theory in China.* London: Croom Helm, 1980.

Tierney, Brian, ed. *The Crisis of Church and State, 1050–1300.* Englewood Cliffs, N.J.: Prentice-Hall, 1964.

Top, Franklin H., ed. *The History of American Epidemiology.* St. Louis, Mo.: C. V. Mosby, 1952.

Tranié, Jean. *La patrie en danger 1792–1793: Les campagnes de la révolution*, vol. 1. Paris: Lavauzelle, 1987.

Treichler, Arnold. *Die Staatliche Pestprophylaxe im Alten Zürich und Diesbezügliche Vereinbarungen mit Anderen Schweizer-Städten und mit dem Ausland*. Zurich: Orell Füssli, 1926.

Trigger, Bruce G. *The Children of Aataentsic: A History of the Huron People to 1660*. Montreal: McGill-Queen's University Press, 1987.

———. *Handbook of North American Indians, Northeast*, vol. 15. Washington, D.C.: Smithsonian Institute, 1978.

Trong, Pham, et al. "A Mixed Pneumonic Bubonic Plague Outbreak in Vietnam." *Military Medicine*, 132 (February 1967):93–97.

Trotter, Yates, Jr., et al. "Asian Influenza in the United States, 1957–58." *The American Journal of Hygiene*, 70 (July 1959):34–50.

Trowell, H. C., and Burkitt, D. P., eds. *Western Diseases: Their Emergence and Prevention*. Cambridge, Mass.: Cambridge University Press, 1987.

Trueta, Joseph; Wilson, A. B. Kinnier; and Agerholm, Margaret. *Handbook on Poliomyelitis*. Springfield, Ill.: Charles C. Thomas, 1956.

Tuchman, Barbara W. *A Distant Mirror: The Calamitous 14th Century*. New York: Knopf, 1978.

Turnbull, C. M. *A History of Singapore, 1819–1988*, 2nd ed. Singapore: Oxford University Press, 1989.

Turtledove, Harry, tr. *The Chronicle of Theophanes*. Philadelphia: University of Pennsylvania Press, 1982.

Twigg, Graham. *The Black Death: A Biological Reappraisal*. London: Batsford Academic and Educational, 1984.

Tyler, Royall. *The Emperor Charles the Fifth*. London: Allen and Unwin, 1956.

Unschuld, Paul U. *Medicine in China: A History of Ideas*. Berkeley: University of California Press, 1985.

Utterstrom, Gustaf. "Some Population Problems in Pre-Industrial Sweden." *Scandinavian Economic History Review*, 2 (1954):103–65.

Van Cleve, Thomas C. "The Fifth Crusade," in *A History of the Crusades*, ed. Kenneth M. Setton. Madison: University of Wisconsin Press, 1969.

van Hartesveldt, Fred R. *The 1918–1919 Pandemic Influenza: The Urban Impact in the Western World*. Lewiston, N.Y.: Mellen Press, 1992.

Van Rooyen, C. E., and Morgan, A. D. "Experimental Work in Egypt." *Edinburgh Medical Journal*, 50 (December 1943):705–20.

Velimirovic, Boris, and Velimirovic, Helga. "Plague in Vienna." *Reviews of Infectious Diseases*, 11 (September–October 1989):808–26.

Veseltear, Arthur J. "The Pneumonic Plague Epidemic of 1924 in Los Angeles." *The Yale Journal of Biology and Medicine*, 47 (March 1974):40–54.

Viswanathan, D. K. *The Conquest of Malaria in India: An Indo-American Cooperative Effort*. Bombay: Company Law Institute Press, 1958.

Vonderlehr, R. A., and Heller, J. R. *The Control of Venereal Disease*. New York: Reynal and Hitchcock, 1946.

Waddy, B. B. "African Epidemic Cerebro-Spinal Meningitis." *The Journal of Tropical Medicine and Hygiene*, 60 (September 1957):179–89.

Wain, Harry. *A History of Preventive Medicine*. Springfield, Ill.: Charles C. Thomas, 1970.

Wallace-Hadrill, J. M. *The Barbarian West: The Early Middle Ages, A.D. 400–1000*. New York: Harper and Row, 1962.

Warner, Oliver. *The Battle of the Nile*. New York: Macmillan, 1960.

Warren, Kenneth S., and Mahmoud, Adel A. F., eds. *Tropical and Geographical Medicine*. New York: McGraw-Hill Information Services, 1990.

Warshaw, Leon J. *Malaria: The Biography of a Killer*. New York: Rinehart, 1949.

Washburn, Wilcomb E. *The Indian in America*. New York: Harper and Row, 1975.

Watson, Sir Malcolm. *African Highway*. London: John Murray, 1953.

Webster, Noah. *A Brief History of Epidemic and Pestilential Diseases*. New York: Burt Franklin, 1970; reprint of 1799 edition.

Wedgwood, C. V. *The Thirty Years War*. New Haven, Conn.: Yale University Press, 1939.

Wen, Yu-Mei; Xu, Zhi-Yu; and Melnick, Joseph L., eds. *Viral Hepatitis in China: Problems and Control Strategies*, Monographs in Virology Series, vol. 19. Basel, Switzerland: S. Karger, 1992.

West, John F. *Faroe: The Emergence of a Nation*. London: C. Hurst, 1972.

Whipple, George C. *Typhoid Fever: Its Causation, Transmission, and Prevention*. New York: John Wiley and Sons, 1908.

White, Geoffrey M., and Lindstrom, Lamont, eds. *The Pacific Theater: Island Representations of World War II*, Pacific Islands Monograph Series, no. 8. Honolulu: University of Hawaii Press, 1989.

Whitting, Philip, ed. *Byzantium: An Introduction*. New York: New York University Press, 1971.

Wilkins, Robert H., and Brody, Irwin A. "Encephalitis Lethargica." *Archives of Neurology*, 18 (March 1968):324–28.

William of Tyre. *A History of Deeds Done beyond the Sea*, tr. Emily Atwater Babcock and A. C. Krey. New York: Columbia University Press, 1943.

Williams, Greer. *The Plague Killers*. New York: Scribner, 1969.

Williams, Ralph Chester. *The United States Public Health Service, 1798–1950*. Bethesda, Md.: Commissioned Officers Association of the United States Public Health Service, 1951.

Williams, Robert R. *Toward the Conquest of Beriberi*. Cambridge, Mass.: Harvard University Press, 1961.

Williman, Daniel, ed. *The Black Death: The Impact of the Fourteenth-Century Plague*. Binghamton, N.Y.: Center for Medieval and Early Renaissance Studies, 1982.

Wilson, F. P. *The Plague in Shakespeare's London*, 2nd ed. Oxford: Clarendon Press, 1963.

Winslow, Charles-Edward Amory. *The Conquest of Epidemic Disease: A Chapter in the History of Ideas*. Princeton, N.J.: Princeton University Press, 1943.

———. *The Evolution and Significance of the Modern Public Health Campaign*. New Haven, Conn.: Yale University Press, 1984.

Winslow, Ola Elizabeth. *A Destroying Angel: The Conquest of Smallpox in Colonial Boston*. Boston: Houghton Mifflin, 1974.

Wohl, Anthony. *Endangered Lives: Public Health in Victorian Britain*. Cambridge, Mass.: Harvard University Press, 1983.

Wong, K. Chimin, and Lien-teh, Wu. *History of Chinese Medicine*. Shanghai: National Quarantine Service, 1936.

Woods, Robert, and Woodward, John, eds. *Urban Disease and Mortality in Nineteenth-Century England*. New York: St. Martin's Press, 1984.

Woodward, Joseph Janvier. *Outlines of the Chief Camp Diseases of the United States Armies as Observed during the Present War*. Philadelphia: J. B. Lippincott, 1863.

Woodward, Llewellyn. *The Age of Reform, 1815–1870*, 2nd ed. Oxford: Clarendon Press, 1962.

Woodward, Ralph Lee. *Central America: A Nation Divided*. New York: Oxford University Press, 1976.

Worcester, Dean C. *The Philippines: Past and Present*. New York: Macmillan, 1930.

Work, Telford H. "Kyasanur Forest Disease: An Infection of Man by a Virus of the RSS Complex in India," in *Proceedings of the Sixth International Congresses on Tropical Medicine and Malaria* (1958).

Work, Telford H., et al. "Virological Epidemiology of the 1958 Epidemic of Kyasanur Forest Disease." *American Journal of Public Health*, 49 (July 1959):869.

World Health Organization. *Dengue Haemorrhagic Fever: Diagnosis, Treatment and Control*. Geneva: World Health Org., 1986.

———. *The Global Eradication of Smallpox*. Geneva: World Health Org., 1980.

———. *Poliomyelitis*. Geneva: World Health Org., 1955.

———. *Weekly Epidemiological Records*. Geneva: World Health Org., 1989–93.

———. *WHO Chronicle*, 33 (January 1979).

Wright, D. G. *Napoleon and Europe*. London: Longman, 1984.

Wright, Harrison M. *New Zealand, 1769–1840: Early Years of Western Contact*. Cambridge, Mass.: Harvard University Press, 1959.

Wright, Ronald. *Stolen Continents: The Americas Through Indian Eyes Since 1492*. Boston: Houghton Mifflin, 1992.

Wrigley, E. A., and Schofield, R. S. *The Population History of England, 1541–1871: A Reconstruction*. Cambridge, Mass.: Harvard University Press, 1981.

Yen, C. "A Recent Study of Cholera with Reference to an Outbreak in Taiwan in 1962." *Bulletin of the World Health Organization*, 30 (1964):811–25.

Zhdanov, V. M., and Antonova, I. V. "The Hong Kong Influenza Virus Epidemic in the USSR." *Bulletin of the World Health Organization*, 41 (1969):381–86.

Zhdanov, V. M., et al. *The Study of Influenza*, tr. from the Russian. Washington, D.C.: U.S. Department of Health, Education and Welfare, 1960.

Ziegler, Philip. *The Black Death*. Harmondsworth, England: Penguin, 1970.

Zinsser, Hans. *Rats, Lice and History*. Boston: Little, Brown, 1935, 1963.

Zuckerman, Arie J. *Human Viral Hepatitis: Hepatitis-associated Antigen and Viruses*. Amsterdam: North-Holland Publishing, 1975.

Zuckerman, Arie J., and Howard, Colin R. *Hepatitis Viruses and Man*. London: Academic Press, 1979.

GEOGRAPHICAL APPENDIX

(Entries are listed chronologically by region.)

AFGHANISTAN See MIDDLE EAST.

AFRICA

Carthaginian Plague of 396 B.C.
Egyptian Plague of 1347–49
Cape Colony and Cape Town Smallpox Epidemic of 1713
Cape Colony and Cape Town Smallpox Epidemic of 1755
Senegalese Yellow Fever Epidemic of 1778
Sierra Leonean Yellow Fever Epidemics of 1815–85
Madagascan Smallpox Epidemic of 1817–18
Tunisian Plague of 1818–20
Egyptian Plague of 1834–35
Tunisian Cholera Epidemic of 1849–50
Angolan Smallpox Epidemic of 1864–65
Mauritian Malaria Epidemic of 1866–68
Tunisian Typhus Epidemic of 1868
Zanzibar Cholera Epidemic of 1869
Ethiopian Typhus Epidemic of 1876
Cairo and Alexandria Diphtheria Epidemics of 1882–86
Cape Colony and Cape Town Smallpox Epidemic of 1882–85
Egyptian Cholera Epidemic of 1883
Ethiopian Smallpox Epidemics of 1886–98
Congolese Sleeping Sickness Epidemic of 1895–1906
Príncipe Sleeping Sickness Epidemic of 1898–1913
Kenyan Smallpox Epidemic of 1897–99
British Typhoid Epidemic in the Boer War
Ugandan-Tanganyikan Sleeping Sickness Epidemic of 1900–1909
South African Pneumonia Epidemics of the Early 1900s
South African Tuberculosis Epidemics of 1906–14
Egyptian Cholera Epidemic of 1902
South-West African Typhoid Epidemic of 1904–07
Ghanian Plague of 1908
Tripoli Cholera Epidemic of 1911
Moroccan Plague of 1911
Chadian Sleeping Sickness Epidemic of 1912–40
Kilimanjaro Plague of 1912
Northern Rhodesian (Zambian) Plague of 1917–18
Ashanti Influenza Epidemic of 1918
Ethiopian Influenza Epidemic of 1918–19
Mauritian Influenza Epidemic of 1919
Mongallan Meningitis Epidemics of 1918–24 and 1926–31

Nigerian Influenza Epidemic of 1918–19
Sierra Leonean Influenza Epidemic of 1918
Malian Relapsing Fever Epidemic of 1921–22
Chadian Smallpox Epidemics of 1922–32
Ashanti Plague of 1924–25
Madagascan Plague of 1924–25
Ghanian Yellow Fever Epidemic of 1926
Durban Dengue Epidemic of 1926–27
Sudanese Relapsing Fever Epidemic of 1926–28
Ugandan Plagues of 1926–31
South African Pneumonia Epidemics of 1926–40
Nigerian Smallpox Epidemic of 1930–35
Madagascan Plague of 1933–37
South African Typhus Epidemics of 1934 and 1935
South African Plagues of 1935 and 1936
Somalian Smallpox Epidemic of 1936
Ghanian Sleeping Sickness Epidemic of 1936–41
Chadian Meningitis Epidemic of 1937–39
South African Diptheria Epidemics of 1938–43
Upper Voltaic Meningitis Epidemic of 1939
Sudanese Yellow Fever Epidemic of 1940
Egyptian Typhus Epidemic of 1940–45
Ugandan Sleeping Sickness Epidemic of 1940–43
Constantine Malaria Epidemic of 1941
Usambara Malaria Epidemic of 1941–42
Kenyan Plague of 1941–42
Tanganyikan Meningitis Epidemic of 1942
Ghanian Tuberculosis Epidemic of 1942–44
Moroccan Typhus Epidemic of 1942–45
Algerian Typhus Epidemic of 1942–44
Egyptian Malaria Epidemic of 1942–44
Senegalese Plague of 1942–44
Egyptian Relapsing Fever Epidemic of 1944–46
Algerian Relapsing Fever Epidemic of 1943–46
Ghanian Meningitis Epidemics of 1945–49
Kenyan Relapsing Fever Epidemic of 1945–46
Moroccan Relapsing Fever Epidemic of 1945–46
Ghanian Smallpox Epidemic of 1945–47
Rhodesian Smallpox Epidemic of 1946–48
Egyptian Cholera Epidemic of 1947
Nigerian Meningitis Epidemics of 1949 and 1950
Tanganyikan Plague of 1951–53
Ghanian Malaria Epidemic of 1952–54
Kenyan Typhoid Epidemic of 1954
Zambian Smallpox Epidemic of 1955
Tanganyikan Influenza Epidemic of 1957
Ethiopian Malaria Epidemic of 1958

Ethiopian Yellow Fever Epidemic of 1960–62
Somalian Malaria Epidemic of 1961
Senegalese Yellow Fever Epidemic of 1965
Guinean Smallpox Epidemic of 1967
Moroccan Meningitis Epidemics of 1967–70
South African Meningitis Epidemics of 1967–72
African and Asian Conjunctivitis Pandemic of 1969–71
Malian Cholera Epidemic of 1970–71
West African Cholera Epidemics of 1970–71
Chadian Cholera Epidemic of 1971
Kenyan Cholera Epidemic of 1974–75
Zairian Ebola Epidemic of 1976
Egyptian Rift Valley Fever Epidemic of 1977
Nigerian Yellow Fever Epidemic of 1986–90
Sudanese Leishmaniasis Epidemic of 1988–93
African Cholera Pandemic of 1989–91
Burundian Meningitis Epidemic of 1992
Zairian Plague of 1992
African AIDS Epidemic (1980s–   )

ANCIENT HISTORY

Philistine Plague (latter 11th century B.C.)
Plague of Xerxes (480 B.C.)
Roman Pestilence of 451 B.C.
Plague of Athens, Great (430–29 B.C.)
Thasian Mumps Epidemic (c. 410 B.C.)
"Cough of Perinthus" (c. 400 B.C.)
Roman Pestilence of 212 B.C.
Libyan Plague of the First Century A.D.
Antonine Plague (A.D. 165–80)
Plague of Cyprian (A.D. 251–66?)
Plague of Justinian (A.D. 542)
Roman Plague of A.D. 590
Roman Plague of A.D. 680
Constantinople Plague of c. A.D. 746–48

ASIA   See CHINA AND INDOCHINA, INDIA, INDONE-SIA AND THE PHILIPPINES, JAPAN AND KOREA, MIDDLE EAST, OCEANIA.

AUSTRALIA and NEW ZEALAND   See also INDONESIA AND THE PHILIPPINES, OCEANIA.

Australian Smallpox Epidemic of 1788–89
New Zealand Epidemics of the 1790s
Sydney Measles Epidemics of the 1800s
New Zealand Scarlet Fever Epidemics
New Zealand Epidemics of 1820–40
New Zealand Measles Epidemics of 1835 and 1854
New Zealand Whooping Cough Epidemics of 1873 and 1907
Australian Scarlet Fever Epidemic of 1875–76
Sydney Smallpox Epidemic of 1881–82
Sydney Influenza Epidemics of 1890–91
Sydney Plague of 1900
New Zealand Poliomyelitis Epidemics
New Zealand Measles Epidemics of 1915–16 and 1938
Australian Murray Valley Encephalitis Epidemics

Australian Influenza Epidemic of 1918–19
New Zealand Influenza Epidemic of 1918–19
Australian Rubella Epidemic of 1938–41
New Zealand Troops Poliomyelitis Epidemic of 1940–41

AUSTRIA   See GERMANY AND AUSTRIA.

BRAZIL   See LATIN AMERICA.

BRITAIN AND IRELAND   See also EUROPE.

Yellow Plague of A.D. 664
Plague of England, Great (1348–50)
Plague of Ireland, Great (1348–51)
Plague of Scotland, Great (1348–50)
English Plagues of the 1400s
English Sweating Sickness Epidemics (1485–1552)
London Plague of 1499–1500
English Plagues of the 1500s
Irish Pestilences of 1519–25
Cambridge Typhus Epidemic of 1522 (Black Assize)
Edinburgh Plague of 1530
Irish Pestilences of 1535–36
London Plague of 1563
Edinburgh Plague of 1568–69
Oxford Typhus Epidemic of 1577 (Black Assize)
Irish Plague of 1574–76
London Plague of 1578
Edinburgh Plague of 1585
Exeter Typhus Epidemic of 1586 (Black Assize)
London Plague of 1593
Edinburgh Plague of 1597
Scottish Plague of 1600–1608
London Plague of 1603
Irish Plague of 1604–05
London Plague of 1625
London Plague of 1636
Oxford Typhus Epidemic of 1643
Reading Typhus Epidemic of 1643
Scottish Plague of 1644–48
Tiverton Typhus Epidemic of 1644
Irish Plague of 1650–51
London Typhus Epidemic of 1661–65
Plague of London, Great (1665)
London Smallpox Epidemics of 1667–68, 1674, and 1681
London Typhus Epidemic of 1685–86
Londonderry and Dundalk Typhus and Dysentery Epidemics of 1689
Irish Typhus Epidemics of 1708–10, 1718–20, and 1728–30
London Typhus Epidemics of 1709–20
London Smallpox Epidemic of 1721
London Typhus Epidemic of 1726–29
Irish Typhus and Dysentery Epidemic of 1740–41
London Typhus Epidemic of 1741–42
London Typhus Epidemic of 1750 (Black Assize)
English Smallpox Epidemic of 1751–53
British Smallpox Epidemic of 1796
British Smallpox Epidemic of 1816–19
English Typhus Epidemic of 1816–19

Irish Typhus and Dysentery Epidemic of 1817–18
Scottish Smallpox Epidemics of 1823–31
English Smallpox Epidemic of 1825–26
British Cholera Epidemic of 1832
Irish Typhus Epidemic of 1836–40
Scottish Typhus Epidemic of 1836–40
English Typhus Epidemic of 1837–38
British Smallpox Epidemic of 1837–40
Irish Typhus and Dysentery Epidemic of 1846–50
English Typhus Epidemic of 1847–48
British Cholera Epidemics of 1848–49 and 1853–54
London Typhus Epidemics of 1862–65
British Cholera Epidemic of 1865–66
British Smallpox Epidemic of 1871–72
British Typhoid Epidemic in the Boer War (1899–1902)
British Smallpox Epidemic of 1901–02
British Influenza Epidemic of 1918–19
British Encephalitis Epidemic of 1919–31
British Influenza Epidemic of 1950–51
British Influenza Epidemic of 1957–58
British Influenza Epidemic of 1968–70

CANADA See also EUROPE, UNITED STATES.

Huron Indian Epidemics of 1634–40
Quebec Yellow Fever Epidemic of 1710
Canadian Smallpox Epidemic, Great (1755–57)
Quebec Smallpox Epidemic of 1776
Canadian Indian Smallpox Epidemic of 1780–82
Canadian Cholera Epidemics of 1832 and 1834
Canadian Indian Smallpox Epidemic of 1837
Canadian Measles Epidemic of 1846–47
Canadian Typhus Epidemic of 1847
Canadian Cholera Epidemic of 1849
Canadian Cholera Epidemic of 1854
Montreal Smallpox Epidemic of 1885
European Influenza Pandemic of 1889–90
Yukon Indian Influenza Epidemic of 1900
British Columbian Epidemics of 1908–13
Canadian Influenza Epidemic of 1918–19

CARIBBEAN See also LATIN AMERICA.

Hispaniola Yellow Fever Epidemic of 1495–96
Hispaniola Smallpox Epidemic of 1507
Hispaniola Smallpox Epidemic of 1518
Barbadian Yellow Fever Epidemic of 1647
Jamaican Yellow Fever Epidemic of 1655
Jamaican Yellow Fever Epidemic of 1691
Havana Yellow Fever Epidemic of 1761–62
Haitian Yellow Fever Epidemic of 1794–98
Haitian Yellow Fever Epidemic of 1802
U.S. and Caribbean Dengue Epidemic of 1826–28
Bahamian Yellow Fever Epidemic of 1862–64
Panamanian Yellow Fever Epidemics of 1880–1904
Havana Yellow Fever Epidemic of 1899–1900
Caribbean Dengue Epidemics of 1963–64 and 1968–69

CENTRAL AMERICA See LATIN AMERICA.

CHINA and INDOCHINA

Asiatic Cholera Pandemic of 1817–23
Chinese Cholera Epidemic of 1820–22
Thai Cholera Epidemic of 1820
Asiatic Cholera Pandemic of 1826–37
Asiatic and European Influenza Pandemic of 1830–31
Asiatic and European Influenza Pandemic of 1836–37
Asiatic Cholera Pandemic of 1846–63
Asiatic Cholera Pandemic of 1865–75
Central Asian Cholera Epidemic of 1870–72
Asiatic Cholera Pandemic of 1881–96
Asiatic Influenza Pandemic of 1889–90
Thai Beriberi Epidemics of 1890–1910
Hong Kong Plague of 1894
Asiatic Cholera Pandemic of 1899–1923
Vietnamese Plagues of the Early 1900s
Chinese Plague of 1917–18
Chinese Influenza Epidemic of 1918
Manchurian Cholera Epidemic of 1919
Manchurian Plague of 1920–21
Manchurian and Mongolian Plagues of 1928–30
Chinese Plague of 1931–32
Chinese Cholera Epidemics of 1937–42
Singapore Beriberi Epidemics of 1942–45
U.S.-British-Chinese Armies' Typhus Epidemics of 1943–45
Chinese Cholera Epidemic of 1945–46
Singapore Bornholm Disease Epidemic of 1946
Peking Pneumonia Epidemics of 1949, 1952–53, and 1958–59
Bangkok Poliomyelitis Epidemic of 1952
Asian Influenza Pandemic of 1957–58
Vietnamese Dengue Epidemics of the 1950s, 1960s, and 1970s
Taiwanese Rubella Epidemics of 1957–58 and 1968–69
Taiwanese Encephalitis Epidemics of 1958–61
Singapore Dengue Hemorrhagic Fever Epidemics (1960s and 1970s)
Asiatic Cholera Pandemic of 1961–75
Taiwanese Cholera Epidemic of 1962
Vietnamese Plagues of the 1960s
Hong Kong Influenza Pandemic of 1968
Burmese Dengue Hemorrhagic Fever Epidemics of 1970 and 1971
Singapore Conjunctivitis Epidemics of 1970–80
Malaysian Poliomyelitis Epidemic of 1971–72
Chinese Dengue Epidemics of 1978–80
Xinjiang (Sinkiang) Hepatitis Epidemic of 1986–88
Shanghai Hepatitis Epidemic of 1988
Russian (Red) Influenza Pandemic of 1977–78

EGYPT See AFRICA.

ENGLAND See BRITAIN AND IRELAND.

ETHIOPIA See AFRICA.

EUROPE   See also ANCIENT HISTORY, BRITAIN AND IRELAND, FRANCE, GERMANY AND AUSTRIA, ITALY, SCANDINAVIA, SPAIN AND PORTUGAL, RUSSIA.

Plague of Justinian (A.D. 542)
Black Death (1347–80s)
European Sweating Sickness Epidemics, Northern (1529)
Thirty Years' War Epidemics (1618–48)
Maltese Plague of 1675–76
European Malaria Epidemic of 1678–82
European Influenza Epidemics of 1708–09, 1712, 1729–30, and 1732–33
European Influenza Epidemics of 1742–43 and 1762
European Influenza Pandemic of 1781–82
European Influenza Pandemic of 1788–89
European Malaria Epidemics of 1805–12 and 1823–27
Maltese Plague of 1813
Asiatic Cholera Pandemic of 1817–23
Asiatic Cholera Pandemic of 1826–37
Asiatic and European Influenza Pandemic of 1830–31
European Influenza Pandemic of 1833
Asiatic and European Influenza Pandemic of 1836–37
Asiatic Cholera Pandemic of 1846–63
European Influenza Pandemic of 1847–48
Plague Pandemic, Third (c. 1850s–1959)
Crimean War Epidemics (1845–56)
European Diphtheria Epidemic of the Late 1850s
Asiatic Cholera Pandemic of 1865–75
European Smallpox Pandemic of 1870–75
Asiatic Cholera Pandemic of 1881–96
European Influenza Pandemic of 1889–90
Asiatic Cholera Pandemic of 1899–96
Serbian Typhus Epidemic of 1914–15
Encephalitis Lethargica (von Economo's Disease) Epidemic of 1915–26
Spanish Influenza Epidemic of 1917–19
Maltese Poliomyelitis Epidemic of 1942–43
Asian Influenza Pandemic of 1957–58
Asiatic Cholera Pandemic of 1961–75
Hong Kong Influenza Pandemic of 1968
Russian (Red) Influenza Pandemic of 1977–78

FRANCE   See also EUROPE.
Frankish Smallpox Epidemic of A.D. 580
Frankish Plagues of the Sixth Century A.D.
Crusader Epidemic at Antioch (1098)
Crusader Epidemic at Adalia (1148)
Crusader Epidemic at Acre (1189)
Crusader Epidemic at Damietta (1218–19)
Crusader Epidemic at Al Mansurah (1250)
Dancing Mania (St. John's Dance, St. Vitus's Dance, Tarantism) (1374, 1518)
French Plagues of 1450–1520
Paris Plague of 1466
French Army Syphilis Epidemic of 1494–95
Strasbourg Dancing Mania (1518)
French Plagues of 1520–1600
French Army Typhus Epidemic of 1528
Charles V's Army Epidemic at Metz (1552)

Plague of Lyon in 1564
Paris Diphtheria Epidemic of 1576
Paris Whooping Cough Epidemic of 1578
French Plagues of 1625–40
Plague of Lyon in 1628–29
Picardy Sweat (1718)
Plague of Marseilles (1720–22)
French Dysentery Epidemic of 1738–42
French Influenza Epidemic of 1740
French Typhus and Typhoid Epidemics of 1740–42
French Dysentery Epidemic of 1779
Prussian Army Dysentery Epidemic of 1792
Napoleon's Army Epidemics in the Near East (1798–1801)
Danzig Typhus Epidemic of 1807
Napoleon's Army Epidemics in Russia (1812–13)
Mainz Typhus Epidemic of 1813–14
French Typhus Epidemics of 1813–14
French Miliary Fever Epidemics of the 1800s
Tours Diphtheria Epidemic of 1818–21
French Cholera Epidemic of 1832–33
French Cholera Epidemics of 1848–49, 1853–54, and 1865–66
Crimean War Epidemics (1854–56)
European Smallpox Pandemic of 1870–75
Spanish Influenza Epidemic of 1917–19
Paris Influenza Epidemic of 1918–19

GERMANY AND AUSTRIA   See also EUROPE, ITALY.

Vienna Plague of 1349
Dancing Mania (St. John's Dance, St. Vitus's Dance, Tarantism) (1374, 1518)
German Plagues of 1462–65
European Sweating Sickness Epidemics, Northern (1529)
German, Austrian, and Swiss Plagues of the 1500s
Joachim's Army Typhus Epidemic of 1542
Maximilian II's Army Typhus Epidemic (1566)
Prussian Plague of 1602
Basel Plague of 1610–11
Thirty Years' War Epidemics (1618–48)
German, Austrian, and Swiss Plagues of 1663–68 and 1675–83
Plague of Vienna, Great (1679)
Augsburg Typhus Epidemic of 1703–04
Danzig Plague of 1709
German Typhus Epidemic of 1734
German Typhus, Typhoid, and Dysentery Epidemics of 1741–43
German Typhus and Dysentery Epidemics of 1757–63
Prussian Army Dysentery Epidemic of 1792
Austrian and Prussian Typhus Epidemics of 1805–07
Danzig Typhus Epidemic of 1807
Prussian Typhus Epidemics of 1812–14
Danzig Typhus Epidemic of 1813
Mainz Typhus Epidemic of 1813–14
German Typhus Epidemics of 1813–14, Northern and Central
German Typhus Epidemics of 1813–14, Southern

German Cholera Epidemics of 1830–90
European Smallpox Pandemic of 1870–75
Hamburg Cholera Epidemic of 1892
Serbian Typhus Epidemic of 1914–15
Encephalitis Lethargica (von Economo's Disease) Epidemic of 1915–26
Marburg Virus Epidemic of 1967

GREECE See ANCIENT HISTORY, EUROPE.

GHANA See AFRICA.

HAITI See CARIBBEAN.

ICELAND See SCANDINAVIA.

INDIA See also CHINA AND INDOCHINA, MIDDLE EAST.

Indian Smallpox Epidemic of 1769–70
Indian Cholera Epidemic of 1781–83
Indian Kala-azar Epidemics, Early (1880s and early 1900s)
Indian Cholera Epidemic of 1817–18
Asiatic Cholera Pandemic of 1817–23
Asiatic Cholera Pandemic of 1826–37
Indian Cholera Epidemic of 1826–27
Asiatic and European Influenza Pandemic of 1830–31
Calcutta Smallpox Epidemics of the 1800s
Asiatic and European Influenza Pandemic of 1836–37
Asiatic Cholera Pandemic of 1846–63
Indian Cholera Epidemic of 1860–61
Indian Cholera Epidemic of 1864–65
Asiatic Cholera Pandemic of 1865–75
Indian Cholera Epidemic of 1867–68
Central Asian Cholera Epidemic of 1870–72
Indian Cholera Epidemic of 1875–77
Punjab Malaria Epidemics of 1878–79
Asiatic Cholera Pandemic of 1881–96
Asiatic Influenza Pandemic of 1889–90
Indian Cholera Epidemic of 1891–92
Indian Plague of 1896–97
Asiatic Cholera Pandemic of 1899–1923
Indian Cholera Epidemic of 1900
Indian Plague of 1904–07
Punjab Malaria Epidemic of 1908
Indian Influenza Epidemic of 1918–19
Sri Lankan (Ceylonese) Malaria Epidemic of 1934–35
Sri Lankan (Ceylonese) Dysentery Epidemic of 1942
Indian Kala-azar Epidemics, Later (1940s, 1950s, and 1970s)
Indian Poliomyelitis Epidemics of World War II (1942–44)
Indian and Burmese Sprue Epidemic of 1943–45
Nicobar Islands Poliomyelitis Epidemic of 1947
Delhi Hepatitis Epidemic of 1955–56
Asian Influenza Pandemic of 1957–58
Indian Influenza Epidemic of 1957–58
Indian Kyasanur Forest Disease Epidemics of 1957–58
Indian Dengue Hemorrhagic Fever Epidemics (1960s)
Asiatic Cholera Pandemic of 1961–75

Indian Cholera Epidemic of 1964–66
Sri Lankan (Ceylonese) Malaria Epidemic of 1968–69
Indian Conjunctivitis Epidemic of 1971
Indian-Bangladeshi Cholera Epidemic of 1971
Bangladeshi Smallpox Epidemic of 1971–73
Indian Smallpox Epidemic of 1973–74
Indian Malaria Epidemic of 1974–75
Indian Encephalitis Epidemic of 1977–78
Maldivian Cholera Epidemic of 1978

INDONESIA AND THE PHILIPPINES See also CHINA AND INDOCHINA, OCEANIA.

Philippine Smallpox Epidemic of 1591
Philippine Cholera Epidemic of 1820–21
Asiatic Cholera Pandemic of 1817–23
Indonesian Cholera Epidemic of 1821
Asiatic Cholera Pandemic of 1826–37
Asiatic Cholera Pandemic of 1846–63
Asiatic Cholera Pandemic of 1865–75
Asiatic Cholera Pandemic of 1881–96
Philippine Cholera Epidemics of 1882–83 and 1888–89
Philippine Plague of 1899–1903
Asiatic Cholera Pandemic of 1899–1923
Ontong Java Island Influenza Epidemics
Philippine Beriberi Epidemics of 1901–02 and 1909
Philippine Cholera Epidemic of 1902–04
Javanese (Indonesian) Plague of 1910–14
Indonesian Influenza Epidemic of 1918
Philippine Influenza Epidemic of 1918–19
Javanese (Indonesian) Plague of 1932–34
Philippine Poliomyelitis Epidemic of 1944–45
Philippine Schistosomiasis Epidemic of 1944–45
Philippine Dengue Epidemics of the 1950s and 1960s
Asiatic Cholera Pandemic of 1961–75
Indonesian Smallpox Epidemics of 1965–67
Hong Kong Influenza pandemic of 1968
Russian (Red) Influenza Pandemic of 1977–78

IRAN See MIDDLE EAST.

IRAQ See MIDDLE EAST.

IRELAND See BRITAIN AND IRELAND.

ITALY See also ANCIENT HISTORY, EUROPE.

Henry IV's Army Epidemics of 1081–83
Cava Typhus Epidemic of 1083
Frederick Barbarossa's Army Epidemic (1167)
Plague of Florence (Black Vomit) (1348)
Dancing Mania (St. John's Dance, St. Vitus's Dance, Tarantism) (1374, 1518)
Plague of Florence in 1417
Florence Dysentery Epidemic of 1425
Florence Plague of 1430
Italian Plagues of 1477–79
French Army Syphilis Epidemic of 1494–95
Italian Typhus Epidemic of 1505

French Army Typhus Epidemic of 1528
Venice Plague of 1575–77
Italian Influenza Epidemic of 1580
Italian Diphtheria Epidemic of 1618
Italian Plagues of 1629–31
Plague of Florence in 1630–33
Italian Plagues of 1656–57
Cremona Diphtheria Epidemic of 1747–48
Dalmatian Plague of 1783–84
Italian Typhus Epidemics of 1796–1800
Livorno-Lucca Yellow Fever Epidemic of 1804
Italian Smallpox Epidemics of 1814
Albenga Meningitis Epidemic of 1815
Italian Typhus Epidemic of 1816–18
Italian Meningitis Epidemics of 1839–45
Italian Cholera Epidemic of 1866–67
Italian Smallpox Epidemic of 1870–72
Italian Cholera Epidemic of 1884–85
Italian Smallpox Epidemic of 1900–02
Italian Whooping Cough Epidemics of 1901–05
Spanish Influenza Epidemic of 1917–19
Italian Smallpox Epidemic of 1920–21
Naples Typhus Epidemic of 1943–44
Italian Typhoid Epidemics of 1950–52
Asian Influenza Pandemic of 1957–58
Hong Kong influenza Pandemic of 1968
Russian (Red) Influenza Pandemic of 1977–78

JAPAN AND KOREA   See also CHINA AND INDO-CHINA.

Japanese Epidemic of A.D. 585–87
Japanese Smallpox Epidemics of the Eighth and Ninth Centuries A.D.
Japanese Smallpox Epidemic of A.D. 735–37
Japanese Smallpox Epidemics of the Tenth Century A.D.
Japanese Epidemic of A.D. 994–95
Japanese Measles Epidemics of A.D. 998–1025
Japanese Syphilis Epidemic of 1512
Japanese Rubella Epidemic of 1684
Japanese Measles Epidemic of 1690–91
Japanese Measles Epidemic of 1708–09
Japanese Measles Epidemic of 1730–31
Japanese Measles Epidemic of 1753
Japanese Measles Epidemic of 1776
Japanese Measles Epidemic of 1803
Asiatic Cholera Pandemic of 1817–23
Korean Cholera Epidemics of 1821–22 and 1895
Japanese Cholera Epidemic of 1822
Japanese Measles Epidemic of 1823–24
Asiatic Cholera Pandemic of 1826–37
Asiatic and European Influenza Pandemic of 1830–31
Asiatic and European Influenza Pandemic of 1836–37
Asiatic Cholera Pandemic of 1846–63
Japanese Cholera Epidemics of 1858–59 and 1862
Japanese Measles Epidemic of 1862
Asiatic Cholera Pandemic of 1865–75
Asiatic Cholera Pandemic of 1881–96
Asiatic Influenza Pandemic of 1889–90
Asiatic Cholera Pandemic of 1899–1923

Japanese Army Beriberi Epidemic of 1904–05
Japanese Encephalitis Epidemics of the 1920s and 1930s
Japanese Dengue Epidemics of 1942–45
Japanese-Korean Typhus Epidemic of 1945–46
Japanese Malaria Epidemic of 1945–46
Korean Hepatitis Epidemic of 1950–51
Korean Hemorrhagic Fever Epidemic of 1951–54
Asian Influenza Pandemic of 1957–58
Japanese Influenza Epidemic of 1957–58
Asiatic Cholera Pandemic of 1961–75

KENYA   See AFRICA.

KOREA   See JAPAN AND KOREA.

LATIN AMERICA   See also CARIBBEAN, EUROPE.

Mexican Smallpox Epidemic of 1520–21
Peruvian Smallpox Epidemic of 1525–27
Brazilian Smallpox Epidemic of 1555–62
Mexican Typhus Epidemic of 1576
Venezuelan Smallpox Epidemic of 1580
Peruvian Smallpox Epidemic of 1585
Brazilian Smallpox Epidemic of 1660
Brazilian Smallpox Epidemic of 1665–66
Guayaquil Yellow Fever Epidemics of 1740, 1743, and 1842
Havana Yellow Fever Epidemic of 1761–62
Colombian Smallpox Epidemic of 1776
Mexico City Smallpox Epidemic of 1779
Mexican-Guatemalan Smallpox Epidemic of 1797
Mexico City Typhus Epidemic of 1813
Mexican Smallpox Epidemic of 1833
Rio de Janeiro Yellow Fever Epidemics of 1849–1902
Panamanian Yellow Fever Epidemics of 1880–1904
Brazilian Plagues of 1899–1988
Havana Yellow Fever Epidemic of 1899–1900
Rio de Janeiro Smallpox Epidemics of 1904 and 1908
Brazilian Smallpox Epidemic of 1905
Ecuadoran Plagues of 1908–88
Venezuelan Yellow Fever Epidemic of 1929
Brazilian Malaria Epidemic of 1938–40
Santiago Meningitis Epidemic of 1941–43
Bolivian Hemorrhagic Fever Epidemic of 1959–64
Brazilian Smallpox Epidemic of 1967–71
Guatemalan Dysentery Epidemic of 1969–70
Peruvian Cholera Epidemic of 1991–92

MALAYSIA   See CHINA AND INDOCHINA, INDONESIA AND THE PHILIPPINES.

MEXICO   See LATIN AMERICA.

MIDDLE EAST

Saudi Arabian Smallpox Epidemic of A.D. 569–71
Syrian Plague of A.D. 638–39
Crusader Epidemic at Antioch (1098)
Crusader Epidemic at Adalia (1148)
Crusader Epidemic at Acre (1189)

Crusader Epidemic at Damietta (1218–19)
Crusader Epidemic at Al Mansurah (1250)
Black Death in the Middle East (1348–49)
Persian Plague of 1772–73
Persian Plague of 1800
Asiatic Cholera Pandemic of 1817–23
Persian Cholera Epidemics of 1821–22
Syrian Cholera Epidemic of 1822–23
Asiatic Cholera Pandemic of 1826–37
Persian Cholera Epidemic of 1829–30
Persian Plague of 1830
Asiatic and European Influenza Pandemic of 1830–31
Mecca Cholera Epidemic of 1831
Persian Influenza Epidemic of 1833
Asiatic and European Influenza Pandemic of 1836–37
Asiatic Cholera Pandemic of 1846–63
Persian Cholera Epidemics of 1846–63
Asiatic Cholera Pandemic of 1865–75
Mecca Cholera Epidemic of 1865
Persian Cholera Epidemics of 1866–70
Central Asian Cholera Epidemic of 1870–72
Asiatic Cholera Pandemic of 1881–96
Asiatic Influenza Pandemic of 1889–90
Asiatic Cholera Pandemic of 1899–1923
Iraqi Schistosomiasis Epidemics of c. 1910–30
Persian Influenza Epidemic of 1918
Afghan Influenza Epidemic of 1918
Pakistani Malaria Epidemic of 1929
Afghan Cholera Epidemics of the 1930s and 1940s
Iranian (Persian) Typhus Epidemic of 1942–44
Syrian Cholera Epidemic of 1947–48
Israeli Leptospirosis Epidemic of 1949–50
Saudi Arabian Malaria Epidemic of 1950–51
Israeli Diphtheria Epidemic of 1950–51
Israeli Poliomyelitis Epidemics of 1950–52
Turkish Influenza Epidemic of 1957–58
Israeli West Nile Fever Epidemics of the 1950s
Asiatic Cholera Pandemic of 1961–75
Afghan Smallpox Epidemic of 1970–72

NETHERLANDS, THE See EUROPE.

NEW ZEALAND See AUSTRALIA AND NEW ZEALAND.

OCEANIA See also AUSTRALIA AND NEW ZEALAND, INDONESIA AND THE PHILIPPINES.

Tahitian Venereal Disease Epidemic of 1768–69
Fiji Islands Epidemics of the Late 1700s and Early 1800s
Samoan Influenza Epidemics of the 1800s
Tahitian Smallpox Epidemic of 1841
South Pacific Islands Dysentery Epidemics of 1843
Hawaiian Smallpox Epidemic of 1853
French Polynesian Measles Epidemic of 1854
Fiji Islands Measles Epidemics of 1875, 1903, and 1911
Gilbert and Ellice Islands Measles Epidemics of 1890 and 1936
Tongan and Samoan Measles Epidemics of 1893

Hawaiian Plague of 1899–1900
Samoan Whooping Cough Epidemics
South Pacific Islands Influenza Epidemic of 1918–19
Southwest Pacific Malaria Epidemics of 1942–45
Southwest Pacific Typhus Epidemics of 1942–45
Guam Encephalitis Epidemic of 1947–48
Guam Mumps Epidemic of 1947–48
French Polynesian Measles Epidemic of 1950–51
Tahitian Poliomyelitis Epidemic of 1951
Solomon Islands Poliomyelitis Epidemic of 1951
Papua New Guinea Influenza Epidemic of 1969–70
Southwest Pacific Dengue Epidemics of the 1970s
Fiji Islands Dengue Epidemics of 1971–73 and 1975
Southwest Pacific Ross River Fever Epidemics of 1979–80

PAKISTAN See INDIA, MIDDLE EAST.

PHILIPPINES See INDONESIA AND THE PHILIPPINES.

PORTUGAL See SPAIN AND PORTUGAL.

RUSSIA See also CHINA AND INDOCHINA, EUROPE, MIDDLE EAST.

Russian Ergotism Epidemic of 1722
Astrakhan Plague of 1727–28
Russian Plague of 1738–39
Napoleon's Army Epidemics in Russia (1812–13)
Astrakhan Cholera Epidemic of 1823
Russian Cholera Epidemic of 1829–31
Crimean War Epidemics (1854–56)
Russian Cholera Epidemic of 1892–93
Russian Cholera Epidemic of 1910
Serbian Typhus Epidemic of 1914–15
Russian Typhus Epidemics of 1914–22
Russian Cholera Epidemics of 1915–22
Russian Influenza Epidemic of 1918–19
Russian Malaria Epidemic of 1922–23
Russian Influenza Epidemics of 1925–50
Russian Influenza Epidemic of 1964–65
Russian Influenza Epidemic of 1968–69
Russian (Red) Influenza Pandemic of 1977–78
Russian Diphtheria Epidemic of 1992–93

SCANDINAVIA See also EUROPE, GERMANY AND AUSTRIA.

Plague of Iceland, Great (1402–04)
Icelandic Plague of 1494–95
European Sweating Sickness Epidemics, Northern (1529)
Icelandic Smallpox Epidemic of 1707–09
Greenlandic Smallpox Epidemic of 1733–34
Scandinavian Epidemics of 1736–39
Swedish Epidemics of the Early 1740s
Finnish Ergotism Epidemics of the 1800s
Faeroe Islands Measles Epidemic of 1846
Stockholm Poliomyelitis Epidemic of 1887
Swedish Poliomyelitis Epidemic of 1905

Swedish Poliomyelitis Epidemic of 1911
Copenhagen Poliomyelitis Epidemic of 1952

SOUTH AFRICA   See AFRICA.

SOUTH AMERICA   See LATIN AMERICA.

SPAIN AND PORTUGAL   See also EUROPE.

Spanish Plagues of the 1400s
Portuguese Plagues of the 1400s
Granada Typhus Epidemic of 1489
Spanish Plagues of the 1500s
Portuguese Plagues of the 1500s
Spanish Diphtheria Epidemics of 1583–1618
Spanish Plagues of 1596–1602
Spanish Plagues of 1637, 1646–52, and 1678–82
Cádiz Yellow Fever Epidemic of 1800
Spanish Yellow Fever Epidemic of 1803–05
Gibraltar Yellow Fever Epidemics of 1804–28
Cádiz Yellow Fever Epidemic of 1810
Barcelona Yellow Fever Epidemic of 1821
Spanish Cholera Epidemic of 1833–34
Spanish Cholera Epidemic of 1854–55
Spanish Cholera Epidemic of 1865
Spanish Cholera Epidemic of 1884–85
Spanish Plagues of 1905 06 and 1923

SRI LANKA   See INDIA.

SWEDEN   See SCANDINAVIA.

SWITZERLAND   See EUROPE, GERMANY AND AUSTRIA.

UNITED STATES   See also CANADA, EUROPE, LATIN AMERICA.

Seneca Indian Measles Epidemic of 1592–96
Massachusetts Smallpox Epidemic of c. 1617–19
Massachusetts Smallpox Epidemic of c. 1633
Connecticut Smallpox Epidemic of 1634
Massachusetts Smallpox Epidemic of 1648–49
Iroquois Indian Smallpox Epidemic of 1662
Boston Smallpox Epidemic of 1666
Boston Smallpox Epidemic of 1677–78
New York Yellow Fever Epidemic of 1668
Charleston Yellow Fever Epidemic of 1699
Boston Smallpox Epidemic of 1702–03
New York Yellow Fever Epidemic of 1702
Charleston Yellow Fever Epidemic of 1706
Boston Smallpox Epidemic of 1721–22

Charleston Yellow Fever Epidemics of 1728 and 1732
New England Diphtheria and Scarlet Fever Epidemics of 1735–40
New York Yellow Fever Epidemics of 1743 and 1745
Boston Smallpox Epidemic of 1763–64
New England Influenza Epidemic of 1789
Charleston Yellow Fever Epidemics of 1792–99
New England Scarlet Fever Epidemic of 1793–95
Philadelphia Yellow Fever Epidemic of 1793
New Haven Yellow Fever Epidemic of 1794
New York Yellow Fever Epidemic of 1795
Omaha Indian Smallpox Epidemic of 1802
U.S. and Caribbean Dengue Epidemic of 1826–28
Oregon Malaria Epidemic of 1829–33
U.S. Cholera Epidemic of 1832
Mandan Indian Smallpox Epidemic of 1837
Blackfoot Indian Smallpox Epidemic of 1837–38
Cayuse Indian Measles Epidemic of 1847
U.S. Cholera Epidemic of 1849
U.S. Dengue Epidemics of 1850–51 and 1878–80
Hawaiian Smallpox Epidemic of 1853
U.S. Civil War Epidemics (1861–65)
U.S. Cholera Epidemic of 1866
Gros Ventre Indian Smallpox Epidemic of 1869
New York Smallpox Epidemics of 1868–75
U.S. Cholera Epidemic of 1873
U.S. Yellow Fever Epidemics of 1878–79
European Influenza Pandemic of 1889–90
Asiatic Influenza Pandemic of 1889–90
Vermont Poliomyelitis Epidemic of 1894
Hawaiian Plague of 1899–1900
San Francisco Plague of 1900–04
U.S. Smallpox Epidemic of 1901–03
San Francisco Plague of 1907–09
New York Poliomyelitis Epidemic of 1907
U.S. Poliomyelitis Epidemic of 1916
Spanish Influenza Epidemic of 1917–19
Los Angeles Plague of 1924–25
U.S. Poliomyelitis Epidemic of 1931
Los Angeles Poliomyelitis Epidemic of 1934
U.S. Poliomyelitis Epidemic of 1942–53
Guam Mumps Epidemic of 1947–48
Asian Influenza Pandemic of 1957–58
U.S. Influenza Epidemic of 1957–58
Houston Encephalitis Epidemic of 1964
U.S. Rubella Epidemic of 1964
New Mexico Plague of 1965
Hong Kong Influenza Pandemic of 1968
U.S. Influenza Epidemic of 1968–69
Philadelphia "Legionaires' Disease" Epidemic (1976)
Russian (Red) Influenza Epidemic of 1977–78
U.S. AIDS Epidemic (1980s–   )

VIETNAM   See CHINA AND INDOCHINA.

INDEX

Boldface page numbers indicate main essays

A

Abenaki (Abnaki) Indians
Huron Indian smallpox (1634-40) 134
Aborigines
Australian smallpox (1788-89) 20
Abraha (Ethiopian prince)
Saudi smallpox (569-71) 284
acquired immunodeficiency syndrome (AIDS) *see* AIDS
Acre (Akko, Israel)
Crusader Epidemic (1189-91) 67-68
acute hemorrhagic conjunctivitis (AHC)
Africa/Asia: (1969-71) 3
India: (1971) 141
acute respiratory disease (ARD)
Russian influenza (1968-69) 277
Adalia (Antalya, Turkey)
Crusader Epidemic (1148) **68**
adenovirus (AV11)
Singapore conjunctivitis (1970-80) 292
Adhemar (bishop of Le Puy)
Crusader Epidemic at Antioch (1089) 69
Adrianampoinimerina (king of Madagascar)
Madagascan smallpox (1817-18) 195
Advance (ship)
Canadian cholera (1849) 47
Aëdes aegypti (mosquito) *see* dengue; yellow fever
Aëdes albopictus (mosquito)
dengue: China (1978-80) 61; Japan (1942-45) 167; U.S./Caribbean (1826-28) 336
Aëdes caballus (mosquito)
Egyptian Rift Valley fever (1977) 82
Aëdes circumluteolus (mosquito)
Egyptian Rift Valley fever (1977) 82
Aëdes cooki (mosquito)
Southwest Pacific dengue (1970s) 299
Aëdes polynesiensis (mosquito)
Fiji Islands dengue (1971-73/75) 103
South Pacific Ross River fever (1979-80) 301
Aëdes pseudoscutellaris (mosquito)
Fiji Islands dengue (1971-73/75) 103
Aëdes rotumae (mosquito)
Fiji Islands dengue (1971-73/75) 103
Aëdes scutellaris (mosquito)
U.S./Caribbean dengue (1826-28) 336
Aëdes tabu (mosquito)
Southwest Pacific dengue (1970s) 299
Aëdes theileri (mosquito)
Egyptian Rift Valley fever (1977) 82
Aëdes vigilax (mosquito)
Southwest Pacific Ross River fever (1979-80) 301
Afghanistan
cholera: (1930s/40s) 1
influenza: (1918) 1
smallpox: (1970-72) **1-2**
Africa *see also specific country (e.g., Ghana)*
AIDS: (1987-) **2-3**
cholera: (1970-71) **354-355**; (1989-91) **3-4**
conjunctivitis: (1969-71) 3
influenza: (1889-90) 16-17, 96-98
Africa (ship)
Sierra Leone influenza (1918) 289
Agramonte, Aristides
Havana yellow fever (1899-1900) 129

AHC *see* acute hemorrhagic conjunctivitis
Ahmed Bey (Tunisian ruler)
Tunisian cholera (1849-50) 328-329
AIDS (acquired immunodeficiency syndrome)
Africa: (1987-) 2-3
United States: (1981-) 333-335
Albemarle, Second Earl of
Havana yellow fever (1761-62) 128
Albengan, Italy
meningitis (1815) **4**
Aleut Indians
Yukon Indian influenza (1900) 357
Alexander III (pope)
Frederick Barbarossa's army epidemic (1167) 106
Alexandria, Egypt
diphtheria (1882-86) **45**
Algeria
malaria: (1941) **64**
relapsing fever: (1943-46) **4-5**
typhus: (1942-44) **5**
Algonquin Indians
Huron Indian smallpox (1634-40) 134
Al Mansurah (El Mansûra, Egypt)
Crusader Epidemic (1250) **68-69**
Amelia (ship)
Philadelphia yellow fever (1793) 243
American Fur Company
Canada smallpox (1837) 48
American Revolution (1775-83)
Quebec smallpox (1776) 265
Andrew of Wyntoun
Scottish plague (1848-50) 259
Angola
smallpox (1864-65) **5-6**
Anopheles culcifacies (mosquito)
Sri Lankan malaria (1934-35) 309
Anopheles funestus (mosquito)
Mauritian malaria (1866-68) 204
South Africa malaria (1929-35) 295
Anopheles gambiae (mosquito) *see* malaria
anthrax 360t
antigenic shift
Spanish influenza (1917-19) 305
Antioch, Syria
Crusader Epidemic (1089) 69-70
Antonine Plague (Plague of Galen) (165-180 A.D.) **6-7**
Apodemus agrarius (mouse)
Korean hemorrhagic fever (1951-54) 181
Apollo 11 disease *see* acute hemorrhagic conjunctivitis (AHC)
Arabian American Oil Company
Saudi malaria (1950-51) 284
Arbuthnot, John
London typhus (1726-29) 191
Archimedes (Greek mathematician)
Roman pestilence (212 B.C.) 270
ARD *see* acute respiratory disease
Arikara Indians
smallpox: Canadian Indians (1780-82) 48; Mandan Indians (1837) 201
Armstrong, Richard
Hawaii smallpox (1853) 130
Arnold, Benedict
Quebec smallpox (1776) 265
Arthur Mervyn (Charles Brockden Brown)
Philadelphia yellow fever (1793) 244
Ashanti (African ethnic group)
influenza: (1918) **7**
plague: (1924-25) **7**
Ashdod, Plague of *see* Philistines
Ashraf, Malik
Black Death in Middle East (1347-1351) 26

Asia *see also specific country (e.g., China)*
cholera: (1817-23) **8**; (1826-37) **8-9**; (1846-63) **9-11**; (1865-75) **11-12**; (1870-72) **54-55**; (1881-96) 12; (1899-1923) **12-14**; (1961-75) **14-15**
conjunctivitis: (1969-71) **3**
influenza: (1781-82) 93-94; (1830-31) **15**; (1836-37) **15-16**; (1889-90) **16-17**; (1957-58) **7-8**
"Asian flu" *see* H2N2 influenza virus
Assiniboin Indians
smallpox: Canadian Indians (1837) 48; Mandan Indians (1837) 201
Astrakhan, Russia
cholera: (1823) **17**
plague: (1727-28) **17-18**
atabrine (drug)
malaria: Southwest Pacific (1942-45) 300
Atalanta (ship)
U.S. cholera (1866) 338
Athens, Greece
Great Plague (430-429 B.C.) **250**
atoxyl (drug)
sleeping sickness: Chad (1912-40) 56; Uganda-Tanganyika (1900-1909) 332
Atsina Indians *see* Gros Ventre Indians
Augsburg, Germany
typhus (1703-04) **18**
aureomycin (drug)
pneumonia: Peking (1949/52-53/58-59) 236
Australia
encephalitis (MEV): (1917-18/22/25-26/51/74) **19**
influenza: (1890-91) 314-315; (1918-19) **18-19**
measles: (1800s) 315
plague: (1900) 316-317
rubella: (1938-41) **19**
scarlet fever: (1875-76) **19-20**
smallpox: (1788-89) **20**
Austria
cholera: (1866-67) 157
plagues: (1349) **351**; (1500s) **115**; (1663-68/75-83) **115-116**
sleeping sickness: (1915-26) 83
typhus: (1805-07) **20-21**
Austro-Prussian War (1866)
Italian cholera (1866-67) 157
Azande (African ethnic group)
Mongallan meningitis (1918-24/26-31) 210
Aztec Indians
Mexico: smallpox (1520-21) 207-208; typhus (1576) 208
AZT (zidovudine)
AIDS: United States (1981-) 334

B

bacillary dysentery (shigellosis)
Guatemala (1969-70) 125
Bacon, Francis
London plague (1593) 186
Oxford typhus (1577) 232
Baguia, Francisco de
Mexico smallpox (1520-21) 207
bag ventilation
Copenhagen polio (1952) 65
Bahamas
yellow fever (1862-64) **22**
Baillou, Guillaume de
Paris: diphtheria (1576) 234; whooping cough (1578) 235
Baldwin, Dwight
Hawaii smallpox (1853) 131
Bangkok, Thailand
polio (1952) **22**
Bangladesh
cholera: (1971) **135-136**
smallpox: (1971-73) **22-23**

Bangla Joy disease *see* acute hemorrhagic conjunctivitis (AHC)
Bantus (African ethnic group)
plagues: South Africa (1935/36) 296
pneumonia: South Africa (1926-40) 296
smallpox: Cape Colony/Cape Town (1882-85) 52
typhoid: South-West Africa (1904-07) 298
typhus: South Africa (1934/35) 297
Barbadas
yellow fever: (1647) **23**; (1691) **23-24**
Barcelona, Spain
yellow fever (1821) **24**
Basel, Switzerland
plague (1610-11) **24-25**
Bede (English chronicler)
Yellow Plague (664 A.D.) 357
Behring, Emil von
Spanish diphtheria (1583-1618) 304
Beijing (Peking), China
pneumonia (1949/52-53/58-59) 236
Bell, A. N.
U.S. smallpox (1901-03) 347
Bell, Hesketh
Uganda-Tanganyika sleeping sickness (1900-09) 332
Belle Brune (ship)
Quebec yellow fever (1710) 265-266
Bellevue Stratford Hotel (Philadelphia)
legionnaires' disease (1976) 242-243
Belsunce, Henri François de
Marseilles plague (1720-22) 259
Bengali, India
smallpox (1769-70) 147
Benoit, Carlos Luis
Philippine cholera (1820-21) 245
beriberi 367t, 368t, 370t
Japanese army: (1904-05) 166
Philippines: (1901-02/09) 244-245
Singapore: (1942-45) 291
Thailand: (1890-1910) 323
Berkeley, George
Irish typhus/dysentery (1740-41) 152
Beveridge, C. E. G.
Sudanese relapsing fever (1926-28) 312
Beveridge, William
European influenza (1847-48) 96
Bidatsu (emperor of Japan)
Japanese epidemic (585-87) 168
bilharziasis *see* schistosomiasis
birds
Indian Kyasanur Forest Disease (1957-58) 144
Black Assize *see* typhus fever
Black Death (1347-1351)
Asia/Europe: **25-26**
Middle East: **26-27**
Blackfoot Indians
smallpox (1837-38) **27**, 49
Black Plague *see* Black Death
Black Vomit *see* Florence, Italy
Blue, Rupert
San Francisco plague (1907-09) 283
Boccaccio, Giovanni
Plague of Florence (1347-48) 253
Boer War (1899-1902)
British army typhoid 42
Bolivia
hemorrhagic fever (1959-64) **27-28**
Bombay, India
plague (1896-97) 145
Bordetella pertussis (bacterium)
whooping cough: Italy (1901-05) 164; Samoa (1849/1907/26/36-37/50) 281

Bornholm disease (pleurodynia) 370t
Singapore (1946) 291
Boston, Massachusetts
smallpox: (1666) **28**; (1677-78) **28-29**; (1702-03) **29**; (1721-22) **29-30**; (1763-64) **30**
Bougainville, Louis Antoine de
Tahitian VD (1768-69) 320
Boylston, Zabdiel
Boston smallpox (1721-22) 30
Bradford, William
Connecticut smallpox (1634) 63, 64
Bradstreet, Simon
Boston smallpox (1666) 28
Brazil
malaria: (1938-40) **30-31**
plagues: (1899-1988) **31-32**
smallpox: (1555-62) **32**; (1660) **32-33**; (1665-66) **33**; (1878) **33-34**; (1904/08) **267-268**; (1905) **34-35**; (1967-71) **35**
yellow fever: (1849-1902) **269**; (1904/08) 267-268
breakbone fever *see* dengue
Bretonneau, Pierre-Fidèle
Tours diptheria (1818-20) 327-328
Brief History of Epidemic and Pestilential Diseases, A (Noah Webster)
New York yellow fever (1668) 219
Britain *see* Great Britain
British Army
cholera: (1854-56) **66-67**
dysentery: (1854-56) **66-67**
scurvy: (1854-56) **66-67**
smallpox: (1871-72) 41
typhoid: (1899-1902) 42
typhus: (1854-56) **66-67**; (1943-45) 335
British Columbia, Canada
typhoid (1908-13) **37**
Broad Street pump (London, England)
cholera (1848-49/53-54) 36
bronchopneumonia
Peking (1949/52-53/58-59) 236
Broussais, François
French cholera (1832-33) 108
Brown, Charles Brockden
Philadelphia yellow fever (1793) 244
Brunswick, Duke of
Prussian army dysentery (1792) 262-263
bubonic plague 360t-372t
Ashanti: (1924-25) 7
Asia/Africa/Latin America (Third Plague Pandemic): (1850-1959) **260-261**
Asia/Europe (Black Death) (Second Plague Pandemic): (1347-1351) 25-26
Astrakhan: (1727-28) 17-18
Australia: (1900) 316-317
Austria: (1349) 351; (1500s) 115; (1663-68/75-83) 115-116, 259-260
Basel: (1610-11) 24-25
Brazil: (1899-1988) 31-32
China: (1931-32) 62
Constantinople: (c. 746-48 A.D.) 64-65
Dalmatia: (1783-84) 71
Danzig: (1709) 72-73
Ecuador: (1908-88) 75-76
Edinburgh: (1530) 76; (1568-69) 76-77; (1585) 77; (1597) 77
Egypt: (1347-49) 80; (1834-35) 80-81
England: (1348-50) 251-252; (1400s) 83-84; (1499-1500) 183; (1500s) 84-85; (1530) 76; (1563) 183-184; (1568-69) 76-77; (1578) 184-185; (1585) 77; (1593) 185-186; (1597) 77; (1603) 186-187; (1625) 187-188; (1636) 188; (1664-65) 256

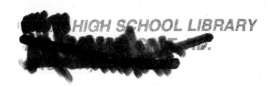